DIET, NUTRIENTS, and BONE HEALTH

DIET, NUTRIENTS, and BONE HEALTH

Edited by
John J.B. Anderson
Sanford C. Garner
Philip J. Klemmer

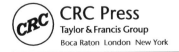

CRC Press
Taylor & Francis Group
Boca Raton London New York

CRC Press is an imprint of the
Taylor & Francis Group, an **informa** business

CRC Press
Taylor & Francis Group
6000 Broken Sound Parkway NW, Suite 300
Boca Raton, FL 33487-2742

First issued in paperback 2019

© 2012 by Taylor & Francis Group, LLC
CRC Press is an imprint of Taylor & Francis Group, an Informa business

No claim to original U.S. Government works

ISBN-13: 978-1-4398-1955-5 (hbk)
ISBN-13: 978-0-367-38229-2 (pbk)

Visit the Taylor & Francis Web site at
http://www.taylorandfrancis.com

and the CRC Press Web site at
http://www.crcpress.com

Contents

PART III   Effects of Life Cycle Changes on Bone

PART IV Race, Ethnicity, and Bone

PART V Osteopenia and Osteoporosis

PART VI   Conclusion

Preface

This expanded and advanced treatise, *Diet, Nutrients, and Bone*, is a follow-up a decade and a half later of our earlier book, *Calcium and Phosphorus in Health and Disease*. Considerable advances in our knowledge and understanding of the roles of nutrients in skeletal development and maintenance have been made since publication of that book in 1996. The current book is an expansion of the earlier one and, in essence, an update. Several new topics, however, have been introduced, whereas greater coverage has been given to other topics. Finally, based on their own research and expertise, an impressive group of scientists has made significant contributions to this offering that is intended for graduate students and established researchers in the bone field and related areas of investigation. Public health aspects of bone health are emphasized in this book, that is, health promotion and disease prevention from a nutritional perspective.

The authors thank the following for their assistance in various aspects of this book: Boyd R. Switzer, Jean C. Brown, and the reference staff of the Health Sciences Library at the University of North Carolina.

John J.B. Anderson
Sanford C. Garner
Philip J. Klemmer

Contributors

John J.B. Anderson
Department of Nutrition
Gillings School of Global Public Health
University of North Carolina
Chapel Hill, North Carolina

Connie W. Bales
Department of Medicine
Duke University School of Medicine
Durham, North Carolina

Susan I. Barr
Department of Food, Nutrition, and Health
University of British Columbia
Vancouver, British Columbia, Canada

Adam D.G. Baxter-Jones
College of Kinesiology
University of Saskatchewan
Saskatoon, Saskatchewan, Canada

Jennifer L. Bedford
Department of Food, Nutrition, and Health
University of British Columbia
Vancouver, British Columbia, Canada

Erika Bono
Department of Human Nutrition
Kansas State University
Manhattan, Kansas

Mona S. Calvo
Office of Applied Research and Safety
    Assessment
Center for Food Safety and Applied
    Nutrition
Laurel, Maryland

Yu-ming Chen
Department of Community and Family
    Medicine
Prince of Wales Hospital
The Chinese University of Hong Kong
Hong Kong, People's Republic of China

Felicia Cosman
Department of Medicine
College of Physicians and Surgeons
Columbia University
New York

and

Regional Bone and Clinical Research Centers
Helen Hayes Hospital
West Haverstraw, New York

R.A. Faulkner
College of Kinesiology
University of Saskatchewan
Saskatoon, Saskatchewan, Canada

Robyn K. Fuchs
Department of Physical Therapy
School of Health and Rehabilitation Sciences
Indiana University
Indianapolis, Indiana

Takuo Fujita
Calcium Research Institute
Katsuragi Hospital
Osaka, Japan

Sanford C. Garner
Integrated Laboratory Systems, Inc.
Durham, North Carolina

Gail R. Goldberg
Nutrition and Bone Health Research Group
MRC Human Nutrition Research
Elsie Widdowson Laboratory
Cambridge, United Kingdom
and
Keneba, The Gambia

Elizabeth Grubert
Department of Epidemiology and Biostatistics
School of Public Health
University at Albany
Rensselaer, New York

Kevin Hannon
Department of Basic Medical Sciences
College of Veterinary Medicine
Purdue University
West Lafayette, Indiana

Suzanne C. Ho
Department of Community and Family Medicine
Prince of Wales Hospital
The Chinese University of Hong Kong
Hong Kong, People's Republic of China

Michael F. Holick
Department of Medicine
Vitamin D, Skin and Bone Research
   Laboratory
Boston University Medical Center
Boston, Massachusetts

Guizhou Hu
Department of Research and Development
Biosignia, Inc.
Durham, North Carolina

Karl L. Insogna
Department of Internal Medicine
Yale University School of Medicine
New Haven, Connecticut

Merja Kärkkäinen
Department of Food and Environmental Sciences
University of Helsinki
Helsinki, Finland

Anne M. Kenney
Allied Health Sciences
University of Connecticut
Storrs, Connecticut

Jane E. Kerstetter
Allied Health Sciences
University of Connecticut
Storrs, Connecticut

Philip J. Klemmer
UNC Kidney Center
University of North Carolina
Chapel Hill, North Carolina

Marjo H.J. Knapen
Maastricht University
and
BioPartner Center Maastricht
Maastricht, the Netherlands

Martin Kohlmeier
Department of Nutrition
University of North Carolina
Chapel Hill, North Carolina

Christel Lamberg-Allardt
Department of Food and Environmental
   Sciences
University of Helsinki
Helsinki, Finland

Susan A. Lanham-New
Nutritional Sciences Division
University of Surrey
Guildford, United Kingdom

Richard D. Lewis
Department of Foods and Nutrition
University of Georgia
Athens, Georgia

Yong Li
Molecular Biosciences
Department of Nutritional Sciences
University of Connecticut
Storrs, Connecticut

Denis M. Medeiros
School of Biological Sciences
The University of Missouri-Kansas City
Kansas City, Missouri

Håkan Melhus
School of Biological Sciences
The University of Missouri-Kansas City
Kansas City, Missouri

Jeri W. Nieves
Department of Epidemiology
Mailman School of Public Health
Columbia University, New York

and

Regional Bone and Clinical Research
    Centers
Helen Hayes Hospital
West Haverstraw, New York

Anna Nordström
Department of Community Medicine and
    Rehabilitation
and
Department of Surgical and Perioperative
    Sciences, Sports Medicine
Umeå University
Umeå, Sweden

Peter Nordström
Department of Surgical and Perioperative
    Sciences, Sports Medicine
and
Department of Community Medicine and
    Rehabilitation
Umeå University
Umeå, Sweden

David A. Ontjes
Department of Medicine
University of North Carolina School of
    Medicine
Chapel Hill, North Carolina

Norman K. Pollock
Department of Pediatrics
Georgia Health Sciences University
Augusta, Georgia

Ann Prentice
Nutrition and Bone Health Research
    Group
MRC Human Nutrition Research
Elsie Widdowson Laboratory
Cambridge, United Kingdom
and
Keneba, The Gambia

Martin M. Root
Department of Nutrition and Health Care
    Management
Appalachian State University
Boone, North Carolina

Clifford J. Rosen
Maine Medical Center Research Institute
Scarborough, Maine

Inez Schoenmakers
Nutrition and Bone Health Research Group
MRC Human Nutrition Research
Elsie Widdowson Laboratory
Cambridge, United Kingdom

Mark F. Seifert
Department of Anatomy and Cell Biology
School of Medicine
Indiana University
Indianapolis, Indiana

Sue A. Shapses
Department of Nutritional Sciences
Rutgers University
New Brunswick, New Jersey

Bonny L. Specker
E.A. Martin Program in Human Nutrition
South Dakota State University
Brookings, South Dakota

Ramu Sudhagoni
E.A. Martin Program in Human Nutrition
South Dakota State University
Brookings, South Dakota

Anna K. Surdykowski
Allied Health Sciences
University of Connecticut
Storrs, Connecticut

Natalie W. Thiex
E.A. Martin Program in Human Nutrition
South Dakota State University
Brookings, South Dakota

Frances A. Tylavsky
Department of Preventive Medicine
University of Tennessee Health Sciences Center
Memphis, Tennessee

Sumithra K. Urs
Maine Medical Center Research Institute
Scarborough, Maine

Cees Vermeer
Maastricht University
and
BioPartner Center Maastricht
Maastricht, the Netherlands

Kate A. Ward
Nutrition and Bone Health Research Group
MRC Human Nutrition Research
Elsie Widdowson Laboratory
Cambridge, United Kingdom

Stuart J. Warden
Department of Physical Therapy
School of Health and Rehabilitation Sciences
Indiana University
Indianapolis, Indiana

John D. Wark
Department of Medicine
University of Melbourne
and
Bone & Mineral Service
Royal Melbourne Hospital
Parkville, Victoria, Australia

Bruce A. Watkins
Department of Nutritional Sciences
University of Connecticut
Storrs, Connecticut

Susan Joyce Whiting
College of Pharmacy and Nutrition
University of Saskatchewan
Saskatoon, Saskatchewan, Canada

Kenlyn R. Young
Department of Nutrition
Meredith College
Raleigh, North Carolina

Part I

Introduction to Diet and Bone

1 Overview of Relationships between Diet and Bone

John J.B. Anderson

CONTENTS

INTRODUCTION

The consumption of adequate amounts of food ingredients, that is, nutrients and phytochemicals, is critical to bone and general health. The typical patterns of eating and living influence skeletal development and the maintenance of bone tissue throughout life. Because bone health depends on a few nutrients not so easily obtained in sufficient quantity from meals over short time spans, the overall dietary pattern of food consumption takes on great importance in making available sufficient amounts of the critical bone-building nutrients. Throughout the millennia, cultures have obtained these essential nutrients without knowledge of nutritional science. In recent years, technologically advanced nations have adopted eating patterns in which traditional foods have been replaced, in part, by overly processed foods. These convenient but less nutritious foods have become common in

Western societies. Disappearing, however, is knowledge about healthier eating behaviors practiced by our ancestors.

Information about the relationships between nutrients, including eating patterns, and bone development and maintenance from birth to late life is reviewed in this chapter. Emphasis is placed on recent research that has enhanced our understandings of diet–bone relationships. Calcium and phosphorus, two critical nutrients needed for the mineralization of the organic matrix of bone, receive greater emphasis than do other nutrients required for bone health. Coverage of osteoporosis and vitamin D deficiency diseases are limited mainly to their nutritional determinants rather than to other risk factors.

This introductory chapter briefly highlights the contributions of dietary patterns and specific nutrients that have significant effects on bone health. Short sections on the roles of individual nutrients are covered in the early part of the chapter, and then integrative aspects of the diet are emphasized later in the chapter. This book provides updates on similar topics covered in our earlier publication (Anderson and Garner, 1996).

NUTRIENTS REQUIRED FOR BONE GROWTH AND BONE MAINTENANCE

Most U.S. citizens are omnivorous in their eating habits, but a small percentage (1% to 5%) of the population is vegetarian in one form or another. A large percentage of the North American population fails to meet the currently recommended guidelines for optimal nutrient intakes; some nutrients are consumed in excess; others, in insufficient or even severely deficient quantities. Of particular concern is that intakes of calcium and vitamin D are lower than recommended by current guidelines (Ervin et al., 2004). Corrections of common deficits, such as of calcium and vitamin D, are well recognized as major adjustments needed by deficient adult and elderly individuals to help them maintain their bone mass. Improvement of deficient intakes of these nutrients in children and adolescents is clearly needed to support skeletal growth and to achieve optimal peak bone mass (PBM) by the end of the growth years. Other nutrient deficits, however, may be equally important (Ilich and Kerstetter, 2000; Nieves, 2005). For example, vitamin K and magnesium are also essential for bone health, and intakes of these by Americans are generally insufficient (less than 70% of Dietary Reference Intake or [DRI]) or even deficient (50% or less). Beyond nutritional deficits, excesses in dietary intakes of total calories (energy), protein, sodium, and phosphorus may have adverse effects on the bones of both children and adults. Nutritional factors affecting the bones health, both positively and negatively, are listed in Table 1.1. Each of these dietary factors and a few other nutrients and phytochemicals are briefly noted in this section as preparation for subsequent chapters.

TABLE 1.1
Nutritional Factors Affecting Bone Health: Beneficial and Adverse Effects

Nutrient	Beneficial Intakes	Adverse When Intakes Are
Calcium	RDA amounts	Too little or too much[a]
Phosphorus	RDA amounts	Too much
Vitamin D	RDA amounts	Too little or too much[b]
Animal protein	~15% of total intake	Too much animal (not plant)
Vitamin K	>RDA amounts	Too little
Sodium	2400 mg (recom. amt.)	Too much
Magnesium	RDA amounts	Too little
Vitamin A	RDA amounts	Too little or too much[b]

Notes: RDA = recommended dietary allowance.

[a] Excessive intakes of calcium may contribute to arterial calcification.

[b] Excessive intakes of vitamin D and vitamin A from supplements may be toxic.

ENERGY

Energy intake and bone mass are positively associated in all life stages. During childhood, energy intakes must be sufficient to support skeletal formation and growth (Ilich et al., 2003). In children, excessive weight gain, that is, overweight or obesity, typically does not favor optimal skeletal growth and has been reported to lead to an increase in fractures, especially of the wrist (Goulding et al., 2000). In adults, however, weight gain from excessive energy intake exerts a positive influence on bone mass, and, conversely, extreme weight loss and/or undernutrition may increase the risk of osteoporosis. Weight loss due to anorexia nervosa or other eating disorders is usually accompanied by bone loss. In anorexic women, bone loss results from the associated estrogen deficiency, as well as suboptimal energy intake. Loss of normal body fat may lead to a reduction in ovarian estrogen production amenorrhea and bone loss (Gordon et al., 2002).

PROTEIN

Bone formation during growth in early life requires sufficient protein intake to form the organic matrix of bone. Both high- and low-protein intakes are detrimental to bone. When a low-protein intake by adults is supplemented with protein (meat) in the face of a low-calcium intake, intestinal calcium absorption may be increased and presumably bone mass may be maintained rather than decreased (Kerstetter et al., 2005; Hunt et al., 2009). On the other hand, in growing children, high dietary intakes of protein, particularly animal protein containing acidic amino acids, may increase urinary calcium losses, leading to suboptimal skeletal growth and bone mass (Zhang et al., 2010). Optimal protein intakes, including that from animal sources, support healthy bone development and maintenance later in life (Promislow et al., 2002b; Ilich et al., 2003). Sufficient protein intake may reduce hip fractures of the elderly (Misra et al., 2009) (see Chapter 15).

CALCIUM

The most calcium-rich food sources of calcium exist as low-fat dairy products. Typical intakes of calcium in the United States are less than the recommended amounts by current guidelines starting during early adolescence. Comparisons of dietary intakes and recommended amounts of calcium for U.S. men and women are listed in Table 1.2. A plant-based diet may be capable of supplying sufficient

TABLE 1.2
Comparisons of Dietary Intakes and Recommended Amounts of Calcium and Phosphorus of U.S. Men and Women

Age, Years	Dietary Intakes		Recommendations	
	Calcium	Phosphorus	Calcium	Phosphorus
14–18	787	1172	1300	1250
19–50	~750	~1245	1000	700
>51	619	1055	1200	700

Source: Ervin, R.B., Wang, C.-Y., Wright, J.D., and Kennedy-Steenson, J. Dietary intake of selected minerals for the United States population: 1999–2000 (*advance data no. 341*). CDC, Vital and Health Statistics, US DHHS, Hyattsville, MD; and Food and Nutrition Board, Institute of Medicine. 1997. *Dietary Reference Intakes for Calcium, Phosphorus, Magnesium, Vitamin D, and Fluoride.* National Academy Press, Washington, DC.

Notes: ~ means imputed data.
See also Chapter 8.

calcium if appropriate foods are selected (Weaver et al., 1999). Calcium from dairy foods may be the best sources for skeletal development (Matkovic et al., 2004; Huncharek et al., 2008). Consumption of calcium-fortified foods taken as part of the regular diet may also effectively optimize or maintain skeletal health (Heaney, 2007). Calcium supplements may increase intake in those who cannot meet their needs by ingesting conventional or calcium-fortified foods alone, but such supplementation in premenarcheal females was effective for only 12 to 18 months (Cameron et al., 2004). These gains, however, may not be maintained after the calcium supplements are stopped, and bone losses may quickly offset the earlier gains, at least in growing children (Johnston et al., 1992). Supplementation alone may not be effective in promoting a gain in bone mass if the individual is already consuming an adequate amount of calcium, that is, near or above recommended intakes; in fact, bone loss may still occur in calcium-supplemented women but at a lower rate than in a comparable group of women on a placebo (Riis et al., 1987). A unified public health strategy is needed to ensure optimal calcium intakes from foods (both natural foods and fortified foods) and, if necessary, supplements in the North American population, while avoiding the excessive amounts that approach the tolerable upper intake levels for calcium (2500 mg/day) and raise the risk of soft tissue and vascular calcification by adults (Food and Nutrition Board, Institute of Medicine, 1997) (see below and Chapters 8 and 34).

PHOSPHORUS

Phosphorus, along with calcium, is present in the skeleton in large amounts as part of bone mineral. Therefore, dietary phosphate is required to support the growth and maintenance of the skeleton. However, the average Western diet rich in processed foods contains greater quantities of this essential element than in previous decades. Concern has been raised about the possible adverse effects of excessive intake rather than those of deficiency of this nutrient (Calvo and Park, 1996). Table 1.2 compares U.S. data for phosphorus intakes with recommended amounts. A few studies have shown that excessive phosphate intake from foods exerts adverse effects on the skeleton (Calvo et al., 1990; Kemi et al., 2008, 2009). In addition, because of the differing absorption efficiencies (70% for phosphorus and 30% for calcium) during adulthood, it is advisable to aim for an intake ratio of about 1:1 (see Chapters 8 and 9 for discussions of the calcium:phosphorus ratio).

MAGNESIUM

Magnesium is another mineral nutrient that has been shown in animal studies to be required for normal bone development and maintenance. Magnesium is not an integral part of bone mineral crystals composed of calcium and phosphorus, that is, hydroxyapatite. Approximately two-thirds of the total 25 g of magnesium in the average human body is bound to bone crystal surfaces. Magnesium supplementation has shown little or no effect in increasing bone mass (Rude et al., 2009). Low magnesium intakes are common among men and women of all ages in North America, primarily because of insufficient consumption of dark green vegetables (see Chapter 14).

VITAMIN D

Dietary vitamin D is converted into one of the essential hormones, 1,25-dihydroxyvitamin D, that, along with parathyroid hormone (PTH), regulates calcium metabolism. The importance of vitamin D in bone metabolism is evident in the diseases of vitamin D deficiency, that is, rickets in children and osteomalacia in adults (Kreiter et al., 2000; Holick, 2007; Stoffman and Gordon, 2009). Rickets results in deformities of bones. Osteomalacia in adults typically leads to osteopenia, fractures, poor fracture healing, and muscle weakness. Many elderly have serum vitamin D concentrations that are below optimal levels because of a decreased consumption of food sources and too little exposure to sunlight, which permits skin production of vitamin D. The cutaneous production of vitamin D decreases with age, as well as a consequence of the use of sun-blocking clothing and creams. Sun exposure is particularly low in northern latitudes during the winter months. Skin production of vitamin D in response to UVB light exposure has, in the past, been the major source of this molecule during the months of UVB penetration of the atmosphere, that is, late spring, summer, and early autumn in the northern hemisphere, whereas at present, dietary sources have taken on more prominence. Today, a large majority of North Americans fail to consume adequate amounts of this essential fat-soluble vitamin (Tylavsky et al., 2005; Holick, 2008) (see Chapter 10).

VITAMIN K

Vitamin K, a micronutrient, is now considered to be protective against the loss of bone mass and osteoporosis because of its role in the maintenance of the organic matrix of bone, through modification of specific amino acids in matrix proteins. Studies in postmenopausal women have shown that vitamin K may have modest beneficial effects on bone turnover and calcium metabolism (Braam et al., 2004). The actions of vitamin K may be responsible for other beneficial effects on the skeleton and calcium metabolism (Booth et al., 2000). At least one other study, however, does not support a benefit of vitamin K on bone mineral density (BMD) or fracture prevention (Binkley et al., 2009) (see Chapter 12).

VITAMIN A

Consumption of vitamin A within recommended levels is considered to be beneficial to bone health, but negative effects can result from either too little or too much vitamin A. Both types of bone cells, osteoblasts and osteoclasts, contain receptors for retinoic acid, which is derived from vitamin A. High vitamin A (retinol) intake may contribute to excessive resorption of bone resulting in bone loss (Promislow et al., 2002a) and even to hip fractures (Feskanich et al., 2002). Consumption of β-carotene, other carotenoids, and lycopene from fruits and vegetables, however, has been shown to have positive effects on bone health that reduce the risk of hip fracture (Sahni et al., 2009a), perhaps through their antioxidant roles (see below) rather than their conversion to retinol (see Chapter 11).

VITAMIN C

Like vitamin K, vitamin C or ascorbic acid plays a major role in maintaining bone health through its effect on modification of bone proteins. Bone matrix, composed of collagen, the major organic component of bone, serves to organize the three-dimensional lamellar structure of bone and is the major determinant of bone strength. Collagen molecules are cross-linked, which increases their strength and thus supports bone strength. Optimal amounts of vitamin C intake at reasonable levels have been shown to reduce the risk of hip fracture (Sahni et al., 2009b). In vitamin C deficiency, the organic structure of bone, that is, cross-linking, may be weakened because of suboptimal cross-linking of bone collagen. Fortunately, deficiency of vitamin C in the United States is rare because of fortification of many foods with vitamin C. Also, vitamin C has an important role as an antioxidant in bone cells, as well as in other cell types of the body's tissues (see below) (see Chapter 14).

ANTIOXIDANT NUTRIENTS

Several antioxidant nutrients naturally occurring in foods act to lower the activity of free radicals in cells and, therefore, help to prolong the lives of the cells, including bone cells. Vitamin C has already been mentioned, but vitamin E, carotenoids and lycopene, selenium, and perhaps another trace element or two have important roles in diminishing the oxidative effects of free radicals—highly reactive oxygen species (Basu et al., 2001; Maggio et al., 2003). Finally, many phytochemicals from a wide variety of plant foods, especially polyphenolic molecules, have similar roles (see Chapter 19).

FLUORIDE

Fluoridation of drinking water has been very effective in reducing dental caries, but studies on the effects of this nutrient in increasing bone mineral content (BMC) and reducing bone fractures have been disappointing. Studies of fluoride have shown that protection is not obtained from the cariostatic levels found in municipal water supplies, that is, 1 ppm. Fluoride supplements at sufficiently high doses (>3 ppm) may even be deleterious to bone because of defects in the mineral phase of bone, causing it to be well mineralized but brittle, that is, hysteresis. At present, supplemental use of fluoride is not recommended for osteoporotic women or others because of the risk of adverse bone effects associated with higher exposures. The Food and Drug Administration is not likely to ever approve of fluoride use in amounts greater than 1 ppm for the intended benefit of bone mass because the quality of bone formed at higher intakes is structurally inferior, and fracture risk may actually be increased (Kleerekoper, 1996) (see Chapter 14).

PHYTOMOLECULES

Phytoestrogens, including soy isoflavones, have been proposed to have osteoprotective actions because of their activation of estrogen receptors in bone cells, especially osteoblasts. These estrogen-like molecules, classified chemically as polyphenols, were reported to have positive effects on bone measurements in postmenopausal women and women with low circulating estrogens compared with those in placebo-treated women in some studies, but more recent studies have failed to support these findings. Isoflavones from soy products may have weak skeletal benefits in postmenopausal women (Arjmandi et al., 2003), but a few recent reports do not support such benefits (Alekel et al., 2010; Wong et al., 2009). In young adult women with normal estrogen status, isoflavones appear to have no effect on bone (Anderson et al., 2002).

SUMMARY

Many nutrients are required for optimal skeletal growth and maturation. The Dietary Reference Intakes of the nutrients, but not of phytomolecules, have been published by the National Academies Press (Food and Nutrition Board, Institute of Medicine, 1997, 2004). Only a few specific recommendations are given in this section, because typically, the quantities are readily available (see also Table 1.2).

CALCIUM AND PHOSPHORUS INTERRELATIONSHIPS

Dietary calcium deficiency or insufficiency among adults is common, but phosphorus deficiency is extremely rare, because practically all natural foods contain phosphorus (see section "Phosphorus" above). Suboptimal phosphorus consumption from foods remains highly unlikely if adequate energy is consumed. Low phosphorus intake, however, may exist in a small percentage (<5%) of elderly living in poverty or near poverty and not consuming enough of foods containing adequate amounts of phosphorus. A very low phosphorus intake may result in hypophosphatemic osteomalacia, which decreases both bone density and bone strength. Supplementation with phosphate salts is not recommended for healthy individuals because high quantities of this mineral are already consumed in diets rich in processed foods in the United States.

Phosphate excess—and calcium deficiency together—tends to increase PTH secretion and thereby decrease skeletal mass and density, partly because phosphate ions are absorbed much more rapidly than calcium ions (Anderson and Talmage, 1973). If chronic, the continuous hyperparathyroidism may lead to osteopenia and osteoporosis (see Chapters 8 and 9 on calcium to phosphorus ratio). Phosphate toxicity resulting from excessive dietary phosphorus is extremely rare in individuals with normal kidney function. The recent decline in the dietary calcium-to-phosphorus ratio over the past several decades to less than 1:1, even as low as 0.5:1, has resulted from a declining consumption of dietary calcium associated with less milk intake and an increase in dietary phosphorus from cola-type beverages and foods processed with phosphate additives.

CALCIUM AND VITAMIN D INTERRELATIONSHIPS

A deficient dietary calcium status has a large impact on the renal production of the hormonal form of vitamin D as well as on the increased serum concentration of PTH. Both of these hormonal adaptations are designed to enhance calcium absorption and release of calcium from bone to reestablish the normal serum concentration of calcium ions. If both dietary intakes of calcium and vitamin D are lower than recommended, too little calcium is absorbed and, thus, less goes into bone mineral (see section "Vitamin D" above). Extreme consequences of a deficiency of these two nutrients are rickets in children and osteomalacia in adults, and each of these diseases is reviewed in later chapters.

NUTRITION AND BONE HEALTH ACROSS THE LIFE CYCLE

Nutrient requirements differ according to the stage of the life cycle. These needs are determined by the greater demands for growth of the skeleton during early life and the requirements to maintain the skeleton once PBM is achieved by about the age of 30 years. The early life accumulation of bone, that is,, the "early gain," yields mean measurements of BMD of the healthy population of 20- to 29-year-old males and females that are used as the standards for comparison with individual bone measurements late in life (see World Health Organization standards for BMD in Chapter 32).

The "later loss" of bone differs between men and women. Accelerated skeletal declines in bone mass and density of women occur characteristically beyond the age of menopause, that is, about aged 50 years, and these declines are associated first with osteopenia and then with osteoporosis. In men, the late-life declines start later, and they typically result in less overall loss prior to death at younger ages than that for women. The combination of the earlier period of life, that is, accumulation of bone mineral in the skeleton, and the later period as one of loss, has been aptly described as the "early gain and later loss" by an observant physical anthropologist (Garn, 1970). These changes in bone mass across the life cycle are illustrated later in this volume.

The accumulation of bone mineral and the eventual loss of that mineral are intimately connected with the activity of living cells within bone. These cells are responsible for the activities of bone modeling (building predominantly), that is, bone formation and bone resorption (degradation), and remodeling (building and turning over the final model) that occur during skeletal development and throughout life. Insufficient intakes of calcium and vitamin D commonly exist among fairly high percentages of the U.S. population, and these high deficits extend across the life cycle, although they are higher in females than those in males (Food and Nutrition Board, 1997). Failure to achieve optimal PBM as a consequence of poor nutrition during the growth years cannot be reversed later in life through increased intakes of calcium and vitamin D.

NUTRITION AND SKELETAL GROWTH FROM BIRTH THROUGH ADOLESCENCE

Provision of an adequate diet containing all of the nutrients required for the development of healthy bones of children is obviously the responsibility of the parents or caretakers. Good nutrition during the postnatal growth years influences greatly the achievement of optimal skeletal growth, which, of course, is governed by genetic potential. Many studies throughout the world have shown that high-quality diets, in terms of protein, energy, and micronutrients, foster good growth of all tissues, including the skeleton. Thus, more affluent youth in developed Western countries and in Japan since the 1950s achieve or approach the mean heights of American children. Calcium and other minerals in the diet are retained in the skeleton, but calcium intake per se has little to do with skeletal growth acceleration. Adequate calcium intake is necessary, but not sufficient in itself, to achieve optimal bone mass. Adequate energy and high-quality protein are the critical nutrients needed for providing the stimulus for organic matrix production as part of skeletal growth from infancy through adolescence. Calcium intakes need to remain reasonably high to increase the mineral content and density of the skeleton both during growth (prepuberty and postpuberty) and in the early postgrowth period of the 20s (young adulthood). This need for calcium is especially evident for females, who consume too little calcium in the United States and most Western nations to accumulate adequate amounts of the mineral. Rapidly growing males in their late adolescent years also need an abundant amount of calcium, perhaps even more than the age-specific DRIs, for an optimal skeletal mass.

The concept of a calcium requirement is complicated by the fact that, often despite somewhat poor dietary calcium intakes, American children have satisfactory skeletal growth if the intakes of energy and protein are satisfactory. At least during the adolescent period of growth, the efficiency of calcium absorption is high, perhaps 60%, to meet the skeleton's needs for calcium in the formation of hydroxyapatite. Optimal development of PBM, however, is achieved by calcium intakes approximating the DRI (1300 mg/day) from dairy products and other calcium-containing foods throughout these early years. Premenarcheal girls (10 to 12 years old) typically have the greatest gains of bone mass and density of any stage of the life cycle because of their rapid growth, and with optimal calcium intakes, they continue gaining bone mass (Bonjour et al., 2001). Positive calcium balance is the rule during the growth phase; zero (or slightly positive) balance exists during the equilibrium phase of the decade of the 20s; and negative calcium balance dominates during the resorptive phases of the postmenopausal and elderly periods of life. A healthy state of calcium balance exists when formation equals resorption over a period of months, that is, zero balance, but after the decade of the 20s, zero balance probably rarely occurs (see Chapter 8).

Skeletal growth in length (height) ceases in adolescent females within approximately 2 to 4 years following menarche (Bonjour et al., 1997; Jackman et al., 1997; Matkovic et al., 2004), whereas in males it continues into the early 20s. As stated above, however, calcium intakes continue to be important because of the accumulation of calcium in hydroxyapatite, the mineral salt in bone, during this early adult phase, sometimes called bone consolidation. Accrual of PBM is not achieved until after both growth in length and postgrowth mineral acquisition have been completed, that is, by approximately 30 years of age. Thus, adequate calcium intakes remain important for both the achievement of PBM and the maintenance of these skeletal tissues during the early adult decades. The age-specific recommended calcium allowances (DRIs) decrease from 1300 mg/day during adolescence to slightly less during adulthood (see Chapter 8). A high-calcium intake later in life, however, does not compensate for a deficient intake during childhood and adolescence.

Nutrition and Bone Changes after Skeletal Growth (Length) Has Ceased

The mineral phase of the compact tissue of long-bone shafts increases its calcium and phosphorus content during this postgrowth period. For example, it has been estimated that young adult women between ages 20 and 30 years may gain an additional 5% to 10% of their skeletal mass over this decade. The widths of the long bones may continue to increase at very low rates throughout much of the remainder of life. Optimal calcium intakes then should maximize an individual's PBM by about 30 years of age. In women, the maintenance of bone mass gained by early adulthood becomes more important with each passing decade after the menopause or equivalent age in males when the loss of bone mass continues, often at an increased rate. In females, an accelerated loss of bone occurs typically within the first decade following menopause.

After growth ceases, physical activity (exercise) and pregnancy/lactation are the major factors that contribute to both higher rates of bone remodeling and increased BMC and BMD until approximately age 40 years (Tylavsky et al., 1989). After that time, both increased remodeling and bone loss typically occur until the age of 50 years, the typical age at the start of the menopausal transition that lasts for approximately a decade.

Nutrition and Skeletal Losses during Late Life

During the decade following menopause, resorption increases relative to formation (referred to as *uncoupling*) in the elderly period of life and contributes to reduced BMC and BMD. Males do not have an equivalent to menopause, and they lose bone gradually during the later decades of life. Mean estimates of calcium intakes of men and women typically are lower than the AI of 1200 mg/day, starting at the age of 50 years.

Slowing the dominance of resorption over formation in the later adult decades may be enhanced by exercise coupled with adequate calcium intake in addition to the use of bone-conserving drugs. Physicians previously prescribed hormone-replacement therapy, consisting of an estrogen and a progestin, during the early menopause, but these drugs may increase the risk of breast, endometrial, or other reproductive cancers, at least in older women. So, now, other drugs prescribed mostly for women to slow the loss of bone mass and density (secondary prevention) have been quite robust (see Chapter 5). Supplemental calcium has been used to slow bone loss by inhibiting PTH release in aged subjects (McKane et al., 1996) and to help maintain bone mass (see Chapter 27).

The precise human requirements for calcium beyond the adolescent growth phase remain uncertain. During late adulthood, when sarcopenia, a decline in muscle mass, commonly accompanies osteopenia, elders have a high prevalence of both low calcium and vitamin D intakes, and supplements may improve bone measurements, that is, BMD, to a modest degree. Calcium supplementation of postmenopausal women has yielded very limited gains in BMD (see Chapters 8 and 32). Too high an intake of calcium, however, may contribute to arterial calcification, especially when renal function declines (see above).

The type of bone tissue that undergoes greater loss with aging is trabecular or cancellous bone, in large part because of greater surface areas. Much of the trabecular tissue is located in the vertebral bodies (spine) and the ends of the long bones (hip and wrist). Many individuals begin to lose height around the age of 50 years because of the shortening of the vertebral height (not the leg height) resulting from compression or even crushing of the vertebrae, particularly those in the lumbar region (lower spine) whose vertebral bodies are high in trabecular bone tissue.

When bone mass declines below a certain low threshold in women within a decade or two after menopause and in men by their 60s and 70s, increased risk of fractures of the vertebrae and hips may occur in these individuals. In addition to dietary and activity factors, many other lifestyle variables contribute to osteoporotic fractures and subsequent survival, especially following hip fractures (see Chapter 32). Because of the high prevalence rates of hip fractures in the elderly, which result in significant mortality and cost for care, osteoporosis has become an enormous public health problem in the United States as well as in practically all other Western nations, especially as these populations are aging. In future decades, virtually all Asian, African, and Latin American countries will be similarly affected. Many reasons can be given for the increasing worldwide rates of osteoporotic hip fractures, but a major demographic factor is the increasing longevity of women and men in economically developed countries because of better nutrition, better health care, and generally improved living conditions. The aging of populations is also occurring in less developed nations, and the age-adjusted rates of osteoporotic fractures are anticipated to increase greatly in these nations.

VEGETARIAN DIETS

Vegetarian diets come in different forms from strict (vegan) through lacto-, ovo-, or lacto-ovo-vegetarian to vegetarian diets with occasional fish. Flexitarians are those who try to eat reasonably cheaply, but on occasion, they may consume some poultry or red meat. Omnivores, of course, consume all groups of foods, and many processed food choices are made within this type of eating behavior. Emphasis in this book is based on results of bone studies of omnivorous eating patterns, although bone mass accumulation and loss appear to be similar in vegetarians.

The few bone studies that have been performed with lacto-ovo-vegetarians and a recent meta-analysis confirm that vegetarians have similar bone measurements at all ages of the life cycle as omnivores—both within normal ranges of BMD during early adulthood—but that the mean measurements appear to be slightly lower for vegetarians (Ho-Pham et al., 2009), although only trivially lower (Lanham-New, 2009). The only prospective study that examined bone changes of elderly lacto-ovo-vegetarians showed that they lost bone mass over 5 years at approximately the same rate as omnivores (Reed et al., 1994).

ROLE OF PHYSICAL ACTIVITY IN BONE DEVELOPMENT AND MAINTENANCE

Over the last decade or so, numerous reports have been published with findings on the beneficial effect of weight-bearing exercise on BMC and BMD. The most beneficial gains resulting from exercise occur in the early periods of life (premenarche in girls and slightly later in boys) (Welch and Weaver, 2005). Benefits of physical activities on the skeleton may occur at any age, although they are less robust after growth has ceased. The elderly show the least gains in BMC or BMD, but nevertheless, they may improve in these measurements as well as in their microarchitectural bone structures of the affected bones (see Chapters 3 and 33). What has recently become evident, however, is that the practices of upper body exercise, walking, and other activities must be continued on a regular basis or any gains of bone mass will be lost. The rates of osteoporotic fractures occurring during the postmenopausal decades have been shown to be greater in nonactive women than those among more active women.

Physical activities exert forces on bone tissue that both enhance development during the bone modeling years and help maintain bone during the bone remodeling years. The benefits of activity on bone from roughly the age of 40 years and beyond have only small or no effects on BMD, but they do increase bone turnover—hence new bone—at critical sites of the skeleton and they may delay fractures at these sites (Dornemann et al., 1997). The combination of exercise plus AIs of calcium and other nutrients contribute to healthy bones.

SUMMARY

A good diet containing all the nutrients at recommended intakes, plus phytochemicals from plant foods, is optimal for bone health, especially during the first two decades of life. A healthy dietary pattern coupled with regular physical activity maximizes skeletal development and PBM, as established for 20- to 29-year-old males and females. Later in life, low bone mass or osteopenia typically precedes the development of osteoporosis by approximately a decade. Osteoporosis reflects the long-term senescence of the skeletal tissues and losses of both bone mass and density, but it may occur prematurely if ovarian production of estrogens ceases because of premature menopause or oophorectomy.

Osteoporosis is a multifactorial disorder with risk factors relating to nutrition; lifestyle, including cigarette smoking; hormonal status; and yet to be determined hereditary determinants. The risk of fracture is related to the degree of osteoporosis and factors related to risks of falls, including balance and agility, and to impairments in vision and cognition. This common bone disease among elders may be delayed—although not avoided—by a good diet, that is, calcium, vitamin D, and other nutrients, plus regular physical exercise, healthy lifestyle behaviors, and drugs. Adequate dietary calcium and vitamin D intakes and reduced consumption of phosphorus, particularly from processed foods and cola-type soft drinks, may help slow the loss of bone mass in the later decades of life by suppressing PTH secretion.

Elders who consume little or no dairy products obtain most of their calcium from breads and baked goods, but not enough calcium exists in these foods to meet the recommended intakes for calcium. Problem nutrients for bone health continue to be too little consumption of calcium and vitamin D and of too much phosphorus (as phosphates) and sodium at all ages of the life cycle.

REFERENCES

Alekel, D.L., Van Loan, M.D., Koehler, K.J., et al. 2010. The Soy Isoflavones for Reducing Bone Loss (SIRBL) study: A 3-year randomized controlled trial in postmenopausal women. *Am J Clin Nutr* 91: 218–230.

Anderson, J.J.B., Chen, X.W., Boass, A., et al. 2002. Soy isoflavones: No effects on bone mineral content and bone mineral density in healthy, menstruating young adult women after one year. *J Am Coll Nutr* 21: 388–393.

Anderson, J.J.B., and Garner, S.C., eds. 1996. *Calcium and Phosphorus in Health and Disease.* CRC Press, Boca Raton, FL.

Anderson, J.J.B., and Talmage, R.V. 1973. The Effect of calcium infusion and calcitonin on plasma phosphate in sham-operated and thyroparathyroidectomized dogs. *Endocrinology* 93: 1222–1226.

Arjmandi, B.H., Khalil, D.A., Smith, B.J., et al. 2003. Soy protein has a greater effect on bone in postmenopausal women. *J Clin Endocrinol Metab* 88: 1048–1054.

Basu, S., Michaelsson, K., Olofsson, H., et al. 2001. Association between oxidative stress and bone mineral density. *Biochem Biophys Res Commun* 288: 275–279.

Binkley, N., Harke, J., Krueger, D., et al. 2009. Vitamin K treatment reduces undercarboxylated osteocalcin but does not alter bone turnover, density, or geometry in healthy postmenopausal North American women. *J Bone Miner Res* 24: 983–991.

Bolland, M.J., Barber, P.A., Doughty, R.N., et al. 2008. Vascular events in healthy older women receiving calcium supplementation: Randomised controlled trial. *BMJ* 336: 262–265.

Bonjour, J.-P., Chevally, T., Ammann, P., et al. 2001. Gain in bone mineral mass in prepubertal girls 3–5 years after discontinuation of calcium supplementation: A follow-up study. *Lancet* 358: 1208–1212.

Bonjour, J.-P., Carrie, A.L., Ferrari, S., et al. 1997. Calcium-enriched foods and bone mass growth in prepubertal girls: A randomized double blind placebo-controlled trial. *J Clin Invest* 99: 1287–1294.

Booth, S.I., Tucker, K.L., Chen, H., et al. 2000. Dietary vitamin K intakes are associated with hip fractures but not with BMD in elderly men and women. *Am J Clin Nutr* 71: 1201–1208.

Braam, L.A., Knapen, M.H., Geusens, P., et al. 2004. Vitamin K_1 supplementation retards bone loss in postmenopausal women between 50 and 60 years of age. *Calcif Tiss Int* 73: 21–26.

Calvo, M.S., Kumar, R., and Heath, H.H., III. 1990. Persistently elevated parathyroid hormone secretion and action in young women after four weeks of ingesting high phosphorus, low calcium diets. *J Clin Endocrinol Metab* 70: 1334–1340.

Calvo, M.S., and Park, Y.K. 1996. Changing phosphorus content of the U.S. diet: Potential for adverse effects on bone. *J Nutr* 126: 1168S.

Cameron, M.A., Paton, L.M., Nowson, C.A., et al. 2004. The effect of calcium supplementation on bone density in premenarcheal females: A co-twin approach. *J Clin Endocrinol Metab* 89: 4916–4922.

Demer, L. A skeleton in the atherosclerotic closet. 1995. *Circulation* 92: 2029–2032.

Dornemann, T.M., McMurray, R.G., Renner, J.B., et al. 1997. Effects of high-intensity resistance exercise on bone mineral density and muscle strength of 40–50 year old women. *J Sports Med Phys Fitness* 37: 246–251.

Ervin, R.B., Wang, C.-Y., Wright, J.D., et al. 2004. Dietary intake of selected minerals for the United States population: 1999–2000 (*advance data no. 341*). CDC, Vital and Health Statistics, US DHHS, Hyattsville, MD, 8 pages.

Feskanich, D., Singh, V., Willett, W., et al. 2002. Vitamin A intake and hip fractures among postmenopausal women. *JAMA* 287: 47–54.

Food and Nutrition Board, Institute of Medicine. 1997. *Dietary Reference Intakes for Calcium, Phosphorus, Magnesium, Vitamin D, and Fluoride.* National Academy Press, Washington, DC.

Food and Nutrition Board, Institute of Medicine. 2004. *Dietary Reference Intakes for Electrolytes and Water.* National Academy Press, Washington, DC.

Garn, S. 1970. *The Early Gain and Late Loss of Cortical Bone: In Nutritional Perspective.* Thomas, C.C., Springfield, IL.

Gordon, C.M., Goodman, E., Emans, S.J., et al. 2002. Physiologic regulators of bone turnover in young women with anorexia nervosa. *J Pediatr* 141: 64–70.

Goulding, A., Taylor, I.E., Jones, F.A., et al. 2000. Overweight and obese children have low bone mass and area for their weight. *Int J Obesity* 24: 627–632.

Heaney, R.P. 2007. Bone health. *Am J Clin Nutr* 85: 300S–303S.

Holick, M.F. 2007. Vitamin D deficiency. *New Engl J Med* 357: 266–281.

Holick, M.F. 2008. Vitamin D: A D-lightful health perspective. *Nutr Rev* 66: S182–S194.

Ho-Pham, L.T., Nguyen, N.D., and Nguyen, T.V. 2009. Effect of vegetarian diets on bone mineral density: A Bayesian meta-analysis. *Am J Clin Nutr* 90: 943–950.

Huncharek, M., Muscat, J., and Kupelnick, B. 2008. Impact of dairy products and dietary calcium on bone-mineral content in children: Results of a meta-analysis. *Bone* 40: 312–321.

Hunt, J.R., Johnson, L.K., and Roughead, Z.K.F. 2009. Dietary protein and calcium interact to influence calcium retention: A controlled feeding trial. *Am J Clin Nutr* 89: 1357–1365.

Ilich, J.Z., Brownbill, R.A., and Tanborini, L. 2003. Bone and nutrition in elderly women: Protein, energy, and calcium as main determinants of bone mineral density. *Eur J Clin Nutr* 57: 554–565.

Ilich, J.Z., and Kerstetter, J.E. 2000. Nutrition in bone health revisited: A story beyond calcium. *J Am Coll Nutr* 19: 715–737.

Jackman, L.A., Millane, S.S., Martin, B.R., et al. 1997. Calcium retention in relation to calcium intake and postmenarcheal age in adolescent females. *Am J Clin Nutr* 66: 327–333.

Johnston, C.C., Jr., Miller, J.Z., Slemenda, C.W., et al. 1992. Calcium supplementation and increases in bone mineral density of children. *New Engl J Med* 327: 82–87.

Kemi, V.E., Karkkainen, M.U.M., Karp, H.J., et al. 2008. Increased calcium intake does not completely counteract the effects of increased phosphorus intake on bone: An acute dose-response study in healthy females. *Br J Nutr* 99: 832–839.

Kemi, V.E., Rita, H.J., Karkkainen, M.U.M., et al. 2009. Habitual high phosphorus intakes and foods with phosphate additives negatively affect serum parathyroid concentration: A cross-sectional study on healthy premenopausal women. *Public Health Nutr* 12: 1885–1892.

Kerstetter, J.E., O'Brien, K.O., Caseria, D.M., et al. 2005. The impact of dietary protein on calcium absorption and kinetic measures of bone turnover in women. *J Clin Endocrinol Metab* 90: 26–31.

Kleerekoper, M. 1996. Fluoride: The verdict is in, but the controversy lingers. *J Bone Miner Res* 11: 565–567.

Kreiter, S.R., Schwartz, R.P., Kirkman, H.N., Jr., et al. 2000. Nutritional rickets in African American breast-fed infants. *J Pediatr* 137: 153–157.

Lanham-New, S.A. 2009. Is "vegetarianism" a serious risk factor for osteoporotic fracture? *Am J Clin Nutr* 90: 910–911.

Maggio, D., Barabani, M., Pierandrei, M., et al. 2003. Marked decreases in plasma antioxidants in aged osteoporotic women: Results of a cross-sectional study. *J Clin Endocrinol Metab* 88: 1523–1527.

Matkovic, V., Landoll, J.D., Badenhop-Stevens, N.E., et al. 2004. Nutrition influences skeletal development from childhood to adulthood: A study of hip, spine, and forearm in adolescent females. *J Nutr* 134: 701S–705S.

McKane, W.R., Khosla, S., Egan, K.S., et al. 1996. Role of calcium intake in modulating age-related increases in parathyroid function and bone resorption. *J Clin Endocrinol Metab* 81: 1699–1703.

Misra, D., Berry, S., Broe, K.E., et al. 2009. Does dietary protein reduce hip fracture risk in elders? The Framingham Osteoporosis Study. *Osteoporos Int* (in press).

Nieves, J.W. Osteoporosis: The role of micronutrients. 2005. *Am J Clin Nutr* 81: 1232S–1239S.

Promislow, J.H.E., Goodman-Gruen, D., Slymen, D.J., et al. 2002a. Retinol intake and bone mineral density in the elderly. *J Bone Miner Res* 17: 1359–1362.

Promislow, J.H.E., Goodman-Gruen, D., Slymen, D.J., et al. 2002b. Protein consumption and bone mineral density in the elderly: The Rancho Bernardo Study. *Am J Epidemiol* 155: 636–644.

Reed, J.A., Tylavsky, F.A., Anderson, J.J.B., et al. 1994. Camparative changes in radial bone density of elderly female lactoovovegetarians and omnivores. *Am J Clin Nutr* 59: 1197S–1202S.

Riis, B., Thomsen, K., and Christiansen, C. 1987. Does calcium supplementation prevent postmenopausal bone loss? A double-blind, controlled clinical trial. *New Engl J Med* 316: 173–177.

Rude, R.K., Singer, F.R., and Gruber, H.E. 2009. Skeletal and hormonal effects of magnesium deficiency. *J Am Coll Nutr* 28: 131–141.

Sahni, S., Hannan, M.T., Blumberg, J., et al. 2009a. Protective effect of total carotenoid and lycopene intake on the risk of hip fracture: A 17-year follow-up from the Framingham Osteoporosis Study. *J Bone Miner Res* 24: 1086–1094.

Sahni, S., Hannan, M.T., Gagnon, D., et al. 2009b. Protective effect of total and supplemental vitamin C intake on the risk of hip fracture—A 17-year follow-up from the Framingham Osteoporosis Study. *Osteoporos Int* 20: 1853–1861.

Stoffman, N., and Gordon, C.M. 2009. Vitamin D and adolescents: What do we know? *Curr Opin Pediatr* 21: 465–471.

Tylavsky, F.A., Bortz, A.D., Hancock, R.L., et al. 1989. Familial resemblance of radial bone mass between premenopausal mothers and their college-age daughters. *Calcif Tissue Int* 45: 265–272.

Tylavsky, F.A., Ryder, K.A., Lyyktikainen, A., et al. 2005. Vitamin D, parathyroid hormone, and bone mass in adolescents. *J Nutr* 135: 2735S–2738S.

Weaver, C.M., Proulx, W.R., and Heaney, R. 1999. Choices for achieving adequate dietary calcium with a vegetarian diet. *Am J Clin Nutr* 70 (Suppl): 543S–548S.

Welch, J.M., and Weaver, C.M. 2005. Calcium and exercise affect the growing skeleton. *Nutr Rev* 63: 361–373.

Zhang, Q., Ma, G., Greenfield, H., et al. 2010. The association between dietary protein intake and bone mass accretion in pubertal girls with low calcium intakes. *Br J Nutr* 103: 714–723.

2 Role of Lifestyle Factors in Bone Health

John J.B. Anderson and Philip J. Klemmer

CONTENTS

INTRODUCTION

Although dietary factors remain the central focus of this book, lifestyle variables are also important determinants of bone health. Therefore, a brief account of the relevant lifestyle factors is provided as background for the later chapters that examine these factors in greater detail.

Several nondietary risk factors that may increase the likelihood of osteoporotic fractures of the skeleton have been identified. These potentially adverse risk factors promote the loss of bone mass that contribute over time to fractures (Table 2.1). Each of these lifestyle variables and environmental factors has a risk by itself, and when coupled with one or more other risk factors, the risk typically increases exponentially. A classic example of multiple risk factors was reported in 1976 by an endocrine specialist in Charleston, SC, who had observed in 36 of his elderly female patients with vertebral fractures that they all exhibited thinness, excessive cigarette smoking, and possibly too much consumption of alcohol (Daniell, 1976). So, thin older (>70) postmenopausal women who have hip fractures will have been at risk over the previous decade or longer before their bone loss becomes clinically apparent by the development of pathologic bone fractures as a result of osteoporosis.

In some instances, a few lifestyle practices may have positive effects on the skeleton and hence the prevention of osteoporosis-related fractures. For example, regular physical activity, including upper body weight exercise, may promote a small improvement in bone mass or at least maintain bone at a steady-state of skeletal integrity. This latter point is especially important in preventing hip fractures because maintenance of a stable bone mineral density at this site yields major benefits. The topic of exercise is covered in other chapters.

The elderly commonly have losses of visual acuity, hearing, muscular strength, and equilibrium, any or all of which may contribute to falls and fractures (see below). The loss of muscle mass, also known as sarcopenia, typically goes hand in hand with osteopenia, or bone mass loss that is not as

TABLE 2.1

Lifestyle or Nondietary Risk Factors for Osteoporosis

Cigarette smoking (any amount, but pack a day more detrimental)

Excessive alcohol consumption (exceeding two drinks a day for men and one drink a day for
  women)

Insufficient physical activity and sedentary lifestyle

Drugs—over-the-counter and prescription [vitamin A, corticosteroids, anabolic steroids, phenytoin
  (Dilantin), proton pump inhibitors, and others]

Falls for many reasons (see Table 2.3)

TABLE 2.2

World Health Organization Definitions of Osteoporosis and Osteopenia: SDs Relative to Means of 20- to 29-Year-Old Controls

Classification	Definition of T Score[a]
Normal BMD	Within ± 1 SD of mean
Osteopenic BMD	Between 1 and 2.5 SDs below mean
Osteoporotic BMD	Greater than 2.5 SDs below mean

[a] T-Score compares the current BMD measurement of adult with
  20- to 29-year-old means.

BMD = bone mineral density; SD = standard deviation.

severe as in osteoporosis. Medications may also affect these same sensory organs and contribute to falls and fractures (see below). The one fracture that should be the focus of fracture prevention is of the hip because an individual with a broken hip has significantly greater morbidity and mortality over the next 6 to 12 months.

The decline in body mass to the point of thinness may be the most important of the acquired risk factors. A decline in lean body mass (LBM) because of inactivity or too little food consumption is a major determinant of bone loss and fracture. Accompanying the leanness from sarcopenia, which translates to an overall decline in muscle strength, is the associated bone loss leading to osteopenia and eventually to osteoporosis, as defined by the World Health Organization (WHO) (Table 2.2). The decline in muscle strain on the skeleton at sites of muscle insertion is typically coupled with decreased bone formation and excessive bone resorption (Ontjes and Anderson, 2009).

NONDIETARY RISK FACTORS CONTRIBUTING TO OSTEOPOROSIS

Each major risk factor for osteopenia and osteoporosis is briefly reviewed in this section. Fractures resulting from osteoporosis in the elderly are associated with a high risk of mortality (Cauley, 2000).

THINNESS AND LOW LBM

Maintenance of LBM, which reflects muscle mass, helps conserve skeletal mass because of the coordinated functions of the musculoskeletal system. Whereas obesity is not recommended for healthy individuals, some fat mass contributes to body mass (and body mass index [BMI]) that places individuals in the healthy weight range (BMI of 18.5 to 24.9). When BMI is below 18.5, individuals are classified as underweight, and underweight means less LBM. Elders with low LBM are at increased risk of fractures, as well as of many other chronic diseases. Low-LBM elders who also smoke tobacco and consume excessive amounts of alcohol have greatly increased risk of hip fractures (see below).

Cigarette Smoking

Cigarette smoking adversely affects practically every organ system of the body, mainly because of oxidative stress and accelerated atherosclerosis. Cigarette smoking may also increase oxidative damage within cells that contributes to reduced cellular functions. In women, cigarette smoking decreases serum estrogen concentrations by stimulating estrogen catabolism in the liver, and it may contribute to an early menopause. Bone loss typically follows declines in serum estrogen concentrations. In older men, current smoking adversely affects fractures of the vertebrae and hips (Jutberger et al., 2010).

Excessive Alcohol Consumption

Too much alcohol has direct deleterious effects on cells of the body, including bone cells. Modest alcohol consumption (two drinks a day by men or one drink a day by women), however, is not considered a risk factor, and these small amounts may actually have a slightly positive effect on bone tissue, as it does in other tissues of the body.

Insufficient Physical Activity

This topic is considered in considerable detail in Chapters 5, 20, and 30. Adequate physical activity when coupled with a healthy dietary pattern contributes to optimal skeletal development early in life and to maintenance later in life. Physical activity may be the most important lifestyle variable for boosting and maintaining bone mass in adult life. The types of beneficial activities include aerobic ones, such as walking, stair climbing, and gardening, but loading exercises, such as lifting weights or other activities, may also improve muscle and bone.

Drug Usage—Over-the-Counter and Prescription Drugs

Excessive or inappropriate use of drugs, whether over-the-counter or prescription drugs, may have detrimental effects on the skeletal system. Vitamin A overuse has long been known to have adverse skeletal effects (see Chapter 11). A classic example of a prescription medication used to treat seizures, Dilantin, exists, and without adequate vitamin D supplementation, individuals taking this drug have been reported to develop vitamin D deficiency and osteomalacia which may cause growth abnormalities in children and pathologic fractures in adults.

Prednisone and other corticosteroid hormones have adverse effects on bone tissue when chronically used over periods of months to years. Osteoporosis is a well-established adverse effect of these agents.

The drug class known as proton pump inhibitors (PPIs) also has adverse effects on calcium metabolism in chronic users. PPIs reduce acid (H+) secretion by gastric cells and the reduced amounts of acid entering the small intestine decrease the absorption of calcium in the more alkaline intestinal fluid. Increased fracture rates have been reported in older patients taking PPIs (Yang et al., 2006).

Illicit recreational drugs may also have adverse effects on bone, mainly because of poor dietary intakes.

Decline of Sensory Perceptions

Limited vision, hearing, or equilibrium contributes to stumbling and falls (see below), which contribute to fractures in fragile elders. Correction of these losses may not be entirely possible, but new medical techniques and therapies may help mitigate these deficits.

Falls

Falling has been established as a major risk factor for skeletal fractures, particularly among the elderly (Tinetti et al., 1988). Lifestyle rather than physical risk factors has been reported to greatly contribute to falls in the elderly (Faulkner et al., 2009). New approaches to preventing falls include home safety measures, such as avoiding throw rugs and loose wire cords, installing hand-hold bars in bathrooms and hallways, improving overhead lighting, and utilizing hip pads. Because poor coordination and balance contribute to falls, any intervention, such as walking-assist devices, helps to reduce fall-related fractures. Falls may also be reduced by avoiding drugs which alter cognitive function, such as sleep aids and tranquilizers, and even excessive alcohol and antihypertensive drugs which may cause orthostatic syncope (falling). Individuals with cognitive decline, memory loss, and Alzheimer's disease may have fewer falls with improved home lighting. Individuals with depression are much more likely to fall than those without.

Low serum vitamin D status, that is, 25-hydroxyvitamin D, has been shown at least in one study to contribute to poor clinical function and balance measurements and to falls, possibly by reducing muscle strength (Shahar et al., 2009). Vitamin D supplementation may reduce the risk of falls (Bischoff-Ferrari et al., 2004, 2009; Close, 2009; Pramyothin et al., 2009). Also, an adequate serum folate concentration has been found to be associated with a reduction in falls (Shahar et al., 2009).

OTHER ADVERSE RISK FACTORS CONTRIBUTING TO THE PATHOGENESIS OF OSTEOPOROSIS

Additional biological risk factors contribute adversely to osteoporosis. Some of these factors relate to declines in organ system functions, particularly kidney function, whereas others relate to general lifestyle, such as inactivity and the consumption of excessive nutrient supplements. Several of these factors are listed in Table 2.3. In essence, these physiological declines result in the loss of bone mass over time (see Chapters 27 and 34).

Individual elderly osteoporotic individuals at high risk of fracture, often referred to as the frail old, need to be placed on effective antiosteoporotic drug therapy. If not, these frail old individuals have approximately a 10% increased risk of death associated with fragility fracture, as reported in one meta-analysis (Bolland et al., 2010). Supplemental dietary calcium and/or vitamin D treatment, although possibly beneficial to bone, has not been shown to have as much of an effect in reducing falls or fractures, and hence deaths, in other meta-analyses (Bischoff-Ferrari, et al., 2005, 2009; Tang et al., 2007), including one that has been withdrawn (Shea et al., 2002).

TABLE 2.3
Adverse Biological Risk Factors Contributing to the Pathogenesis of Osteoporosis

Thinness with low lean body mass (<18.5 BMI for low lean body mass)
Age-related functional (organ system) declines
   Low estrogen status: hypogonadism, early oophorectomy, premature menopause
   Androgen deficiency
   Sarcopenia
   Osteopenia
Low bone mass at any age (relative to age-appropriate norms)
Decline of sensory functions

SUMMARY

Several major nondietary risk factors or lifestyle variables that may increase the risk of fractures are briefly highlighted. Both nondietary and dietary risk factors take on greater significance in elderly subjects, whether they have already had a vertebral or hip fracture or not. Fragility fractures in osteoporotic elderly subjects resulting because of falls are a major reason for the high morbidity and mortality among this age group. Strategies designed for the prevention of fractures need to include consideration of all of these identified risk factors and any others that may arise.

REFERENCES

Bischoff-Ferrari, H.A., Dawson-Hughes, B., Staehelin, H.B., et al. 2009. Fall prevention with supplemental and active forms of vitamin D: A meta-analysis of randomized controlled trials. *BMJ* 339: 3692–3703.

Bischoff-Ferrari, H.A., Dawson-Hughes, B., Willett, W.C., et al. 2004. Effect of vitamin D on falls: A meta-analysis. *JAMA* 291: 1999–2006.

Bischoff-Ferrari, H.A., Willett, W.C., Wong, J.B., et al. 2005. Fracture prevention with vitamin D supplementation: A meta-analysis of randomized controlled trials. *JAMA* 293: 2257–2264.

Bolland, M.J., Grey, A.B., Gamble, G.D., et al. 2010. Effect of osteoporosis treatment on mortality: A meta-analysis. *J Clin Endocrinol Metab* 95: 1174–1181.

Cauley, J.A. 2000. Risk of mortality following clinical fractures. *Osteoporos Int* 11: 556–561.

Close, J.C.T. 2009. Falls in older people: Risk factors, assessment and intervention. *IBMS BoneKEy* 6: 368–384.

Daniell, H.W. 1976. Osteoporosis of the slender smoker. *Arch Intern Med* 136: 298–304. [This classic paper was based on one endocrinologist's clinical practice.]

Faulkner, K.A., Cauley, J.A., Studenski, S.A., et al. 2009. Lifestyle predicts falls independent of physical risk factors. *Osteoporos Int* 20: 2025–2034.

Jutberger, H., Lorentzon, M., Barrett-Connor, E., et al. 2010. Smoking predicts incident fractures in elderly men: Mr OS Sweden. *J Bone Miner Res* 25: 1010–1016.

Ontjes, D.A., and Anderson, J.J.B. 2009. Nutritional and pharmacologic aspects of osteoporosis. In *Handbook of Clinical Nutrition and Aging,* Bales, C.W., and Ritchie, C.S., eds. Humana Press, Springer Science, New York.

Pramyothin, P., Techasurungkul, S., Lin, J. et al. 2009. Vitamin D status and falls, frailty and fractures among postmenopausal Japanese women living in Hawaii. *Osteoporos Int* 20: 1955–1962.

Shahar, D., Levi, M., Kurtz, I., et al. 2009. Nutritional status in relation to balance and falls in the elderly. *Ann Nutr Metabol* 54: 59–66.

Shea, B., Wells, G.A., Cranney, A., et al. 2002. Meta-analysis of calcium supplementation for the prevention of postmenmopausal osteoporosis. *Endocr Rev* 23: 552–559.

Tang, B.P.M., Eslick, G.D., Nowson, C., et al. 2007. Use of calcium or calcium in combination with vitamin D supplementation to prevent fractures and bone loss in people aged 50 years and older: A meta-analysis. *Lancet* 370: 657–666.

Tinetti, M.E., Speechley, M., and Gintner, S.M. 1988. Risk factors for falls among elderly persons living in the community. *New Engl J Med* 319: 1701–1707.

Yang, Y., Lewis, J., Epstein, S., et al. 2006. Long-term proton pump inhibitor therapy and risk of hip fracture. *JAMA* 296: 2947–2953.

3 Bone Marrow and Stem Cell Recruitment

Sumithra K. Urs and Clifford J. Rosen

CONTENTS

INTRODUCTION

In the past decade, it has become clear that the skeleton is integrated with other metabolic tissues and that the skeletal microenvironment, which includes not only bone cells but also hematopoietic precursors, adipocytes, endothelial, and stem cells, is critical for regulating the process of bone remodeling. The niche that is established at various locales throughout the marrow requires the maintenance of all these cell types to preserve skeletal mass and respond to stressors that may be genetic, environmental, or pharmacologic. Diet also plays a critical role in maintaining the health of the niche and influences the exit of stem cells from a quiescent to active state and their eventual differentiation. In this review, we discuss the origin of bone cells, their relationship to other marrow components, and the effects of diet on the proliferation and differentiation of these cells.

BONE CELL ORIGIN

Bone-forming cells arise from a common progenitor cell type, the mesenchymal stem cells (MSCs), located in bone marrow. MSCs are multipotent stem cells that can differentiate into a variety of cell types including osteoblasts, chondrocytes, myocytes, and adipocyte (Pei and Tontonoz, 2004; Hong et al., 2005; Lin et al., 2008; Shockley et al., 2009). The lineage commitment of the MSCs depends on vital cues and delicate alterations in the microenvironment of the bone marrow niche in the form of signaling molecules, growth factors, and hormones that can affect their differentiation. These changes can occur as autocrine, paracrine, or endocrine signals and have a profound impact on the lineage preferences of the MSCs. Bone resorbing cells arise from hematopoietic precursors, and their differentiation is dependent on signals from MSCs that are undergoing differentiation.

The major types of bone cells typically found in the bone marrow include osteoblasts, osteocytes, osteoclasts, and osteoprogenitor cells. (1) Osteoblasts, commonly called bone-forming cells, secrete osteoid, which forms the bone matrix. The process of mineralization of that matrix is also controlled by osteoblasts. Surprisingly, these cells are terminally differentiated and are unable to divide. (2) Osteocytes, which are mature osteoblasts, no longer secrete matrix, yet they are surrounded by it. These cells are responsible for maintaining skeletal metabolism through a series of canaliculi projecting from their cell body. They participate in nutrient/waste exchange via blood vessels and signaling of osteoblasts and resting cells. Their resting metabolic rate is low, and they contain few mitochondrial, but they are biologically active. (3) Osteoclasts, which are large, multi-nucleated cells, concentrate in the endosteum and function in the resorption and degradation of existing bone. (4) Osteoprogenitors are immature progenitor cells that have the capacity to divide and differentiate into osteoblasts or other mesenchymal cells.

MOLECULAR REGULATION OF BONE FORMATION

Bone formation is a tightly regulated process characterized by a sequence of events starting from commitment of osteoprogenitor cells, their differentiation into preosteoblasts, and eventually maturity of osteoblasts that synthesize the collagenous bone matrix, which is progressively mineralized. These processes are tightly regulated by transcription factors and cytokines that play a pivotal role in initiating gene transcription and supporting osteoblastogenesis (Figure 3.1). Several key factors are responsible for the full differentiation of MSCs, including the following:

1. RUNX2/Cbfa1 (Runt-related transcription factor 2/core-binding factor-1) is the first transcription factor and perhaps the most important member of Runt family transcription factors expressed in mesenchymal cells at the onset of skeletal development and present throughout osteoblast differentiation; Runx2 stimulates early MSC differentiation but late in the process may downregulate osteoblast differentiation (Marie, 2008).
2. Osterix (Osx) is a zinc finger transcription factor specifically expressed by osteoblasts and an early marker of osteogenesis; it is vitally important for osteoblast maturation and acts downstream of Runx2 (Nakashima et al., 2002).
3. AP1, the activator protein 1 (AP-1), a transcription factor, is a heterodimeric protein composed of proteins belonging to the c-Fos, c-Jun, ATF, and JDP families. This family

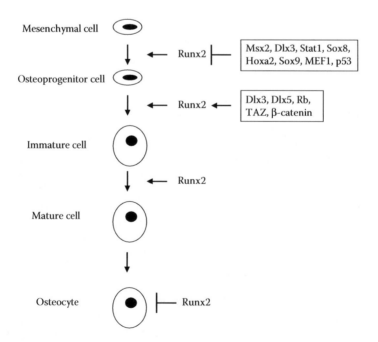

FIGURE 3.1 Schematics of transcriptional regulation of osteogenesis occurring in the bone marrow.

regulates gene expression in response to a variety of stimuli, including cytokines, growth factors, stress, and bacterial and viral infections. AP-1 controls a number of cellular processes in the osteoblast differentiation scheme including differentiation, proliferation, and apoptosis (Hess et al., 2001).

4. ATF4/CREB2 (activating transcription factor 4) belongs to a family of DNA-binding proteins that includes the AP-1 family of transcription factors, cAMP-response element binding proteins (CREBs) and CREB-like proteins. ATF4 transcription factor is known to play a role in osteoblast differentiation along with RUNX2 and Osterix. ATF4 enhances bone formation by favoring amino acid import and collagen synthesis in osteoblasts, a function requiring its phosphorylation by RSK2 (Elefteriou et al., 2006). Further, CCAT/enhancer binding protein beta also promotes osteoblast differentiation by enhancing Runx2 activity with ATF4 (Tominaga et al., 2008). Terminal osteoblast differentiation, represented by matrix mineralization, can be significantly inhibited by the inactivation of JNK, and JNK inactivation downregulates expression of ATF4 and subsequently matrix mineralization, making ATF4 a critical factor in osteogenesis.

5. A recently recognized transcription factor is TAZ, the transcriptional coactivator with a PDZ motif acting as an important coactivator with the potential to bind to two critical transcription factors in the mesenchymal population, Runx2 and PPARγ. TAZ binding to Runx2 promotes osteogenesis, whereas binding to PPARg represses adipogenesis by suppressing PPARγ activation, thus playing an important role in balancing MSC differentiation (Hong et al., 2005; Hong and Yaffe, 2006; Rosen and MacDougald, 2006; Hong et al., 2009).

Apart from these transcription factors, β-catenin, an intracellular subunit of the cadherin protein complex, is implicated as an integral component in the Wnt signaling pathway controlling bone formation and bone mass. Interaction of Wnt proteins with Frizzled and LRP5/6 coreceptors leads to inhibition of GSK-3-mediated β-catenin phosphorylation, resulting in β-catenin accumulation and translocation to the nucleus, binding to LEF/TCF transcription factors, and activation of downstream genes (Hay et al., 2009). Inactivation of β-catenin blunts osteoblast differentiation from mesenchymal progenitors, indicating that β-catenin plays an essential role in osteoblast differentiation in vivo. Interactions between β-catenin and Runx2 are also essential for BMP9-induced osteogenic differentiation of MSCs by BMP9 (Tang et al., 2008). Other factors include the Homeobox proteins (Msx1, Msx2, Dlx5, and Dlx6), which function as transcriptional repressors during embryogenesis through interactions with components of the core transcription complex and other homeoproteins. These may also have roles in limb-pattern formation; craniofacial development, particularly odontogenesis; and tumor growth inhibition. Mutations in homeobox 7 have been associated with nonsyndromic cleft lip with or without cleft palate (Boersma et al., 1999).

Peroxisome-proliferator-activated receptor gamma 2 (PPARγ2), CCAAT/enhancer-binding proteins (C/EBPs) delta, helix-loop-helix (HLH) proteins (Id and Twist), basic helix-loop-helix (bHLH), and transcription factors TRPS-1 (Piscopo et al., 2009) and Hey1 (Sharff et al., 2009) have all been implicated in cell lineage determination and differentiation and are critical components of osteogenesis in the bone marrow. These transcription factors and proteins are regulated by other factors such as parathyroid hormone (PTH), estrogen, glucocorticoids, vitamin D, bone morphogenetic protein (BMP-2, 9), and the growth factors TGF-β, IGF-1, FGF-2, and FGF-18.

LIFE CYCLE CHANGES IN BONE MARROW CELL PRODUCTION

The most common factors influencing the dynamics of BM cell populations are diseases, drugs, and aging. As previously mentioned, MSCs residing in the bone marrow not only are a crucial cellular components in the microenvironment influencing the commitment and differentiation of osteogenesis, adipogenesis, and osteoclastogenesis but also are vital for supporting hematopoiesis (Guo et al., 2000). Active hematopoiesis itself is an essential requirement for maintaining skeletal homeostasis in the bone marrow niche. Clinical and experimental observations have revealed a reciprocal relationship between hematopoiesis and MSCs differentiation in the bone marrow (Shockley et al., 2007; Rodriguez et al., 2008; Shockley et al., 2009). In the normal bone marrow where active hematopoiesis takes place, the marrow appears red. In contrast, when hematopoietic tissues are damaged by irradiation or chemotherapeutic drugs, or otherwise impaired during the aging process, adipocytes begin to expand and accumulate lipid, and ultimately, the marrow takes on a yellow appearance. Lipid accumulation actively suppresses hematopoietic progenitor proliferation and osteoblast differentiation. Serum from aging women has been found to have an inhibitory effect on osteoblast differentiation but not on adipocyte differentiation (Abdallah et al., 2006). Because osteoblasts and adipocytes share an inverse relationship, especially in the bone marrow, the influence of adipocytes in the bone marrow itself becomes a critical determinant of skeletal remodeling (Rosen et al., 2009; Rosen and Klibanski, 2009). Comparison of the number and function of hematopoietic stem and progenitor cells in adipocyte-rich bone marrow with adipocyte-poor bone marrow identified a decrease in absolute numbers of hematopoietic progenitor cells. A decrease in the numbers of hematopoeitic progenitor cells relative to adipocytes in the adipocyte-rich bone marrow suppressed hematopoiesis (Naveiras et al., 2009). In addition, cell-cycle activities of hematopoietic stem and progenitor cells also vary between adipocyte-rich and adipocyte-poor bone marrow, with the hematopoietic cells staggering in the G0 phase in adipocyte-rich marrow (Sugimura and Li, 2009). Some of the factors that modulate MSCs and hematopoietic stem cells (HSCs) by initiating a proinflammatory immune response are Dlk-1/FA-1 (Delta like-1/fetal antigen-1) (Abdallah et al., 2007) and proinflammatory cytokines, such as interleukin 1 (IL-1beta) and tumor necrosis factor alpha (TNF-alpha), which also inhibit osteogenic differentiation and bone repair during inflammation (Lacey et al., 2009).

AGING

Bone mass is maintained through a delicate balance between bone formation and resorption. During growth, bone formation exceeds resorption, and total bone mass increases. As adulthood progresses, the balance shifts and resorption exceeds formation. Bone is lost beginning early in adulthood and continues unabated into old age. Bone mass is maintained through a balance between osteoblast and osteoclast activity. Osteoblasts themselves regulate the number and activity of osteoclasts through expression of RANKL, osteoprotegerin (OPG), and macrophage-colony stimulation factor (M-CSF). Aging increases osteoclastogenesis and is accompanied by increased expression of RANKL and M-CSF expression, increased stromal/osteoblastic cell-induced osteoclastogenesis, and expansion of the osteoclast precursor pool. Aging results in decrease of proproliferative, antiapoptotic, and functional responses of growth factor signaling (IGF-1) with impaired receptor activation and signal transduction through MAPK (ERK½) and PI3K (AKT) pathways (Cao et al., 2005, 2007). Monocyte/macrophage population, as judged by expression of CD11b, increases with age by about 30%. The transcription factor hypoxia-inducible factor (HIF) plays an important role in maintenance of oxygen homeostasis and has an anabolic function in cartilage and bone development. Expression of HIF-1alpha is reduced with aging, thereby impairing the response to ischemia and production of angiogenic cytokines like VEGF (Wang et al., 2007; Shomento et al., 2009). Interestingly, hypoxia also induces an adipocyte-like phenotype, but not the expression of adipogenic markers (Fink et al., 2004). Aging is also associated with enhanced generation of reactive oxygen species (ROS) in the marrow which are generated in response to increased activity of enzymes like Alox12 and15. Fatty acid products, prostaglandins, and other products, such as HODE, can bind to PPARγ and enhance adipocyte differentiation (Jilka, R.L. 2002 personal communication).

Growth hormone (GH) is an important physiological regulator of bone growth and remodeling. Osteoblasts and chondrocytes have receptors for GH, and addition of GH increases cell proliferation and osteoblast differentiation while suppressing bone marrow lipid accumulation. A recent study showed that GH replacement in hypophysectomized (HYPOX) rats could reverse bone loss and mineralizing perimeter, along with bone marrow adiposity and precursor pool size (Menagh et al., 2009).

However, PTH can also reverse the inhibitory effect of HYPOX on mineralizing perimeter but has no effect on marrow adiposity. Insulin-like growth factor (IGF-1) can accelerate bone marrow stem cell mobilization by paracrine activation of stromal-cell-derived factor SDF-1alpha/CXCR4 and contributes to MSC stimulation. Most of these molecules identified as modulators are growth factors and cytokines acting via the MAPK signaling pathway (Haider et al., 2008). Some genes like Dlk-1/Pref-(Delta-like 1/preadipocyte factor-1) and Zfp512 control adipocyte and osteoblast differentiation (Abdallah et al., 2004; Wu et al., 2009a). Dlk-1/Pref-1 acts by inhibiting mineralization, and new bone formation by inhibiting expression of known bone gene markers like Collagen 1 (Col1), alkaline phosphatase (ALP), and osteocalcin (OC), whereas zinc finger protein 512 (Zfp512) inhibits Runx2/Cbfa1 and suppresses transition of osteoprogenitor cells to immature and mature osteoblasts. Furthermore, Pref-1 has been implicated in bone marrow adiposity and low BMD in anorexia nervosa patients (Fazeli et al., 2009). Recently, negative regulators for osteoblast differentiation, such as integrin and noggin, have been recognized. Although there is a sufficient pool of osteoprogenitor cells in the bone marrow, it is possible that not all of these stem cells mature to form the osteoblasts that mediate bone formation. Furthermore, the microenvironment modulates every step of osteogenesis and adipogenesis occurring in the bone marrow milieu. While some in vitro studies have suggested that inhibition of the adipocyte differentiation pathway leads to enhanced osteoblastogenesis, this has not been supported by in vivo studies. However, early B-cell factor-1 (Ebf-1), a transcription factor expressed in MSCs and essential for B-cell fate specification and function has been reported to induce both osteogenesis and adipogenesis (Hesslein et al., 2009). Dozens of factors, including systemic, local, and inherent changes in the bone cell population, likely contribute to age-related bone loss. Whether the changes in stromal/osteoblastic cell function and osteoclast precursor number reflect inherent cell senescence or whether the extracellular milieu in the process of aging alters the metabolic activity of the maturing preosteoblast–osteoclast remains to be determined.

On the other hand, bone marrow stromal cells also support osteoclast differentiation and express receptor activator of NF-kB ligand (RANKL) (Takagi and Kudo, 2008). Some bone marrow stromal cell lines, for example, TSB cell lines, support osteoclast differentiation and differentiate into osteoblasts, suggesting that osteoblast precursor cells can support osteoclast differentiation. Osteoclast inhibitory lectin (OCIL), a type II C-type lectin that binds to NK-cell-associated receptor Nkrp1d and sulfated glycosaminoglycans, is expressed by several cell types found in bone and inhibits osteoclast differentiation and osteoblast mineralization (Nakamura et al., 2007). Certain growth factor deficiencies like vitamin B12 deficiency can stimulate osteoclastogenesis, which manifests in the form of loss of bone mass during aging (Vaes et al., 2009). In sum, a balance of stimulatory and inhibitory signals determines MSC progression through a particular lineage and continued regeneration.

DRUGS

The use of nonsteroidal anti-inflammatory drugs (NSAIDs) is ubiquitous in contemporary medical practice as highly effective adjuncts for the amelioration of postoperative pain. NSAIDs act through inhibition of cyclooxygenase (COX-2) enzymes and therefore diminish prostaglandin production. However, eicosanoids (prostaglandins) are intimately involved in the modulation of bone metabolism and favor bone anabolism. Inhibition of cyclooxygenase-2 downregulates osteoclast and osteoblast differentiation while favoring adipocyte differentiation (Kellinsalmi et al., 2007). Insulin and/or glycemic status can also regulate osteogenesis. The consequences of diabetes and insulin treatment on bone formation and osteoblastogenesis show decreases in new bone formation. Insulin treatment can restore bone formation to levels observed in nondiabetic controls; however, it fails to exert a significant decrease in adipogenesis. RUNX2 and several RUNX2 target genes, including matrix metalloproteinase-9, ALP, integrin binding sialoprotein, Dmp1, Col1a2, Phex, VDR, osteocalcin, and osterix, are significantly downregulated during insulin deficiency, hyperglycemia, and diabetic conditions; all these contributing to diabetic bone diseases (Fowlkes et al., 2008). Rosiglitazone, a commonly used antidiabetic thiazolidinedione class of drug, has also been found to decrease bone formation and increase adipocyte and osteoclast numbers (Ali et al., 2005).

DIETARY AND OTHER INFLUENCES ON BONE MARROW CELL PRODUCTION

Numerous nutrients and dietary components, ranging from macronutrients to micronutrients as well as bioactive food ingredients, influence bone health. Many of the nutrients and food components can potentially have a positive or negative impact on bone health (Table 3.1). They can affect bone turnover by various mechanisms, including alterations of bone structure, rates of bone metabolism, and responsiveness to endocrine and/or paracrine signals. These dietary factors range from inorganic minerals (e.g., calcium, magnesium, phosphorus, sodium, potassium, and various trace elements) and vitamins (vitamins A, D, E, K, C, and certain B vitamins) to macronutrients, such as protein and fatty acids. In addition, the relative proportions of these dietary factors derived from different types of diets (vegetarian vs. omnivorous) may also affect bone health and bone marrow cell production. In recent years, a number of bioactive food components have been proposed as being beneficial for bone health (Bonjour, 2005; Cashman, 2007). Below, several of those nutrients and their relationship to stromal cell differentiation are examined.

Calcium is critical for normal growth and development of the skeleton and is essential for achieving optimal peak bone mass. Adequate calcium also modifies the rate of bone loss associated with aging. Over the past decade, convincing evidence has emerged with respect to the effects of dietary calcium on bone health across several age groups. Calcium in food sources generally is present as salts or associated with other dietary constituents in the form of complexes of calcium ions (Ca^{2+}). Calcium must be released in an ionized soluble form to be absorbed both by passive diffusion and by active transport mediated by vitamin D through transcellular and paracellular pathways (Cashman, 2007). Ionic calcium regulates chemotaxis of selective bone marrow cells through the Ca-sensing receptor CaR and CXCR4, an important receptor

TABLE 3.1
Nutritional Factors That Influence Bone

Beneficial Nutrient Factors	Potentially Detrimental Environmental Factors
Calcium	Excess alcohol
Copper	Excess caffeine
Zinc	Excess sodium
Fluoride	Excess fluoride
Magnesium	Excess/insufficient proteins
Phosphorus	Excess phosphorus
Potassium	Excess/insufficient vitamin A
Vitamin C	Excess n-6 PUFA
Vitamin D	
Vitamin K	
B vitamins	
n-3 fatty acids	
Proteins	
Whey-derived peptides	
Phytoestrogens	
Nondigestable oligosaccharides (especially inulin-type fructans)	

Source: Adapted from Cashman, K.D., *J Nutr* 137: 2507S–2512S, 2007.

promoting stem cell mobilization and homing (Wu et al., 2009). Dietary zinc reduces osteo-clast resorption and increases osteoblast differentiation, matrix maturation, and mineralization (Hadley et al., 2009).

Among the vitamins, vitamin D is found naturally in very few foods; however, endogenous synthesis of vitamin D occurs when skin is exposed to UV radiation (290–320 nm) from sunlight. Vitamin D deficiency is characterized by inadequate mineralization, or demineralization, of the skeleton. In children, severe vitamin D deficiency results in rickets, whereas in adults, it leads to a mineralization defect in the skeleton causing osteomalacia. In addition, secondary hyperparathyroidism associated with low vitamin D status enhances mobilization of calcium from the skeleton. Vitamin D deficiency contributes to osteoporosis through less efficient intestinal absorption of calcium, increased bone loss, muscle weakness, and a weakened bone microstructure. Supplemental vitamin D can significantly reduce the risk of fracture in older people. Recently, BM-MSCs were shown to have the molecular machinery to metabolize and respond to vitamin D, wherein circulating 25OH-vitamin D signaling is amplified through IGF-1 upregulation and induced 1-alpha hydroxylase (CYP27B1). These processes also potentiate osteoblast differentiation by IGF-1 (Zhou et al., 2009).

Vitamin K is a fat-soluble molecule essential for promoting the activity of Gla proteins in bone and elsewhere. Osteocalcin, a bone-specific protein, is gamma carboxylated by vitamin K. The circulating concentration of carboxylated versus uncarboxylated osteocalcin reflects the relative level of vitamin K nutritional status. In some studies, low vitamin K has been shown to be an indicator of hip fracture and a predictor of BMD. Relatively high-dose vitamin K_1 supplementation (1 mg/day) for 3 years, if coadministered with calcium, magnesium, zinc, and vitamin D, reduced postmenopausal bone loss (Braam et al., 2003a, 2003b) and improved hematopoietic functions (Miyazawa and Aizawa, 2004), although no evidence from other studies supports a role for vitamin K in reducing fracture risk. Consumption of fish or n-3 fatty acids protects not only against cardiovascular and autoimmune disorders, but these long-chain n-3 fatty acids have beneficial effects on bone mineral density and bone accrual (Hogstrom et al., 2007) and they may decrease bone resorption markers (Sun et al., 2003; Griel et al., 2007).

Estrogen deficiency is a major contributory factor to the development of osteoporosis in women, and estrogen and/or hormone replacement therapy (HRT), bisphosphonates, calcitonin, and raloxifene, as well as calcium and vitamin D supplementation, are the mainstays for prevention of bone loss in postmenopausal women. Recently, as a consequence of poor uptake and adherence of HRT as well as potential concerns over an increased risk of malignancy and other side effects associated with the use of HRT, attention has focused on the dietary phytoestrogens. Dietary phytoestrogens are nonsteroidal isoflavones naturally occurring in foods of plant origin (especially soy-based foods) that structurally resemble natural estrogens and compete with them for binding estrogen receptors. One such isoflavone is soy-derived genistein, which when supplemented (56 mg/day) significantly increased BMD in the femur and lumbar spine; these effects appeared to be of similar magnitude as those achieved with HRT in early postmenopausal women (Morabito et al., 2002). These compounds have been shown in vitro to have prodifferentiation effects on the preosteoblasts (Morris et al., 2006). However, large randomized placebo-controlled trials in postmenopausal women are just now finishing and will determine if a role for the isoflavones in the prevention of osteoporosis materializes.

Factors that negatively regulate bone and marrow functions include oxidized low density lipoproteins, which have a direct inhibitory effect on differentiation of preosteoblasts and MSCs by inhibition of alkaline phosphatase activity, collagen I processing, and mineralization. These regulatory factors operate through a mitogen-activated protein (MAP) kinase-dependent pathway to direct progenitor marrow stromal cells to undergo adipogenic instead of osteogenic differentiation (Chu et al., 2009). Furthermore, along the same lines, a low carbohydrate–high fat (LC–HF) diet has been found to impair longitudinal growth, BMD, and mechanical properties, possibly mediated by reductions in circulating IGF-1 (Bielohuby et al., 2009). This finding was surprising and has lowered enthusiasm among advocates of an LC–HF diet, particularly because serum bone formation markers as well as expression of transcription factors influencing osteo-blastogenesis are reduced with this diet. On the other hand, a high-fat diet can also decrease can-cellous bone mass in certain circumstances (Cao et al., 2009). A balanced diet combined with adequate exercise is the best recommendation for a proper functioning of the body and main-taining a balance in the bone marrow stromal cells for cell recruitment and balance between resorption and formation.

SUMMARY

Although knowledge about the bone marrow niche has grown dramatically in the last decade, many unanswered questions remain. The precise relationship between adipogenesis and osteo-genesis remains to be clarified; similarly bone cell development is essential for hematopoiesis, but the factors that coordinate that response are not fully defined. The effects of dietary compo-nents on marrow cellular processes are important, yet the model systems are not perfect, and the randomized trials for nutrients other than calcium are lacking. Even the actions of vitamin D are controversial, and the effects of this hormone/vitamin on marrow elements need further clarifica-tion. Significant research imperatives relative to dietary factors and the bone marrow niche need further examination.

REFERENCES

Abdallah, B.M., Boissy, P., Tan, Q., et al. 2007. Dlk1/FA1 regulates the function of human bone marrow mesen-chymal stem cells by modulating gene expression of pro-inflammatory cytokines and immune response-related factors. *J Biol Chem* 282: 7339–51.

Abdallah, B.M., Haack-Sorensen, M., Fink, T., et al. 2006. Inhibition of osteoblast differentiation but not adi-pocyte differentiation of mesenchymal stem cells by sera obtained from aged females. *Bone* 39: 181–8.

Abdallah, B.M., Jensen, C.H., Gutierrez, G., et al. 2004. Regulation of human skeletal stem cells differentiation by Dlk1/Pref-1. *J Bone Miner Res* 19: 841–52.

Ali, A.A., Weinstein, R.S., Stewart, S.A., et al. 2005. Rosiglitazone causes bone loss in mice by suppressing osteoblast differentiation and bone formation. *Endocrinology* 146: 1226–35.

Bielohuby, M., Matsuura, M., Herbach, N., et al. 2009. Short Term exposure to low-carbohydrate/high fat diets induces low bone mineral density and reduces bone formation in rats. *J Bone Miner Res* Aug 4. Epub ahead of print.

Boersma, C.J., Bloemen, M., Hendriks, J.M., et al. 1999. Homeobox proteins as signal transduction inter-mediates in regulation of NCAM expression by recombinant human bone morphogenetic protein-2 in osteoblast-like cells. *Mol Cell Biol Res Commun* 1: 117–24.

Bonjour, J.P. 2005. Dietary protein: An essential nutrient for bone health. *J Am Coll Nutr* 24: 526S–36S.

Braam, L.A., Knapen, M.H., Geusens, P., et al. 2003a. Vitamin K1 supplementation retards bone loss in post-menopausal women between 50 and 60 years of age. *Calcif Tissue Int* 73: 21–6.

Braam, L.A., Knapen, M.H., Geusens, P., et al. 2003b. Factors affecting bone loss in female endurance athletes: A two-year follow-up study. *Am J Sports Med* 31: 889–95.

Cao, J.J., Gregoire, B.R., and Gao, H. 2009. High-fat diet decreases cancellous bone mass but has no effect on cortical bone mass in the tibia in mice. *Bone* 44: 1097–104.

Cao, J.J., Kurimoto, P., Boudignon, B., et al. 2007. Aging impairs IGF-I receptor activation and induces skeletal resistance to IGF-I. *J Bone Miner Res* 22: 1271–9.

Cao, J.J., Wronski, T.J., Iwaniec, U., et al. 2005. Aging increases stromal/osteoblastic cell-induced osteoclasto-genesis and alters the osteoclast precursor pool in the mouse. *J Bone Miner Res* 20: 1659–68.

Cashman, K.D. 2007. Diet, nutrition, and bone health. *J Nutr* 137: 2507S–12S.

Chu, L., Hao, H., Luo, M., et al., 2009. Ox-LDL modifies the behavior of bone marrow stem cells and impairs their endothelial differentiation via inhibition of Akt phosphorylation. *J Cell Mol Med.* Epub ahead of print.

Elefteriou, F., Benson, M.D., Sowa, H., et al. 2006. ATF4 mediation of NF1 functions in osteoblast reveals a nutritional basis for congenital skeletal dysplasiae. *Cell Metab* 4: 441–51.

Fazeli, P.K., Bredella, M.A., Misra, M., et al. 2009. Preadipocyte factor-1 is associated with marrow adipos-ity and bone mineral density in women with anorexia nervosa. *J Clin Endocrinol Metab.* Epub ahead of print.

Fink, T., Abildtrup, L., Fogd, K., et al. 2004. Induction of adipocyte-like phenotype in human mesenchymal stem cells by hypoxia. *Stem Cells* 22: 1346–55.

Fowlkes, J.L., Bunn, R.C., Liu, L., et al. 2008. Runt-related transcription factor 2 (RUNX2) and RUNX2-related osteogenic genes are down-regulated throughout osteogenesis in type 1 diabetes mellitus. *Endocrinology* 149: 1697–704.

Griel, A.E., Kris-Etherton, P.M., Hilpert, K.F., et al. 2007. An increase in dietary n-3 fatty acids decreases a marker of bone resorption in humans. *Nutr J* 6: 2.

Guo, Z., Tang, P., Liu, X., et al. 2000. Mesenchymal stem cells derived from human bone marrow support hematopoiesis in vitro. *Zhongguo Shi Yan Xue Ye Xue Za Zhi* 8: 93–6.

Hadley, K.B., Newman, S.M., and Hunt, J.R. 2009. Dietary zinc reduces osteoclast resorption activities and increases markers of osteoblast differentiation, matrix maturation, and mineralization in the long bones of growing rats. *J Nutr Biochem.* Epub ahead of print.

Haider, H., Jiang, S., Idris, et al. 2008. IGF-1-overexpressing mesenchymal stem cells accelerate bone marrow stem cell mobilization via paracrine activation of SDF-1alpha/CXCR4 signaling to promote myocardial repair. *Circ Res* 103: 1300–8.

Hay, E., Laplantine, E., Geoffroy, V., et al. 2009. N-cadherin interacts with axin and LRP5 to negatively regulate Wnt/beta-catenin signaling, osteoblast function, and bone formation. *Mol Cell Biol* 29: 953–64.

Hess, J., Porte, D., Munz, C., et al. 2001. AP-1 and Cbfa/runt physically interact and regulate parathyroid hormone-dependent MMP13 expression in osteoblasts through a new osteoblast-specific element 2/AP-1 composite element. *J Biol Chem* 276: 20029–38.

Hesslein, D.G., Fretz, J.A., Xi, Y., et al. 2009. Ebf1-dependent control of the osteoblast and adipocyte lineages. *Bone* 44: 537–46.

Hogstrom, M., Nordstrom, P., and Nordstrom, A. 2007. n-3 Fatty acids are positively associated with peak bone mineral density and bone accrual in healthy men: The NO2 Study. *Am J Clin Nutr* 85: 803–7.

Hong, D., Chen, H.X., Xue, Y., et al. 2009. Osteoblastogenic effects of dexamethasone through upregulation of TAZ expression in rat mesenchymal stem cells. *J Steroid Biochem Mol Biol* 116: 86–92.

Hong, J.H., Hwang, E.S., Mcmanus, M.T., et al. 2005. TAZ, a transcriptional modulator of mesenchymal stem cell differentiation. *Science* 309: 1074–8.

Hong, J.H., and Yaffe, M.B. 2006. TAZ: A beta-catenin-like molecule that regulates mesenchymal stem cell differentiation. *Cell Cycle* 5: 176–9.

Kellinsalmi, M., Parikka, V., Risteli, J., et al. 2007. Inhibition of cyclooxygenase-2 down-regulates osteoclast and osteoblast differentiation and favours adipocyte formation in vitro. *Eur J Pharmacol* 572: 102–10.

Lacey, D.C., Simmons, P.J., Graves, S.E., et al. 2009. Proinflammatory cytokines inhibit osteogenic differentiation from stem cells: Implications for bone repair during inflammation. *Osteoarthritis Cartilage* 17: 735–42.

Lin, Y.F., Jing, W., Wu, L., et al. 2008. Identification of osteo-adipo progenitor cells in fat tissue. *Cell Prolif* 41: 803–12.

Marie, P.J. 2008. Transcription factors controlling osteoblastogenesis. *Arch Biochem Biophys* 473: 98–105.

Menagh, P., Turner, R., Jump, D., et al. 2009. Growth hormone regulates the balance between bone formation and bone marrow adiposity. *J Bone Miner Res.* Epub ahead of print.

Miyazawa, K., and Aizawa, S. 2004. Vitamin K2 improves the hematopoietic supportive functions of bone marrow stromal cells in vitro: A possible mechanism of improvement of cytopenia for refractory anemia in response to vitamin K2 therapy. *Stem Cells Dev* 13: 449–51.

Morabito, N., Crisafulli, A., Vergara, C., et al. 2002. Effects of genistein and hormone-replacement therapy on bone loss in early postmenopausal women: A randomized double-blind placebo-controlled study. *J Bone Miner Res* 17: 1904–12.

Morris, C., Thorpe, J., Ambrosio, L., et al. 2006. The soybean isoflavone genistein induces differentiation of MG63 human osteosarcoma osteoblasts. *J Nutr* 136: 1166–70.

Nakamura, A., Ly, C., Cipetic, M., et al. 2007. Osteoclast inhibitory lectin (OCIL) inhibits osteoblast differentiation and function in vitro. *Bone* 40: 305–15.

Nakashima, K., Zhou, X., Kunkel, G., et al. 2002. The novel zinc finger-containing transcription factor osterix is required for osteoblast differentiation and bone formation. *Cell* 108: 17–29.

Naveiras, O., Nardi, V., Wenzel, P.L., et al. 2009. Bone-marrow adipocytes as negative regulators of the haematopoietic microenvironment. *Nature* 460: 259–63.

Pei, L., and Tontonoz, P. 2004. Fat's loss is bone's gain. *J Clin Invest* 113: 805–6.

Piscopo, D.M., Johansen, E.B., and Derynck, R. 2009. Identification of the GATA factor TRPS1 as a repressor of the osteocalcin promoter. *J Biol Chem* 284: 31690–703.

Rodriguez, J.P., Astudillo, P., Rios, S., et al. 2008. Involvement of adipogenic potential of human bone marrow mesenchymal stem cells (MSCs) in osteoporosis. *Curr Stem Cell Res Ther* 3: 208–18.

Rosen, C.J., Ackert-Bicknell, C., Rodriguez, J.P., et al. 2009. Marrow fat and the bone microenvironment: Developmental, functional, and pathological implications. *Crit Rev Eukaryot Gene Expr* 19: 109–24.

Rosen, C.J., and Klibanski, A., 2009. Bone, fat, and body composition: Evolving concepts in the pathogenesis of osteoporosis. *Am J Med* 122: 409–14.

Rosen, E.D., and MacDougald, O.A. 2006. Adipocyte differentiation from the inside out. *Nat Rev Mol Cell Biol* 7: 885–96.

Sharff, K.A., Song, W.X., Luo, X., et al. 2009. Hey1 basic helix-loop-helix protein plays an important role in mediating BMP9-induced osteogenic differentiation of mesenchymal progenitor cells. *J Biol Chem* 284: 649–59.

Shockley, K.R., Lazarenko, O.P., Czernik, P.J., et al. 2009. PPARgamma2 nuclear receptor controls multiple regulatory pathways of osteoblast differentiation from marrow mesenchymal stem cells. *J Cell Biochem* 106: 232–46.

Shockley, K.R., Rosen, C.J., Churchill, G.A., et al. 2007. PPARgamma2 regulates a molecular signature of marrow mesenchymal stem cells. *PPAR Res* 2007: 81219.

Shomento, S.H., Wan, C., Cao, X., et al. 2009. Hypoxia-inducible factors 1alpha and 2alpha exert both distinct and overlapping functions in long bone development. *J Cell Biochem.* Epub ahead of print.

Sugimura, R., and Li, L., 2009. Shifting in balance between osteogenesis and adipogenesis substantially influences hematopoiesis. *J Mol Cell Biol.* Epub ahead of print.

Sun, D., Krishnan, A., Zaman, K., et al. 2003. Dietary n-3 fatty acids decrease osteoclastogenesis and loss of bone mass in ovariectomized mice. *J Bone Miner Res* 18: 1206–16.

Takagi, K., and Kudo, A. 2008. Bone marrow stromal cell lines having high potential for osteoclast-supporting activity express PPARgamma1 and show high potential for differentiation into adipocytes. *J Bone Miner Metab* 26: 13–23.

Tang, N., Song, W.X., Luo, J., et al. 2008. BMP9-induced osteogenic differentiation of mesenchymal progenitors requires functional canonical Wnt/beta-catenin signaling. *J Cell Mol Med.* Epub ahead of print.

Tominaga, H., Maeda, S., Hayashi, M., et al. 2008. CCAAT/enhancer-binding protein beta promotes osteoblast differentiation by enhancing Runx2 activity with ATF4. *Mol Biol Cell* 19: 5373–86.

Vaes, B.L., Lute, C., Blom, H.J., et al. 2009. Vitamin B$_{12}$ deficiency stimulates osteoclastogenesis via increased homocysteine and methylmalonic acid. *Calcif Tissue Int* 84: 413–22.

Wang, Y., Wan, C., Deng, L., et al. 2007. The hypoxia-inducible factor alpha pathway couples angiogenesis to osteogenesis during skeletal development. *J Clin Invest* 117: 1616–26.

Wu, M., Hesse, E., Morvan, F., et al. 2009a. Zfp521 antagonizes Runx2, delays osteoblast differentiation in vitro, and promotes bone formation in vivo. *Bone* 44: 528–36.

Wu, Q., Shao, H., Darwin Eton, D., et al. 2009. Extracellular calcium increases CXCR4 expression on bone marrow-derived cells and enhances pro-angiogenesis therapy. *J Cell Mol Med.* Epub ahead of print.

Zhou, S., Leboff, M.S., and Glowacki, J. 2009. Vitamin D metabolism and action in human bone marrow stromal cells. *Endocrinology.* Epub ahead of print.

4 Skeletal Tissues and Mineralization

Sanford C. Garner and John J.B. Anderson

CONTENTS

INTRODUCTION

The skeleton conducts a number of essential functions for maintenance of life in vertebrates, some of which involve the obvious rigid structure provided by bone and others that result from the dynamic organization of bone at the microscopic level. Bone provides both mechanical support for the body, including attachment for locomotor muscles, and protection for portions of soft tissue, such as brain, spinal cord, heart, and lungs. In addition, all blood cell formation or hematopoiesis takes place in the bone marrow. A less obvious function of bone is that it serves as a metabolic reservoir for calcium and other minerals. A constant exchange of ions of calcium (Ca), phosphate (inorganic phosphorus or Pi), and other mineral elements occurs between bone mineral surfaces and extracellular fluid in bone tissue. This constant ebb and flow of Ca and Pi is the result primarily of the active exchange of these minerals that occurs at the interface of bone mineral surfaces with the extracellular fluid and secondarily of the remodeling processes within bone that renew bone microstructure throughout life. As described by Talmage and others based on the pioneering concepts of William F. Neuman, the control of free calcium ion concentration in the extracellular fluids is primarily regulated at the mineralized bone surfaces (Talmage and Talmage, 2006, 2007; Talmage and Mobley, 2008, 2009). The processes involved the regulation of the solubility of hydroxyapatite, which would otherwise result in an equilibrium between bone mineral and the fluid passing over it that would lower plasma calcium below the concentration necessary to maintain the normal function of mammalian tissue.

Bone can be described at several levels. Bone may be considered first as a structural material, a mixture of organic matrix and inorganic (mineral) materials. Bone may also be viewed at the level of a mechanical device, with a characteristic resistance to bending, to compression, and to fracture. At a gross physical (organ) level, long bones such as the leg or arm bones may be separated into anatomical regions of epiphysis, metaphysis, and diaphysis. The total bone structure also consists of an arrangement of trabecular and cortical bone. Bone microstructure, that is, the mixture of trabecular and cortical bone in different bones or in different portions of the same bone, may be equally, if not more, important than the absolute amount of bone mineral in determining strength and resistance to fracture. The structural analysis of bone is beyond the scope of this chapter, but the reader is referred to references (Evans, 1973; Currey, 1984; Albright and Skinner, 1987; Lanyon, 1992; Mammone and Hudson, 1993) for additional information.

At the microscopic or histological (tissue) level, bone consists of osteoblasts and osteoclasts that create and destroy bone, respectively. Bone as a metabolic entity serves as a storage reservoir for minerals, especially Ca and phosphorus (P), but also for other macrominerals and trace minerals. As a dynamic part of the body's response to changing availability of these minerals, bone mineral is essential for maintaining Ca and Pi concentrations in the extracellular fluid compartment within limits acceptable for numerous functions essential to the continued well-being of the individual. Bone also undergoes extensive changes during growth, in response to physical exercise, and during maintenance of skeletal tissues throughout the life cycle.

BONE AS AN ORGAN

Bone is considered a component of the body's connective tissue, but together with teeth and cartilage, it shares the ability to add mineral to the underlying organic matrix of collagen and noncollagenous proteins, that is, to become calcified. All bone consists of mineral (hydroxyapatite) deposited within an organic (collagen) matrix. The mineral alone is hard, rigid, and brittle and is effective mainly in resistance to compression. The collagen matrix on the other hand remains flexible and is mainly tension resistant, that is, strong, reducing fractures. In combination, the organic and inorganic components of bone produce a material that is one-third the weight but ten times as flexible and with approximately equal tensile strength as that of cast iron (Albright and Skinner, 1987).

STRUCTURE

Bone is organized into two types of structure that are intermixed within each bone (Clarke, 2008). These structures are compact (cortical) bone, which forms the shafts of the long bones and the outer surface of almost all bones, and trabecular bone, also called cancellous or spongy bone, which fills the ends of the shafts of the long bones as well as forming most of the structure of the vertebrae (Figure 4.1). Most of the volume occupied by compact bone consists of calcified matrix (~80%), whereas only a small portion (~15%) of trabecular bone volume is calcified; the space between the trabeculae is often filled with bone marrow, especially early in life, and later fat cells become prominent in this space.

GROSS ANATOMY

Anatomists separate bone into two types, the flat bones, such as skull bones, scapula, mandible, and ilium, and the long bones, such as tibia, femur, and humerus. The long bones consist of three anatomic divisions, as illustrated in Figure 4.1. The inner surface of the bone is called the endosteum, and the outer surface, the periosteum. The shaft, or diaphysis, is a hollow cylinder of compact bone. The ends of the bone are known as the epiphyses and consist of a thin cortical layer of compact bone surrounding a region of trabecular bone. The metaphysis is a tapering, transitional region between the epiphysis and the diaphysis containing both cortical and trabecular bone. The epiphysis and metaphysis are separated by a plate of hyaline cartilage called the epiphyseal growth plate (or physis). The growth plate is the site at which elongation of the long bones occurs by proliferation of chondrocytes, cartilage-forming cells. Calcification of this cartilaginous area at puberty results in closure of the growth plate and cessation of longitudinal growth (Cormack, 1987; Fawcett, 1994).

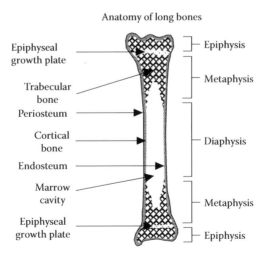

Anatomy of long bones

FIGURE 4.1 Anatomy of long bones. The long bones, i.e., the tibia, femur, humerus, and radius, are divided anatomically to three segments: the epiphyses, the metaphyses, and the diaphysis. The composition of cortical and trabecular bone varies as one moves from segment to segment.

BONE AS TISSUE

Bone tissue contains a number of different cell types that perform the functions necessary to build and maintain bone structure and carry out the homeostatic functions of bone. Thus, there are osteoblasts, which are responsible for formation of bone; cells derived from the osteoblasts that are present in mature bone; and osteoclasts, which are capable of resorbing bone tissue during turnover of bone. In addition to the cellular components of bone tissue, the majority of bone tissue consists of hydroxyapatite (see section "Chemical Structure" below) crystals deposited within a protein matrix that consists primarily of type I collagen. However, the other protein constituents of bone organic matrix are quite varied, and the role of many of these molecules remains to be discovered.

MICROSCOPIC ANATOMY OF BONE CELLS

Bone cells can be divided into two general types, bone-forming cells and bone-resorbing cells, which are derived from different osteoprogenitor cells. The bone-forming cells, or osteoblasts, are believed to give rise to related cell types with different functions in bone, for example, the osteocyte and the resting osteoblast, or bone-lining cell. The osteoclast is the major cell responsible for bone resorption (see Chapter 3).

Bone-Forming Cells (Osteoblasts)

The osteoblasts are derived from mesenchymal cells and are related to fibroblasts and the cells forming the walls of blood vessels (Figure 4.2). Preosteoblasts are found in the tissue layers near bone-forming surfaces. They are elongated cells lacking the full ability of the mature osteoblasts to synthesize bone matrix proteins, but they retain the ability to divide.

Osteoblasts are bone-forming cells that secrete collagen to form the osteoid or unmineralized bone matrix and also regulate the processes that initiate mineralization. Osteoblasts are metabolically active

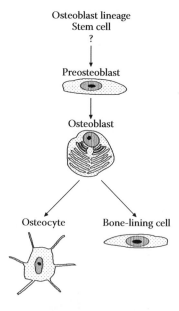

FIGURE 4.2 Osteoblast lineage. The osteoblast is derived from the same stem cell population that gives rise to mesenchymal cells, including fibroblasts; however, the source of these stem cells has not been identified. Once the stem cell differentiates to the preosteoblast, the daughter cells of this line are committed to osteoblastic development. The fate of osteoblasts once bone has been formed is threefold: (1) they may undergo apoptosis; (2) remain on the surface of the bone as biosynthetically inactive bone-lining cells; or (3) completely enclose themselves in bone, forming an osteocyte.

cells and are characterized by an abundant rough endoplasmic reticulum and Golgi apparatus for synthesis and export of proteins (Figure 4.2). These cells also express characteristic membrane proteins, particularly the enzyme alkaline phosphatase, which has been proposed as a regulator of mineralization for many years, although its function remains undefined. Osteoblasts possess receptors for two of the major Ca and bone-regulating hormones, parathyroid hormone (PTH) and 1,25-dihydroxyvitamin D [1,25(OH)$_2$D]. It is generally accepted that the major effects of these hormones on maintenance of plasma Ca and on bone turnover are controlled via osteoblastic cells (see Chapter 6).

Osteoblast-Derived Cells of Mature Bone

Osteoblasts give rise to two cell types within bone that maintain some osteoblastic characteristics but no longer synthesize collagen for formation of new bone.

Osteocytes

Osteocytes are the most common type of bone cells, making up 90% of the total number of cells in bone. These bone cells that lie within small cavities or lacunae are completely surrounded by bone. They are osteoblasts that have surrounded themselves with matrix and remain connected with each other and with cells on the bone surface by gap junctions at the ends of thin processes that pass through thin tubular channels or canaliculi. The canaliculi provide a passageway for the diffusion of nutrients from extracellular fluid to these cells. Osteocytes also have the capability of resorbing bone by a process known as osteocytic osteolysis. These cells have a role in the control of bone remodeling (Henriksen et al., 2009), but a full understanding of the importance of the osteocytic activities awaits further research.

Bone-Lining Cells

Bone-lining cells are also called resting osteoblasts or surface osteocytes. As the names imply, these cells are osteoblast-like cells that are no longer actively forming bone but are not completely surrounded by bone. These lining cells are central to maintenance of blood Ca levels, perhaps by actively pumping Ca ions from the bone fluid compartment to the extracellular fluid compartment. Although it is likely that these cells represent another developmental stage of the osteoblast, similar to the osteocyte, it has been suggested that these cells are formed directly from preosteoblasts, which they resemble histologically. It has been demonstrated that the bone-lining cells can be stimulated to differentiate into active osteoblasts.

Bone-Resorbing Cells (Osteoclasts)

Osteoclasts are multinucleated, giant cells that are capable of resorbing both bone mineral and matrix (Blair et al. 1993). The osteoclasts are formed from cells of the monocyte–phagocyte lineage (Figure 4.3). The cellular lineage of the osteoclast was defined in experiments with the disease osteopetrosis, a condition of dense bone growth without osteoclastic remodeling. Animal models with this disease either lack the mononuclear precursor cells or these cells fail to respond to the cytokines that signal cell proliferation and maturation. In either case, the number of functional osteoclasts is insufficient to resorb substantial amounts of bone, and hence, bone turnover is significantly depressed in osteopetrosis. (This disease in humans also may result from defects in the machinery of acidification [Stark and Savarirayan, 2009].)

The osteoclast resorbs bone in a region of attachment of the cell to the bone surface where the cell membrane is elaborately folded, resulting in the characteristic appearance of this area called the "ruffled border" (Figure 4.4; Henriksen et al., 2008; Boyce et al., 2009). Bone resorption involves the lowering of the pH in the region between the osteoclast and the bone surface through secretion of hydrogen ions (H$^+$), which are generated within the osteoclasts by carbonic anhydrase II (the same enzyme that is present in H$^+$ (acid)-secreting cells of the stomach and kidney). The site of bone resorption is separated from the surrounding tissue by a ring of contractile proteins, the sealing zone, which is formed by actin filaments anchored through integrins to the bone surface. Within this zone, the bone surface is exposed to low pH and concentrated lysosomal enzyme activity, leading to

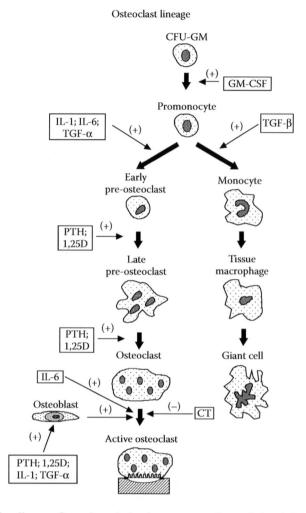

FIGURE 4.3 Osteoclast lineage. Osteoclasts derive from a stem cell population (colony-forming unit–granulocyte–macrophage or CFU-GM) that is capable of giving rise to osteoclasts or monocytes/macrophages. CFU-GM is stimulated by the granulocyte–macrophage colony-stimulating factor to differentiate into premonocytes. The premonocyte may commit to either the osteoclastic or monocytic pathway under the stimulus of local factors (cytokines), including interleukin-1 (IL-1), interleukin-6 (IL-6), and transforming growth factor-β (TGF-β) for the osteoclastic lineage and transforming growth factor-α for the monocytic lineage. Further development of the osteoclastic cell is stimulated by PTH and 1,25-dihydroxyvitamin D, which may act directly on the differentiating osteoclasts or may act through the osteoblast. Other cytokines, such as IL-1 and TGF-β, also stimulate resorptive activity through the osteoblast. The active osteoclast may also be regulated directly through stimulatory cytokines such as IL-6 and by inhibitory agents such as the circulating peptide CT.

the description of this region as a "secondary lysosome." However, Blair et al. (1993) have pointed out that the ability of the osteoclast to acidify the region of bone adjacent to the ruffled border vastly exceeds the transport of H^+ into cytoplasmic lysosomes.

CHEMICAL STRUCTURE

Although bone is organized into different structural components, at the molecular level, all bone tissues share a common composition. Bone consists of an inorganic or mineral phase composed primarily of hydroxyapatite crystals deposited within an organic phase of cross-linked collagen fibers.

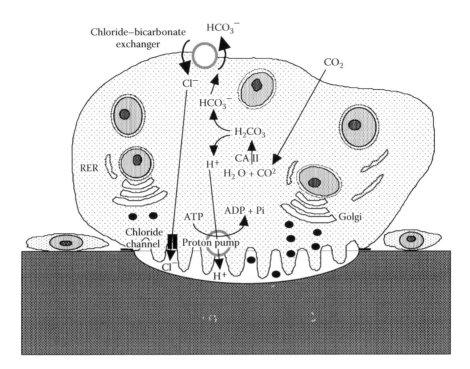

FIGURE 4.4 Osteoclast. The principal, and perhaps the only, bone-resorbing cell is the osteoclast. This multinucleated cell forms a "sealing zone" with the bone surface that allows a local area of bone to be exposed to low pH, which is produced by active pumping of hydrogen ions into the resorption pit, and a high concentration of proteolytic enzymes, which are released from lysosomes into the area of resorption.

The mineral phase provides stiffness and resistance to compression, whereas the organic phase gives the bone strength and resistance to breaking. Together, this composite structure has both rigidity and resistance to fractures. Hydroxyapatite has the chemical structure $Ca_{10}(PO_4)_6(OH)_2$ and makes up approximately 60%–65% of bone by weight. Type I collagen fibers make up 90% of total bone proteins. When bone is first formed as part of a newly modeled bone or as part of the repair of a fracture, the collagen fibers are randomly oriented, and this bone is referred to as woven bone. However, as bone is remodeled during growth or as part of normal bone turnover, the collagen fibers are laid down in parallel arrays that are visible under polarized light as layers within the bone. Thus, this mature bone is referred to as lamellar (layered) bone.

COLLAGEN AND NONCOLLAGENOUS PROTEINS OF BONE MATRIX

As stated above, type I collagen makes up approximately 90% of bone matrix protein. The remaining 10% of total bone proteins consists of a mixture of proteins that are either synthesized by osteoblasts or are serum derived (Termine, 1988). Whether the serum-derived proteins play a role in bone metabolism or whether they are simply trapped during the formation of bone matrix is not known. The remaining noncollagenous proteins of bone matrix (Table 4.1) are synthesized primarily by osteoblasts, and less so by osteoclasts. These additional matrix proteins, which function as either structural or chemical signaling proteins, can be divided into four general classes:

Cell-Attachment Proteins

Cell attachment is mediated by the family of proteins that constitute the integrins. Integrins are membrane-spanning proteins that recognize the amino acid sequence Arg–Gly–Asp (RGD) in extracellular proteins. Bone cells synthesize four proteins, that is, fibronectin, thrombospondin,

TABLE 4.1
Possible Functions of Noncollagenous Proteins of Bone Matrix

Noncollagenous Protein of Bone Matrix	Possible Function
Thrombospondin	Cell attachment
Fibronectin	Cell attachment
Bone sialoprotein	Cell attachment
Osteopontin	Cell attachment
Proteoglycan I (biglycan)	Unknown
Proteoglycan II (decorin)	Unknown
Osteonectin	Calcium binding
Osteocalcin	Calcium binding
Matrix Gla protein	Unknown
Insulin-like growth factor-1	Growth related
Platelet-derived growth factor	Growth related
Transforming growth factor-β	Growth related

osteopontin, and bone sialoprotein (BSP), that are part of the extracellular matrix and serve as sites for cell attachment. Only BSP is confined primarily to bone, whereas the other proteins are found in many nonskeletal connective tissues.

Proteoglycans

Proteoglycans consist of a central core protein to which acidic polysaccharide side chains are attached. The side chains or glycosaminoglycans in bone are primarily chondroitin sulfate and heparin sulfate. The proteoglycans may facilitate osteoblast interaction with cell-attachment and other proteins, but their function remains unknown.

γ-Carboxylated (Gla) Proteins

The bone Gla proteins contain γ-carboxylated glutamine residues that are the product of a vitamin-K-dependent enzymatic process. The addition of the second carboxyl group to the side chain of the glutamine residue produces a binding site for Ca ions. Ca ions are essential cofactors in the function of γ-carboxylated proteins of the blood-clotting cascade, and the ability of the bone Gla proteins to bind Ca plays a role in the regulation of bone mineralization (Krüger et al., 2009). Osteocalcin, a bone Gla protein, is found only in bone, where its synthesis by osteoblasts is regulated by $1,25(OH)_2D$. The serum concentration of osteocalcin is often regarded as a marker for bone turnover. A second γ-carboxylated protein, matrix Gla protein, is found in both bone and cartilage.

Growth-Related Proteins

Growth-related proteins represent the largest number of different protein molecules found in bone. In addition to the insulin-like growth factors (IGF-1 and IGF-2), bone also contains TGF-$_{\beta1-5}$ and other proteins secreted by osteoblasts that stimulate osteoblast growth in a paracrine/autocrine manner (Hauschka et al., 1988). One role suggested for these factors after they are liberated by osteoclastic action has been in the recruitment of osteoblasts to areas of bone resorption.

Other osteoblast-derived proteins found in bone matrix include alkaline phosphatase and osteonectin, a glycoprotein that makes up approximately 2% of bone protein in developing bone. Alkaline phosphatase has long been associated with osteoblasts and its synthesis, and secretion of this enzyme by these cells is considered a marker of bone formation. The function of alkaline phosphatase in bone cell biology, however, must be considered unknown. Osteonectin (also called secreted protein acidic and rich in cysteine or SPARC) is found in both proliferating bone and in growing tissues and is the most abundant noncollagenous protein in bone (Kapinas et al., 2009). This glycoprotein promotes osteoblast differentiation and supports cell survival, as well as likely plays a role in maintaining the balance between bone resorption and formation.

BONE FORMATION

All bone is formed by deposition of hydroxyapatite crystals within a collagen matrix. However, the process by which the collagen matrix is laid down differs according to the two major types of bone formation, intramembranous and endochondral bone formation (bone modeling on a cartilaginous structure) (Deschaseaux et al., 2009).

INTRAMEMBRANOUS BONE FORMATION

The flat bones of the skull, the jaw, and the ribs are formed by intramembranous bone formation. In this process, mesenchymal cells differentiate directly into preosteoblasts and then into osteoblasts in areas of highly vascular embryonic connective tissue. The bone matrix synthesized by these cells is randomly oriented (or woven), and calcification is accomplished in irregular patches rather than in the orderly fashion seen in remodeling bone. Eventually, this bone is remodeled to form lamellar bone.

ENDOCHONDRAL BONE FORMATION (BONE MODELING)

The long bones are formed de novo by calcification of a cartilaginous structure that serves as a model for the new bone. Cartilage is formed by chondroblasts, cells that are derived from prechondroblasts arising from the same mesenchymal cells that form osteoblasts. The chondrocytes secrete a collagen matrix, eventually enclosing themselves into lacunae. Because cartilage consists primarily of collagen fibers and is not rigid, chondrocytes can continue to enlarge and divide, expanding the lacunar spaces. Cartilage also expands at the periphery by appositional (circumferential) growth.

Cartilage is an avascular tissue, and the cells receive their nutrients by diffusion through the fluid surrounding the collagen fibers. Invasion of the cartilage by blood vessels initiates the process of mineralization of the organic matrix. As a result of the reduced diffusion of nutrients to the chondrocytes after mineralization, these cells begin to die. Not all chondrocytes are destroyed during initial calcification of the bone model, however. At each end of the bone, a layer of epiphyseal cartilage remains (see Figure 4.1), and this epiphyseal growth plate serves as the site of bone formation for elongation during growth. As chondrocytes proliferate, the oldest layers begin to calcify. This calcified cartilage is resorbed by osteoclasts, leaving calcified longitudinal septa. Osteoblasts form additional woven bone on these septa to form trabeculae of the primary spongiosa. As additional remodeling of these trabeculae takes place, lamellar bone replaces the woven bone and secondary spongiosa is formed.

The epiphyseal cartilage calcifies after puberty as a result of increases at that time of estrogens in females and testosterone in males. Epiphyseal closure occurs at an earlier age in females, resulting in earlier cessation of longitudinal growth. Delayed puberty, for almost any reason except undernutrition, results in elongation of the long bones and increased height in both females and males.

MINERALIZATION

Bone mineralization involves the formation of hydroxyapatite crystals within calcifying cartilage or newly laid down organic matrix (osteoid) in remodeling bone or new, woven bone. Two distinct mechanisms operate to deposit mineral in bone (Bonucci, 1971; Skinner, 1979; Termine et al., 1980). In lamellar bone formed during remodeling, mineral is deposited in association with the tightly spaced collagen fibrils and associated noncollagenous proteins. In the more open environment of randomly oriented collagen fibrils in cartilage and in woven bone, mineralization is characterized by matrix vesicles that provide a site for hydroxyapatite crystal formation (Anderson et al., 2005; Nahar et al., 2008). These 50- to 200-nm diameter membrane-invested vesicles are formed by exocytosis from the plasma membrane of chondrocytes and osteoblasts. Crystallization eventually produces a crystal larger than the original vesicle and the vesicle is destroyed. Thus, the earliest bone formation either in endochondral bone formation or in woven bone proceeds by vesicle-driven mineralization.

When bone matrix is first synthesized, it requires a period of time before mineralization can occur. Thus, sites of active bone formation are marked by a layer of unmineralized bone matrix, or osteoid, that is not yet calcified. It is not known whether this delay is due to removal of inhibitors of crystal formation or to formation of proteins that are necessary for initiation of mineralization. However, about 5 to 10 days after new matrix is laid down, an initial, rapid phase of bone mineralization is initiated (Bala et al., 2009), which results in mineralization at about 50% to 70% of the maximum level eventually achieved. A secondary phase follows this and is characterized by a slow, gradual maturation of the mineral component that takes up to 30 months to complete.

Several inhibitors of bone mineralization have been identified, including pyrophosphate and phosphoproteins associated with calcified tissues (Termine et al., 1980; Orimo, 2010). The rate of mineralization appears to be related to the presence of these inhibitor molecules. Pyrophosphate is generated by NPP1 and is transported out of the cell by ANKH. The pyrophosphate is hydrolyzed by tissue nonspecific alkaline phosphatase to remove the inhibition and provide inorganic phosphate, which promotes mineralization.

Bone modeling adapts structure to loading by changing bone size and shape and removes damage and so maintains bone strength. Remodeling is initiated by damage-producing osteocyte apoptosis, which signals the location of damage via the osteocyte–canalicular system to endosteal lining cells that form the canopy of a bone remodeling compartment (BRC). Molecular signaling within the BRC between precursors, mature cells, cells of the immune system, and products of the resorbed matrix titrates the birth, work, and lifespan of this remodeling machinery to either remove or form a net volume of bone (see also Chapter 3).

BONE RESORPTION

Bone resorption is defined as removal of both bone mineral and organic matrix to produce a cavity in the bone structure, that is, a resorption pit or Howship's lacuna. This process is carried out primarily by the osteoclast (Figure 4.3). Osteoclasts remove bone in a regulated fashion essential for both the remodeling process and for reconfiguring bone during the modeling process in endochondral bone formation. The major difference in osteoclastic regulation in these two processes is the time-dependent coupling of bone resorption with bone formation that is a characteristic of bone remodeling and the simultaneous, but physically separated, resorption and formation during modeling. Molecular signals regulate the activity of bone cell precursors and the mature bone cells to determine the extent of bone resorption and formation in the remodeling process (Seeman, 2009).

Once bone is dissolved beneath the osteoclast, the Ca and Pi ions and amino acids resulting from protein hydrolysis are removed from the resorption pit (Howship's lacunae) by several possible mechanisms: (1) translocation of individual components through the cytoplasm; (2) bulk transfer of these products via endocytotic vesicles; or (3) release of products when the osteoclast detaches along the sealing zone. The last mechanism is supported by microscopic evidence that osteoclasts are capable of moving along the surface of bone and forming multiple resorption pits. This suggests that the osteoclast is capable of continued bone resorption, but local factors may regulate the maximum size of a given resorption pit.

Resorption of bone on the surface of either trabecular or compact bone results in excavation of shallow Howship's lacuna. However, in compact bone, a group of osteoclasts may continue to resorb bone deep into the compact bone, forming a cylindrical opening through the bone; this cylindrical structure is known as an osteon or Haversian system. Osteoblasts will line the surface of this

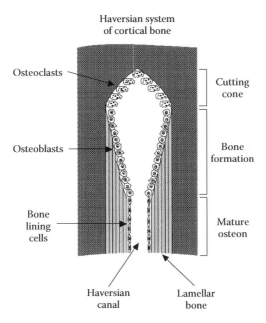

FIGURE 4.5   Haversian systems. The Haversian systems (osteons) of compact bone are formed when a "cutting cone" of several osteoclasts excavates an area of bone. At the reversal zone between the cutting cone and area of bone formation, osteoblasts move in and begin replacing the bone with concentric layers of lamellar bone. An opening is left through the center of the Haversian canal through which blood vessels and nerves pass.

cylinder and lay down new bone in concentric rings until they have filled the excavation except for a central region through which blood vessels and nerves extend (Figure 4.5).

The activity of the osteoclasts is stimulated by PTH and vitamin D, whereas osteoclasts are inhibited by calcitonin (CT) and estrogens. Thus, the regulation of osteoclastic activity by these hormones is believed to be mediated by cytokines secreted by the osteoblasts (McSheehy and Chambers, 1986). Osteoblasts are responsive to both PTH and vitamin D and are believed to produce factors with osteoclast osteoclast-resorption-stimulating activity that are either secreted into the surrounding extracellular fluid or are bound to the cell membrane of the osteoblast (or extracellular matrix) and affect the osteoclasts via direct contact with the cell (Fuller et al., 1991).

BONE REMODELING

During growth, the bones must be constantly reshaped to maintain their optimal shape for support. As elongation occurs, the protuberance of the epiphysis must be reduced by osteoclastic resorption as this volume is filled first by the metaphyseal region and eventually by the cylindrical diaphysis (Figure 4.6). In growing bone, bone resorption and formation take place in separate regions of the bone, with formation exceeding resorption, so that gains in bone mass occur as part of early-life skeletal development.

In mature bone, osteoblastic bone formation occurs only at sites of osteoclastic activity and ideally results in replacement of the exact quantity of bone removed by resorption (Figure 4.7). When bone formation fails to keep pace with bone resorption, a net decrease in bone mass results; osteoporosis is marked by such a discrepancy between removal of bone and its replacement. The rate of bone turnover is much higher in trabecular bone, where approximately 25% of bone is resorbed and replaced annually, whereas there is only about 3% of cortical bone turnover each year (Manolagas and Jilka, 1995).

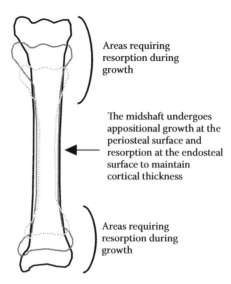

FIGURE 4.6 Reshaping of a long bone during growth (modeling). During growth, the bones must be reshaped to maintain the bone model. The outer aspect of the epiphysis is resorbed as the bone length increases at the epiphyseal plate. The midshaft undergoes both resorption on the endosteal surface and growth on the periosteal surface and maintain a similar cortical thickness as the diameter of the bone increases. The process of modeling is distinct from that of remodeling (Figure 4.7), in which the resorption of bone and its subsequent formation are tightly coupled at individual sites.

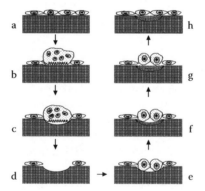

FIGURE 4.7 Coupling of remodeling in Howship's lacunae. Remodeling of bone is a multistep process beginning with (a) activation at an area of bone surface covered by bone-lining cells. (b) Osteoclast(s) are recruited to this site and (c) excavate a resorption pit (Howship's lacuna). During the (d) reversal phase, the osteoclast moves away from the resorption pit and (e) osteoblasts move in and (f) begin replacing the resorbed bone with new layers of bone. (g) Once this process is complete and the bone tissue has been completely restored, (h) the osteoblasts are replaced by quiescent bone-lining cells again. (Talmage, R.V., Grubb, S.A., and VanderWiel, C.J. 1983. Physiologic processes in bone. In *The Musculoskeletal System: Basic Processes and Disorders*, Wilson, F. C., ed., 2nd ed., Chapter 8. J.B. Lippincott Co., Philadelphia.)

THE BONE MULTICELLULAR UNIT AND BONE REMODELING

The concept of bone remodeling was advanced by Frost (1963). He later introduced the concept of the bone multicellular unit for the multicellular sequence of changes in bone that resulted in renewal of bone matrix and mineral in distinct units.

As the organic matrix ages, it becomes brittle and weak and undergoes microfractures. Bone remodeling replaces it with new matrix. This process of remodeling of mature bone consists of a predictable and ordered sequence of bone resorption followed by bone formation, and it can be divided into the following three stages:

1. Activation of osteoclasts
2. Resorption by osteoclasts
3. Formation by osteoblasts

The periods of resorption and formation are also separated by a period sometimes called the reversal phase, as osteoclasts are replaced by osteoblasts at the resorption site.

REGULATION OF BONE REMODELING

The processes of bone remodeling also are involved in the response of bone to strain, such as repeated exercise, that results in greater bone mass and in stronger bone, and remodeling is essential for the healing of bone fractures. Although bone remodeling could occur in a random fashion, intersecting the site of microfracture damage by chance, a process has been described whereby bone cells, particularly osteocytes, act as mechanosensors to regulate these activities so that areas of damage are replaced preferentially (Robling and Turner, 2009).

The process by which osteoblasts replace the bone removed from the bone surface is closely regulated or coupled (Martin et al., 2009) (see Chapter 3). The regulation of bone remodeling requires interactions between bone-resorbing and bone-forming cells. Experiments with isolated osteoblasts and osteoclasts have demonstrated that osteoclasts alone are not responsive to stimulation; however, when cocultured with osteoblasts, addition of PTH or $1,25(OH)_2D$ can promote bone resorption by osteoclasts. In addition, exposing osteoclasts to medium conditioned by osteoblasts stimulated by PTH or $1,25(OH)_2D$ has a similar stimulatory effect on bone resorption. Therefore, osteoblasts must synthesize a factor that promotes bone resorption by the osteoclast. Numerous proteins are present in bone along with collagen. Several of these are large glycoprotein molecules that likely serve primarily structural function. Many soluble proteins, however, are also incorporated into mineralized bone at the time of matrix formation. As discussed above (see the section on noncollagenous proteins of bone matrix), protein growth factors secreted by osteoblasts or adsorbed from plasma are almost always present in mature bone. Liberation of these factors during bone resorption may serve as signals for the recruitment of osteoblasts to resorption sites.

The local factors that are secreted by osteoblasts and other cells of the bone marrow or stromal cells are proteins known collectively as cytokines (Chambers, 1988; Mundy, 1992; Roodman, 1993). Cytokines may either stimulate osteoclastic bone resorption or inhibit resorption and stimulate bone formation. Factors in the local environment of bone that stimulate osteoclastic bone resorption include interleukin-1, transforming growth factors-α (TGF-α), tumor necrosis factor-α (TNF-α), and interleukin-6. Bone resorption is inhibited by TGF-α, γ-interferon, and interleukin-4. Because these agents are secreted by cells of the lymphocyte and macrophage lineages, bone marrow is a rich source for these peptides.

Osteoblast regulation of proliferation of osteoclast precursors is regulated by macrophage colony-stimulating factor, which is secreted by the osteoblast. The receptor activator of NFκB (RANK) ligand (RANKL) is a member of the TNF superfamily that is expressed on the membrane of osteoblasts and activates receptor RANK on osteoclast precursors (Yavropoulou and Yolos, 2008; Seeman, 2009). Osteoblasts can also inhibit osteoclast formation through osteoprotegerin, a secreted protein that acts as a decoy receptor for RANKL.

The investigation of the role of cytokines in bone remodeling and in the regulation of bone cell metabolism will be greatly accelerated in the near future by the development of specific animal models with selected deletion or overexpression of specific cytokines and/or their receptors. In many cases, researchers may be able to target specifically these mutations to cells of bone, or they may mutate the genes for these proteins in all cells.

LIFESTYLE EFFECTS

A few topics relating to bone formation and maintenance require special emphasis.

Peak Bone Mass Accrual

At some time during the third decade of life, individuals will have accumulated the largest amount of bone tissue they will have at any time during their lifetime. This peak bone mass is a critical factor in contributing to the risk of osteoporotic fracture later in life. The attainment of peak bone mass by about the age of 30 years depends on the genetic inheritance of an individual, on nutrition from the prenatal period through adulthood, and on physical activity.

Effect of Exercise (Strain) on Bone

As discussed in Chapter 5 of this volume, mechanical stress on bone influences skeletal adaptation, an effect that may be particularly important during the growth of the skeleton in early life and in the aged. Considerable evidence supports a role for mechanical loading (strain) or gravitational force in maintaining bone mass (Rubin and Lanyon, 1984). Individuals that are confined to long-term bed rest or that have participated in space flights lose bone. If bones are not subjected to load through mechanical usage, normal bone mass development will be limited to about 30% to 50% of normal, and even the cross-sectional shape of the long bones will fail to develop normally (Robling and Turner, 2009).

Bone mineral density (BMD) in the spine of postmenopausal women can be increased by aerobic, weight-bearing, and resistance exercises (Iwamoto et al., 2009). Although extensive loss of bone can be observed in a relatively short period of time with inactivity or weightlessness (Donaldson et al., 1970; Vogel et al., 1977), the gain in bone mass with exercise is much smaller. Comparison of bone mineral content (BMC) and BMD in young adult women suggests that increased physical activity may offset, at least in part, an inadequate dietary Ca intake (Metz et al., 1993).

Studies in experimental animal models generally support the concept that the response to mechanical loading is a local one and does not affect other bones, including the contralateral limb (Sugiyama et al., 2009). The adaptive response affects both the cortical and trabecular bone. Mechanical loading signals changes in bone cells that produce biochemical and eventually structural changes in bone (Robling and Turner, 2009). As theorized over 100 years ago by Julius Wolff, bone adjusts its structure to adapt to the loads placed upon it.

AGING AND OSTEOPOROSIS

Aging is generally associated with a net loss of bone tissue at all skeletal sites. The bone appears normal, and excessive osteoclasts cannot be found, but too little bone, or osteopenia, exists. Thus, bone is more susceptible to fracture, especially the trabecular bone tissue. Osteoporotic fractures occur most commonly to the vertebrae, distal radius and ulna (wrist), proximal femur (hip), or humerus (upper arm).

Bone loss in aging occurs mainly from the endosteal surface of the cortex, which would result in thinning and weakening of the structure; however, exercise can increase the rate of periosteal bone formation (Seeman, 2009) (see Chapter 5). This periosteal increase can result in a bone with larger diameters of both the internal and external part of the cross-section, but the mechanical strength of the bone is maintained.

ASSESSMENT OF BONE MASS AND BONE TURNOVER

A great need exists for accurate methods of assessing bone mass and bone turnover for either diagnosis in subjects who are believed to be at risk for bone loss or assessment of treatment modalities in those who have already lost bone. Although the most accurate information on bone quality and bone remodeling activity at a particular site can be obtained by bone histomorphometry, the invasive nature of this procedure limits its usefulness in diagnosis and treatment of bone disorders. Although X-rays can be used to provide some information about gross changes in bone structure, the need to measure much smaller changes in BMC or BMD has led to the development and refinement of instruments that can be used to noninvasively determine bone quality in a particular area with continually improving accuracy and reproducibility. Another goal has been to reduce the exposure to radiation as low as possible. Several general types of these instruments are discussed below.

Although BMC and/or BMD can be measured with accuracy and reproducibility approaching 1%–2%, this provides information only on the current status of the bone, not on changes in bone formation and resorption that can be related to treatment. Some of the molecules that are present in blood and/or urine are discussed below as possible markers for the dynamic processes occurring within the bone.

BONE HISTOMORPHOMETRY

The most accurate estimates of bone mass are obtained by direct sampling of the bone, for example, transiliac bone biopsy, followed by biochemical and histological analyses. Because of the invasive nature of this procedure, which requires removal of a cylindrical core of bone through the iliac crest, it is not in routine use. However, as a research tool, this procedure can provide valuable information about the rates of bone formation and turnover when bone is labeled *in vivo* with tetracycline, fluorescein, or other fluorescent markers of bone mineralization. Together with well-established staining techniques for bone, these fluorescent compounds can be used to measure the actual bone turnover rate during the period of study and define the status of the population of bone cells in the region examined. These methods are frequently used to assess bone abnormalities in patients with chronic kidney disease because of the effects of renal failure on bone health (Ott, 2008).

IN VIVO MEASUREMENTS OF BMC AND BMD

The need to assess BMC and/or BMD in large numbers of individuals has prompted the development of several noninvasive methods that give quantitative results, as opposed to qualitative estimates from standard X-rays. The ideal for a useful method of measuring bone densitometry is a technique that is both accurate, that is, that provides an estimate of bone mass or density that is very close to the true value, and precise, that is, being able to measure reproducibly the same site in the skeleton. Because of the relatively slow rate of change in bone mass during most of the life cycle, precision in the range of 1%–2% is necessary to measure meaningful changes in bone mass or density even when studies extend over a year or more. Older methods, such as radiographic absorptiometry, single-photon absorptiometry, and dual-photon absorptiometry, have largely been replaced.

Dual-Energy X-Radiographic Absorptiometry

Dual-energy X-radiographic absorptiometry (DXA) was an important advance in the diagnosis of osteoporosis by measurement of BMD when it was first introduced in routine clinical practice in 1987 (Blake and Fogelman, 2009). DXA is generally considered the best method for diagnosing osteopenia or osteoporosis on the basis of the World Health Organization (WHO) *T*-score definition of osteopenia as $-2.5 < T < 1.0$ and osteoporosis as -2.5. The *T* score is calculated based on the mean BMD for healthy young adults (aged 20–29 years). In addition to the usefulness of DXA in diagnosing osteoporosis, its BMD results also can be used to predict fracture risk, to target therapies against fractures, and to monitor the response to those treatments.

The basic principle of DXA is that it utilizes two monoenergetic X-rays (gamma photons) that are generated by an X-ray machine and then focuses on a target tissue site for a short period. A machine-driven tracking system allows the source to move across (laterally) different sites of interest or the entire body from head to toes. One of the X-rays is harder, and the other is soft. The harder

X-ray is stopped to a large extent by the skeletal (mineralized) tissue, whereas most of the soft X-rays are stopped by the soft tissue, including fat. The algorithm uses the weight, height, sex, and age of the individual, as well as the X-ray attenuation data for calculating BMC or BMD, fat mass, and lean body mass, exclusive of bone, that is, a three-compartment model of body composition. DXA instruments are typically found in radiology departments of hospitals where radiation safety is carefully monitored. The radiation dosages to subjects with either of these methods are very low, for example, the amount received by a person flying at 40,000 ft from New York to Denver or about a tenth of the radiation dose of a standard chest X-ray.

Babies, small infants, and even pregnant women can be measured with the DXA technique because of the low radiation doses, but of course, an experimental study measuring the bone mass of pregnant women would be almost impossible to do.

Bone

Measurements of BMC and BMD using DXA are considered very accurate (3% to 4%) for normal-weight or thin individuals, but not for heavily muscled and obese subjects because of the greater attenuation by increased mass from soft tissues. Precision, however, remains good (2%) for all subjects. Measurements of the axial skeleton can be made with this method, as well as those of the appendicular skeleton. In addition, total body measurements from head to toe (or neck to toe) can be made. A special arm attachment (device) permits separate measurement of the radius and ulna. These measurements can be done quite rapidly (fast mode) or more slowly.

Fat

Therefore, the normalized data set used for comparison does not apply to very obese individuals (>50% body mass) or to sick patients who have lost much of their lean tissue, who may also be dehydrated, or who may have shifts of water (fluid) from blood to extravascular fluid compartments. The potential pitfalls of using DXA have not so dampened the enthusiasm of investigators that they are discarding this method; to the contrary, they are trying different ways to improve the method for evaluating body fat under conditions of excessive obesity.

Quantitative Computed Tomography

Although quantitative computed tomography (QCT) was introduced in the mid-1970s, it is less widely used than DXA (Adams, 2009). QCT does have several advantages, including the ability to measure cortical and trabecular BMD separately, in providing a measurement related to the volume of bone rather than the cross-sectional area and in providing information on geometric and structural characteristics of the bone that contribute to its strength. QCT requires a slightly higher radiation dose compared with DXA, but it is similar to the spinal radiographs that are used to diagnose osteoporosis. The technique, however, is only used routinely for estimating vertebral bone density, especially of the lumbar region of the spine. Comparison of single measurements using QCT and DXA cannot be made, and QCT cannot be used for calculation of the WHO T-score definitions of osteopenia and osteoporosis, but multiple measurement trends can be used for comparison.

Other Methods

Another method for the assessment of BMD and diagnosis of osteoporosis is quantitative ultrasound, which has advantages of low cost and lack of ionizing radiation compared with DXA and QCT (Guglielmi and de Terlizzi, 2009). Positron emission tomography has been proposed as a method for detection of microdamage in bone, but results have only been reported in a rodent study (Li et al., 2005). Initial results with a microindentation method for *in vivo* measurement of the mechanical properties of bone tissue were reported in 2010 (Diez-Perez et al., 2010).

Summary

The best experimental use of these bone-densitometric machines is for prospective investigations of BMC and BMD in the same individuals using the same machines and operators to limit errors, such as geometry, positioning, and operator differences. DXA has become the method of choice for experimental studies because of its wide availability, high precision, and ease of use, despite some disadvantages of linear density estimates. Furthermore, the low dose of radiation of DXA machines makes them quite safe.

Bone Markers in Blood and Urine

The importance of balanced bone resorption and formation in maintenance of bone health has resulted in continued efforts by researchers and clinicians to find molecules in urine or plasma that reflect bone resorption and/or formation (Delmas, 1993). These markers of bone turnover are likely to change over short periods, for example, hours or days, as opposed to the months or years required for the changes in bone mass or density (described above). Thus, these methods can be used to follow therapeutic intervention in metabolic bone diseases such as osteoporosis (Garnero, 2009). Candidates for these markers are molecules that reflect the enzymatic activities of osteoblasts or osteoclasts or the products resulting from the breakdown of bone tissue.

Markers of Bone Formation

Alkaline phosphatase is an enzyme that is characteristic of osteoblasts, and an increase in the bone-specific isoenzyme, such as b-s ALP, reflects the rate of osteoblastic bone formation. Total blood alkaline phosphatase measurement, however, is less useful because the synthesis of isozymes of alkaline phosphatase in liver, gastrointestinal tract, and other tissues makes measurement and interpretation of changes difficult.

Osteocalcin, also known as bone Gla protein, is one of the proteins that make up bone matrix along with collagen, although its function is not known (see Chapter 12). Synthesis of this protein is dependent on vitamin K. Like collagen and alkaline phosphatase, osteocalcin is synthesized by the osteoblasts, and its blood levels may reflect the level of bone formation.

Another molecule, procollagen type I N-terminal propeptide (PINP), is one of two propeptides (the other is C-terminal propeptide [PICP]) synthesized as part of type 1 procollagen that are cleaved by specific proteases to produce the mature type 1 collagen molecule. PICP is cleared more quickly than PINP (Lüftner et al., 2005). Newer markers for bone formation include BSP, osteopontin, periostin, and urinary midmolecule osteocalcin fragments (Garnero, 2009).

Markers of Bone Resorption

Hydroxyproline is a modified amino acid that is unique to collagen and is measurable in both blood and urine. When collagen is degraded during bone resorption, the hydroxyproline residues are released from the protein and are not reused. Therefore, the amount of hydroxyproline in the blood and/or urine reflects the level of osteoclastic bone resorption, assuming no alteration in turnover of other tissues containing collagen.

Osteoclasts synthesize a tartrate-resistant acid phosphatase (TRAP) that may be measured in blood. Changes in serum concentrations of TRAP may be reflective of bone resorption by osteoclasts.

Mature collagen contains cross-links between adjacent protein molecules. These pyridinoline and deoxypyridinilone intermolecular cross-links can be measured in urine and in some cases in serum, and they are indicative of resorption of collagen molecules because the cross-links are not hydrolyzed before excretion. However, collagen molecules other than bone collagen contain significant amounts of pyridinoline cross-links.

The N-terminal (NTX) and C-terminal (CTX) telopeptides are generated from the collagen I molecule by cathepsin K digestion, whereas carboxy-terminal cross-linked telopeptide (CCX-MMP) and carboxy-terminal telopeptide of type I collagen (ICTP) are generated by matrix-metal-loproteases (MTX).

Additional candidates for markers of bone resorption are tartrate-resistant acid phosphatase (TRACP5) and cathepsin K (Garnero, 2009). TRACP5 is a subform specific to osteoclasts, and cathepsin K is a bone-resorbing enzyme expressed selectively in osteoclasts.

Summary

Bone markers, although useful for estimating changes in turnover, have not yet been shown to be as accurate as would be desirable. Because this area of understanding is being actively investigated, better use of these markers should emerge in the future.

SUMMARY

As an organ, bone can be described by its anatomic location, shape, and function. The organization of bone into cortical and trabecular microstructure is essential for the supportive and metabolic functions provided by the skeleton. At the tissue level, bone contains several different types of cells that are responsible for bone formation (osteoblasts) and bone resorption (osteoclasts) during both growth and maintenance of the skeleton.

Although bone appears externally to be an unchanging structure, its microenvironment is remarkably dynamic. Not only does bone undergo microscopic remodeling processes that are constantly replacing small packets of bone throughout the skeleton, but at the chemical level, bone is constantly exchanging Ca and Pi with extracellular fluid and ultimately with the plasma.

The regulation of Ca homeostasis is complex, involving interactions with kidney and gut and with hormonal factors, especially PTH and vitamin D. The control of bone turnover is even more complex as circulating hormones known to affect bone, including PTH, vitamin D, CT, and estrogen, change in their concentrations. The roles of local bone factors, for example, cytokines, growth factors, and noncollagenous matrix proteins, in the regulation of bone formation and remodeling are only now beginning to be elucidated.

Once the bone matures and the individual attains peak bone mass, a phenomenon that generally occurs between 20 and 29 years of age for different parts of the skeleton, the maintenance of bone health is dependent on the balance between bone resorption and formation. When formation fails to replace the same amount of bone removed by osteoclastic resorption, bone mass decreases. In late life, the resulting low bone mass or osteopenia is eventually evidenced as osteoporosis when an increase in fracture risk occurs. Current research suggests that physical activity and adequate nutrition during periods of bone accretion and bone maintenance contribute to attaining optimal peak bone mass, as well as to minimizing the rate of loss with aging in older individuals.

REFERENCES

Adams, J.E. 2009. Quantitative computed tomography. *Eur J Radiol* 71: 415–424.
Albright, J.A., and Skinner, H.C.W. 1987. Bone: Structural organization and remodeling dynamics. In *The Scientific Basis of Orthopaedics*, Albright, J.A. and Brand, R.A., eds. Appleton & Lange, Norwalk, CT, 161 pp.
Anderson, H.C., Garimella, R., and Tague, S.E. 2005. The role of matrix vesicles in growth plate development and mineralization. *Frontiers Biosci* 10: 822–837.
Bala, Y., Farley, D., Delmas, P.D., et al. 2009. Time sequence of secondary mineralization and microhardness in cortical and cancellous bone from ewes. *Bone* 46: 1204–1212.
Blair, H.C., Schlesinger, P.H., Ross, F.P., et al. 1993. Recent advances toward understanding osteoclast physiology. *Clin Orthop Rel Res* 294: 7–22.
Blake, G.M., and Fogelman, I. 2009. The clinical role of dual energy X-ray absorptiometry. *Eur J Radiol* 71: 406–414.
Bonucci, E. 1971. The locus of initial calcification in cartilage and bone. *Clin Orthop Rel Res* 78: 108–139.
Boyce, B.F., Yao, Z., and Xing, L. 2009. Osteoclasts have multiple roles in bone in addition to bone resorption. *Crit Rev Eukar Gene Exp* 19: 171–180.
Chambers, T.J. 1988. The regulation of osteoclastic development and function. In *Cell and Molecular Biology of Vertebrate Hard Tissues, Ciba Foundation Symposium 136*, Evered, D. and Harnett, S., eds. Wiley, Chichester, UK, pp. 92–107.
Clarke, B. 2008. Normal bone anatomy and physiology. *Clin J Am Soc Nephro* 3(Suppl 3): S131–S139.
Cormack, D.H. 1987. Bone. In *Ham's Histology*, Cormack, D. H., ed. J.B. Lippincott Co., London, 273 pp.

Currey, J. 1984. *The Mechanical Adaptations of Bones*. Princeton University Press, Princeton, NJ, 294 pp.

Delmas, P.D. 1993. Biochemical markers of bone turnover I: Theoretical considerations and clinical use in osteoporosis. *Am J Med* 95(Suppl 5A): 11S–16S.

Deschaseaux, F., Sensébé, L., and Heymann, D. 2009. Mechanisms of bone repair and regeneration. *Trends Mol Med* 15: 417–429.

Diez-Perez, A., Güerri, R., Nogues, X., et al. 2010. Microindentation for in vivo measurement of bone tissue mechanical properties in humans. *J Bone Miner Res* 25: 1877–1885. DOI 10.1002/jbmr.73.

Donaldson, C.L., Hulley, S.B., Vogel, J.M., et al. 1970. Effect of prolonged bed rest on bone mineral. *Metabolism* 1: 1071–1084.

Evans, F.G. 1973. *Mechanical Properties of Bone*, Charles C Thomas, Springfield, IL, 322 pp.

Fawcett, D.W. 1994. Bone. In *Bloom and Fawcett: A Textbook of Histology*, Fawcett, D. W., ed. Chapman & Hall, New York, 194 pp.

Frost, H.M. 1963. *Bone Remodelling Dynamics*. Charles C Thomas, Springfield, IL, 175 pp.

Fuller, K., Gallagher, A.C., and Chambers, T.J. 1991. Osteoclast resorption-stimulating activity is associated with the osteoblast cell surface and/or the extracellular matrix. *Biochem Biophys Res Commun* 181: 67–73.

Garnero, P. 2009. Bone markers in osteoporosis. *Curr Ostoporosis Rep* 7: 84–90.

Guglielmi, G., and de Terlizzi, F. 2009. Quantitative ultrasound in the assessment of osteoporosis. *Eur J Radiology* 71: 425–431.

Hauschka, P.V., Chen, T.L., and Mavrakos, A.E. 1988. Polypeptide growth factors in bone matrix. In *Cell and Molecular Biology of Vertebrate Hard Tissues, Ciba Foundation Symposium 136*, Evered, D. and Harnett, S., eds. Wiley, Chichester, UK, 207 pp.

Henriksen, K, Neutzky-Wulff, A.V., Bonewald, L.F., et al. 2009. Local communication on and within bone controls bone remodeling. *Bone* 44: 1026–1033.

Henriksen, K., Sørensen, M.G., Jensen, V.K., et al. 2008. Ion transporters involved in acidification of the resorption lacuna in osteoclasts. *Calcif Tissue Int* 83: 230–242.

Iwamoto, J., Sato, Y., Takeda, T., et al. 2009. Effectiveness of exercise in the treatment of lumbar spinal stenosis, knee osteoarthritis, and osteoporosis. *Aging Clin Exp Res* (Epub ahead of print).

Kapinas, K., Kessler, C.B., and Delaney, A.M. 2009. mIR-29 suppression of osteonectin in osteoblasts: Regulation during differentiation and by canonical Wnt signaling. *J Cell Biochem* 108: 216–224.

Krüger, T., Westenfeld, R., Schurgers, L., et al. 2009. Coagulation meets calcification: The vitamin K system. *Int J Artif Organs* 32: 67–74.

Lanyon, L.E. 1992. Control of bone architecture by functional load bearing. *J Bone Min Res* 7(Suppl 2): S369–S375.

Li, J., Miller, M.A., Hutchins, G.D., et al. 2005. Imaging bone microdamage in vivo with positron emission tomography. *Bone* 37: 819–824.

Lüftner, D., Jozereau, D., Schildhauer, S., et al. 2005. PINP as serum marker of metastatic spread to the bone in breast cancer patients. *Anticancer Res* 25: 1491–1500.

Mammone, J.F., and Hudson, S.M. 1993. Micromechanics of bone strength and failure, *J Biomechanics* 26: 439–446.

Manolagas, S.C. and Jilka, R.L. 1995. Bone marrow, cytokines, and bone remodeling. Emerging insights into the pathophysiology of osteoporosis. *New Engl J Med* 335: 305–311.

Martin, T., Gooi, J.H., and Sims, N.A. 2009. Molecular mechanisms coupling bone formation to resorption. *Crit Rev Eukaryot Gene Expr* 19: 73–88.

McSheehy, P.M.J., and Chambers, T.J. 1986. Osteoblastic cells mediate osteoclastic responsiveness to parathyroid hormone. *Endocrinology* 118: 824–828.

Metz, J.A., Anderson, J.J.B., and Gallagher, P.N., Jr. 1993. Intakes of calcium, phosphorus, and protein, and physical-activity level are related to radial bone mass in young adult women. *Am J Clin Nutr* 58: 537–542.

Mundy, G.R. 1992. Cytokines and local factors which affect osteoclast function, *Int J Cell Cloning* 12: 215–222.

Nahar, N.N., Missana, L.R., Garimella, R., et al. 2008. Matrix vesicles are carriers of bone morphogenetic proteins (BMPs), vascular endothelial growth factor (VEGF), and noncollagenous matrix proteins. *J Bone Miner Metab* 26: 514–519.

Orimo, H. 2010. The mechanism of mineralization and the role of alkaline phosphatase in health and disease. *J Nippon Med Sch* 77: 4–12.

Ott, S.M. 2008. Histomorphometric measurements of bone turnover, mineralization, and volume. *Clin J Am Soc Nephrol* 3(Suppl 3): S151–S156.

Robling, A.G., and Turner, C.H. 2009. Mechanical signaling for bone modeling and remodeling. *Crit Rev Eukar Gene Exp* 19: 319–338.

Roodman, G.D. 1993. Role of cytokines in the regulation of bone resorption, *Calcif Tissue Int* 53(Suppl 1): S94–S98.

Rubin, C.T., and Lanyon, L.E. 1984. Regulation of bone formation by applied dynamic loads. *J Bone Jt Surg* 66-A: 397–402.

Seeman, E. 2009. Bone modeling and remodeling. *Crit Rev Eukar Gene Exp* 19: 219–233.

Skinner, H.C.W. 1979. Bone: Mineralization. In *The Scientific Basis of Orthopaedics*, Albright, J. A., and Brand, R. A., eds. Appleton & Lange, Norwalk, CT, 199 pp.

Stark, Z., and Savarirayan, R. 2009. Osteoporosis. *Orphanet J Rare Diseases* 4: http://www.ojrd.com/content/4/1/5.

Sugiyama, T., Price, J.S., and Lanyon, L.E. 2009. Functional adaptation to mechanical loading in both cortical and cancellous bone is controlled locally and is confined to the loaded bones. *Bone* 46: 314–331.

Talmage, R.V., Grubb, S.A., and VanderWiel, C.J. 1983. Physiologic processes in bone. In *The Musculoskeletal System: Basic Processes and Disorders*, Wilson, F. C., ed., 2nd ed., Chapter 8. J.B. Lippincott Co., Philadelphia.

Talmage, R.V., and Mobley H.T. 2008. Calcium homeostatis: Reassessment of the actions of parathyroid hormone. *Gen Comp Endocrinol* 156: 1–8.

Talmage, R.V., and Mobley H.T. 2009. The concentration of free calcium in plasma is set by the extracellular action of noncollagenous proteins and hydroxyapatite. *Gen Comp Endocrinol* 162: 245–250.

Talmage, R.V., and Talmage, D.W. 2006. Calcium homeostasis: Solving the solubility problem. *J Musculoskelet Neuronal Interact* 6: 402–407.

Talmage R.V., and Talmage D.W. 2007. Calcium homeostasis: How bone solubility relates to all aspects of bone physiology. *J Musculoskelet Neuronal Interact* 7: 108–112.

Termine, J.D. 1988. Non-collagen proteins in bone. In *Cell and Molecular Biology of Vertebrate Hard Tissues, Ciba Foundation Symposium 136*, Evered, D. and Harnett, S., eds. Wiley, Chichester, UK, 178 pp.

Termine, J.D., Eanes, E.D., and Conn, K.M. 1980. Phosphoprotein modulation of apatite crystallization, *Calcif Tissue Int* 31: 247–251.

Vogel, J.M., Whittle, W.M., Smith, M.C., et al. 1977. Bone mineral measurement, experiment M078. In *Biomedical Results from Skylab*, Pool, S.L., ed. Administration, National Aeronautics and Space Administration, GPO, Washington, DC, 183 pp.

Yavropoulou, M.P., and Yovos, J.G. 2008. Osteoclastogenesis—current knowledge and future perspectives. *J Musculoskelet Neuronal Interact* 8: 204–216.

5 Optimizing the Skeletal Benefits of Mechanical Loading and Exercise

Stuart J. Warden and Robyn K. Fuchs

CONTENTS

INTRODUCTION

Osteoporosis is a prominent and growing problem characterized by a reduction in bone strength and consequent increase in the risk for low-trauma fractures. Key determinants of bone strength and thus fracture risk include the amount of bone material present (quantity), and the spatial distribution (structure) and intrinsic properties (quality) of this material. There is clear evidence for a genetic contribution to these bone properties, with heritability estimates ranging from 60% to 90%, depending on the skeletal property and site assessed (Peacock et al., 2002). The remaining variance in bone properties is accounted for by other factors.

Nondominant   Dominant

Control

Thrower

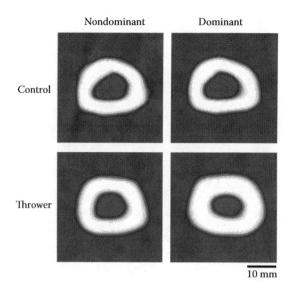

10 mm

FIGURE 5.1   The skeletal effects of mechanical loading and exercise are eloquently observed in individuals playing sports that expose their dominant upper extremity to mechanical overload. The images depict the structural features of the midshaft humerus in the nondominant and dominant upper extremities of a sedentary control individual and throwing (baseball) athlete, as acquired using peripheral quantitative computed tomography. Note the larger bone with thicker cortex in the dominant upper extremity of the thrower when compared with the nondominant upper extremity and the upper extremities in the control individual. (Reprinted from *Bone*, 45, Warden, S.J., et al., 931–41, 2009, with permission from Elsevier.)

The skeleton's primary function is mechanical wherein it provides internal support to enable the force of gravity to be countered and presents attachment sites to allow muscle forces to generate motion at specialized bone-to-bone linkages. Given this mechanical role, it follows teleologically that skeletal tissue responds and adapts to its prevailing mechanical environment. This phenomenon is loosely referred to as Wolff's law, named after the German anatomist/surgeon Julius Wolff who suggested that the form of bone is related to mechanical stress by a mathematical law (Wolff, 1892).

Although basic tenets of Wolff's law contain inaccuracies (Pearson and Lieberman, 2004), the general concept that bone adapts to its mechanical environment is widely accepted. Genetics may impact the magnitude of this adaptation with studies utilizing animal models demonstrating genotype influences on skeletal mechanosensitivity (Robling and Turner, 2002; Robling et al., 2007); however, co-twin studies and studies investigating bone health within individuals who unilaterally overload one extremity have confirmed that mechanical loading in the form of exercise is an important genetic-independent factor influencing skeletal properties (Figure 5.1) (Huddleston et al., 1980; Iuliano-Burns et al., 2005; MacInnis et al., 2003; Warden et al., 2009).

This chapter discusses mechanical loading features that influence skeletal adaptation and the response of the skeleton to the mechanical loading associated with exercise during two critical phases of the life span—growth and aging. Included is a discussion of the contribution of nutrition and pharmaceutical agents to mechanically induced skeletal adaptation during growth and aging, respectively.

MECHANICAL LOADING FEATURES INFLUENCING SKELETAL ADAPTATION

SKELETAL ADAPTATION IS INFLUENCED BY LOAD MAGNITUDE

Animal studies introducing controlled loading to the skeleton have provided a wealth of knowledge regarding mechanical loading features contributing to skeletal adaptation. Initially, these studies

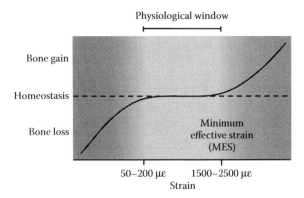

FIGURE 5.2 Adaptation of the skeleton to mechanical loading according to Frost's mechanostat theory. Frost mechanostat theory predicted mechanical strains to fall between two effective strain levels—the minimum effective strain (MES), speculated to be in the vicinity of 1500 to 2500 με (Frost, 1987) and a lower effective strain level, suggested to be approximately 50–200 με. When mechanical strains fell within this "physiological window," bone resorption during remodeling equaled formation, resulting in mineral homeostasis and no bone adaptation. When mechanical usage caused strain levels to fall outside the window, an imbalance between resorption and formation was predicted. Bone loss (net mineral loss) was predicted for strains below the lower effective strain level (50–200 με), whereas bone gain (net mineral gain) was predicted for strains above the MES (1500–2500 με). For extremely high strains, microscopic trauma (microdamage) was predicted.

identified load magnitude as a key factor determining adaptation. When discussing the magnitude of loads applied to the skeleton, the internal strain that the bone experiences is most relevant. Strain refers to the change in length per unit length of a structure and is typically expressed in terms of microstrain (με) in bone because of its small value. Bone strains during usual activities of daily living range from 400 to 1500 με, although activities involving high impact loads result in higher strains (Burr et al., 1996). For bone to respond and adapt to an external load, the microstrain engendered within the bone needs to surpass a certain threshold that is greater than what is typically experienced (Rubin and Lanyon, 1985; Turner et al., 1994b).

The importance of strain to skeletal mechanoresponsiveness was recognized by the pioneering work of Dr. Harold M. Frost who developed a mathematical model for describing the response of bone to mechanical loading—Frost's mechanostat theory (Frost, 1987). This theory described a negative feedback control system where bone was maintained such that everyday mechanical strains fell between two effective strain levels—the minimum effective strain (MES), speculated to be in the vicinity of 1500 to 2500 με, and a lower effective strain level, suggested to be approximately 50–200 με (Frost, 1987, 1990). The combination of these two strain levels created a "physiological window" wherein mechanical strains within the window resulted in mineral homeostasis, whereas strains below and above the window resulted in net mineral loss and gain, respectively (Figure 5.2).

Skeletal Adaptation Is Enhanced with Novel Mechanical Loading

Frost's mechanostat theory provided a quantum advance in understanding bone adaptation to loading, yet it was not without limitations (Martin, 2000; Turner, 1999). In particular, the theory assumed that bone cells were somehow preprogrammed with a MES value which set the threshold for a skeletal response. However, it is now understood that the MES must vary both between and within bones; otherwise, relatively nonloaded bones (i.e., cranium) and sites (i.e., along the neutral axis in a bending bone) would constantly be in states of net mineral loss. Such loss of bone tissue does not occur because bone cell mechanosensitivity is plastic.

Plasticity forms the foundation of the cellular accommodation theory. The theory agrees that mechanosensitive cells must contain some strain threshold above which a mechanical signal can elicit a cellular response yet argues that the threshold is not a set value, rather is a product of local strain history (Turner, 1999). The cellular accommodation theory assumes that when a strain threshold is surpassed, the mechanosensor cells gradually accommodate to the new state, either by cytoskeletal reorganization or by change of the extracellular microenvironment. Given that bone adaptation is error driven (Lanyon, 1992), the bone response is then proportional to the difference between the new strain and the ever-changing set point, rather than being directly related to the absolute magnitude of the new strain induced by a loading stimulus. Therefore, adaptation to mechanical loading is greatest when strains differ most from usual strains (i.e., when novel loads are introduced). Preliminary evidence to support the cellular accommodation theory has been provided experimentally with bone formation in a mechanical loading study closely resembling the theory's predicted results, but not those predicted by Frost's mechanostat theory (Schriefer et al., 2005).

SKELETAL ADAPTATION IS INFLUENCED BY HOW FAST LOADS ARE INTRODUCED

Bone adaptation to a loading stimulus is not dependent on strain magnitude alone, as indicated by the observation that dynamic loading induces significantly greater adaptation than if the same strain magnitudes are held statically (Lanyon and Rubin, 1984; Robling et al., 2001b). The preferential response of bone to dynamic stimuli, combined with its greater adaptation to increased strain magnitude, suggests that a bone's adaptive response to loading is influenced by how fast strain is introduced. This relationship has been confirmed experimentally with higher strain rates generating greater bone adaptation (Mosley and Lanyon, 1998; Turner et al., 1994a, 1995a).

As strain rate is the product of strain magnitude and loading frequency, it fits that increasing either component may contribute to the magnitude of bone adaptation. Frequency refers to the number of loading cycles per second. A positive relationship between loading frequency and cortical bone adaptation exists, with increasing loading frequency beyond a threshold of 0.5 Hz generating progressively greater adaptation (Hsieh and Turner, 2001; Turner et al., 1994a, 1995a; Warden and Turner, 2004).

SKELETAL ADAPTATION IS GREATEST WITH BRIEF YET OFTEN MECHANICAL LOADING

Further features influencing the skeletal adaptive response to loading include the duration of loading and length of rest between loading bouts. Extending the duration of loading does not necessarily yield proportional increases in bone mass (Rubin and Laynon, 1984; Umemura et al., 1997). As loading duration increases, the bone formation response tends to fade as the mechanosensitive cells accommodate to the prevailing environment. The decline in adaptation with ongoing loading cycles fits a logarithmic relationship such that after only 20 back-to-back loading cycles, bone has lost more than 95% of its mechanosensitivity (Turner and Robling, 2003). These observations indicate that loading programs do not need to be long to induce meaningful adaptation and, in addition, that bone cells need time to resensitize between loading bouts to be responsive to future loading bouts. The amount of rest time required between loading bouts depends on the nature of the loading stimulus. For instance, including a few seconds rest between consecutive loading cycles will result in greater bone adaptation than if the same strain stimulus is introduced with no rests in back-to-back cycles (Robling et al., 2001a; Srinivasan et al., 2002). Rests of a number of hours between consecutive loading bouts also result in greater bone adaptation than if the same strain stimulus is introduced in back-to-back bouts (Robling et al., 2000, 2002a, 2002b).

SKELETAL ADAPTATION IN RESPONSE TO MECHANICAL LOADING IS SITE SPECIFIC

As the response of bone to mechanical loading is highly stimulus specific, it follows that its adaptive response is also highly site specific. This site specficity has been confirmed in individuals

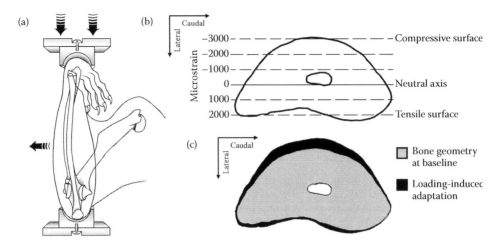

FIGURE 5.3   The adaptive response of bone to mechanical loading is site specific such that only those regions within a bone that experience sufficient microstrain will adapt. (a) Schematic diagram of the rodent ulna axial compression model. The distal forelimb is fixed between upper and lower cups. When force is applied to one of the cups, the ulna is caused to bow laterally. (b) The bending of the ulna under axial compression generates medial surface compression and lateral surface tension at the midshaft. There is no strain along the axis through which the bone is bending (neutral axis). (c) Loading of rat ulnas for 16 weeks using the axial compression model causes new bone to be formed on surfaces of high strain (medial and lateral surfaces). There is minimal new bone formation near the neutral axis (caudal and cranial surfaces) where there is the least microstrain during loading. (Data from Robling, A.G., et al., *J Bone Miner Res*, 17, 1545–54, 2002.)

playing sports that expose their dominant upper extremity to mechanical overload, with only the loaded bones undergoing adaptation (Figure 5.1) (Haapasalo et al., 1996; Huddleston et al., 1980; Jones et al., 1977; Warden et al., 2009). The site-specific nature of bone adaptation to mechanical loading can be localized further than the individual bone level. Long bones are curved such that they bend when axially loaded. Bending results in the exposure of different regions within the bone cross-section to different levels of microstrain. Only those regions within the bone that experience sufficient strain stimulus adapt, as clearly observed in the adaptive response to loading in the rodent ulna axial compression model (Figure 5.3).

IMPLICATIONS OF MECHANICAL LOADING FEATURES INFLUENCING SKELETAL ADAPTATION

Knowledge of the loading characteristics conducive to skeletal adaptation enables the development of appropriate interventions aimed at optimizing skeletal health (Turner and Robling, 2003; Warden et al., 2004). Specifically, exercises should introduce novel, high-magnitude, rapid strains at the specific sites and in the specific directions that adaptation is desired. Unfortunately, in humans, it is unknown what magnitude of external loading is required to induce a certain strain level or what range of strain magnitudes and rates result in adaptation at specific sites. Although these questions are easily examined in animal models, they are difficult to answer in humans due to difficulties in measuring bone strain in vivo. Laboratory-based studies have attached strain gauges to bone surfaces in humans to assess strains during various activities (Milgrom, 2001); however, measurements have only been performed in a small subgroup of the population and on localized sections of a few bones. It is important to appreciate that bone strains quantified at a specific skeletal location may not correspond to strains engendered at distant sites, in alternate bones, or in the wider population. Finite element models have been developed to model bone strains in response to given loads; however, these models remain in their infancy.

Despite limitations in assessing bone loading, activities with high magnitude and rapid loading are known to result in higher strain magnitudes and rates. For example, the limited strain gauge data available do show that activities such as jumping and running result in greater bone strain magnitudes and rates than those of lower load and slower loading rate activities such as walking (Milgrom, 2001). Based on clinical and randomized control trial data, it is known that individuals involved in high and rapid load activities (i.e., jumping and running) exhibit greater lower extremity bone adaptation than that of individuals who are not (Guadalupe-Grau et al., 2009). Thus, exercises involving high magnitude and rapid loads are more conducive of skeletal adaptation.

Exercises may include endurance activities, such as distance running; however, given the desensitization of the skeleton to prolonged loading and preference of the skeleton for novel short-duration loading, activities should also include jumping and landing activities and rapid changes in direction, such as occur during basketball, volleyball, soccer, and gymnastics. These activities expose the skeleton to short-duration, high-magnitude, rapid loading in multiple novel directions, and all have been associated with significant skeletal adaptation (Nichols et al., 2007).

SKELETAL BENEFITS OF EXERCISE DURING GROWTH

GROWTH PRESENTS A "WINDOW OF OPPORTUNITY"

Growth is an opportune time to take advantage of the skeletal benefits of exercise due to the highly plastic skeletal state presented. Growth is primarily characterized by bone modeling, which involves spatially independent osteoblast-mediated bone formation and osteoclast-mediated bone resorption. These processes function to add or remove bone tissue on previously quiescent bone surfaces to effectively alter bone quantity and structure. Exercise during this period primarily influences the skeleton by stimulating de novo bone formation. Mechanical signals are transmitted to the bone surface via osteocyte signaling whereby they stimulate the differentiation of precursor cells into osteoblasts to transform the periosteal cellular layer from a quiescent to an osteogenic cell layer. As a result, periosteal mineral apposition increases, with formation rates rising largely due to alterations in the amount of bone surface undergoing formation.

Observational and longitudinal cohort studies have demonstrated that children and adolescents who lead more physically active lifestyles typically have 10%–15% greater bone mass than that of their peers (Bailey et al., 1999; Janz et al., 2006; Tobias et al., 2007). These data are supported by prospective randomized controlled trials that have demonstrated that weight-bearing exercise in children and adolescents increases bone mass at loaded sites (lower extremities and spine) by up to 5% in <2 years (Hind and Burrows, 2007). The skeletal advantage of exercising during growth has also been eloquently shown in racquet sport players who began training during prepuberty and early puberty. Specifically, girls who began playing before puberty had more than twofold greater differences in bone mass between their playing and nonplaying arms, compared with those who began playing postpuberty (Figure 5.4) (Kannus et al., 1995). This bilateral difference has subsequently been confirmed by others (Bass et al., 2002; Ducher et al., 2009) and supports the presence of a "window of opportunity" during prepuberty and early puberty where the skeleton is most amenable to the influences of mechanical loading and exercise (MacKelvie et al., 2002).

EXERCISE DURING GROWTH OPTIMIZES PEAK BONE MASS

The skeleton appears most receptive to the benefits of exercise during growth; however, reduced bone strength and the concomitant increase in the risk for low-trauma fractures is predominantly an age-related phenomenon (Warden and Fuchs, 2009). This age-related disconnection raises the question as to whether exercise-induced bone changes during growth persist into adulthood when they would be most advantageous in reducing fracture risk (Warden et al., 2005a). The traditional doctrine is that exercise during growth adds extra mineral to maximize peak bone mass, with the

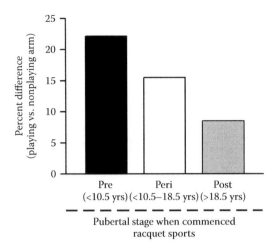

FIGURE 5.4 The growing skeleton is more responsive to mechanical loading than is the adult skeleton. This study of competitive female racquet sport players showed that those who started playing at an earlier age (several years before menarche [Pre]) had more than two times as much differential (playing vs. nonplaying arm) in mineral accrual than that of players who started playing during their adult years [Post]. (Data from Kannus, P., et al., *Ann Intern Med*, 123, 27–31, 1995.)

hypothesis being that the accrual of more bone mineral when young provides greater reserves against both the bone loss and compromised bone strength that develops during aging (Rizzoli et al., 2010). This hypothesis is logical considering that (1) approximately 95% of the adult skeleton is formed by the end of adolescence (Bailey et al., 1999; Bonjour et al., 1991); (2) approximately 25%–30% of the adult bone mineral is accrued during the 2–3 years around puberty (Bailey et al., 1999; Slemenda et al., 1994); (3) exercise enhances growth-related bone accrual and peak bone mass (Valimaki et al., 1994); (4) fracture risk during aging doubles for each standard deviation of bone lost from mean peak bone mass (Johnell et al., 2005); and (5) the onset of osteoporosis has been predicted to be delayed by 13 years, with a 10% increase in peak bone mass (Hernandez et al., 2003).

EXERCISE-INDUCED OPTIMIZATION OF PEAK BONE MASS IS NOT MAINTAINED LONG-TERM

Numerous studies have explored the sustainability of exercise-induced bone mass benefits acquired during growth. Follow-up assessments of former participants in randomized controlled trials have documented that cessation of an osteogenic exercise program is associated with short-term maintenance of exercise-induced bone mass benefits (Fuchs and Snow, 2002; Gunter et al., 2008; Kontulainen et al., 2002). However, these benefits do not appear to persist long-term. For instance, Gunter et al. (2008) demonstrated a jumping exercise intervention to increase bone mass by 3.6% in the exercise group compared with controls, but this difference declined by over 60% (to 1.4%) in the 7 years following intervention cessation (Figure 5.5a). The bone mass difference between groups remained statistically significant at 7 years, and the rate of loss of the intervention benefit appeared to decline over time; however, supplementary evidence provided by Karlsson et al. (2000) suggests that the bone mass benefit of exercise during growth ultimately disappears. These investigators demonstrated that exercise in the form of soccer playing conferred high peak bone mass, but its cessation resulted in accelerated bone loss during nonplaying aging (Figure 5.5b).

CONVENTIONAL IMAGING TECHNIQUES DO NOT ADEQUATELY DETERMINE SKELETAL BENEFITS OF EXERCISE

The loss of the bone mass benefits induced with exercise during growth suggests that the skeletal changes generated by exercise when young do not persist into adulthood when they may influence

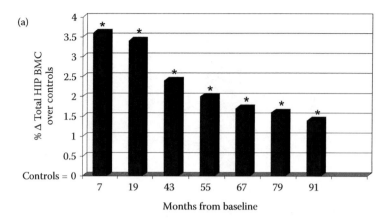

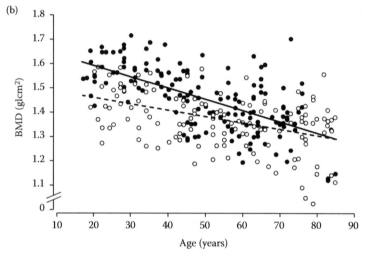

FIGURE 5.5 Exercise-induced optimization of bone quantity is not maintained long-term. (a) Jumping exercise intervention in growing children increased total hip bone mass by 3.6% in the exercise group compared with that in controls, but this difference declined to 1.4% in the 7 years following intervention cessation. (b) Former soccer players (closed circles) achieved a higher lower extremity peak bone mass but had more rapid loss of bone quantity with aging than controls (open circles). (*Panel (a)* Reproduced from Gunter, K., A.D. Baxter-Jones, R. L. Mirwald, et al. *J Bone Miner Res* 23:986–93, with permission from American Scciety of Bone and Mineral Research; *Panel (b)* Reprinted from *The Lancet*, 355, Karlsson, M.K., et al. Exercise during growth and bone mineral density and fractures in old age, 469–70, 2000, with permission from Elsevier.)

osteoporotic fracture risk. However, this conclusion is based on studies that used dual-energy x-ray absorptiometry (DXA) to assess the sustainability of the skeletal benefits of exercise. DXA is the gold standard in the clinical assessment of bone health and provides a picture of overall bone status, but it has limitations in assessing bone strength and fracture risk. Considerable overlap in DXA-derived measures has been found between people who fracture and those who do not (Stone et al., 2003). Also, DXA-derived measures only explain a fraction of the observed reduction in the risk for fracture associated with osteoporosis drug therapies (Cummings et al., 2002).

A prominent reason for the limited usefulness of DXA scans is that bone strength, and the consequent risk for fracture, is dependent upon not only bone quantity but also bone structure. DXA does not provide an adequate measure of bone structure as it is a planar measurement and has low spatial resolution. These features allow DXA to provide a two-dimensional areal analysis of bone; however, this areal analysis can lead to size-related artifacts when compared with a true three-dimensional

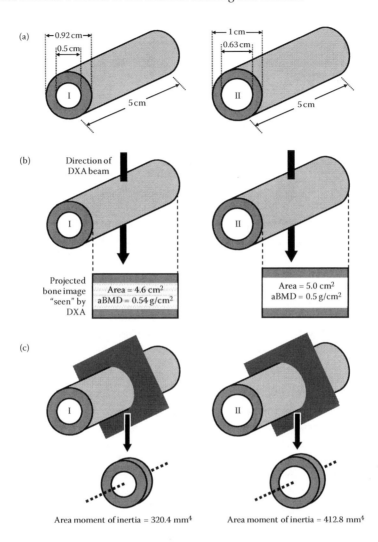

FIGURE 5.6 Schematic illustration of the limitation of dual-energy x-ray absorptiometry (DXA) measures of bone and the influence of structural properties on bone strength. (a) The two bones (I and II) have the same bone mineral content (BMC = 2.5 g), volumetric bone mineral density (BMD = 1063 mg/cm³), and cortical area (0.47 cm²). The only difference between the bones is the distribution of the bone material from the middle of the bone, with the material of bone II being more distant. (b) DXA assessment of the two bones would indicate that the bones have equivalent BMC (2.5 g) and that bone I has a higher areal BMD (aBMD). This results from the fact that bone I has a smaller projected bone area on DXA and DXA-derived BMD is derived as BMC divided by projected bone area. Thus, it may be concluded following assessment of these two bones using DXA that they have equivalent strength (because of their equivalent BMC) or that bone I is stronger (because of its greater aBMD). (c) Bone II is structurally bigger than bone I, as evident by its greater periosteal circumference (3.14 cm vs. 2.89 cm) and total cross-sectional area (0.78 cm² vs. 0.66 cm²). Despite both bones having the same cortical bone cross-sectional area and BMC, the bone material in II is distributed further from the neutral axis than in I, as evident by its greater area moment of inertia (412.8 mm⁴ vs. 320.4 mm⁴). This results in bone II possessing 29% greater resistance to bending than that of bone I purely because of a difference in its structure rather than material properties.

analysis (Figure 5.6). As DXA does not adequately assess bone structure, it is particularly limited when assessing bone changes, or their maintenance, induced by mechanical loading. Mechanical loading associated with exercise predominantly influences bone structure rather than mass as the way of improving bone strength.

EXERCISE DURING GROWTH ENCOURAGES STRUCTURAL OPTIMIZATION

Exercise during growth adds extra material to loaded sites to effectively increase the quantity of bone present; however, mechanical loading associated with exercise generates disproportionate increases in bone strength. For instance, it has been demonstrated in animal models that very small (<10%) changes in bone mass generated via mechanical loading result in very large (>60%) increases in skeletal mechanical properties (Robling et al., 2002a; Warden et al., 2005b). These gains result from the site-specific deposition of new bone tissue to regions where mechanical demands are greatest.

The net result of site-specific deposition of new bone is structural optimization of the skeleton whereby bone material is distributed in such a way that it is better positioned to resist external loads. Typically, this relocation involves new bone being laid down as far as possible from the respective axis of bending or rotation, as observed in clinical trials whereby exercise during growth, especially before puberty, caused new bone to be preferentially laid down on the periosteal (outer) surface of loaded bones (Bass et al., 2002; Ducher et al., 2009; Kontulainen et al., 2003). Such site-specific accrual of new bone is functionally important as it increases bone mass and bone strength where they are needed most while not excessively increasing the overall mass (quantity) of the skeleton.

EXERCISE-INDUCED STRUCTURAL OPTIMIZATION MAY LAST LIFELONG

Exercise-induced gains in bone mass appear to decline following exercise cessation; however, mechanisms exist for exercise-induced structural benefits to remain intact until senescence where they may have antifracture benefits. Age-related loss of bone quantity is principally mediated by endocortical and not periosteal surface changes (Figure 5.7a) (Ahlborg et al., 2003). During aging, progressive periosteal bone apposition occurs, but this circumferential gain is unable to sustain bone quantity because of the more rapid loss of endosteal bone, particularly during the menopausal transition. The net result is progressive structural decay and skeletal weakening during aging. As exercise during growth primarily induces periosteal adaptation and aging is not associated with loss of bone from the periosteal surface, the enhanced structure induced by exercise during growth may remain intact and have antifracture properties later in life (Figure 5.7b).

The hypothesis for sustainability of the skeletal benefits of exercise is supported by an animal study which found that mechanical-loading-induced changes in bone structure and strength, but not quantity, persist lifelong following the cessation of the loading during growth (Warden et al., 2007). Further support is provided by clinical evidence demonstrating that former athletes >60 year of age have lower risk of fragility fractures than that of matched controls (Nordstrom et al., 2005). These data indicate that loading during growth can have antifracture benefits through induced structural changes, independent of any lasting effects on bone quantity.

CONTRIBUTION OF NUTRITION TO MECHANICALLY INDUCED SKELETAL ADAPTATION DURING GROWTH

Nutrition is a key factor for skeletal development and determines whether the necessary building blocks are available for optimal growth. Thus, it is logical to hypothesize that the anabolic response of the skeleton to mechanical loading depends on the availability of essential nutrients. A number of randomized controlled trials in children have confirmed this by demonstrating significant interactions between calcium intake and the skeletal response to exercise (Bass et al., 2007; Specker and Binkley, 2003). In these studies, exercise and calcium supplementation introduced in isolation did

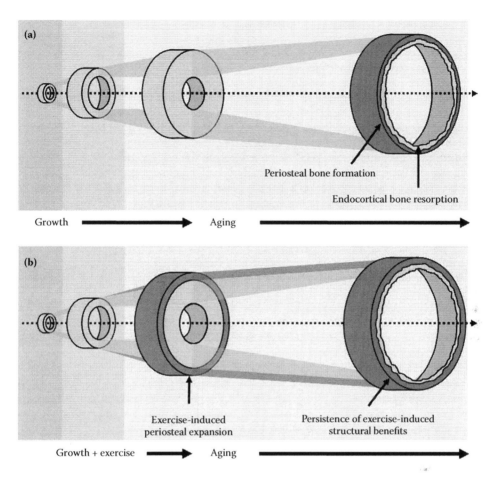

FIGURE 5.7 Bone structural changes associated with aging and exercise. (a) Bone loss during aging occurs primarily via bone resorption on the endocortical surface. There is concomitant bone formation on the periosteal surface, which helps to maintain bone structure, but this is insufficient to maintain bone mass. (b) Exercise during growth facilitates periosteal bone formation, which optimizes bone structure. As bone loss during aging occurs from the inside out, the enhanced structure induced by exercise during growth has the potential to remain intact irrespective of age-related changes in bone mass. (Reproduced from Warden, S.J., and Fuchs, R.K. *Br J Sports Med* 43:885–7, 2009, with permission from BMJ Publishing Group Ltd.)

not influence the skeleton, but when introduced simultaneously, the interventions generated significant skeletal benefits. The bone adaptation suggests that calcium intake needs to be higher than minimally required for growth for the skeletal benefits of exercise to be permitted. The importance of optimal nutrition was confirmed by way of meta-analysis, which concluded that exercise only had a beneficial skeletal effect in the presence of high calcium intakes (>1000 mg/day) (Specker, 1996).

The adequacy of dietary calcium intake has been most extensively studied in terms of the permissive role of nutrition on the skeletal effects of exercise; however, the availability of other nutrients may also play a significant role. In particular, sufficient intake of protein has been linked with the skeletal effects of exercise. The relationship between adequate protein and bone has been shown to be independent of energy intake and calcium intake. Chevalley et al. (2008) demonstrated that protein intake higher than the usual recommended dietary allowance enhanced the positive skeletal effects of exercise before the onset of pubertal maturation. The mechanism for this permissive effect of protein is not clear but may relate to insulin-like growth factor, which is crucial for both muscle and bone tissue development.

EFFECTS OF EXERCISE ON THE AGING SKELETON

Focus Shifts to Maintaining Bone Health and
Protecting Skeleton from Excessive Load

While exercise is best understood in terms of its anabolic effects on bone modeling during growth, it also has a significant role in the mature skeleton. The primary tissue-level process taking place in the mature skeleton is bone remodeling. Remodeling involves the temporally and spatially coordinated actions of osteoclasts and osteoblasts who work in teams to remove and replace discrete, measurable "packets" of bone. During aging, a negative bone balance exists such that more bone is resorbed than is replaced by each team of cells. The result is a progressive net loss of bone mineral and the potential development of osteoporosis. Exercise during aging may limit the loss by reducing the amount of bone resorbed or increasing the amount of bone formed by each team of cells. However, the anabolic effect of exercise during remodeling appears negligible relative to its effects on bone formation during modeling. The limited gain in bone during adulthood has been demonstrated in animal studies which show that the adult skeleton has a lesser anabolic response to mechanical loading than the growing skeleton (Turner et al., 1995b). Instead, exercise during aging appears to exert its primary skeletal effects by reducing bone resorption. The suppression of bone resorption is most clearly evident when exercise levels fall below customary levels, such as during disuse where accelerated remodeling mainly on endosteal and trabecular surfaces contributes to a 0.5%–1% loss of bone mass per month (Pavy-Le Traon et al., 2007).

The ability to perform highly osteogenic exercises (i.e., dynamic, high-impact loading) is limited in adults due to these types of loads being associated with a risk for osteoarthritis, bone microdamage, and stress fractures. Consequently, exercise of the adult skeleton typically involves activities with low- or moderate-impact loads, such as walking, running, aerobic exercise, resistance training, and stair climbing. The introduction of low- or moderate-impact loads to the adult skeleton has been met with variable success in modifying bone mass, with maximal increases being around 2%–3%; however, systematic review and meta-analysis of randomized controlled trial evidence have confirmed that low- or moderate-impact loads are effective in reducing age-related bone loss (Bérard et al., 1997; Bonaiuti et al., 2002; Wallace and Cumming, 2000; Wolff et al., 1999). Likewise, maintaining a consistent loading regimen preserves exercise-induced bone mass changes in animals (Shimamura et al., 2002; Wu et al., 2004) and humans (Heinonen et al., 1999) and offsets the loss of bone associated with aging in humans (Martyn-St James and Carroll, 2009). Thus, exercise in the adult skeleton should be encouraged as a means of preventing bone loss and maintaining bone health.

In addition to maintaining bone health, overwhelming evidence exists that continued exercise throughout life has significant, bone-mass-independent, antifracture benefits. Reports have consistently shown that persons with a current or previous history of low activity levels have a higher incidence of hip fractures than that of persons with a higher activity level. In the Study of Osteoporotic Fractures trial, which longitudinally followed 9,704 women aged 65 years or older for 4 years, there was a 30% reduction in hip fracture risk associated with frequent walking (Cummings et al., 1995). Likewise, in a separate study, walking for at least 4 hours/week among women who did no other exercise was associated with a 41% lower risk of hip fracture compared with that of women who walked for less than 1 hour/week (Feskanich et al., 2002). The reason for the beneficial antifracture effects of exercise on the older skeleton despite its somewhat limited ability to produce significant changes in bone mass may relate to the multifactorial cause of bone fractures. Although low bone mass has been established as an important predictor of fracture risk, the results of many studies indicate that clinical risk factors related to risk of fall also serve as important predictors of fractures (Cummings et al., 1995; Geusens et al., 2002). Only 5%–10% of falls result in fracture; however, 95% of hip fractures result from falls. By way of its beneficial effects on muscle strength, balance, and proprioception, exercise may reduce the risk for falling and, consequently, the risk for fracture by protecting the aging skeleton from excessive loads.

EXERCISE MAY AUGMENT SKELETAL BENEFITS OF PHARMACEUTICAL AGENTS FOR OSTEOPOROSIS

Exercise may be used as an adjunct to pharmaceutical agents for preventing and/or treating osteoporosis. This hypothesis stems from preliminary evidence suggesting that exercise combined with either antiresorptive or anabolic pharmaceutical agents produces additive or even synergistic benefits to bone health. Animal studies using ovariectomized rats investigated whether the reduced endosteal and trabecular bone resorption associated with the use of antiresorptive agents combined with the enhanced periosteal bone formation associated with exercise enhanced bone health more than the introduction of either modality alone did (Fuchs et al., 2007; Tamaki et al., 1998). Tamaki et al. (1998) found etidronate and treadmill running to have independent beneficial effects on midshaft and distal femoral bone mineral density (BMD), whereas Fuchs et al. (2007) found independent beneficial effects for alendronate and treadmill running on midshaft femur mechanical properties. These findings indicate that, at a minimum, bisphosphonates and exercise may have additive beneficial effects. However, both studies also found statistical interactions between the modalities for some measures. These latter findings indicate that combined treadmill running and bisphosphonate therapy induced greater benefits than predicted by the summation of their observed individual effects. These results suggest some form of synergy between exercise and antiresorptive pharmaceutical agents wherein one of the interventions magnifies the effect of the other.

A number of clinical studies have explored the role of combined exercise and antiresorptive therapy on bone health (Fuchs and Warden, 2008). These studies provide some supportive, albeit inconclusive, evidence for synergistic or at least additive effects between the two modalities. Primarily, Braith et al. (2003, 2007) investigated the combined effects of alendronate and resistance training on glucocorticoid-induced osteoporosis following lung or heart transplant in two separate studies. In both studies, participants treated with combination therapy had superior improvements in BMD than those of people treated with alendronate alone. Although these data suggest an additive or even synergistic beneficial effect of combination therapy, this conclusion could not be substantiated as an exercise-alone treated group was not investigated. Chilibeck et al. (2002) and Uusi-Rasi et al. (2003) addressed this limitation by performing randomized controlled trials designed to elicit both the additive and interactive effects of exercise and antiresorptive therapies on bone health in postmenopausal women. Neither study was able to find additive or interactive effects between the treatments for any skeletal measure; however, the resistance exercise program implemented by Chilibeck et al. (2002) was unable to elicit an independent effect, indicating that it may have been inadequately osteogenic, whereas Uusi-Rasi et al. (2003) observed antiresorptive therapy to increase distal tibial bone mass and jumping exercise to increase distal tibial polar section modulus, suggesting that the two interventions had additive effects in optimizing bone health.

While preliminary clinical evidence supporting the combined introduction of exercise and antiresorptive agents for optimizing bone health during aging has been reported, no such evidence currently exists for the combined introduction of exercise and anabolic pharmaceutical agents. However, a number of preclinical cell- and animal-based studies have yielded interesting observations when exploring the combined effects of mechanical loading and parathyroid hormone (PTH) therapy. As both mechanical loading and PTH primarily target bone-forming osteoblasts, their simultaneous introduction may allow one modality to enhance the response of osteoblasts to the effects of the other modality. Such synergy appears to be present with PTH sensitizing the osteogenic response of osteoblasts to mechanical loading, possibly by enhancing the mobilization of intracellular calcium (Ryder and Duncan, 2001). When PTH was introduced prior to or at the commencement of mechanical loading in animal-based studies, synergy between the two modalities occurred such that their individual osteogenic effects were magnified (Kim et al., 2003; Li et al., 2003). These synergistic effects indicate a need for clinical studies investigating the combined effects of PTH and exercise. In designing these studies, a priori consideration needs to be given to the timing of the interventions. PTH has a short half-life (75 minutes) and reaches maximal serum concentrations within 15–45 minutes following subcutaneous injection (Lindsay et al., 1993). Exercise should be performed during this period immediately following PTH administration to optimize any synergistic effects between the treatments. Such timing is not as critical when exploiting synergy between bisphosphonates and exercise due to the prolonged skeletal half-life of the former (Khan et al., 1997; Mitchell et al., 1999).

SUMMARY

Mechanical loading of the skeleton by way of exercise is an important intervention for the reduction in bone strength and consequent increase in the risk for low-trauma fractures associated with aging. Early in life, especially around puberty, exercise should be promoted to develop a skeleton with the most ideal structural design. The hope is that this design persists long-term to have antifracture benefits later in life. Exercises early in life that may facilitate structural optimization of the skeleton include impact activities introducing high magnitude loads at rapid rates in multiple directions, such as those experienced during participation in basketball and gymnastics. As nutrition is permissive of the skeletal effects of exercise, adequate availability of essential nutrients is necessary to enable structural optimization to occur.

The objective of exercise during aging shifts towards preserving bone quantity so as to enter late adulthood with maximal bone stock and protecting the skeleton during late adulthood from excessive loads. Exercises during these phases may include low- or moderate-impact loads, such as walking, running, aerobic exercise, resistance training, and stair climbing. Consideration when prescribing these exercises during aging should be given to their coupling with pharmaceutical agents for preventing and/or treating osteoporosis. By appropriately timing exercise following drug administration, bone health may be optimized above that associated with either intervention in isolation.

ACKNOWLEDGMENTS

This contribution was made possible by support from the National Institutes of Health (R01 AR057740 and R15 AR056858 [S.J.W.]; K01 AR054408 [R.K.F.])

REFERENCES

Ahlborg, H.G., Johnell, O., Turner, C.H., et al. 2003. Bone loss and bone size after menopause. *New Engl J Med* 349:327–34.

Bailey, D.A., McKay, H.A., Mirwald, R.L., et al. 1999. A six-year longitudinal study of the relationship of physical activity to bone mineral accrual in growing children: The university of Saskatchewan bone mineral accrual study. *J Bone Miner Res* 14:1672–9.

Bass, S.L., Naughton, G., Saxon L., et al. 2007. Exercise and calcium combined results in a greater osteogenic effect than either factor alone: A blinded randomized placebo-controlled trial in boys. *J Bone Miner Res* 22:458–64.

Bass, S.L., Saxon, L., Daly, R.M., et al. 2002. The effect of mechanical loading on the size and shape of bone in pre-, peri-, and postpubertal girls: A study in tennis players. *J Bone Miner Res* 17:2274–80.

Bérard, A., Bravo, G., and Gauthier, P. 1997. Meta-analysis of the effectiveness of physical activity for the prevention of bone loss in postmenopausal women. *Osteoporos Int* 7:331–7.

Bonaiuti, D., Shea, B., Iovine R., et al. 2002. Exercise for preventing and treating osteoporosis in postmenopausal women. *Cochrane Database Syst Rev*:CD000333.

Bonjour, J.P., Theintz, G., Buchs, B., et al. 1991. Critical years and stages of puberty for spinal and femoral bone mass accumulation during adolescence. *J Clin Endocrinol Metab* 73:555–63.

Braith, R.W., Conner, J.A., Fulton, M.N., et al. 2007. Comparison of alendronate vs alendronate plus mechanical loading as prophylaxis for osteoporosis in lung transplant recipients: A pilot study. *J Heart Lung Transplant* 26:132–7.

Braith, R.W., Magyari, P.M., Fulton, M.N., et al. 2003. Resistance exercise training and alendronate reverse glu-cocorticoid-induced osteoporosis in heart transplant recipients. *J Heart Lung Transplant* 22:1082–90.

Burr, D.B., Milgrom, C., Fyhrie, D., et al. 1996. In vivo measurement of human tibial strains during vigourous activity. *Bone* 18:405–10.

Chevalley, T., Bonjour, J.P., Ferrari, S., et al. 2008. High-protein intake enhances the positive impact of physical activity on BMC in prepubertal boys. *J Bone Miner Res* 23:131–42.

Chilibeck, P.D., Davison, K.S., Whiting, S.J., et al. 2002. The effect of strength training combined with bispho-sphonate (etidronate) therapy on bone mineral, lean tissue, and fat mass in postmenopausal women. *Can J Physiol Pharmacol* 80:941–50.

Cummings, S.R., Karpf, D.B., Harris, F., et al. 2002. Improvement in spine bone density and reduction in risk of vertebral fractures during treatment with antiresorptive drugs. *Am J Med* 112:281–9.

Cummings, S.R., Nevitt, M.C., Browner, W.S., et al. 1995. Risk factors for hip fractures in white women. *N Engl J Med* 332:767–73.

Ducher, G., Daly, R., and Bass, S. 2009. The effects of repetitive loading on bone mass and geometry in young male tennis players: A quantitative study using magnetic resonance imaging. *J Bone Miner Res* 24:1686–92.

Feskanich, D., Willett, W., and Colditz, G. 2002. Walking and leisure-time activity and risk of hip fracture in postmenopausal women. *JAMA* 288:2300–6.

Frost, H.M. 1987. Bone "mass" and the "mechanostat": A proposal. *Anat Rec* 219:1–9.

Frost, H.M. 1990. Skeletal structural adaptations to mechanical usage (SATMU): 2. Redefining Wolff's law: The bone remodeling problem. *Anat Rec* 226:414–22.

Fuchs, R.K., Shea, M., Durski, S.L., et al. 2007. Individual and combined effects of exercise and alendronate on bone mass and strength in ovariectomized rats. *Bone* 41:290–6.

Fuchs, R.K., and Snow, C.M.. 2002. Gains in hip bone mass from high-impact training are maintained: A ran-domized controlled trial in children. *J Pediatr* 141:357–62.

Fuchs, R.K., and Warden, S.J. 2008. Combination therapy using exercise and pharmaceutical agents to opti-mize bone health. *Clinic Rev Bone Miner Metab* 6:37–45.

Geusens, P., Autier, P., Boonen, S., et al. 2002. The relationship among history of falls, osteoporosis, and frac-tures in postmenopausal women. *Arch Phys Med Rehabil* 83:903–6.

Guadalupe-Grau, A., Fuentes, T., Guerra, B., et al. 2009. Exercise and bone mass in adults. *Sports Med* 39:439–68.

Gunter, K., A. D. Baxter-Jones, R. L. Mirwald, et al. 2008. Impact exercise increases BMC during growth: An 8-year longitudinal study. *J Bone Miner Res* 23:986–93.

Haapasalo, H., Sievänen, H., Kannus, P., et al. 1996. Dimensions and estimated mechanical characteristics of the humerus after long-term tennis loading. *J Bone Miner Res* 11:864–72.

Heinonen, A., Kannus, P., Sievanen, H., et al. 1999. Good maintenance of high-impact activity-induced bone gain by voluntary, unsupervised exercises: An 8-month follow-up of a randomized controlled trial. *J Bone Miner Res* 14:125–8.

Hernandez, C.J., Beaupre, G.S., and Carter, D.R. 2003. A theoretical analysis of the relative influences of peak BMD, age-related bone loss and menopause on the development of osteoporosis. *Osteoporos Int* 14:843–7.

Hind, K., and Burrows, M. 2007. Weight-bearing exercise and bone mineral accrual in children and adoles-cents: A review of controlled trials. *Bone* 40:14–27.

Hsieh, Y.F., and Turner, C.H. 2001. Effects of loading frequency on mechanically induced bone formation. *J Bone Miner Res* 16:918–24.

Huddleston, A. L., Rockwell, D., Kulund, D.N., et al. 1980. Bone mass in lifetime tennis athletes. *JAMA* 244:1107–9.

Iuliano-Burns, S., Stone, J., Hopper, J.L., et al. 2005. Diet and exercise during growth have site-specific skeletal effects: A co-twin control study. *Osteoporos Int* 16:1225–32.

Janz, K.F., Gilmore, J.M., Burns, T.L., et al. 2006. Physical activity augments bone mineral accrual in young children: The Iowa Bone Development study. *J Pediatr* 148:793–9.

Johnell, O., Kanis, J.A., Oden, A., et al. 2005. Predictive value of BMD for hip and other fractures. *J Bone Miner Res* 20:1185–94.

Jones, H., Priest, J., Hayes, W., et al. 1977. Humeral hypertrophy in response to exercise. *J Bone Joint Surg Am* 59:204–7.

Kannus, P., Haapasalo, H., Sankelo, M., et al. 1995. Effect of starting age of physical activity on bone mass in the dominant arm of tennis and squash players. *Ann Intern Med* 123:27–31.

Karlsson, M.K., Linden, C., Karlsson, C., et al. 2000. Exercise during growth and bone mineral density and fractures in old age. *Lancet* 355:469–70.

Khan, S.A., Kanis, J.A., Vasikaran, S., et al. 1997. Elimination and biochemical responses to intravenous alendronate in postmenopausal osteoporosis. *J Bone Miner Res* 12:1700–7.

Kim, C.H., Takai, E., Zhou, H., et al. 2003. Trabecular bone response to mechanical and parathyroid hormone stimulation: The role of mechanical microenvironment. *J Bone Miner Res* 18:2116–25.

Kontulainen, S.A., Kannus, P.A., Pasanen, M.E., et al. 2002. Does previous participation in high-impact training result in residual bone gain in growing girls? One year follow-up of a 9-month jumping intervention. *Int J Sports Med* 23:575–81.

Kontulainen, S., Sievanen, H., Kannus, P., et al. 2003. Effect of long-term impact-loading on mass, size, and estimated strength of humerus and radius of female racquet-sports players: A peripheral quantitative computed tomography study between young and old starters and controls. *J Bone Miner Res* 18:352–9.

Lanyon, L.E. 1992. Control of bone architecture by functional load bearing. *J Bone Miner Res* 7(Suppl. 2):S369–S375.

Lanyon, L.E., and Rubin, C.T. 1984. Static vs dynamic loads as an influence on bone remodelling. *J Biomech* 17:897–905.

Li, J., Duncan, R.L., Burr, D.B., et al. 2003. Parathyroid hormone enhances mechanically induced bone formation, possibly involving L-type voltage-sensitive calcium channels. *Endocrinology* 144:1226–33.

Lindsay, R., Nieves, J., Henneman, J., et al. 1993. Subcutaneous administration of the amino-terminal fragment of human parathyroid hormone-(1–34): Kinetics and biochemical response in estrogenized osteoporotic patients. *J Clin Endocrinol Metab* 77:1535–9.

MacInnis, R.J., C. Cassar, C. A. Nowson, et al. 2003. Determinants of bone density in 30- to 65-year-old women: A co-twin study. *J Bone Miner Res* 18:1650–6.

MacKelvie, K.J., K. M. Khan, and H. A. McKay. 2002. Is there a critical period for bone response to weight-bearing exercise in children and adolescents? A systematic review. *Br J Sports Med* 36:250–7.

Martin, R.B. 2000. Toward a unifying theory of bone remodelling. *Bone* 26:1–6.

Martyn-St James, M., and Carroll, S. 2009. A meta-analysis of impact exercise on postmenopausal bone loss: The case for mixed loading exercise programmes. *Br J Sports Med* 43:898–908.

Milgrom, C. 2001. The role of strain and strain rates in stress fractures. In *Musculoskeletal Fatigue and Stress Fractures*, edited by D. B. Burr and C. Milgrom, 119–29. Bota Raton, Florida: CRC Press.

Mitchell, D.Y., Heise, M.A., Pallone, K.A., et al. 1999. The effect of dosing regimen on the pharmacokinetics of risedronate. *Br J Clin Pharmacol* 48:536–42.

Mosley, J.R., and Lanyon, L.E. 1998. Strain rate as a controlling influence on adaptive modeling in response to dynamic loading of the ulna in growing male rats. *Bone* 23:313–8.

Nichols, D.L., Sanborn, C.F., and Essery, E.V. 2007. Bone density and young athletic women. An update. *Sports Med* 37:1001–14.

Nordstrom, A., Karlsson, C., Nyquist, F., et al. 2005. Bone loss and fracture risk after reduced physical activity. *J Bone Miner Res* 20:202–7.

Pavy-Le Traon, A., Heer, M., Narici, M.V., et al. 2007. From space to Earth: Advances in human physiology from 20 years of bed rest studies (1986–2006). *Eur J Appl Physiol* 101:143–94.

Peacock, M., Turner, C.H., Econs, M.J., et al. 2002. Genetics of osteoporosis. *Endocr Rev* 23:303–26.

Pearson, O.M., and Lieberman, D.E. 2004. The aging of Wolff's "law": Ontogeny and responses to mechanical loading in cortical bone. *Am J Phys Anthropol* Suppl 39:63–99.

Rizzoli, R., Bianchi, M.L., Garabedian, M., et al. 2010. Maximizing bone mineral mass gain during growth for the prevention of fractures in the adolescents and the elderly. *Bone* 46:294–305.

Robling, A.G., Burr, D.B., and Turner, C.H. 2000. Partitioning a daily mechanical stimulus into discrete loading bouts improves the osteogenic response to loading. *J Bone Miner Res* 15:1596–1602.

Robling, A.G., Burr, D.B., and Turner, C.H.. 2001a. Recovery periods restore mechanosensitivity to dynamically loaded bone. *J Exp Biol* 204:3389–99.

Robling, A.G., Duijvelaar, K.M., Geevers, J.V., et al. 2001b. Modulation of appositional and longitudinal bone growth in the rat ulna by applied static and dynamic force. *Bone* 29:105–13.

Robling, A.G., Hinant, F.M., Burr, D.B., et al. 2002a. Improved bone structure and strength after long-term mechanical loading is greatest if loading is separated into short bouts. *J Bone Miner Res* 17:1545–54.

Robling, A.G., Hinant, F.M., Burr, D.B., et al. 2002b. Shorter, more frequent mechanical loading sessions enhance bone mass. *Med Sci Sports Exerc* 34:196–202.

Robling, A.G., and Turner, C.H. 2002. Mechanotransduction in bone: Genetic effects on mechanosensitivity in mice. *Bone* 31:562–9.

Robling, A.G., Warden, S.J., Shultz, K.L., et al. 2007. Genetic effects on bone mechanotransduction in congenic mice harboring bone size and strength quantitative trait loci. *J Bone Miner Res* 22:984–91.

Rubin, C.T., and Laynon, L.E. 1984. Regulation of bone formation by applied dynamic loads. *J Bone Joint Surg Am* 66:397–402.

Rubin, C.T., and Lanyon, L.E. 1985. Regulation of bone mass by mechanical strain magnitude. *Calcif Tissue Int* 37:411–7.

Ryder, K.D., and Duncan, R.L. 2001. Parathyroid hormone enhances fluid shear-induced [Ca2+]i signaling in osteoblastic cells through activation of mechanosensitive and voltage-sensitive Ca2+ channels. *J Bone Miner Res* 16:240–8.

Schriefer, J.L., Warden, S.L., Saxon, L.K., et al. 2005. Cellular accomodation and the response of bone to mechanical loading. *J Biomech* 38:1838–45.

Shimamura, C., Iwamoto, J., Takeda, T., et al. 2002. Effect of decreased physical activity on bone mass in exercise-trained young rats. *J Orthop Sci* 7:358–63.

Slemenda, C.W., Reister, T.K., Hui, S.L., et al. 1994. Influences on skeletal mineralization in children and adolescents: Evidence for varying effects of sexual maturation and physical activity. *J Pediatr* 125:201–7.

Specker, B., and Binkley, T. 2003. Randomized trial of physical activity and calcium supplementation on bone mineral content in 3- to 5-year-old children. *J Bone Miner Res* 18:885–92.

Specker, B.L. 1996. Evidence for an interaction between calcium intake and physical activity on changes in bone mineral density. *J Bone Miner Res* 11:1539–44.

Srinivasan, S., Weimer, D.A., Agans, S.C., et al. 2002. Low-magnitude mechanical loading becomes osteogenic when rest is inserted between each load cycle. *J Bone Miner Res* 17:1613–20.

Stone, K.L., Seeley, D.G., Lui, L.Y., et al. 2003. BMD at multiple sites and risk of fracture of multiple types: Long-term results from the Study of Osteoporotic Fractures. *J Bone Miner Res* 18:1947–54.

Tamaki, H., Akamine, T., Goshi, N., et al. 1998. Effects of exercise training and etidronate treatment on bone mineral density and trabecular bone in ovariectomized rats. *Bone* 23:147–53.

Tobias, J.H., Steer, C.D., Mattocks, C.G., et al. 2007. Habitual levels of physical activity influence bone mass in 11-year-old children from the United Kingdom: Findings from a large population-based cohort. *J Bone Miner Res* 22:101–9.

Turner, C.H. 1999. Toward a mathematical description of bone biology: The principal of cellular accommodation. *Calcif Tissue Int* 65:466–71.

Turner, C.H., Forwood, M.R., and Otter, M.W. 1994a. Mechanotransduction in bone: Do bone cells act as sensors of fluid flow? *FASEB J* 8:875–8.

Turner, C.H., Forwood, M.R., Rho, J.-Y., et al. 1994b. Mechanical loading thresholds for lamellar and woven bone formation. *J Bone Miner Res* 9:87–97.

Turner, C.H., Owan, I., and Takano, Y. 1995a. Mechanotransduction in bone: Role of strain rate. *Am J Physiol* 269:E438–42.

Turner, C.H., and Robling, A.G. 2003. Designing exercise regimens to increase bone strength. *Exerc Sport Sci Rev* 31:45–50.

Turner, C.H., Takano, Y., and Owan, I. 1995b. Aging changes mechanical loading thresholds for bone formation in rats. *J Bone Miner Res* 10:1544–9.

Umemura, Y., Ishiko, T., Yamauchi, T., M, et al. 1997. Five jumps per day increase bone mass and breaking force in rats. *J Bone Miner Res* 12:1480–5.

Uusi-Rasi, K., Kannus, P., Cheng, S., et al. 2003. Effect of alendronate and exercise on bone and physical performance of postmenopausal women: A randomized controlled trial. *Bone* 33:132–43.

Valimaki, M.J., Karkainen, M., Lamberg-Allardt, C., et al. 1994. Exercise, smoking and calcium intake during adolescence and early adulthood as determinants of peak bone mass. *BMJ* 309:230–5.

Wallace, B.A., and Cumming, R.G. 2000. Systematic review of randomized trials of the effect of exercise on bone mass in pre- and postmenopausal women. *Calcif Tissue Int* 67:10–8.

Warden, S.J., Bogenschutz, E.D., Smith, H.D., et al. 2009. Throwing induces substantial torsional adaptation within the midshaft humerus of male baseball players. *Bone* 45:931–41.

Warden, S.J., and Fuchs, R.K. 2009. Exercise and bone health: Optimising bone structure during growth is key, but all is not in vain during ageing. *Br J Sports Med* 43:885–7.

Warden, S.J., Fuchs, R.K., Castillo, A.B., et al. 2007. Exercise when young provides lifelong benefits to bone structure and strength. *J Bone Miner Res* 22:251–9.

Warden, S.J., Fuchs, R.K., Castillo, A.B., et al. 2005a. Does exercise during growth influence osteoporotic fracture risk later in life? *J Musculoskelet Neuronal Interact* 5:344–6.

Warden, S.J., Fuchs, R.K., and Turner, C.H. 2004. Steps for targeting exercise towards the skeleton to increase bone strength. *Eura Medicophys* 40:223–32.

Warden, S.J., Hurst, J.A., Sanders, M.S., et al. 2005b. Bone adaptation to a mechanical loading program significantly increases skeletal fatigue resistance. *J Bone Miner Res* 20:809–16.

Warden, S.J., and Turner, C.H. 2004. Mechanotransduction in cortical bone is most efficient at loading frequencies of 5–10 Hz. *Bone* 34:261–70.

Wolff, I., van Croonenberg, J.J., Kemper, H.C.G., et al. 1999. The effect of exercise training programs on bone mass: A meta-analysis of published controlled trials in pre- and postmenopausal wmoen. *Osteoporos Int* 9:1–12.

Wolff, J. 1892. *Das Gesetz der Transformation der Knochen*. Bei Hirschwald, Leipzig.

Wu, J., Wang, X.X., Higuchi, M., et al. 2004. High bone mass gained by exercise in the growing male mice is increased by subsequent reduced exercise. *J Appl Physiol* 97:806–10.

6 Hormone Actions in the Regulation of Calcium and Phosphorus Metabolism

David A. Ontjes

"The constancy of the internal environment is the condition for free and independent life."

**Claude Bernard, in
"Lectures on the Phenomena
of Life Common to Animals
and Plants" (1878)**

CONTENTS

BODY CALCIUM AND PHOSPHORUS: HOMEOSTASIS AND BALANCE

This chapter discusses the role of the endocrine system in regulating calcium homeostasis and calcium and phosphate balance. Hormones are the primary agents responsible for sustaining a number of essential conditions within our internal environment. These include plasma concentrations of glucose, amino acids, sodium, potassium, and not least, calcium ions.

In this chapter, calcium homeostasis refers to the processes by which a constant concentration of ionized calcium is maintained in the extracellular fluid. The distribution of calcium between bone and other body compartments is in a dynamic equilibrium and is closely regulated by several hormones, the most important of which are parathyroid hormone (PTH) and calcitriol. Calcium balance refers to the processes leading to the gain or loss of all calcium from the entire body pool. Because most of the calcium pool resides in bone, calcium balance is synonymous with the net gain or loss of mineralized bone over time. In the hierarchy of conditions essential for survival, a constant concentration of ionized calcium commonly takes precedence over maintenance of an optimal bone mass. Some of the circumstances in which bone mass is sacrificed to maintain calcium homeostasis are discussed later in this chapter.

NEED FOR CALCIUM HOMEOSTASIS

A constant concentration of ionized calcium in the extracellular fluid is essential for several vital processes including the stability and permeability of plasma membranes. Consequently, the normal concentration of ionized calcium measured in plasma is narrow, ranging from 1.12 to 1.23 mmol/L

(4.48 to 4.92 mg/dL). A reduction in the extracellular calcium concentration increases the permeability of cell membranes to sodium and increases the excitability of muscle and nerve tissues, causing nerve discharge and muscle contraction. The resulting clinical manifestation in humans with hypocalcemia is tetany. Extracellular calcium ions can bind to a G-protein-linked calcium-sensing receptor (CaSR) in parathyroid, renal epithelial, and other cells to control cellular function directly in these tissues. In addition to its role in the normal mineralization of bone matrix, extracellular calcium also activates numerous extracellular enzymes and clotting factors.

Intracellular calcium is sequestered within mitochondria, endoplasmic reticulum, or sarcoplasmic reticulum, where its release can be stimulated by the activation of a number of cell-surface receptors by several hormones and neurotransmitters. In cells, calcium ions act as a second messenger by interacting with a large number of key enzymes and other proteins governing muscle contraction, microtubule and microfilament assembly, and membrane permeability.

DISTRIBUTION OF BODY CALCIUM AND PHOSPHORUS

The body of an average adult contains approximately 1 kg of calcium, 99% of which is deposited in bone as hydroxyapatite. About 1% of the calcium in bone is rapidly exchangeable with that in the extracellular fluid. The remainder may be mobilized more slowly when conditions require. The overall distribution is shown in Table 6.1.

Approximately 85% of total body phosphorus resides in bone in the form of hydroxyapatite and 15% in soft tissues. In contrast to calcium, extraskeletal phosphorus is located primarily within cells where it may serve as a component of numerous complex organic molecules, such as nucleic acids and phospholipids, or in free ionic form as HPO_4^{2-} or $H_2PO_4^-$. The concentration of extracellular phosphate ions is influenced by many of the same hormones that regulate extracellular calcium ions. However, extracellular phosphorus concentration is much less tightly regulated than that of calcium, with normal concentrations ranging from 0.87 to 1.45 mmol/L (2.7 to 4.5 mg/dL).

ORGANS IMPORTANT IN REGULATING CALCIUM AND PHOSPHORUS BALANCE

Gastrointestinal Tract

Gastrointestinal Calcium Absorption

The gastrointestinal (GI) tract governs entry of both calcium and phosphorus into the body and plays an important role in overall calcium balance. Calcium is absorbed in its ionized form, mainly

---

TABLE 6.1
Distribution of Calcium in Body Tissues

In bone	1000 g (99%)
Non-labile hydroxyapatite	999 g
Labile skeletal calcium pool	1 g
In extracellular fluid	1 g (0.1%)
Plasma	0.2 g (48% ionized; 46% protein bound; 6% complexed)
In cells	1 g (0.1%)

Source: Bringhurst, F.R., and Leder, B.Z. 2006. Regulation of calcium and phosphate homeostasis. In *Textbook of Endocrinology*, DeGroot, L.J., and Jameson, J.L., eds., 5th ed., Chapter 74. Elsevier Saunders, Philadelphia.

in the duodenum and jejunum. Insoluble salts of calcium are not well absorbed. Absorption occurs by two processes, one that is active and saturable and a second that is passive and nonsaturable. The saturable process is mediated by calcium-binding proteins existing in the duodenum and upper jejunum. One of these binding proteins, known as TRPV6, exists in the highest concentration on the apical cell surface in intestinal endothelial cells (den Dekker et al., 2003). The expression of the TRPV6 gene is stimulated by $1,25(OH)_2D_3$ or calcitriol, acting through the vitamin D receptor. The TRPV6 protein appears to facilitate the movement of calcium ions through the apical brush border and across the endothelial cell membrane by formation of a selective calcium channel.

Once calcium has entered the intestinal endothelial cell, it must be transported through the cytoplasm and moved out of the cell into the extracellular compartment against an electrochemical gradient. Transport across the cytoplasm is carried out by a cytosolic protein known as calbindin D_{9K}. Once calcium ions reach the basolateral membrane, they dissociate from calbindin and are actively extruded out of the cell by high-affinity membrane Ca^{2+}-ATPases to diffuse into the extracellular fluid and enter the portal circulation (Bronner et al., 1986). The expression of the calbindin gene and the activity of membrane Ca^{2+}-ATPases are also governed by the vitamin D receptor in intestinal endothelial cells. Thus, calcitriol is the primary regulator of the active, saturable component of intestinal calcium transport (Bringhurst and Leder, 2006). This pathway accounts for most of the calcium transport occurring when calcium ion concentrations within the intestinal lumen are low. The efficiency of the active pathway can be regulated up or down, depending on the availability of dietary calcium and the prevailing need to maintain calcium homeostasis.

The jejunum and ileum also provide for a passive, nonsaturable movement of calcium across the intestinal lumen through paracellular channels (Karbach, 1992). This mechanism predominates in delivering calcium from the gut to the systemic circulation under conditions where the intraluminal concentration of calcium is high, as for example in subjects taking oral calcium supplements. Vitamin D may also play a role in enhancing this process as well, although the mechanism is unclear.

At the same time that absorption of calcium is occurring in the upper GI tract, there is a movement of calcium into the intestinal lumen in the form of bile and other digestive juices. These endogenous intestinal secretions normally contain 100 to 200 mg of calcium per day and are little affected by dietary or serum calcium. Net absorption represents the difference between active and passive calcium absorption and endogenous intestinal secretions.

The efficiency of calcium absorption can vary greatly from 5% to 70% under different conditions in the same individual. The relationships between dietary calcium intake and absorption are illustrated in Figure 6.1. Under conditions of dietary calcium restriction and with adequate supplies of vitamin D, active absorption is maximized. At higher calcium intakes, passive absorption plays an increasing role. As the calcium supply increases, the overall efficiency of calcium absorption decreases, whereas the total amount of calcium absorbed continues to increase, but at a slower rate. At dietary calcium intakes below approximately 200 mg/day, the obligatory excretion of calcium from endogenous intestinal secretions exceeds the absorption of calcium from the upper GI tract so that the gut actually becomes a source of net calcium loss.

Gastrointestinal Phosphorus Absorption

The average dietary intake of phosphorus is 800–900 mg/day, usually exceeding the minimum requirement of 400 mg/day. Normally, about 70% of dietary phosphorus is absorbed in the duodenum and proximal jejunum. In the jejunum, a saturable, active, sodium-dependent process is responsive to vitamin D and a nonsaturable process is thought to represent passive paracellular transport. The active process is mediated by a sodium phosphate transporter in the luminal brush border of intestinal epithelial cells. Calcitriol stimulates the active process by increasing the expression of the transporter. Thus, both calcium and phosphorus absorption are stimulated by calcitriol. In contrast to calcium absorption, however, the basal absorption of phosphate in the absence of vitamin D is much higher, suggesting that the passive paracellular mechanism plays a more dominant role (Cross et al., 1990).

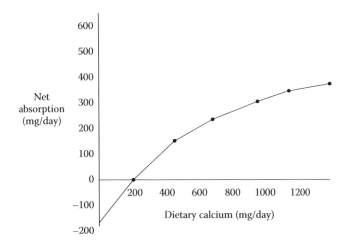

FIGURE 6.1 Model relationship of dietary calcium intake and net gastrointestinal absorption of calcium in a healthy young individual. Note that the efficiency of absorption declines as dietary calcium intake increases. At dietary calcium intakes of less than ~200 mg/day, net absorption becomes negative due to fecal loss of calcium from intestinal secretions.

Kidney

Renal Calcium Excretion

At normal rates of glomerular filtration, 7000 to 10,000 mg of ionized calcium is delivered to the proximal renal tubules each day, yet only 100–300 mg is ultimately excreted in the urine. Approximately 98% of the filtered calcium load is normally reabsorbed at various sites along the nephron. About 60% to 70% is absorbed in the proximal tubules, and another 20% to 25% is absorbed in the loop of Henle, mainly by passive paracellular diffusion. In contrast, the 8% to 10% absorbed in the distal tubule is hormonally controlled and involves transcellular transport mechanisms. Epithelial cells in the distal tubules possess transport proteins similar to those seen in the intestinal epithelium where calcium is also actively absorbed. These proteins include an epithelial calcium channel, TPRV5, which is closely homologous to TPRV6 in the gut, a calcium-binding protein, calbindin D, basolateral calcium ATPases, and a basolateral Na$^+$/Ca^{++} exchanger. Similar to the process in the gut, calcium penetrates into the tubular epithelial cell through a TPRV5 calcium channel, moves across the cytoplasm bound to a calbindin protein, and is finally extruded against a gradient by the Na$^+$/Ca^{++} exchanger and calcium ATPase located in the basolateral membrane (Hoenderop et al., 2002; Loffing and Kaissling, 2003).

The regulation of calcium reabsorption in the nephron is a complex process involving both hormones and divalent cations. PTH is the main regulator of calcium absorption in the distal nephron. It increases calcium absorption in the distal tubules through several mechanisms including activating the TRPV5 channel, increasing calbindin expression, and increasing the affinity for calcium of basolateral Ca^{2+}-ATPases (Hoenderop et al., 2002). Calcitriol augments the action of PTH, apparently by further increasing the expression of TRPV5, calbindin, and plasma-membrane-associated Ca^{2+}-ATPases (Hoenderop et al., 2001).

Calcium ion itself plays a role in the control of calcium reabsorption in those portions of the nephron possessing a CaSR. The ascending limb of the loop on Henle possesses CaSRs that are activated by the binding of calcium ions present in the tubular fluid. At this site in the nephron, activation of the CaSR results in a reduction of calcium and sodium transport and a decrease in urinary concentrating ability. Thus, a rise in serum Ca^{2+} concentration tends to be buffered by increased renal excretion of calcium and a more dilute urine (Tfelt-Hansen and Brown, 2005). This self-regulatory process can occur independently of PTH and calcitriol. Inactivating mutations in the CaSR tend to cause hypercalcemia due in part to impaired renal clearance of calcium in a syndrome known as familial hypocalciuric hypercalcemia (FHH) (Brown, 2007). The CaSR is also present in bone and parathyroid cells, where it plays an important regulatory role, as discussed later in this chapter.

Renal Phosphate Excretion

Eighty-five percent of the phosphorus present in the plasma is in the form of free ions, HPO_4^{2-} and $H_2PO_4^-$ or complexed with sodium as $NaHPO_4^-$ and is thus ultrafiltrable at the renal glomerulus. The control of serum phosphate is accomplished mainly by alterations in the renal reabsorption of phosphate filtered at the glomerulus. At normal glomerular filtration rates, the filtered load of phosphate is 4,000 to 6,000 mg/day. With varying dietary phosphate intake, the reabsorption of phosphate from the glomerular filtrate can vary widely, from 70% to 95%. The fractional excretion of phosphate in the urine, determined by the ratio of phosphate to creatinine clearance, typically ranges from 10% to 15%. Most of the filtered phosphate is reabsorbed by the proximal tubule in an active process requiring sodium ions. At least three separate Na–P cotransporters have been identified at various locations on the nephron. The type II Na–P cotransporter accounts for most of the transport in the proximal tubule and is involved in the regulation of phosphate transport by PTH. A substantial part of the regulation of the renal handling of phosphate is dependent on the ambient concentration of PTH. Increased serum PTH rapidly leads to decreased expression of the type II Na–P cotransporter and thus to reduced phosphate reabsorption. Ablation of the gene coding for the type IIa Na–P cotransporter in mice results in a loss of 70% of proximal phosphate transport and loss of regulation by both PTH and dietary phosphorus intake (Murer et al., 2000).

Renal phosphate excretion is highly responsive to variations in dietary phosphorus intake. With restricted intake, a rapid increase in the tubular reabsorption of phosphate follows, and conversely with a high intake, there is a decrease. Some of the adaptations of the kidney to variations in dietary phosphate intake occur independently of PTH. The mechanisms of this PTH-independent regulation are incompletely understood. However, one of the likely mediators is FGF-23, a member of the fibroblast growth factor (FGF) family of proteins with potent phosphaturic effects. FGF-23 is produced by certain tumors occurring in hypophosphatemic patients with tumor-induced osteomalacia (Shimada et al., 2001). In other patients with the autosomal dominant form of hypophosphatemic rickets, mutations may occur in the FGF-23 gene, rendering the FGF-23 molecule more resistant to proteolytic cleavage. This resistance leads to augmented FGF-23 activity in the kidney with increased phosphate excretion and an abnormally low serum phosphate.

Bone

The role of osteoblasts and osteoclasts in the deposition and resorption of bone mineral is discussed in detail in the preceding chapter (see Chapter 5). The hydroxyapatite composed of bone mineral contains 6 mmol of phosphate for every 10 mmol of calcium (approximately 1 mg of phosphorus for 2 mg calcium). The estimated quantity of calcium released daily by osteoclastic bone resorption is 250 to 500 mg/day. Significantly higher estimates of calcium flux have been derived from calcium isotope studies measuring the movement of calcium between the extracellular fluid pool and the fluid enclosed by bone lining cells (Talmage et al., 1976). One of the well-known effects of PTH is to stimulate bone resorption through osteoclastic activity. This effect is most likely achieved indirectly through the actions of cytokines. Mature osteoclasts do not have PTH receptors. Furthermore, osteoclast-mediated release of calcium from bone into the extracellular fluid is too slow to serve the need for minute-to-minute maintenance of a constant extracellular concentration of ionized calcium. PTH in fact does act to increase extracellular calcium concentration within minutes, but the mechanisms for this rapid action are not entirely understood. PTH receptors exist on bone lining cells, osteocytes, and osteoblasts. Following fibroblast growth factor (PTH) administration, there is a rapid entry of calcium from the bone surface into bone lining cells and osteocytes followed by a net movement of calcium into the extracellular fluid (Talmage et al., 1976).

Osteoclasts are directly inhibited by calcitonin, a hormone secreted by parafollicular cells located in the thyroid gland in mammals. Intravenous administration of calcitonin to rats, rabbits, and

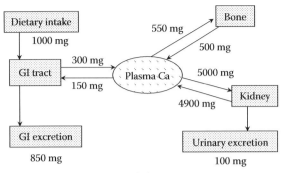

FIGURE 6.2 Optimal calcium balance in a healthy young adult. The numbers represent the estimated flux of calcium in milligrams per day in the gastrointestinal tract, kidney, and bone assuming an optimal dietary intake of calcium and normal hormonal regulation of calcium homeostasis.

humans produces a rapid decrease in serum calcium, mediated primarily by a decreased release of ionized calcium from bone. Osteoclasts do have calcitonin receptors. After exposure to calcitonin in vitro, these cells show almost immediate changes in structure accompanied by a reduction in their resorptive activity (Chambers et al., 1985). The pharmacologic effects of calcitonin are clinically useful in treating hypercalcemia in patients, but it is doubtful that calcitonin plays a physiological role in regulating calcium homeostasis in man. Thyroidectomized subjects lacking calcitonin have no recognizable impairment in regulating their serum calcium levels. Furthermore, subjects with persistently high serum levels of calcitonin, due to calcitonin-secreting thyroid tumors (medullary thyroid carcinoma), have no significant derangements in calcium homeostasis.

Overall Requirements for Positive Calcium Balance

To achieve a steady increase in bone mass during childhood or to maintain a healthy bone mass during adulthood, the GI tract, the kidney, and bone tissue must all function effectively under normal hormonal regulation. In addition, a sufficient dietary intake of calcium must exist. The basic elements required for a positive calcium balance are illustrated in Figure 6.2. In an optimal state with a daily calcium intake of 1000 mg, approximately 30% or 300 mg of the ingested calcium might be absorbed. Of this amount, 150 mg would be secreted back into the intestinal lumen, leading to a loss of 850 mg/day in the stool. Thus, the net gain of body calcium from the intestinal tract would be 150 mg. Approximately 5000 mg of ionized and free calcium would be filtered at the renal glomeruli, and 4900 mg would be reabsorbed back into the plasma leading to a net loss of 100 mg/day in the urine. The combined loss of calcium in the stool and the urine might therefore total 950 mg/day. The estimated flux of calcium into and out of mineralized bone might be on the order of 500 mg/day. In an optimal situation, as illustrated in Figure 6.2, total calcium intake would exceed output by 50 mg/day, with the net gain being deposited in bone. Obviously diseases causing derangements in the function or control of the GI tract, the kidney, or bone itself can interfere with the delicate balance between calcium intake and loss. Some of these conditions are discussed in the sections below, dealing with the regulation of calcium metabolism by individual hormones.

PTH–VITAMIN D ENDOCRINE SYSTEM AND CALCIUM HOMEOSTASIS

PTH

PTH is the primary endocrine mediator of calcium homeostasis. The actions of PTH are enhanced and in some cases mediated by calcitriol, the active form of vitamin D.

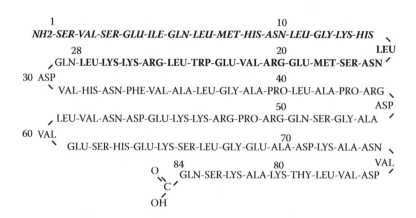

FIGURE 6.3 Amino acid sequence of human PTH. The first 13 amino acids of the N-terminus are sufficient for partial biological activity, whereas the first 34 amino acids provide full biological activity. (Data from Keutmann, H.T., et al., *Biochemistry*, 17, 5723–5729, 1978.)

Structure and Biosynthesis of PTH

PTH is a polypeptide hormone containing 84 amino acids, as shown in Figure 6.3. Biosynthesis occurs in parathyroid epithelial cells where the PTH gene encodes a larger precursor known as pre-pro-PTH. The precursor has an additional 29 amino acids at the amino-terminus of PTH, which are removed by the action of proteolytic enzymes before mature PTH is secreted. The intracellular processing of pre-pro-PTH occurs in two steps. In the first step, occurring in the endoplasmic reticulum, a signal peptidase removes the "pre" or leader sequence to yield pro-PTH. In the second step, occurring in the Golgi apparatus, a second peptidase removes the "pro" sequence before PTH is packaged into secretory granules to await secretion. Normally, the precursor forms of mature PTH are not secreted.

Forms of Circulating PTH

PTH 1-84, commonly referred to as intact PTH, is the main secretory product of the parathyroid glands. Normally, PTH 1–84 accounts for approximately 5%–30% of all PTH peptides in the circulation. The intact hormone has a plasma half life of only 2 to 4 minutes, being rapidly broken down by peptidases in the liver and kidney to form amino-terminal and carboxy-terminal fragments. Amino-terminal fragments containing only the first 13 amino acids of the structure of intact PTH 1-84 are still able to activate the PTH receptor and display biological activity. These amino-terminal fragments are very rapidly cleared from the circulation and constitute less than 10% of circulating PTH peptides. The carboxy-terminal fragments do not bind to the usual PTH receptors and lack a hypercalcemic effect. Carboxy-terminal peptides of PTH have a plasma half life five to ten times longer than that of intact PTH and can constitute 70% to 90% of all PTH peptides in the circulation.

Assay of Circulating PTH

PTH in the circulation is measured by radioimmunoassays using antibodies directed against antigenic sites located in either the amino-terminus or carboxy-terminus of intact PTH. The most commonly used assays for assessing PTH secretion in human subjects employ two antibodies, one directed at the amino-terminus and a second directed at the carboxy-terminus. In these assays, the carboxy-terminal antibody is typically bound to a solid support such as a polystyrene bead and then is exposed to a serum sample containing both intact PTH and various fragments. All polypeptides containing the carboxy-terminal amino acid sequence bind to the solid support. The PTH peptides bound to the solid support are then exposed to the second amino-terminal antibody, which is prelabeled with [125]Iodine or a chemiluminescent molecule allowing detection of the bound antibody.

Generally, such "sandwich" assays detect only the intact, biologically active PTH molecule, containing both carboxy-terminal and amino-terminal antigens (Wood, 1992).

PTH-Related Peptide

A paracrine factor produced by a variety of cell types and known as PTH-related peptide (PTHrP) has structural similarities to PTH. In the fetus, PTHrP plays a physiological role in directing placental calcium transfer. Normally, PTHrP does not play a significant role in controlling calcium homeostasis, but when secreted in large quantities by certain malignant tumors, it can cause hypercalcemia by stimulating calcium release from bone. PTHrP is the humoral factor most frequently associated with the hypercalcemia of malignancy (Stewart, 2005). PTHrP and PTH share a similar amino-terminal sequence capable of interacting with and stimulating a common receptor in bone tissue. The PTHrP gene is distinct from the PTH gene, and unlike PTH, its expression is not regulated by serum ionized calcium. The carboxyl-terminal sequences of PTH and PTHrP are quite dissimilar. Thus, PTHrP is not measured in most radioimmunoassays for intact PTH.

ACTIONS OF PTH

PTH increases serum calcium by promoting the release of calcium from bone, by stimulating calcium reabsorption by the distal tubules of the kidney, and indirectly by promoting GI calcium absorption through the mediation of calcitriol (see Figure 6.4). Concurrent with these effects on calcium homeostasis, PTH increases phosphorus release from bone and increases urinary phosphate excretion. The net effect is usually a decrease in serum phosphorus concentration provided that renal responsiveness is normal.

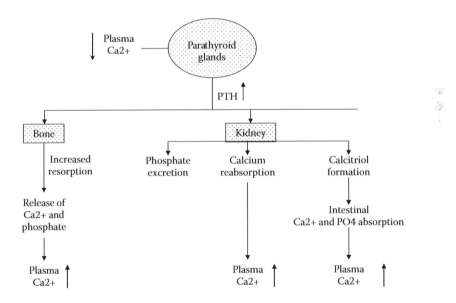

FIGURE 6.4   The response of the PTH–calcitriol regulatory system to hypocalcemia. A decline in serum Ca²⁺ directly stimulates PTH secretion by the parathyroid glands. PTH acts on bone to cause immediate release of exchangeable Ca²⁺ from the bone compartment into the extracellular fluid. Later increased calcium absorption by osteoclasts releases additional calcium as well as phosphorus. PTH acts on the kidney to increase calcium flux from the glomerular filtrate back into the extracellular fluid and to increase phosphate excretion, thus increasing serum calcium and reducing serum phosphorus concentrations. At the same time, PTH action on the kidney increases the synthesis of calcitriol, which in turn stimulates more active absorption of calcium from the gastrointestinal tract. The net movement of Ca²⁺ into the extracellular fluid by the combination of these effects restores the serum calcium concentration to normal.

PTH Receptors and Intracellular Messengers

PTH receptors of several types exist in various tissues in the body. The classical receptor, PTH1R, mediates the actions of PTH on bone and kidney. This receptor binds both PTH and PTHrP and recognizes the common N-terminal sequence of both ligands. PTH1R is heavily expressed not only in bone and kidney, but it is also present in other tissues such as breast, skin, heart, blood vessels, and pancreas where its function is unknown. Binding of PTH to PTH1R activates multiple intracellular signaling pathways, including the adenylate cyclase–cyclic AMP system. PTH1R is a 500-amino-acid protein located in the cell membrane with its ligand-binding region oriented toward the external cell surface. Like a number of other peptide hormone receptors, the intracellular domain of PTH1R binds G protein subunits that in turn transduce the hormone signal into cellular responses involving intracellular second messengers. Studies with cloned PTH1R indicate that the receptor can be coupled to more than one G protein and that other second messengers, in addition to cAMP, may be involved in the cellular response. Other mediators include the phospholipase C-protein kinase C system, which promotes increased intracellular concentrations of inositol triphosphate and diacylglycerol (Juppner et al., 2006). Although it is unclear which of these systems is paramount in regulating calcium homeostasis, an experiment of nature suggests that the cyclic AMP system may be the most critical. In patients with a genetic disorder known as pseudohypoparathyroidism, a mutation in the stimulatory G protein subunit, $G_s\alpha$, leads not only to a failure of PTH to generate cAMP in bone and kidney cells but also to a condition of chronic hypocalcemia and hyperphosphatemia. Patients with this mutation fail to show a rise in serum calcium or an increase in urinary cAMP and phosphate after the administration of PTH (Thakker and Juppner, 2006).

Actions of PTH on Bone

PTH acts on bone to release calcium in two phases. The most immediate effect is to release calcium ions from a bone reservoir that is readily available and in equilibrium with the extracellular fluid. PTH increases the availability of Ca and P in the bone fluid compartment, a response mediated primarily by bone lining cells (Talmage, 1967). Within minutes after exposure to PTH, and before osteoclasts can be involved, there is a rise in extracellular Ca^{2+} concentration. The mechanism of this effect is still unknown.

The later effects of PTH on osteoblasts and osteoclasts vary according to the concentration of PTH and the duration of exposure. Most evidence indicates that osteoblasts, but not mature osteoclasts, express PTH receptors (Murray et al., 2005), yet the action of osteoclasts is ultimately required for bone resorption. The prevailing view today is that the initial effect of PTH on bone cells is on osteoblasts, which have been shown to have a high density of PTHR1 receptors and to respond with a rapid increase in cAMP and inositol triphosphate. When exposed to low, intermittent concentrations of PTH, osteoblastic cells show increased maturation and bone-forming activity. With higher PTH concentrations and more prolonged exposure, osteoclast activation occurs and bone resorption is accelerated. The signal promoting this effect is probably mediated by cytokines stimulated by the action of PTH on osteoblasts and acting on osteoclasts through paracrine mediators. RANK is a cell-surface receptor expressed in osteoclast precursors that controls osteoclast maturation and activation. RANK ligand, a cell-surface protein from cells of the osteoblast lineage, binds to RANK and activates it. Osteoprotegerin (OPG), another protein secreted by osteoblasts, acts as a decoy receptor for RANK ligand, binding it and preventing it from activating RANK. PTH increases the expression of RANK ligand in osteoblastic cells and reduces the expression of OPG, thus promoting the activation of osteoclasts (Ma et al., 2001; Huang et al., 2004). Administration of OPG blocks the calcemic action of exogenous PTH in vivo. The functions of these mediators in bone cell biology are discussed more thoroughly in Chapters 3 and 4. The end result of prolonged, high concentrations of PTH is an increase in osteoclast numbers and activity accompanied by a reduction in the quantity of calcium and phosphorus stored in bone as hydroxyapatite.

Other PTH receptors, including receptors recognizing the C-terminal portion of intact PTH as well as circulating C-terminal fragments, have been described in bone and other tissues. Distinct receptors for the C-terminus of PTH (CPTHRs) have been identified in both bone and renal tissues. The biological significance of these receptors is still unclear. However, in vivo studies suggest that CPTHRs may have a calcium-lowering effect, whereas in vitro studies on bone cells and tissues suggest that they exert antiresorptive effects (Murray et al., 2005).

Actions of PTH on Kidney

Tubular Handling of Calcium and Phosphorus

PTH acts on PTH1R receptors in the kidney tubules to stimulate calcium reabsorption and to inhibit phosphate reabsorption. The distal tubule is the site where calcium reabsorption is actively regulated. As discussed earlier, PTH increases calcium reabsorption from the distal tubular fluid by mediating the activity of several transport proteins including the TRPV5 channel, calbindin, and Ca^{2+}-ATPase (Hoenderop et al., 2002). Thus, when the serum concentration of Ca^{2+} declines, the resulting rise in serum PTH increases the reabsorption of calcium from distal tubular fluid and less calcium is excreted in the urine, correcting the hypocalcemia (Figure 6.4). The opposite sequence of events occurs when the serum concentration of Ca^{2+} rises. In addition, an elevated serum calcium acts directly on renal CaSRs to increase calciuresis (Hebert, 1996).

PTH is also the major hormone controlling renal phosphate handling. It acts to inhibit mainly proximal but also distal tubular reabsorption of phosphate by affecting the activity of phosphate transport proteins, as discussed earlier. In the proximal tubule, the main effect of PTH is to decrease the activity of the sodium phosphate cotransporter (Murer et al., 2000).

PTH Effects on Calcitriol Synthesis

An additional important effect of PTH on the kidney is to stimulate the expression of 1-alpha hydroxylase in the proximal tubule, thus promoting the conversion of 25-hydroxyvitamin D to 1,25-dihydroxyvitamin D (calcitriol). The factors affecting the interconversion of vitamin D metabolites are discussed in detail in Chapter 10. In the presence of normally functioning kidneys, a decline in serum calcium leads to an increase in serum PTH followed by increased serum calcitriol and an increase in the GI absorption of calcium and phosphorus (Figure 6.4).

Basis of Use of PTH as Antiosteoporosis Drug

Paradoxically, PTH can act either as an anabolic agent, promoting bone formation, or as a catabolic agent, promoting bone resorption, depending on its concentration and the duration of tissue exposure. When present at low concentrations for intermittent, brief intervals, the predominant effect of PTH, or its active analogs, is the stimulation of osteoblast activation and bone formation. When present in continuous high concentrations, the dominant effects of PTH are to promote RANK ligand expression by osteoblasts and to activate osteoclasts to resorb bone (Ma et al., 2001). Teriparatide (PTH 1–34), a synthetic peptide consisting of the amino-terminal 34 amino acids of PTH, has been shown in clinical trials to promote increased bone density and to reduce fracture risk in postmenopausal women and men with osteoporosis. Teriparatide, when given in low doses (20 mcg) by subcutaneous injections once a day, is therefore an effective antiosteoporosis drug (Neer et al., 2001; Cosman and Lindsay, 2008).

CONTROL OF PTH SECRETION

The concentration of extracellular ionized calcium regulates PTH secretion by a typical negative feedback effect on parathyroid cells. The relationship between serum ionized calcium and serum intact PTH is characterized by a sigmoidal curve, as shown in Figure 6.5. The midpoint on the steepest portion of the curve represents the concentration of ionized calcium at which PTH secretion is half maximal and represents the set point at which serum calcium tends to be maintained. In normal individuals, a decrease of as little as 0.1 mg/dL in serum ionized calcium leads to a rapid increase in PTH secretion, whereas an increase leads to rapid lowering (Brown, 1983). The most

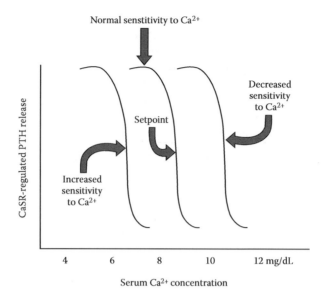

FIGURE 6.5 The relationship of PTH secretion to serum calcium concentration. The center curve shows the normal relationship, where the set point of half-maximal secretion is equal to a normal serum calcium concentration of approximately 9 mg/dL. The curve on the left shows an increased sensitivity to inhibition by calcium, as might be seen in a gain-of-function mutation in the CaSR. The curve on the right shows decreased sensitivity, as might be seen in an inactivating mutation in the CaSR in patients with familial hypocalciuric hypercalcemia or in some parathyroid adenomas.

immediate effect of hypocalcemia on parathyroid cells, occurring within minutes, is exocytosis of preformed PTH from secretory vesicles into the extracellular fluid. This is followed within hours by an increase in PTH gene expression, and within days to weeks by proliferation of parathyroid cells (Naveh-Many et al., 1989). The latter effects involve increased PTH gene expression and parathyroid cell hyperplasia and are also activated under conditions where extracellular concentrations of calcitriol are low.

Role of Calcium Sensing Receptor in Regulating PTH Secretion

The CaSR is a large cell-surface protein expressed in multiple tissues, including the parathyroid glands, kidneys, osteoblasts, and osteoclasts. The proposed structure of the CaSR in human parathyroid glands is shown in Figure 6.6. This receptor is the primary mediator of the negative feedback effect of ionized calcium on PTH secretion. The CaSR is highly expressed on the surface of parathyroid chief cells, where it senses small variations in calcium concentration. Binding of Ca^{2+} to the CaSR is thought to cause dimerization of monomeric CaSR in the cell membrane and to inhibit adenylate cyclase through action on a G protein. Reduced intracellular levels of cAMP then lead to reduced PTH secretion, although the pathways are not fully known. The CaSR also activates intracellular phospholipases, probably indirectly through a protein-kinase-C-mediated mechanism (Diaz and Brown, 2006).

Role of Calcitriol in Regulating PTH Secretion

The parathyroid glands possess vitamin D receptors that mediate a negative feedback of active vitamin D metabolites on PTH secretion. Calcitriol acts on parathyroid cells to downregulate the expression of the PTH gene, leading to a decrease in PTH messenger RNA and decreased PTH synthesis (Naveh-Many et al., 1989). Calcitriol also induces increased expression of the CaSR in parathyroid tissue, thereby increasing the sensitivity of parathyroid cells to inhibition by Ca^{2+} (Dusso et al., 2005). In chronic renal failure, prolonged deficiency of calcitriol leads to reduced CaSR

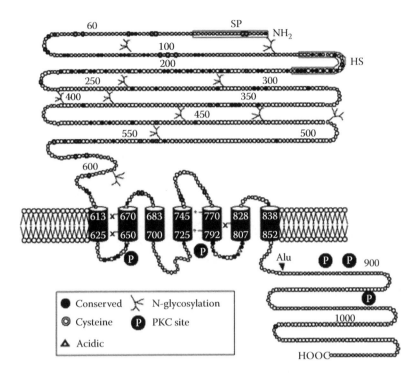

FIGURE 6.6 Schematic representation of the proposed structure of the bovine calcium-sensing receptor. The amino acid sequence from 1–600 resides in the extracellular compartment outside the parathyroid cell plasma membrane and interacts directly with calcium ions. The transmembrane sequence from 613 to 852 is hydrophobic and resides within the cell membrane, whereas the C-terminal sequence resides within the cell. SP denotes a signal peptide that is cleaved in the process of biosynthesis. HS denotes hydrophobic substance. (Reproduced with permission from Brown, E.M., G. Gamba, D. Riccardi, et al. *Nature*, 366, 578, 1993.)

levels, requiring markedly higher Ca^{2+} levels to suppress PTH secretion and parathyroid cellular hyperplasia.

Other Ions Affecting PTH Secretion

Hyperphosphatemia stimulates PTH secretion and parathyroid cell hyperplasia, primarily by inducing a decline in the serum concentration of Ca^{2+}. At high serum phosphorus concentrations, calcium ions move from the extracellular compartment into tissues, resulting in lower concentrations of Ca^{2+} to inhibit PTH secretion. Evidence exists that chronic hyperphosphatemia, as seen in chronic renal failure, can stimulate PTH secretion and parathyroid gland hyperplasia by a direct action on parathyroid cells (Slatopolsky et al., 1996). Other cations including magnesium, aluminum, and strontium bind to the CaSR, but their affinity is much lower than that of calcium so that their effects on PTH secretion are minimal under normal conditions.

Drugs Affecting PTH Secretion

Lithium is widely used as a mood-stabilizing drug for the treatment of bipolar disorders. From 10% to 25% of patients on chronic lithium therapy develop mild hypercalcemia and inappropriately high serum PTH concentrations (Kallner and Petterson, 1995). Lithium induces an abnormal response of parathyroid cells to calcium in vitro where the Ca^{2+}–PTH response curve is shifted to the right, causing a higher set point for calcium inhibition (Brown, 1981). In lithium-treated human subjects, there is also a rightward shift of the response curve, suggesting altered calcium sensing at the level of the CaSR (Haden et al., 1997).

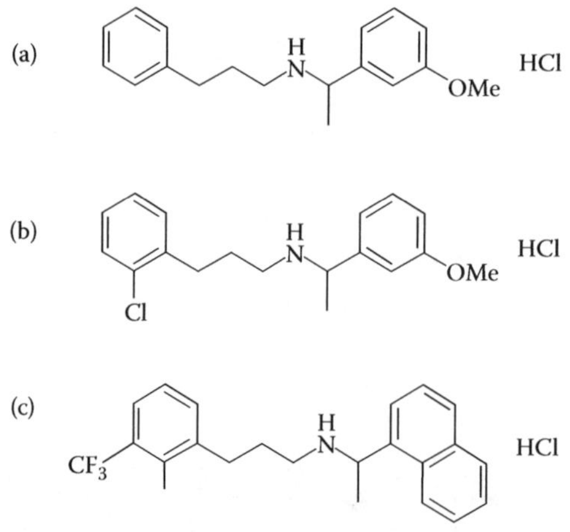

FIGURE 6.7 Chemical structure of three phenylalkylamine calcimimetic compounds. (a) NPS R-467. (b) Tecalcet hydrochloride, a first-generation calcimetic compound. (c) Cinacalcet, a second-generation calcimimetic compound. (Adapted from Nagano, N., *Pharmacol Ther*, 109, 339–365, 2006.)

Calcimimetics

Following the identification and sequencing of the CaSR, pharmaceutical research has focused on finding compounds that might interact with the receptor and either stimulate it (calcimimetics) or inhibit it (calcilytics). Calcimimetics would be expected to "trick" the CaSR into responding as it would in the presence of increased Ca^{2+} and therefore reduce PTH secretion. Several calcimimetics have been described and tested, but only one such compound is currently approved in the United States for use as a drug in human subjects. Cinacalcet is a phenylalkylamine compound with the structure shown in Figure 6.7. In patients with both primary and secondary hyperparathyroidism, cinacalcet is effective in reducing serum PTH concentrations (Nagano, 2006). In one trial involving subjects with primary hyperparathyroidism, there was no improvement in bone mineral density (BMD), although both serum calcium and PTH concentrations were reduced (Peacock et al., 2009). This is a promising field of pharmaceutical research where new compounds are under active investigation.

DISEASES CAUSED BY ABNORMAL PTH SECRETION OR ACTION

Primary Hyperparathyroidism

Primary hyperparathyroidism is diagnosed in patients whenever serum concentrations of both ionized calcium and PTH are abnormally elevated. Secondary hyperparathyroidism refers to conditions in which serum PTH levels are appropriately elevated in response to low serum concentrations of calcium or active vitamin D metabolites. The differences between primary and secondary hyperparathyroidism in terms of clinical laboratory findings are illustrated in Figure 6.8.

Primary hyperparathyroidism is the most common cause of hypercalcemia in the United States. This condition is most frequently caused by a benign parathyroid adenoma having a higher than normal set point for negative feedback control by Ca^{2+}. Less frequently, the condition is caused by primary hyperplasia of all of the parathyroid glands. The mechanism of inappropriate PTH secretion involves a decreased sensitivity of individual parathyroid cells to calcium, an increase in the number of parathyroid cells, or a combination of both. The cells in most parathyroid adenomas are monoclonal, suggesting that a mutation has occurred in a key growth-controlling gene. The gene mutations implicated in causing inappropriate cell proliferation are the subject of several reviews (Hendy, 2000; Arnold et al., 2002; Brown, 2002) and will not be discussed in detail here.

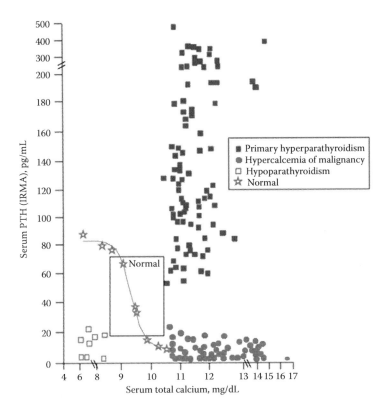

FIGURE 6.8 Serum PTH and calcium concentrations in various disease states. The normal range is illustrated by the sigmoid curve in the box. Serum PTH and calcium are both elevated in patients with primary hyperparathyroidism and are both low in patients with hypoparathyroidism. In patients with the hypercalcemia of malignancy, calcium is elevated but immunoreactive PTH is low because PTHrP is not recognized by most clinical immunoassays for PTH. (Adapted from Haden, S.T., et al., *Clin Endocrinol*, 52, 329–338, 2000.)

Hypercalcemia of Malignancy

As discussed above, PTHrP is produced in large quantities by some malignant tumors, particularly those of squamous cell origin. In other malignancies, hypercalcemia may be mediated by other humoral factors, particularly tumor-produced cytokines (Stewart, 2006). Still, other tumors, particularly lymphomas, express the gene for 1-alpha hydroxylase and are associated with excessive production of calcitriol. In patients having tumor-associated hypercalcemia, serum levels of intact PTH are almost always low (see Figure 6.8). Ectopic production of PTH by nonparathyroid tumors is very rare.

Congenital or Acquired Abnormalities of CaSR

The density of extracellular CaSRs is known to be reduced in some parathyroid adenomas and may account in part for a decreased sensitivity to calcium feedback control (Kifor et al., 1996, Cetani et al., 2000). In a few uncommon but very informative familial disorders, both activating and inactivating mutations in the CaSR account for the observed abnormalities in calcium homeostasis. Inactivating mutations are responsible for a syndrome called familial hypocalciuric hypercalcemia in which the set point of the PTH response curve to serum Ca^{2+} is shifted to the right (see Figure 6.5). Higher concentrations of Ca^{2+} are required to inhibit PTH secretion, resulting in hypercalcemia with inappropriately normal or elevated serum PTH. In patients with FHH, reduced activity of the CaSR in the kidney results in reduced tubular clearance of calcium, causing hypocalciuria.

In contrast, activating mutations of the CaSR cause an increased sensitivity of parathyroid cells to inhibition by Ca^{2+} and hypocalcemia of varying severity (Brown, 2007).

Acquired diseases associated with autoantibodies to the CaSR may affect calcium homeostasis by either activating or inactivating the receptor. Some patients with autoimmune hypoparathyroidism have anti-CaSR antibodies capable of activating the receptor, thus inhibiting PTH secretion, whereas a few patients with hypercalcemia apparently have antibodies that may inactivate the receptor, causing hyperparathyroidism (Gavalas et al., 2007; Pelletier-Morel et al., 2008; Brown, 2009).

Hypoparathyroidism and Pseudohypoparathyroidism

A deficiency of either PTH itself or an inability to respond to PTH causes hypocalcemia and hyperphosphatemia (Levine, 2006). Primary hypoparathyroidism, an absolute deficiency of PTH, may be caused by an autoimmune disease in which parathyroid cells are damaged or destroyed by autoantibodies. More commonly, the parathyroid glands are inadvertently destroyed by surgical procedures on the thyroid gland or by radiation therapy directed at malignant tumors in the neck. Patients with primary hypoparathyroidism present with hypocalcemia, often accompanied by symptoms of muscle cramps or tetany and an inappropriately low serum level of intact PTH.

Patients with what is known as pseudohypoparathyroidism secrete PTH normally but have hypocalcemia due to target organ resistance to the actions of PTH. Detailed knowledge about the mechanisms of PTH resistance in patients with pseudohypoparathyroidism has provided greater insight into the mechanisms of action of PTH at the cellular level. Several variants of this syndrome have been described, but in the most common type, the defect is an inherited abnormality of the G protein ($G_s\alpha$) linking the PTHR1 receptor to adenylate cyclase and cAMP formation (Levine, 2006). The G protein defect results in a failure of PTH to stimulate cAMP formation in bone and kidney cells. As one might expect, patients with pseudohypoparathyroidism have hypocalcemia and hyperphosphatemia with serum PTH levels that are generally high or high–normal.

STEROID HORMONES AND BONE METABOLISM

A number of hormones do not play a direct role in maintaining calcium homeostasis, as does PTH, but do affect overall calcium balance in important ways. A deficiency (or in some cases an excess) of these hormones can lead to skeletal changes resulting in metabolic bone disease. Several classes of steroid hormones, including estrogens, androgens, and glucocorticoids, have important skeletal effects. In addition, thyroid hormones and certain pituitary hormones, especially growth hormone (GH), play a role in promoting bone growth and maturation. The purpose of this section will be to discuss the role of these hormones in bone metabolism and their role in the pathogenesis or treatment of osteoporosis.

GENERAL FEATURES OF STEROID HORMONE ACTION

Steroid hormones are derivatives of cholesterol synthesized by the gonads or the adrenal cortex. During the reproductive years, the principal steroid products of the ovaries are estradiol and progesterone. In men, the principal testicular steroid is testosterone. All steroid hormones are believed to have a common mechanism of action, as depicted in Figure 6.9. Typically, the steroid ligand circulates in the plasma in association with a binding protein. It dissociates from the binding protein to cross the cell membrane and bind to a specific cytoplasmic receptor within the cell. As a result, the receptor–steroid complex usually forms an active dimer that migrates to the cell nucleus and interacts with genomic DNA to regulate the expression of various steroid-responsive genes. Ultimately, the concentrations of proteins encoded by these genes are altered, leading to a cellular response. Steroid receptors belong to a family of related proteins with similar structure, each having its own preference for binding steroids of a particular class. Each receptor class has a ligand-binding region for attachment of the preferred steroid and a nuclear-binding region which interacts

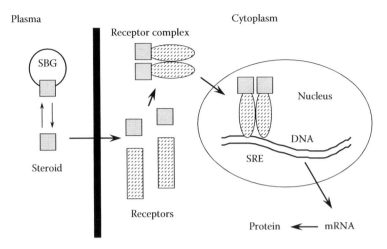

FIGURE 6.9   General mechanism of action for steroid hormones. The steroid ligand dissociates from its specific steroid-binding globulin (SBG) in plasma to enter the target cell by diffusion. Once inside the cell, the steroid binds to an intracellular receptor that is specific for each class of steroid hormones. The steroid–receptor complexes associate to form active dimmers and then enter the cell nucleus where they bind to the DNA of steroid-responsive genes at specific steroid response elements (SREs). Binding results in either enhancement or suppression of gene expression, resulting in alterations in the amounts of messenger RNA (mRNA) and protein formed. (From Ontjes, D.A., The role of estrogens and other steroid hormones in bone metabolism, in *Calcium and Phosphorus in Health and Disease*, Anderson, J.J.B., and Garner, S.C., eds., CRC Press, Boca Raton, FL. With permission.)

with specific nucleotide sequences in the DNA of steroid-responsive genes. The general structure of steroid receptors is illustrated in Figure 6.10. Note that the receptors for vitamin D and thyroid hormones are also members of the same family (Tsai and O'Malley, 1994).

ESTROGENS

Sources of Estrogens in Women and Men

The natural estrogens produced by the ovary are estradiol, estrone, and estriol (see Figure 6.11). Estradiol is the major secretory product of the ovary in women of child-bearing age and accounts for most of the estrogenic activity in the circulation. Estrone and estriol are weaker estrogens and are mainly produced by extragonadal conversion from estradiol in the liver. During pregnancy, large quantities of estrogens are produced by the placenta. Estradiol is synthesized in the body by conversion from testosterone by aromatization of the A ring of the steroid nucleus. This conversion is favored in the ovary, where the concentration of the aromatase enzyme is high, but also occurs to a minor degree in the testes. Testosterone may also be converted to estradiol in nongonadal tissues possessing an aromatase enzyme. After menopause, ovarian production of estradiol virtually ceases, but peripheral production from adrenal androgens continues, yielding mainly the weaker estrogen, estrone, as shown in Figure 6.12.

In addition to the natural estrogens, there are a large number of synthetic estrogens, developed specifically by the pharmaceutical industry for use as oral contraceptives and for estrogen replacement therapy. The most commonly used synthetic estrogen is ethinyl estradiol, a compound having approximately 50 times the potency of natural estradiol when administered orally (Figure 6.11). Not all compounds having estrogenic activity are steroids—they need only to be able to bind to and activate the estrogen receptor to have estrogenic activity. An example of such a compound is diethylstilbestrol, also shown in Figure 6.11. Estrogen-like compounds may occur in nature in various foods, including soy protein, where two compounds, genistein and daidzein, have weak estrogenic activity.

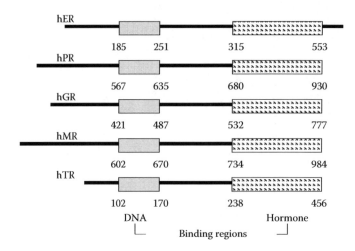

FIGURE 6.10 Structure of the family of steroid hormone receptors. The domains responsible for binding to the steroid ligand to the steroid response elements of genomic DNA are indicated. The structure of the hormone binding domain confers specificity for binding of the steroid class. Human estrogen receptor (hER), human progestin receptor (hPR), human glucocorticoid receptor (hGR), human mineralocorticoid receptor (hMR), and human thyroid hormone receptor (hTR) are shown. (From Ontjes, D.A., The role of estrogens and other steroid hormones in bone metabolism, in *Calcium and Phosphorus in Health and Disease*, Anderson, J.J.B., and Garner, S.C., eds., CRC Press, Boca Raton, FL. With permission.)

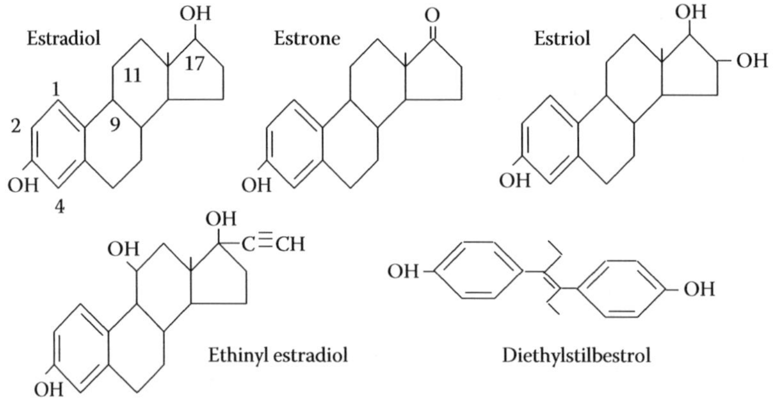

FIGURE 6.11 Structures of natural and synthetic compounds having estrogen activity. Estradiol, estrone, and estriol are all naturally produced. Ethinyl estradiol and diethylstilbesetrol are synthetic estrogens given orally as drugs.

Effects of Estrogen on Bone Metabolism and Calcium Balance

As early as the 1940s, Fuller Albright showed that postmenopausal women were in negative calcium balance and that estrogen administration could correct the negative balance (Riggs et al., 2002). Estrogens, like other steroid hormones, act through specific intracellular receptors that are capable of regulating the expression of specific genes. High-affinity estrogen receptors have been found in all tissues usually considered to be targets for estrogen action including the oviducts, endometrium, and breast. Bone cells also contain estrogen receptors. Two types of estrogen receptors have been identified; estrogen receptor-alpha (ER-alpha) and estrogen receptor-beta (ER-beta). Both types of receptors are found in osteoblasts, whereas ER-alpha is also present in osteoclasts. Studies in knockout mice indicate that animals lacking the ER-alpha receptor but not the ER-beta receptor are short and have lower femoral bone densities (Couse and Korach, 1999; Vidal et al., 2000).

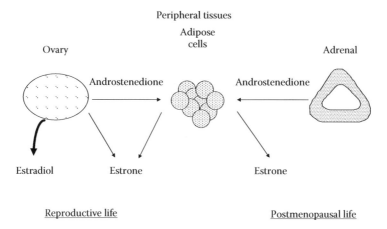

FIGURE 6.12   Sources of estrogens in women during reproductive life and after menopause. Estradiol is the main estrogen produced by the ovaries during reproductive life. Both before and following menopause, the ovaries and the adrenal glands produce the weak androgen, androstenedione, which is converted in peripheral tissues to the weak estrogen, estrone. Estrone is the main circulating estrogen in postmenopausal women.

Estrogens tonically inhibit bone resorption mainly by influencing the cytokine network described earlier. More than one cytokine appears to be involved. There is good evidence that estrogen deficiency leads to the increased production of TNF-alpha and IL-1, both of which can stimulate RANK ligand synthesis and activate osteoclasts (Manolagos, 2000; Weitzmann and Pacifici, 2006). Other studies implicate a role for TNF-beta, OPG, and IL-6. An additional effect of estrogen deficiency may be reduced bone formation by osteoblasts. Both IL-7 and TNF-alpha, whose production is known to be increased in estrogen deficiency, have been shown to decrease the activity of osteoblasts.

Whatever the cellular mechanisms may be, the net effect of estrogen deficiency is an increase in overall bone resorption and a failure of new bone formation to keep up—hence, a loss of bone mineral. Typically, the earliest phase of trabecular bone loss begins in the perimenopausal period when serum estrogen levels begin to decline and accelerate at menopause. This is followed by a period of slower bone loss involving both trabecular and cortical bone (Riggs et al., 2008). The accelerated phase lasts for 4–8 years before decelerating back to a slower continuous rate of loss characteristic of aging. During the accelerated phase, bone loss in one large cohort of women averaged 5.6% for the vertebrae and 2.9% for the proximal femur over a period of 4 years (Sowers et al., 2006). At the same time that bone density is being lost, changes occur in bone microstructure that further impair its strength. In trabecular bone, there is a disproportionate loss of structural cross struts and in cortical bone increased porosity, leading to increased risk of fragility fractures.

Most of the effects of estrogen deficiency are exerted directly on bone cells, but adverse extraskeletal effects may also contribute (Riggs et al., 2008). During the accelerated phase of bone loss, calcium ions move out of bone into the extracellular space, slightly increasing serum calcium concentrations. This results in a slight suppression of PTH secretion and consequently a reduced rate of calcitriol formation. Lower levels of PTH allow an increased loss of calcium in the urine, due to reduced renal tubular reabsorption of calcium, whereas lower levels of calcitriol lead to reduced absorption of calcium and phosphorus from the GI tract. The overall effects of estrogen deficiency on calcium balance are illustrated in Figure 6.13.

Effects of Estrogen Administration on Osteoporosis

In normal women, the loss of bone mass usually accelerates at menopause, coinciding with the onset of menopausal symptoms such as hot flashes and vaginal dryness. Early metabolic studies

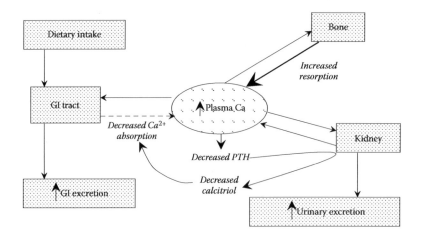

Net negative calcium balance

FIGURE 6.13   Results of estrogen deficiency on calcium balance. The primary effect of estrogen deficiency is accelerated bone resorption, leading to a net movement of Ca^{2+} from bone to serum. The slightly increased concentration of serum Ca^{2+} inhibits PTH secretion resulting in a decreased synthesis of calcitriol by the kidney. The reduction in calcitriol leads to reduced gastrointestinal absorption of calcium from the diet. The overall effect is a net negative calcium balance.

in postmenopausal women showed that a negative calcium balance could be prevented by estrogen administration (Albright, 1947). Later, when techniques for measuring bone density became available, it became apparent from a number of clinical trials that estrogens could indeed prevent the loss of bone mass and in some cases even increase it. None of these trials were large enough to give conclusive results about the effects of estrogen on fracture risk. Estrogen replacement therapy became a widespread clinical practice, not only for the relief of menopausal symptoms, but because of the widely held opinion that postmenopausal estrogens could prevent osteoporosis and reduce the risk of coronary heart disease. This practice changed with the publication of the findings of the Women's Health Initiative (WHI) clinical trial. The WHI trial compared the effects of long-term therapy with estrogen plus progestin versus placebo in over 16,000 postmenopausal women. The WHI treatment regimen included 0.625 mg of conjugated equine estrogens and 2.5 mg of medroxyprogesterone given daily. As expected, hip fractures were significantly reduced in the treated subjects (relative risk 0.66; confidence interval 0.45–0.98). However, the risk of several adverse outcomes was increased in the estrogen–progestin-treated group, including myocardial infarction, breast cancer, stroke, and pulmonary embolism. All cause mortality was not significantly affected. The investigators in this study concluded that the net benefits of hormone replacement therapy did not justify its use in most postmenopausal women (Roussouw et al., 2002). As a result of this study, no estrogen product is approved by the Food and Drug Administration in the United States for the treatment of postmenopausal osteoporosis, only for prevention.

Many investigators have published short-term studies of bone density outcomes using treatment regimens differing from those used in the WHI trial. Doses of conjugated estrogens as low as 0.3 mg/day are effective in preserving bone density (Lindsay et al., 2005). There is also evidence that estrogens and calcium are interactive. The addition of a calcium supplement can make a dose of 0.3 mg of conjugated estrogens as effective as a higher dose of 0.625 mg/day (Ettinger et al., 1987). Whether alternative doses of estrogen or the use of different progestins might decrease long-term fracture risk without having the same adverse effects as the WHI trial is unknown.

TABLE 6.2
Activity Spectrum of Selective Estrogen Receptor Modulators

Compound	Clinical Use	Antiestrogen Effects	Proestrogen Effects
Clomiphene	Fertility drug	Hypothalamus/pituitary	Uterus, breast
Tamoxifen	Breast cancer drug	Hypothalamus/pituitary	Uterus
		Breast	Bone
			Serum lipids
Raloxifene	Antiosteoporosis drug	Hypothalamus/pituitary	Bone
		Breast cancer	Serum lipids

SELECTIVE ESTROGEN RECEPTOR MODULATORS

General Properties of Selective Estrogen Receptor Modulators

A wide variety of compounds are capable of interacting with estrogen receptors. Complete estrogen agonists, such as estradiol itself, activate estrogen receptors in all tissues of the body that are normally estrogen responsive. These tissues include not only bone but also the endometrium, breast, and the hypothalamus where a negative feedback of estrogens normally inhibits gonadotropin secretion by the pituitary gland. To have an agonist or proestrogen effect in a specific tissue, a ligand must first bind to the estrogen receptor in that tissue. It must then cause a conformational change in the receptor, leading to receptor dimerization and interaction with DNA at estrogen response elements in specific genes. Only when all of these conditions are fulfilled does the estrogen-like ligand succeed in modifying the expression of the targeted genes. Selective estrogen receptor modulators (SERMs) are compounds that can bind to estrogen receptors in multiple target tissues but can only act as agonists in a limited subset of tissues by activating the receptors. In other tissues, SERMs can act as estrogen antagonists by binding to estrogen receptors, but failing to activate them can block the effects of natural active estrogens. The main effects of several SERMs in current clinical use are summarized in Table 6.2. Clomiphene has been used for many years as a drug to promote fertility in women. Its main therapeutic action is on estrogen receptors in the hypothalamus. These receptors mediate the normal negative feedback effect of estrogens on pituitary secretion of luteinizing hormone (LH) and follicle stimulating hormone (FSH). By inhibiting these receptors, the usual negative feedback is blocked and gonadotropin secretion is increased, thereby stimulating ovulation. Tamoxifen is a drug used primarily as an adjuvant in the treatment of breast cancer. It functions as an estrogen antagonist in breast tissue, inhibiting the estrogen-dependent stimulation of tumor growth in breast cancers having estrogen receptors.

Biological Effects of Raloxifene

Raloxifene is a SERM used primarily for the treatment of osteoporosis. Its mechanism of action is well understood from X-ray crystallographic studies comparing the conformation of the estrogen receptor after binding either estradiol or raloxifene (Brzozowski et al., 1997; Prince et al., 2008). The binding of raloxifene to the estrogen receptor causes displacement of a C-terminal helix in the receptor, leading to interference with the binding of coactivator proteins that are necessary for estrogen effects in certain tissues (breast) but not in others (bone). Thus, the estrogen receptor is effectively blocked in breast tissue but is activated in bone. Studies in rats and monkeys suggest that raloxifene has effects similar to estradiol in inhibiting bone loss after oophorectomy. Both raloxifene and estrogen inhibit increases in osteoclast number and bone turnover as well as the reduction in bone strength seen after oophorectomy (Turner et al., 1994).

Raloxifene has no significant effects on the endometrium but acts as an estrogen antagonist in breast tissue and as an estrogen agonist in the liver, where it reduces synthesis of low-density lipoprotein cholesterol and increases the synthesis of certain clotting factors.

Effects of SERMs in Treatment of Osteoporosis

Both tamoxifen and raloxifene have similar effects of bone, but only raloxifene has been approved by the U.S. Food and Drug Administration for the treatment of osteoporosis. In the largest clinical fracture trial with raloxifene (the MORE Trial), 7705 postmenopausal women with low bone densities received either raloxifene, 60 or 120 mg/day, or a placebo and were followed for 36 months (Ettinger et al., 1999). Women receiving raloxifene had significantly fewer new vertebral fractures than those of control women, regardless of the dose or presence of prior vertebral fractures. Among the women receiving 60- and 120-mg raloxifene, the 3-year risk of vertebral fracture was 6.6% and 5.4%, respectively, compared with a risk of 10.1% in the placebo group. There was no difference among the groups in the incidence of hip or nonvertebral fractures. In the MORE trial and another large clinical trial primarily examining the effects of raloxifene on coronary artery disease (Barrett-Connor et al., 2006), no reduction in coronary events was seen. In both trials, the incidence of invasive breast cancer was reduced in the raloxifene-treated women, whereas the incidence of venous thromboembolic disease was increased.

A number of other compounds with estrogen-like activity on bone are known and are being actively investigated as potential drugs for the prevention and treatment of osteoporosis, breast cancer, and possibly coronary disease.

ANDROGENS

Sources in Men and Women

Androgenic steroids are produced in the gonads and adrenal glands of both men and women. Testosterone, the most potent androgen, is the major steroid secreted by the testes. Much smaller quantities of testosterone are produced by the ovaries, and by the adrenal glands in both sexes. The adrenal glands secrete large quantities of weak androgens, mainly androstenedione and dehydroepiandrosterone. These weak androgens can be converted by peripheral tissues into small quantities of testosterone. Thus, in adult men, over 90% of circulating androgen activity is produced directly by the testes in the form of testosterone. In adult women, circulating androgen activity is much lower and is derived equally from ovarian and adrenal sources. The pathways for peripheral interconversion of androgenic steroids are illustrated in Figure 6.14. Most of the testosterone produced in the

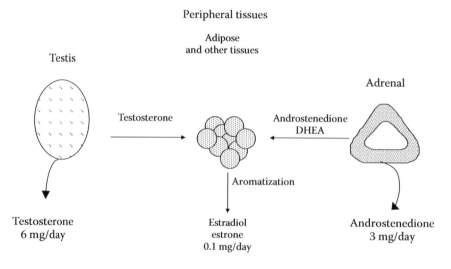

FIGURE 6.14 Sources of circulating androgens and estrogens in the adult male. The most potent androgen, testosterone, is produced directly in large amounts by the testes. Weaker androgens, including androstenedione and dehydroepiandrosterone, are produced by the adrenal glands. Both testosterone and androstenedione may be aromatized in peripheral tissues to small quantities of estradiol and other estrogens.

ovaries is aromatized to estradiol before it is secreted. Testosterone is also aromatized in peripheral tissues to estradiol in both sexes. Aromatase enzyme activity is widely present in a number of tissues, including adipose cells, hepatocytes, and even bone cells. In the normal male, approximately 15% of circulating estrogen is produced by the testes, whereas the other 85% is produced by peripheral metabolism (Gennari et al., 2004).

The clinical importance of aromatase activity for bone health in men is demonstrated by the effect of congenital aromatase deficiency on bone development and bone mass. In males with aromatase deficiency, there is a delay in skeletal development during puberty, lack of epiphysial closure, and osteopenia or osteoporosis. These skeletal defects are similar to those seen in males with a congenital deficiency of ER-alpha and imply that at least part of the effects of testosterone on bone may be mediated by the conversion of testosterone to estrogen (Smith et al., 1994; Gennari et al., 2004).

Effects of Testosterone on Bone Metabolism and Calcium Balance

The administration of testosterone to orchiectomized animals can stimulate bone formation and inhibit bone resorption. Although a part of this effect may be due to the peripheral conversion of testosterone to estrogen, there is good evidence that testosterone itself has direct effects on bone. An androgen receptor (AR) has been identified in a number of cell types and cloned (Chang et al., 1988; Lubahn et al., 1988). The AR is a typical member of the steroid hormone receptor family, with an overall structure and mode of action resembling that of the estrogen receptor. A high-affinity AR is present in osteoblastic cells of both men and women. These receptors bind other natural and synthetic androgens as well as testosterone, but they do not bind estrogens, progesterone, or glucocorticoids. ARs are also expressed in osteocytes, bone stromal cells, and osteoclasts (Wiren, 2008). The level of AR expression in osteoblasts increases as osteoblasts mature, suggesting that a key action of androgens occurs in mature, mineralizing osteoblasts. The effects of androgens on osteoblasts, as observed in tissue culture experiments, are complex and biphasic. Early exposure promotes osteoblast proliferation and maturation, but continued exposure can promote decreased cell viability and apoptosis.

In isolated osteoclasts, androgens reduce bone resorption and reduce the stimulatory effects of PTH. It is likely that part of the inhibitory effect of androgens on bone resorption is mediated by the RANK ligand–OPG system through actions on osteoblasts. Increased expression of OPG mRNA occurs after the exposure of osteoblasts to testosterone in tissue culture (Chen et al., 2004). Other cytokines originating in osteoblasts may also be involved. Androgens, as well as estrogens, inhibit the expression of interleukin-6 (IL-6) by osteoblast cells. IL-6 is another cytokine associated with the activation of osteoclast activity (Wiren, 2008). The release of tonic inhibitory effects of androgens on osteoclastic activity may explain the rapid increase in bone resorption rates seen after orchiectomy in experimental animals.

Effects of Androgen on Osteoporosis in Men

Testosterone deficiency can occur as a result of congenital defects, as an acquired disease, or as a natural result of aging. In aging men, changes gradually occur in the hypothalamic–pituitary–gonadal axis, leading to decreased serum concentrations of total and free testosterone. Levels of free biologically active testosterone decline more than those of total testosterone do as a result of increasing levels of sex hormone binding globulin (SHBG) occurring with age. In the Baltimore Longitudinal Study of Aging, the fraction of men who were hypogonadal increased with each decade, as shown in Figure 6.15 (Harman et al., 2001). In men aged 80 years and older, the prevalence of hypogonadism was approximately 50% as measured by total testosterone and nearly 90% as measured by the free testosterone index (total testosterone/SHBG). Despite these significant declines, it is unclear whether testosterone deficiency is the dominant factor responsible for the increasing occurrence of osteoporosis in elderly men. Some cross-sectional studies have failed to show an association

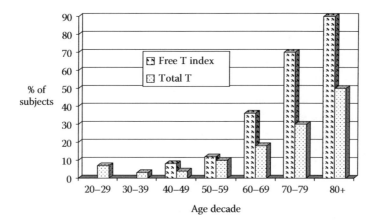

FIGURE 6.15 Increasing prevalence of hypogonadism in aging men. Bar height indicates the percent of men in each 10-year interval with total testosterone <325 ng/dL or free testosterone index below 0.153 nmol/nmol (below the normal range for each test). The number of men who were hypogonadal by either criterion increased after the age of 50 years. More men were hypogonadal by the free testosterone index than by total testosterone after the age of 50 years. (Data from Harman, S.M., et al., *J Clin Endocrinol Metab*, 86, 724–731. 2001.)

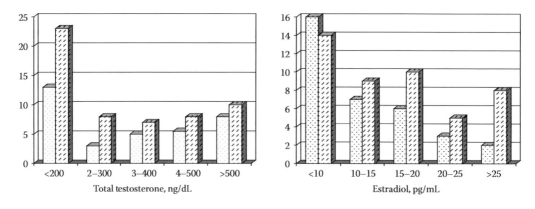

FIGURE 6.16 Percentage of osteoporosis (*T*-score < 2.5, dotted bars) and rapid bone loss (>3% per year, cross-hatched bars) in relation to serum total testosterone and estradiol in men aged 65 years and older. The prevalence of low bone density and rapid bone loss both increase as estradiol concentration declines. Low bone density is also associated with the lowest testosterone concentrations of less than 200 ng/dL. (Data from Fink, H.A., et al., *J Clin Endocrinol Metab*, 91, 3908–3915, 2006.)

between low bone density and serum testosterone levels in older men after adjusting for other factors such as age, body mass index, and estrogen levels. In one large longitudinal study of 2447 men over the age of 65 years, the prevalence of osteoporosis of the hip increased as total or bioavailable estradiol levels declined (Fink et al., 2006). In the same study, there was also an increased incidence of osteoporosis in men whose total testosterone levels were less than 200 ng/dL, but no increasing risk of osteoporosis as testosterone declined above this threshold (see Figure 6.16). One interpretation of these data would be that estrogens are more directly involved than are testosterone in the maintenance of bone health in elderly men. Very low testosterone levels below 200 ng/dL could still have an adverse effect by lowering estradiol formation through a reduced peripheral conversion of testosterone to estrogen.

In young men with testosterone deficiency, testosterone replacement clearly increases BMD whether the testosterone deficiency is due to a congenital defect or acquired disease. In one study of 72 men with hypogonadism, testosterone replacement for up to 16 years led to a sustained

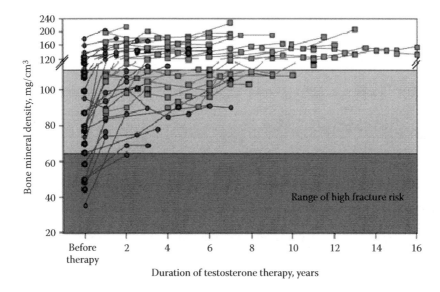

FIGURE 6.17 Changes in spinal bone density in hypogonadal men receiving testosterone. Increases in bone mineral density, as measured by quantitative computed tomography, are shown in 23 men receiving long-term testosterone therapy. The data show measurements made before initiation of testosterone therapy and follow-up measurements made after 2 years of testosterone therapy. The greatest increase in bone density occurred in the first year of therapy. (Data from Behre, H.M., et al., *J Clin Endocrinol Metab*, 82, 2386–2390, 1997.)

improvement in BMD in the lumber spine, as measured by quantitative computed tomography (see Figure 6.17). The mean bone density increased from 95 to 120 mg/cm³ in the first year of treatment (Behre et al., 1997). None of the observational studies in younger men have been placebo-controlled trials with a sufficient number of subjects to demonstrate a reduction in fracture risk.

Clinical trials testing the effects of testosterone on BMD in older men have yielded mixed results. In one study of 108 men over the age of 65 years, using transdermal testosterone hip and spine bone density improved no more in the treated subjects than in the placebo group (Snyder et al., 1999). The mean serum testosterone in this trial was 367 ng/dL (still within the normal range). In another trial using intramuscular testosterone in a group of 70 men whose mean testosterone was <350 ng/dL (below the normal range), spine and hip densities were significantly improved in the treated group (Amory et al., 2004). The difference in results may be accounted for by the differences in initial testosterone concentration in the two studies or possibly by differences in the mode of testosterone administration. None of the clinical trial data in older men are sufficient to judge whether any form of testosterone therapy is effective in reducing fractures. Because of the continuing uncertainties regarding therapeutic effectiveness in elderly men, testosterone should probably be used for the treatment of osteoporosis only in combination with other proven drugs, such as bisphosphonates and teriparatide, in subjects where the serum testosterone is clearly low.

GLUCOCORTICOIDS

The adrenals secrete several types of steroids including glucocorticoids, mineralocorticoids, and androgens. Adrenal androgens have been discussed earlier in the sections on estrogens and androgens. The glucocorticoids, typified by cortisol, are essential for life because of their physiological roles in supporting vital functions such as the maintenance of blood pressure and normal glucose homeostasis. A temporary increase in the secretion of cortisol is part of the normal response of the body to stress. At high concentrations, glucocorticoids can suppress the inflammatory and immune responses of the body to a variety of injurious stimuli. Glucocorticoids do not play a significant physiological role in calcium homeostasis, but at persistent high concentrations, they do promote a strongly negative calcium balance. Thus, a chronic excess of cortisol or other more potent synthetic glucocorticoids is an important risk factor for the development of osteoporosis.

Sources of Glucocorticoids and Causes of Glucocorticoid Excess

More than 70 years ago, Harvey Cushing described osteoporosis in patients with pituitary tumors and adrenal hyperplasia. Patients with endogenous overproduction of cortisol (Cushing's syndrome) usually have either adrenocorticotropin (ACTH)-producing pituitary tumors or cortisol-producing tumors of the adrenal glands. Osteoporosis in such patients can be prevented by appropriate therapy designed to reduce cortisol secretion. Endogenous Cushing's syndrome is relatively uncommon. Unfortunately, iatrogenic Cushing's syndrome, due to the administration of exogenous glucocorticoids by physicians, occurs quite frequently. Very potent synthetic glucocorticoids such as prednisone, methylprednisolone, and dexamethasone are widely used for treating a variety of inflammatory and immune-mediated diseases in patients with no underlying abnormalities in adrenal function. An estimated 0.2%–0.5% of the population of the United States is using glucocorticoids chronically at any given time (Adler et al., 2008). Examples of some of the conditions typically treated with glucocorticoids are listed in Table 6.3.

Effects of Glucocorticoid Excess on Bone Metabolism and Calcium Balance

Direct Effects on Bone Cells

Glucocorticoids at supraphysiologic concentrations directly inhibit osteoblastic activity by interacting with cytoplasmic glucocorticoid receptors. In adult bone, glucocorticoid receptors are present in pre-osteoblast/stromal cells and osteoblasts (Abu et al., 2000). The predominant effect is reduced bone formation. There is a reduced expression of procollagen genes and reduced synthesis

TABLE 6.3
Uses of Glucocorticoids for Treating Inflammatory and Immune-Mediated Diseases

Disease Category	Examples
Allergic diseases	Acute hypersensitivity reactions
	Serum sickness
	Allergic drug reactions
Blood dyscrasias	Acute leukemias, lymphomas
	Autoimmune thrombocytopenia
	Autoimmune hemolytic anemias
Collagen vascular diseases	Rheumatoid arthritis
	Systemic lupus erythematosis
	Temporal arteritis
	Polymyalgia rheumatica
Gastrointestinal diseases	Ulcerative colitis
	Crohn's disease
Pulmonary diseases	Asthma
	Chronic obstructive pulmonary disease
Renal diseases	Autoimmune glomerulitis
Neurological diseases	Multiple sclerosis
	Myasthenia gravis
Skin disorders	Allergic dermatitis (various types)
	Pemphigus and other bullous diseases
	Poison ivy and other exposures
Transplantation medicine	Patients with heart, lung, kidney, or
	liver transplants

of collagen and other matrix proteins. Osteoblast proliferation is inhibited, and there is increased osteoblast and osteocyte apoptosis, leading to a reduced number of active osteoblasts (Weinstein et al., 1998).

Glucocorticoids increase bone resorption, probably through indirect mechanisms. Mature osteoclasts do not have glucocorticoid receptors and are not directly responsive, but glucocorticoids still increase overall osteoclastic activity by promoting osteoclast proliferation (Kaji et al., 1997). They suppress the synthesis of OPG, an inhibitor of osteoclast differentiation, and stimulate the synthesis of RANK ligand by pre-osteoblast/stromal cells (Khosla, 2001).

Extraskeletal Effects of Glucocorticoids on Calcium Balance

High concentrations of glucocorticoids exert indirect effects on bone metabolism through several other mechanisms in intact humans. They decrease the synthesis of androgens and estrogens primarily by inhibiting the secretion of hypothalamic gonadotropin-releasing hormone and pituitary gonadotropins. They decrease the GI absorption of calcium without impairing the production of calcitriol or binding to its intestinal receptors. The mechanism for this effect is poorly understood. However, in rats, glucocorticoids reduce the resistance to passive paracellular calcium diffusion, resulting in increased serosal-to-mucosal backflux (Yeh et al., 1984). This "leakage" of calcium into the intestinal lumen may account for a reduced net absorption from the GI tract, although calcitriol-mediated absorption is not impaired. High serum concentrations of glucocorticoids also tend to increase urinary excretion of calcium. This effect may be due in part to an increase in the filtered load of calcium (Lemann et al., 1970) but may also be due to a decrease in renal tubular calcium reabsorption. In patients with hyperparathyroidism and a high filtered load of calcium, administration of glucocorticoids causes marked hypercalciuria (Breslau et al., 1982).

The effects of high concentrations of glucocorticoids on bone cells as well as the extraskeletal effects on the GI tract and the kidney are summarized in Figure 6.18. The combined actions on bone, gut, and kidney can result in a rapid decrease in bone mass and a negative overall calcium balance.

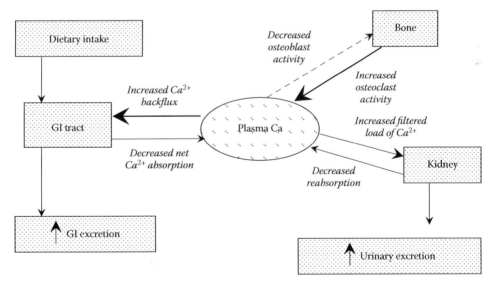

FIGURE 6.18   Results of glucocorticoid excess on calcium balance. The primary effect is on osteoblasts leading to reduced osteoblast numbers and reduced synthesis of bone matrix proteins. Osteoclast numbers and activity are increased. Reduced bone formation and increased bone resorption lead to a decrease in bone mass. Net gastrointestinal absorption of calcium is decreased, whereas urinary excretion of calcium is increased, also contributing to the net negative calcium balance.

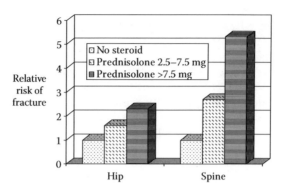

FIGURE 6.19 Effects of low-dose prednisolone on bone. The relative risk of both spine and hip fractures increases progressively, with daily prednisolone doses beginning with as little as 2.5–7.5 mg/day. This dose of prednisolone is equivalent to 12.5–37.5 mg/day of hydrocortisone. (Data from van Staa, T.P., et al., *Arthritis Rheum*, 48, 3224–3229, 2003.)

Glucocorticoid-Induced Osteoporosis

Glucocorticoid-induced osteoporosis is the most common form of drug-induced osteoporosis. Depending on the glucocorticoid dose, there is typically a loss of 1.5%–3% of bone mass during the first 6 months of therapy (Adler et al., 2008). Trabecular bone is initially most affected, followed by a loss of cortical bone. After 2 years of continuous therapy, the rate of bone loss slows to 1.5%–3% per year but continues at a higher rate than normal for the age and sex of the patient. Fractures increase within the first 6 months of therapy and may even precede measurable changes in bone density. Several studies have observed that fractures begin to occur at a higher BMD threshold in patients with glucocorticoid-induced osteoporosis than that in patients with typical postmenopausal osteoporosis (van Staa et al., 2003; Kanis et al., 2004). This suggests that alterations in bone "quality" or microarchitecture may precede changes in overall bone mass.

A safe dose of glucocorticoid low enough to avoid the increased risk of osteoporosis has never been clearly established. In an observational study of 240,000 glucocorticoid-treated patients in the United Kingdom, there was a trend toward increased hip and spine fractures even at "physiological" doses of prednisolone of 2.5 to 7.5 mg/day, as shown in Figure 6.19. Cumulative glucocorticoid dose over time appears to be the most important predictor of bone loss (van Staa et al., 2007). Limited information on alternate day therapy suggests that this regimen is not necessarily protective of bone (Gluck et al., 1981).

Fracture Risk Reduction in Glucocorticoid-Induced Osteoporosis

Glucocorticoids were first used over 60 years ago to treat inflammatory diseases. Although other anti-inflammatory and immunosuppressant drugs are now available, these drugs also have significant associated side effects. In the future, it is likely that glucocorticoids will continue to be widely used because of their low cost and therapeutic effectiveness. Several approaches should be effective in reducing fracture risk in patients requiring long-term glucocorticoid therapy. First, the dose of glucocorticoid should be reduced as quickly as possible to the lowest amount required to maintain control of the underlying disease. Topical or regional steroid administration is often a feasible alternative when the disease process is locally confined, for example, to the bronchial tree, a localized area of skin, or a single joint. Topical administration of glucocorticoid derivatives that are designed to act locally and to be poorly absorbed into the general circulation can yield therapeutic benefits and minimize systemic side effects. Lifestyle modifications including exercise and nutrition are effective in reducing the risk of fractures in patients who are expected to take systemic glucocorticoids for a period of 6 months or more. Smoking cessation, increased weight-bearing exercise, and reduction in alcohol intake are examples of modifiable risk factors that can reduce fracture risk, even in patients continuing on glucocorticoid therapy.

Dietary Supplementation

All guidelines for the prevention of glucocorticoid-induced osteoporosis recommend calcium intakes of at least 1200 mg/day. To achieve this, calcium supplements are usually required because the diets of most glucocorticoid users are insufficient in calcium. In addition, vitamin D supplements should be administered to maintain serum levels of 25-hydroxyvitamin D of at least 30 ng/mL. For most adults over the age of 50 years, the required amount will be at least 1000 IU/day of vitamin D3. Some patients with less efficiency in absorbing the vitamin will require more. This means that vitamin D therapy should be guided by actual serum measurements in individual patients and not by a predetermined dose. A number of clinical trials have used more active vitamin D derivatives such as alfacalcidiol and calcitriol to prevent bone loss in patients on long-term glucocorticoids. Meta-analyses of these trials have concluded that virtually all vitamin D analogs are more effective in reducing fracture risk than no vitamin D therapy at all (de Nijs et al., 2004; Richy et al., 2005). Regardless of the type of vitamin D preparation used, hip fracture rates remained high, especially in patients over 50 years old or with previous fragility fractures, suggesting that dietary supplementation, although useful, was not sufficient for alleviating all risks.

Antiosteoporosis Drugs

The availability of effective antiosteoporosis drugs, particularly the bisphosphonates, has greatly changed the management of patients on chronic glucocorticoid therapy. Several bisphosphonates, including alendronate, risedronate, and zoledronate, have been shown to protect against bone loss in patients on glucocorticoids and are approved by the Food and Drug Administration for this indication (Adler et al., 2008). Fracture risk reduction in trials with alendronate and risedronate ranged from 38% to 90%.

Teriparatide (synthetic PTH 1-34) is also an effective agent in reducing fracture risk. In a 3-year clinical trial comparing the effects of teriparatide versus those of alendronate in 428 subjects with glucocorticoid-induced osteoporosis, both treatments significantly increased BMD, but teriparatide had a greater effect (Saag et al., 2009). Fewer subjects in the teriparatide group had new vertebral fractures than did subjects in the alendronate group (1.7% vs. 7.7%, $P = .007$). There was no difference in the incidence of new nonvertebral fractures.

Sex steroid replacement may be appropriate for some patients. Estrogen replacement reverses or stabilizes bone loss in postmenopausal women on long-term glucocorticoids (Lukert and Raisz, 1990), although there is no information documenting a beneficial effect on fracture risk. As discussed earlier in the section on estrogen therapy, there are potential adverse effects from long-term estrogen replacement therapy that argue against the use of estrogens as first-line therapy when other effective agents are available. Testosterone replacement in men with glucocorticoid-induced hypogonadism is also effective in reducing bone loss. In one study of 15 asthmatic men on long-term glucocorticoid therapy, there was a 5% improvement of bone density in the lumbar spine after treatment for 12 months with intramuscular injections of testosterone (Reid et al., 1996).

Guidelines for Dietary and Drug Management

Based on the available evidence of fracture risk and the effects of various interventions, several organizations have issued guidelines for the prevention and treatment of glucocorticoid-induced osteoporosis. The American College of Rheumatology recommends that all patients receiving the equivalent of ≥5 mg/day of prednisone for 3 months or having a BMD *T*-score below −1.0 receive the following:

1. Calcium and vitamin D supplementation (1000 to 1500 mg/day and 800 IU/day, respectively).
2. Bisphosphonate therapy using an approved drug at the standard dose. Caution should be used in administering bisphosphonates to premenopausal women who might become pregnant. If bisphosphonates are not tolerated, the use of teriparatide or calcitonin should be considered.
3. Replacement of testosterone in men if deficient.
4. Annual measurement of BMD for follow-up.

THYROID HORMONES AND BONE METABOLISM

Introduction

The thyroid gland produces two closely related hormones, thyroxine (T4) and triiodothyronine (T3). These hormones act on nuclear receptors belonging to the same family as the steroid hormone receptors and control the expression of thyroid-hormone-responsive genes in multiple body tissues, including bone. Both T4 and T3 are derived from thyroglobulin, an iodinated glycoprotein that is synthesized by thyroid follicular cells within the gland. The uptake of iodine by thyroid cells, the synthesis of thyroglobulin, and the cleavage and release of T4 and T3 are all controlled by thyroid-stimulating hormone (TSH) from the pituitary gland.

The thyroid gland secretes virtually 100% of circulating T4 but only 20% of circulating T3. The remaining 80% of T3 is derived from T4 by conversion in peripheral tissues, particularly the liver, where an enzyme (5′-deiodinase) removes an iodine atom from the outer ring of T4 to yield T3. An alternative enzyme (3′-deiodinase) removes an alternative iodine atom, yielding an inactive isomeric product known as reverse T3. The sources of circulating T4, T3, and reverse T3 are illustrated in Figure 6.20. Over 99% of T4 and T3 in the circulation are bound to thyroid-binding globulin and other binding proteins produced by the liver.

A classical negative feedback relationship exists between circulating levels of T4 and T3 and pituitary secretion of TSH, which operates to maintain constant concentrations of both thyroid hormones within the circulation. When serum concentrations of free T3 and T4 rise, due to either endogenous thyroid secretion or to administration of exogenous thyroid hormones, pituitary TSH secretion is inhibited, resulting in decreased thyroid secretion. Small increases in thyroid hormone supply can be buffered by decreased stimulation by TSH up to a point. With further increases in supply, serum concentrations of T3 and T4 eventually rise. Thus, patients with mild hyperthyroidism typically have a suppressed serum TSH but maintain T3 and T4 concentrations within the normal range. Such patients have few symptoms and are described as having "subclinical hyperthyroidism." Patients with more severe hyperthyroidism typically have not only suppressed serum TSH but also elevated serum levels of T3 and T4.

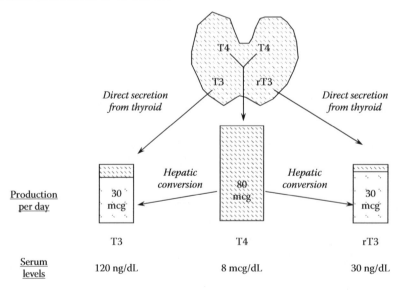

FIGURE 6.20 Sources of thyroid hormones in the circulation. The thyroid gland is the sole source of T4 (levothyroxine). The thyroid secretes smaller quantities of T3 (3,5,3′-triiodothyronine) and reverse T3 (3,3′,5′-triiodothyronine). The majority of circulating T3 and reverse T3 are produced in the liver from T4 by either a 5′-deiodinase (for T3) or a 5-deiodinase (reverse T3). T3 has a higher affinity for the thyroid hormone receptor than T4. Reverse T3 is biologically inactive.

Thyroid hormones act on virtually every tissue in the body. There are two thyroid hormone receptor isoforms, TRα and TRβ. Both receptors are expressed in most tissues, but their levels of expression vary depending on the organ. TRα is most abundantly expressed in the brain, kidney, gonads, muscle, heart, and bone, whereas TRβ is more highly expressed in pituitary and liver. T3 is bound with 10–15 times greater affinity to both receptors than is T4, explaining its greater potency. Once thyroid hormone binds to its intracellular receptor, the receptors bind together as dimers and interact with thyroid hormone response elements in the promoter regions of target genes leading to either increased or decreased gene expression.

Actions on Skeletal Tissue

Thyroid hormones play a role in skeletal growth and maturation and are necessary for normal chondrocyte development (Baran, 2008). The mechanisms of action are complex and still incompletely understood. T4 and T3 regulate heparin sulfate proteoglycan expression in the growth plate during endochondral bone formation and play a role in bone maturation. After bone growth is completed, thyroid hormones increase the activity of both osteoblasts and osteoclasts. T3 can act on osteoblast cells in vitro, increasing their overall activity in part through mediation of growth factors including insulin-like growth factor-I (IGF-I) and fibroblast growth factor (FGF) (Pepene et al., 2001). Circulating IGF-I levels are decreased in patients with hypothyroidism, who typically show decreased rates of bone formation. T3 also increases osteoclast activity. The effect may be mediated in part by the RANK–RANK ligand system through effects on osteoblasts but could also represent a more direct action. T3 increases the expression of c-fos mRNA in osteoclast precursors, suggesting a mechanism independent of RANK ligand–RANK interaction (Kanatani et al., 2004).

Effects of Thyroid Hormone Excess on Bone Health

Overt untreated hyperthyroidism is associated with accelerated bone remodeling, reduced bone density, and an increased fracture rate. Although bone formation rates are increased, bone resorption is increased even further so that there is a net efflux of calcium and phosphorus from bone. PTH secretion is inhibited, and urinary calcium excretion is increased. If urinary clearance of the added calcium load is insufficient to maintain calcium homeostasis, hypercalcemia can develop. Histomorphometric studies of the bone remodeling cycle in hyperthyroid subjects have shown a pronounced shortening of the 200-day length of the normal cycle by as much as 50%. Because osteoclastic and osteoblastic activities are out of balance, significant bone loss occurs with every completed cycle (Eriksen, 1986). In hypothyroid patients, the length of the cycle can double.

The degree of bone loss in several studies of patient cohorts with long-term hyperthyroidism is in the range of 10%–20%. Some studies have shown partial recovery of bone density after thyroid hormone levels are reduced by appropriate treatment (Nielsen et al., 1979; Rosen and Adler, 1992; Diamond et al., 1994; Karga et al., 2004). The risk of fractures is also increased in hyperthyroidism. In one prospective cohort study of 686 white women over the age of 65 years, those with hyperthyroidism were identified by the presence of a low TSH of less than 0.1 mU/L (normal 0.4–4.5 mU/L). (In this subgroup of women, excess circulating thyroid hormones had suppressed serum TSH levels by the negative feedback relationship discussed above.) The relative risks of hip and vertebral fractures were increased in the hyperthyroid subjects by factors of 3.6 and 4.5, respectively, after a mean follow-up of 3.7 years (Bauer et al., 2001).

It is still unclear how severe and prolonged hyperthyroidism must be in order for adverse skeletal effects to occur. Many patients being treated with thyroid hormone for hypothyroidism actually become mildly hyperthyroid, due to excessive thyroid hormone administration. Typically, these patients have a moderately suppressed serum TSH and a serum T4 still within the normal range. Most of them have no symptoms of hyperthyroidism and are considered to have subclinical hyperthyroidism (see above). Several studies have shown that postmenopausal women with subclinical hyperthyroidism have accelerated bone loss (Ross et al., 1987; Lehmke et al., 1992; Franklyn et al., 1994), but adverse effects have been less apparent in premenopausal women and men. One meta-analysis suggested a significant reduction in bone mass only in postmenopausal women (Faber and Galloe, 1994), whereas a second meta-analysis showed adverse effects in premenopausal women as well (Uzzan et al., 1996). Fracture rates have been increased in some studies of patients with iatrogenic subclinical hyperthyroidism (Bauer et al., 2001; Flynn et al., 2010) but not in all (Leese et al., 1992). The risk is probably related not only to the severity and duration of TSH suppression but also to the age of the patients studied. Subclinical hyperthyroidism poses a greater risk for elderly women than it does for premenopausal women or men. Clearly, thyroid hormone replacement therapy per se does not increase the risk of fracture if not given in excess.

In summary, hyperthyroidism has a deleterious effect on bone health proportionate to its severity and duration. Most patients with a suppressed serum TSH and elevated serum T3 and T4 (overt hyperthyroidism) should be treated promptly to reduce their thyroid hormone levels to normal. In patients with only a suppressed TSH who have no symptoms of hyperthyroidism (subclinical hyperthyroidism), immediate therapy may not be required unless the patient has other risk factors for osteoporosis. Postmenopausal women with subclinical hyperthyroidism should be treated because of the prevailing clinical evidence that they are more likely to suffer bone loss and fractures if their mild hyperthyroidism is left untreated.

GROWTH HORMONE AND IGF-I

Introduction

GH is most critical to bone health during childhood and adolescence when it plays a primary role in promoting linear bone growth. GH acts together with other hormones, including sex steroids and thyroid hormone, to promote formation and development of the growth plate and new bone formation. The rate of growth is most rapid during fetal life, and again at puberty, when a growth spurt typically occurs. GH secretion normally peaks during adolescence and then declines steadily during adult life. By middle age, GH secretion rates are typically only 15% of the rates during puberty (Melmed and Jameson, 2006).

GH is a 191-amino-acid polypeptide whose secretion is controlled by two hypothalamic factors, growth hormone releasing hormone (GHRH) and somatostatin. GHRH and somatostatin are both secreted by specific hypothalamic neurons and transported to the anterior pituitary gland via portal blood vessels where they interact with specific receptors on GH-producing cells. GHRH, the dominant hypothalamic factor controlling GH secretion, has a stimulatory effect, whereas somatostatin has an inhibitory effect. The production and release of GHRH and somatostatin in the hypothalamus are controlled by a complex variety of CNS stimuli, including sleep, exercise, and hypoglycemia. Plasma concentrations of GH vary throughout the day, depending on the balance between the effects of GHRH and somatostatin at any given time. Peak levels are typically seen at night within an hour after the onset of deep sleep. The main factors involved in the regulation of GH secretion are illustrated in Figure 6.21.

GH circulates in the plasma bound to a GH-binding protein with a structure similar to that of the extracellular domain of the GH receptor. To interact with its receptor, GH first dissociates from the binding protein and then binds to the extracellular domain of the receptor in target tissues. Receptor binding induces dimerization of GH–receptor complexes followed by signaling through the JAK/STAT intracellular pathway. The activated STAT proteins translocate to the cell nucleus where they modulate the expression of GH-responsive genes. The metabolic effects of GH action in addition to linear growth in children include nitrogen retention with enhanced lean body mass and lipolysis with decreased fat mass in both children and adults (Melmed and Jameson, 2006).

Most of the growth-promoting effects of GH on peripheral tissues are exerted via IGF-I. IGF-I is a polypeptide with some structural similarities to insulin, but with distinct receptors. It is

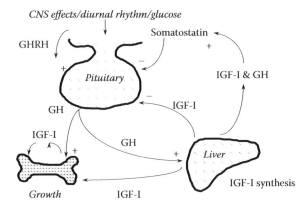

FIGURE 6.21 The complex control of growth hormone and insulin-like growth factor I secretion. GH is secreted by the anterior pituitary under the influence of two hypothalamic hormones. GHRH is stimulatory, and somatostatin is inhibitory for GH release. GH acts on target tissues including liver and bone to stimulate the synthesis and release of IGF-I. IGF-I may act locally to promote mitogenesis in its tissue of origin, as in bone, or may be secreted into the circulation, as from the liver. Circulating IGF-I exerts a negative feedback directly on the pituitary gland to downregulate GH secretion. Together, IGF-I and GH also act on the hypothalamus to stimulate somatostatin secretion, thereby reducing GH secretion by the pituitary. GHRH and somatostatin secretion is regulated by a number of other physiological variables mediated by the central nervous system, including sleep, stress, and the prevailing blood glucose concentration.

a potent mitogenic agent produced by multiple tissues under the influence of GH. Most of the IGF-I in plasma originates from the liver and acts as a circulating growth factor. IGF-I can also be produced directly by bone and connective tissue cells and act locally on neighboring cells to promote growth. Under normal conditions, there is a close correlation between circulating levels of IGF-I and GH. Patients with a deficiency of GH will typically have low plasma levels of both GH and IGF-I.

IGF-I participates together with GHRH and somatostatin in the feedback regulation of GH secretion (see Figure 6.21). When IGF-I levels rise, GH secretion normally tends to fall. In a rare condition known as Laron dwarfism involving a loss-of-function mutation in the GH receptor, IGF-I is not produced. Patients with this condition have short stature in spite of normal or high GH levels because their peripheral tissues fail to respond to GH.

IGF-I is a single-chain polypeptide with 70 amino acids. It is structurally distinct from IGF-II, a related peptide that also has mitogenic activity, but is not GH dependent. IGF-I in the circulation is mostly bound to serum IGF binding proteins (IGFBPs). These binding proteins serve as a storage reservoir, prolonging the half life of circulating IGF and affecting its distribution among various tissues. The most important binding protein is IGFBP-3, whose synthesis is also stimulated by GH (Rosen and Niu, 2008).

The IFG-I receptor is structurally homologous to the insulin receptor and the IGF-II receptor but has a higher affinity for IGF-I than for insulin or IGF-II. This receptor has intrinsic tyrosine kinase activity which is critical for second messenger generation after IGF-I binding occurs. Intracellular signaling involves the JAK/STAT and mitogen-activated protein kinase (MAPK) pathways (Rosen and Niu, 2008). When activated, the IGF-I receptor has antiapoptotic effects in several cell types, including osteoblasts and osteocytes (Le Roith et al., 1997).

Effects of GH and IGF-I on Bone Metabolism

The overall effects of GH on bone are anabolic in adults as well as in children. However, the effects of GH on bone remodeling are complex because there are both circulating and local sources of IGF-I that may interact with bone cells. In vitro both GH and IGF-I have mitogenic effects on osteoblastic cell lines. GH induces the local synthesis of IGF-I by bone cells. The mitogenic effects of GH on osteoblasts can be blocked by the addition of specific monoclonal antibodies to IGF-I (Mohan and Baylink, 1991). IGF-I is mitogenic when added to cultures of rodent preosteoblasts, rapidly increasing the expression of the protooncogene c-fos (Merriman et al., 1990). IGF-I can increase collagen synthesis, alkaline phosphatase activity, and osteocalcin production in osteoblasts and can act as an antiapoptotic factor for differentiated osteoblasts (Rosen and Niu, 2008).

Although a major effect of IGF-I is exerted on osteoblasts, it also plays a role in the coupling of osteoblast activity with osteoclast recruitment and activation, either directly through the IGF-I receptor or through the RANK–RANK ligand pathway (Mochizuki et al., 1992; Rubin et al., 2002). Both in vitro and in vivo, the absence of IGF-I impairs osteoclast recruitment and activation (Wang et al., 2006).

The effects of GH deficiency on skeletal development and growth in children are clear cut. Linear bone growth is impaired and skeletal maturation is usually retarded. Children with GH deficiency have low bone mass, as measured by techniques such as single-photon absorptiometry (Wuster et al., 1992).

In adults, the skeletal effects of GH deficiency are more difficult to define than those in children. This is due in part to the fact that serum GH and IGF-I levels normally decline with aging. In adults, severe GH deficiency usually occurs in association with panhypopituitarism and is accompanied by deficiencies of gonadal and adrenal steroids as well as thyroid hormone. In such patients, the frequent underreplacement of estrogen and testosterone, as well as the possibility of overreplacement with glucocorticoids and thyroid hormone, make it more difficult to identify skeletal effects due solely to GH deficiency. With these reservations in mind, there is much evidence suggesting that adult GH deficiency is associated with low bone turnover osteoporosis and increased fracture risk (Guistina et al., 2008; Rosen and Niu, 2008). Several cross-sectional studies of adults with GH deficiency have found lumbar spine BMD reduced in comparison with those of age- and sex-matched controls (Johansson et al., 1992; Holmes et al., 1994; Colao et al., 1999) and fracture rates increased (Wuster et al., 2001). Bone biopsies from adult males with GH deficiency show decreased osteoid and mineralizing surfaces, suggesting that impaired bone formation plays a dominant role (Bravenboer et al., 1996).

Evidence that declining GH secretion causes bone loss in healthy older adults is more conflicted. Some investigators studying older adults without evidence of pituitary disease have found a significant relationship between bone mass and serum levels IGF-I. In the Framingham Heart Study, there was a strong correlation between the lowest quintile for serum IGF-I and BMD of the spine and hip (Langlois et al., 1998). In males, correlations between low BMD and low concentrations of IGF-I and IGFBP-3 have been reported by several investigators (Ljunghall et al., 1992; Kurland et al., 1997). In one study of young men with idiopathic osteoporosis and low serum IGF-I, dynamic tests of GH secretion were normal, suggesting that factors other than GH deficiency may have been responsible for the low IGF-I levels (Kurland et al., 1998). Others have concluded that even in adults with well-documented GH deficiency, a deleterious effect on BMD is apparent only in younger individuals. Beyond the age of 60 years, no differences were noted between the bone density scores of patients with a history of GH deficiency and control subjects (Murray et al., 2004). In summary, strong evidence supports that GH deficiency plays a role in the pathogenesis of osteopenia in younger subjects with clear-cut pituitary deficiency. However, in other subjects without a history of pituitary disease, where correlations between low BMD and low IGF-I may exist, it is still unclear whether GH deficiency plays a critical role.

Therapy for Osteoporosis

GH replacement therapy using recombinant human growth hormone (rhGH) is now an accepted standard of care for children with GH deficiency. The results in terms of skeletal growth and improvement in BMD have been quite successful. In one observational study, 26 GH-deficient children were given rhGH for 12 months. During that period, the bone density scores (Z-scores) were normalized in nearly 50% of subjects (Saggese et al., 1993). In children with short stature due to causes other than GH deficiency, GH treatment has not improved BMD despite increases in lean body mass (Rosen and Niu, 2008).

In GH-deficient adults, GH replacement therapy causes an increase in serum IGF-I and in lean body mass within 2 weeks. Markers of bone metabolism, including serum osteocalcin and urinary hydroxyproline, routinely increase. The effects of GH replacement on bone density have varied depending on the age and sex of the patients and the dose of GH administered. In one of the few randomized, placebo-controlled clinical trials using "physiological" doses of GH to normalize serum IGF-I, spine BMD increased by nearly 4% in men but did not improve significantly in women. Neither men nor women showed significant improvement in hip BMD (Snyder et al., 2007). Thus far, no clinical trials of sufficient size to examine fractures as a clinical outcome have been reported.

Only a few small trials of GH therapy have been reported in osteoporotic patients without preexisting GH deficiency. The results of these trials, some of which included combinations of GH with antiresorptive agents, have been inconclusive. Likewise, there have been only limited short-term trials testing the effects of recombinant IGF-I administration to adults with osteopenia. In one group of women with anorexia nervosa and low bone mass, IGF-I therapy for 9 months increased spine BMD by 1.1%, whereas a combination of IGF-I and estrogen yielded a 1.8% increase. Subjects receiving placebo experienced bone loss over the same period (Grinspoon et al., 2002).

Currently, therapy with GH and IGF-I holds promise for the treatment of osteoporosis, particularly in subjects with well-defined GH deficiency. These agents are not currently approved for the treatment of osteoporosis because of their high cost, potential long-term side effects, and lack of demonstrated efficacy in fracture reduction. Active therapeutic research with anabolic agents is ongoing and may yield more favorable results in the future, particularly in combination with antiresorptive drugs.

SUMMARY AND CONCLUSIONS

The maintenance of a constant concentration of calcium ions in the extracellular fluid is of critical importance in most multicellular organisms. In man, calcium homeostasis is regulated primarily by the endocrine system through the actions of PTH and 1,25-dihydroxyvitamin D (calcitriol). PTH secretion is regulated by a negative feedback of calcium ions acting through a CaSR in the plasma membrane of parathyroid cells and by a negative feedback of calcitriol acting to inhibit the synthesis of PTH mRNA. In the presence of reduced dietary intake of calcium and vitamin D, serum concentrations of PTH are typically elevated and renal conversion of 25-hydroxyvitamin D to calcitriol is stimulated. Conversely, an excess of dietary calcium or vitamin D downregulates both PTH secretion and calcitriol synthesis.

The most important organs mediating calcium homeostasis are the GI tract, the kidney, and bone itself, which contains 99% of the calcium in the human body. GI absorption of dietary calcium is largely dependent on the presence of calcitriol. Under conditions where the dietary intake of calcium is limited, increased renal synthesis of calcitriol promotes more efficient absorption of calcium and phosphorus by the GI tract. Calcium deprivation also leads to hormonally mediated adjustments in the renal handling of calcium and phosphorus. Increased secretion of PTH stimulates increased renal tubular reabsorption of calcium from the glomerular filtrate, conserving calcium and helping to maintain calcium homeostasis.

Bone cells, primarily osteocytes and bone lining cells, mediate a rapid flux of calcium ions between bone and the extracellular fluid under the influence of PTH. Osteoclasts mediate a slower process of calcium resorption from hydroxyapatite. Bone lining cells, osteocytes, and osteoblasts (but not osteoclasts) have PTH receptors. PTH has a complex, biphasic effect on bone mineral content and calcium balance. One of the earliest effects of PTH is a direct stimulation of osteoblasts resulting in increased bone formation. A more delayed effect, seen with sustained high concentrations of

PTH, consists of an activation of osteoclasts resulting in increased bone resorption. The longer-term effect of PTH on bone resorption is not due to the direct action of PTH on osteoclasts but is mediated by cytokines including the RANK–RANK ligand system. The differing responses of bone cells to short-term and long-term PTH exposure explain why patients with primary hyperparathyroidism due to PTH-secreting parathyroid tumors tend to lose bone mass, whereas patients given intermittent injections of active PTH analogs gain bone mass.

Several other hormones, although not primarily involved in maintaining calcium homeostasis, have significant effects on calcium balance and bone health. Estrogens play an important role in maintaining bone mass in both women and men largely by inhibiting bone resorption. In menopausal women, and also in elderly men, serum levels of estrogen decline, leading to increased bone loss and an increased risk of osteoporosis. The administration of estrogen or SERMs to postmenopausal women can increase BMD and reduce fracture risk.

Testosterone and other androgens promote bone formation by acting directly on ARs located on osteoblasts. Testosterone is also aromatized to estradiol in peripheral tissues and can thus have indirect estrogen-like effects on bone. The administration of testosterone to young men with testosterone deficiency clearly promotes increased bone mass, but the skeletal benefits in elderly men are less certain.

Glucocorticoids, including a number of synthetic derivatives used to suppress inflammatory and immune-mediated diseases, have deleterious effects on bone health. When administered at higher doses for several months, glucocorticoid derivatives lead to a loss of bone mass, largely through their direct inhibitory effects on osteoblast activity. They also reduce net calcium absorption from the GI tract. Glucocorticoid-induced osteoporosis is the most common form of drug-induced osteoporosis. Not only bone mineral content, but also bone microarchitecture is adversely affected, leading to increased fracture risk at a higher threshold of BMD. Dietary supplementation with calcium and vitamin D, as well as the use of bisphosphonates and other antiosteoporosis drugs, are effective in reducing fracture risk in patients who must be continued on glucocorticoid therapy.

Thyroid hormones, T3 and T4, play a physiological role in skeletal growth and maturation. In adult life, thyroid hormones increase the activity of both osteoblasts and osteoclasts, probably acting both directly and through cytokine mediators. At excessive thyroid hormone concentrations, bone resorption is typically increased disproportionately to bone formation, leading to reduced bone mass. The bone remodeling cycle is shortened. The risk of fracture is most significant in postmenopausal women, who already have a tendency to lose bone more rapidly. For this reason, it is particularly important to correct hyperthyroidism and to avoid overtreatment of hypothyroidism in postmenopausal women.

GH and IGF-I have significant anabolic effects on the skeleton. The growth-promoting effects on GH are mediated by IGF-I, a polypeptide produced in peripheral tissues under the influence of GH. GH plays a critical role in promoting linear bone growth and overall bone mass in childhood. During adult life, GH secretion and serum concentrations of IGF-I decline progressively with increasing age. Adults with severe GH deficiency due to pituitary disease typically have a low bone mass with evidence of impaired bone formation. It is less clear whether naturally declining GH secretion in older adults plays a critical role in the development of senile osteoporosis. Several small clinical trials of GH therapy in osteoporotic patients have been reported, but as yet none have demonstrated fracture reduction. Further evidence of efficacy will be required before GH, IGF-I, and related anabolic peptides can be approved as therapeutic agents for the treatment of osteoporosis.

REFERENCES

Abu, E.O., Horner, A., Kusec, V., et al. 2000. The localization of the functional glucocorticoid receptor in human bone. *J Clin Endocrinol Metab* 85: 883–889.

Adler, R.A., Curtis, J., Weinstein, R.S., et al. 2008. Glucocorticoid-induced osteopororosis. In *Osteoporosis*, 3rd Edition, Marcus, R., Feldman, D., Nelson, D.A., and Rosen, C.J., eds. Elsevier Academic Press, Burlington, MA, Chapter 44, 1135–1166.

Albright, F. 1947. Osteoporosis. *Ann Intern Med* 27: 861–882.

Amory, J.K., Watts, N.B., Easley, K.A., et al. 2004. Exogenous testosterone or testosterone with finasteride increases bone mineral density in older men with low serum testosterone. *J Clin Endocrinol Metab* 89: 503–510.

Arnold, A., Shattuck, T.M., Mallya, S.M., et al. 2002. Molecular pathogenesis of primary hyperparathyroidism. *J Bone Miner Res* 17 (Suppl 2): N30–N36.

Baran, D. 2008. Thyroid hormone and the skeleton. In *Osteoporosis*, 3rd Edition, Marcus, R., Feldman, D., Nelson, D.A., and Rosen, C.J., eds. Elsevier Academic Press, Burlington, MA, Chapter 48, 1195–1202.

Barrett-Connor, E., Mosca, L., Collins, P., et al. 2006. Effects of raloxifene on cardiovascular events and breast cancer in postmenopausal women. *New Engl J Med* 355: 125–137.

Bauer, D.C., Ettinger, B., Nevitt, M.C., et al. 2001. Risk for fracture in women with low serum levels of thyroid-stimulating hormone. *Ann Intern Med* 134: 561–568.

Behre, H.M., Kliesch, S., Leifke, F., et al. 1997. Long term effects of testosterone therapy on bone mineral density in hypogonadal men. *J Clin Endocrinol Metab* 82: 2386–2390.

Bravenboer, N., Holzmann, P., De Boer, H, et al. 1996. Histomorphometric analysis of bone mass and bone metabolism in growth hormone deficient adult men. *Bone* 18: 551–557.

Breslau, N.A., Zerwekh, J.E., Nicar, M.J., et al. 1982. Effects of short term glucocorticoid administration in primary hyperparathyroidism: Comparison to sarcoidosis. *J Clin Endocrinol Metab* 54: 824–830.

Bringhurst, F. R., and Leder, B.Z. 2006. Regulation of calcium and phosphate homeostasis. In *Textbook of Endocrinology*, 5th Edition, DeGroot, L.J., and Jameson, J.L., eds. Elsevier Saunders, Philadelphia, Chapter 74, 1465–1498.

Bronner, F., Pannu, D., and Stein, W.D. 1986. An analysis of intestinal calcium transport across rat intestine. *Am J Physiol* 250: G561–G569.

Brown, E.M. 1981. Lithium induces abnormal calcium-regulated PTH release in dispersed bovine parathyroid cells. *J Clin Endocrinol Metab* 52: 1046–1048.

Brown, E.M. 1983. Four parameter model of the sigmoidal relationship between PTH release and extracellular ionized calcium in normal and abnormal parathyroid tissue. *J Clin Endocrinol Metab* 56: 572–581.

Brown, E.M. 2002. The pathophysiology of primary hyperparathyroidism. *J Bone Miner Res* 17 (Suppl 2): N24–N29.

Brown, E.M. 2007. The calcium-sensing receptor: Physiology, pathophysiology and CaR-based therapeutics. *Subcell Biochem* 45: 139–167.

Brown, E.M. 2009. Anti-parathyroid and anti-calcium sensing receptor antibodies in autoimmune hypoparathyroidism. *Endocrinol Metab Clin North Am* 38: 437–445.

Brown, E.M., Gamba, G., Riccardi, D., et al. 1993. Cloning and characterization of an extracellular Ca^{2+}-sensing receptor. *Nature* 366: 575–580.

Brzozowski, A.M., Pike, A.C., Dauter, Z., et al. 1997. Molecular basis of agonism and antagonism in the oestrogen receptor. *Nature* 389: 753–758.

Cetani, F., Picone, L., Cerrai, P., et al. 2000. Parathyroid expression of calcium-sensing receptor protein and in vivo parathyroid hormone–Ca(2+) set-point in patients with primary hyperparathyroidism. *J Clin Endocrinol Metab* 85: 4789–4794.

Chambers, T.J., McSheehy, P.M., Thomson, B.M., et al. 1985. The effect of calcium regulating hormones and prostaglandins on bone resorption by osteoclasts disaggregated from neonatal rabbit bones. *Endocrinology* 116: 234–239.

Chang, C., Kokontis, J., and Liao, S. 1988. Structural analysis of complementary DNA and amino acid sequences of human and rat androgen receptors. *Proc Nat Acad Sci (USA)* 85: 7211–7215.

Chen, Q., Kaji, H., Kanatani, M., et al. 2004. Testosterone increases osteoprotegerin mRNA expression in mouse osteoblast cells. *Horm Metab Res* 36: 674–678.

Colao, A., Di Somma, C., Pivonello, R., et al. 1999. Bone loss is correlated to the severity of growth hormone deficiency in adult patients with hypopituitarism. *J Clin Endocrinol Metab* 84: 1919–1924.

Cosman, F., and Lindsay, R.L. 2008. Treatment with PTH peptides. In *Osteoporosis*, 3rd Edition, Marcus, R., Feldman, D., Nelson, D.A., and Rosen, C.J., eds. Elsevier Academic Press, Burlington, MA, Chapter 78, 1793–1808.

Couse, J.F., and Korach, K.S. 1999. Estrogen receptor null mice: What have we learned and where will they lead us? *Endocrinol Rev* 20: 358–417.

Cross, H.S., Debiec, H., and Peterlik, M. 1990. Mechanism and regulation of intestinal phosphate absorption. *Miner Electrolyte Metab* 16: 115–124.

de Nijs, R.N., Jacobs, J.W., Algra A., et al. 2004. Prevention and treatment of glucocorticoid-induced osteoporosis with active vitamin D3 analogs: A review with meta-analysis of randomized controlled clinical trials including organ transplantation studies. *Osteoporos Int* 15: 589–602.

den Dekker, E., Hoenderop, J.G., Nilius, B., et al. 2003. The epithelial calcium channels, TRPV5 & TRPV6: From identification towards regulation. *Cell Calcium* 33: 497–507.

Diamond, T., Vine, J., Smart, R. et al. 1994. Thyrotoxic bone disease in women: A potentially reversible disorder. *Ann Intern Med* 120: 8–11.

Diaz, R. and Brown, E.M. 2006. Familial hypocalciuric hypercalcemia and other disorders dud to calcium-sensing receptor mutations. In *Endocrinology*, 5th Edition, DeGroot, L.J., and Jameson, J.L., eds. Elsevier Saunders, Philadelphia, Chapter 81, 1595–1609.

Dusso, A.S., Brown, A.J., and Slatopolsky, E. 2005. Vitamin D. *Am J Physiol* 289: F8–F28.

Eriksen, E.F. 1986. Normal and pathological remodeling of human trabecular bone: Three dimensional reconstruction of the remodeling sequence in normals and in metabolic bone disease. *Endocrinol Rev* 7: 379–408.

Ettinger, B., Black, D.M., Mitlak, B.H., et al. 1999. Reduction of vertebral fracture risk in post-menopausal women with osteoporosis treated with raloxifene: Results from a 3-year randomized clinical trial. Multiple Outcomes of Raloxifene Evaluation (MORE). *JAMA* 282: 637–645.

Ettinger, B., Genant, H.K., and Cann, C.E. 1987. Postmenopsusal bone loss is prevented by treatment with low-dosage estrogen with calcium. *Ann Intern Med* 106: 40–45.

Faber, J., and Galloe, A.M. 1994. Changes in bone mass during prolonged subclinical hyperthyroidism due to L-thyroxine treatment: A meta analysis. *Eur J Endocrinol* 130: 350–356.

Fink, H.A., Ewing, S.K., Ensrud, K.E., et al. 2006. Association of testosterone and estradiol deficiency with osteoporosis and rapid bone loss in older men. *J Clin Endocrinol Metab* 91: 3908–3915.

Flynn, R.W., Bonellie, S.R., Jung, R.T., et al. 2010. Serum thyroid-stimulating hormone concentration and morbidity from cardiovascular disease and fractures in patients on long-term thyroxine therapy. *J Clin Endocrinol Metab* 95: 186–193.

Franklyn, J., Betteridge, J., Holder, R., et al. 1994. Bone mineral density in thyroxine treated females with or without a previous history of thyrotoxicosis. *Clin Endocrinol* 41: 425–432.

Gavalas, N.G., Kemp, E.H., Krohn, K.J., et al. 2007. The calcium-sensing receptor is a target of autoantibodies in patients with autoimmune polyendorrine syndrome type 1. *J Clin Endocrinol Metab* 92: 2107–2114.

Gennari, L., Nuti, R., and Bilezekian, J. 2004. Aromatase activity and bone homeostasis in men. *J Clin Endocrinol Metab* 89: 5898–5907.

Gluck, O.S., Murphy, W.A., Hahn, T.J., and Hahn, B. 1981. Bone loss in adults receiving alternate day glucocorticoid therapy. *Arthritis Rheum* 24: 892–898.

Grinspoon, S., Thomas, L., Miller, K., et al. 2002. Effects of recombinant human IGF-I and oral contraceptive administration on bone density in anorexia nervosa. *J Clin Endocrinol Metab* 87: 2883–2891.

Guistina, A., Mazziotti, G., and Canalis, E. 2008. Growth hormone, insulin-like growth factors, and the skeleton. *Endocr Rev* 29: 535–559.

Haden, S.T., Brown, E.M., Hutwitz, S., et al. 2000. The effects of age and gender on parathyroid hormone dynamics. *Clin Endocrinol* 52: 329–338.

Haden, S.T., Stoll, A.L., McCormick, S., et al. 1997. Alterations in parathyroid hormone dynamics in lithium-treated subjects. *J Clin Endocrinol Metab* 82: 2844–2848.

Harman, S.M., Metter, E.J., Tobin, J.D., et al. 2001. Longitudinal effects of aging on serum total and free testosterone levels in healthy men. Baltimore Longitudinal Study of Aging. *J Clin Endocrinol Metab* 86: 724–731.

Hebert, S.C. 1996. Extracellular calcium-sensing receptor: Implications for calcium and magnesium handling in the kidney. *Kidney Int* 50: 2129–2139.

Hendy, G.N. 2000. Molecular mechanisms of primary hyperparathyroidism. *Rev Endocr Metab Disord* 1: 297–305.

Hoenderop, J.G., Muller, D., Van Der Kemp, A.W., et al. 2001. Calcitriol controls the epithelial calcium channel in kidney. *J Am Soc Nephrol* 12: 1342–1349.

Hoenderop, J.G., Nilius, B., and Bindels, R.J. 2002. Molecular mechanism of active Ca^{2+} reabsorption in the distal nephron. *Annu Rev Physiol* 64: 529–549.

Holmes, S.J., Economouu, G., Whitehouse, R.W., et al. 1994. Reduced bone mineral density in patients with adult onset growth hormone deficiency. *J Clin Endocrinol Metab* 78: 669–674.

Huang, J.C., Sakata, L.L., Pfleger, M., et al. 2004. PTH differentially regulates expression of RANKL and OPG. *J Bone Miner Res* 19: 235–244.

Johansson, A.G., Burman, P., Westermark, K., et al. 1992. The bone mineral density in acquired growth hormone deficiency correlates with circulating levels of insulin-like growth factor I. *J Internal Med* 232: 447–452.

Juppner, H., Gardella, T.J., Brown, E.M., et al. 2006. Parathyroid hormone and parathyroid hormone-related peptide in the regulation of calcium homeostasis and bone development. In *Endocrinology*, 5th Edition, DeGroot, L., and Jameson, J.L., eds. Elsevier Saunders, Philadelphia, Chapter 71, 1377–1417.

Kaji, H., Sugimoto, T., Kanatani, M., et al. 1997. Dexamethasone stimulates osteoclast-like cell formation by directly acting on hemopoietic blast cells and enhances osteoclast-like cell formation stimulated by parathyroid hormone and prostaglandin E-2. *J Bone Miner Res* 12: 734–741.

Kallner, G., and Petterson, U. 1995. Renal thyroid and parathyroid function during lithium treatment: Laboratory tests in 207 people treated for 1–30 years. *Acta Psychiatr Scand* 91: 48–51.

Kanatani, M., Sugimoto, T., Sowa, H., et al. 2004. Thyroid hormone stimulates osteoclast differentiation by a mechanism independent of RANKL–RANK interaction. *J Cell Physiol* 201: 17–25.

Kanis, J.A., Johansen, H.K., Oden, A., et al. 2004. A meta-analysis of prior corticosteroid use and fracture risk. *J Bone Miner Res* 19: 893–899.

Karbach, U. 1992. Paracellular calcium transport across the small intestine. *J Nutr* 122: 672–677.

Karga, H., Papapetrou, P.D., Korakovouni, A., et al. 2004. Bone mineral density in hyperthyroidism. *Clin Endocrinol (Oxf)* 61: 466–472.

Keutmann, H.T., Sauer, M.M., Hendy, G.N., et al. 1978. The complete amino acid sequence of human parathyroid hormone. *Biochemistry* 17: 5723–5729.

Khosla, S. 2001. The OPG/RANKL/RANK system. *Endocrinology* 142: 5050–5055.

Kifor, O., Moore, F.D., Jr., Wang, P., et al. 1996. Reduced immunostaining for the extracellular Ca^{2+}-sensing receptor in primary and uremic secondary hyperparathyroidism. *J Clin Endocrinol Metab* 81: 3130–3131.

Kurland, E.S., Chan, F.K., Rosen, C.J., et al. 1998. Normal growth hormone secretory reserve in men with idiopathic osteoporosis and reduced circulating levels of insulin-like growth factor-I. *J Clin Endocrinol Metab* 83: 2576–2579.

Kurland, E.S., Rosen, C.J., Cosman, F., et al. 1997. Insulin-like growth factor-I in men with idiopathic osteoporosis. *J Clin Endocrinol Metab* 82: 2799–2805.

Langlois, J.A., Rosen, C.J., Visser, M., et al. 1998. Associations between insulin-like growth factor I and bone mineral density in older women and men: The Framingham Heart Study. *J Clin Endocrinol Metab* 83: 4257–4262.

Le Roith, D. Parrizas, M., and Blakesley, V.A. 1997. The insulin-like growth factor-I receptor and apoptosis. Implications for the aging process. *Endocrine* 7: 103–105.

Leese, G.P., Jung, R.T., Guthrie, C., et al. 1992. Morbidity in patients on L-thyroxine: A comparison of those with a normal TSH to those with a suppressed TSH. *Clin Endocrinol* 37: 500–503.

Lehmke, J., Bogner, U., Felsenberg, D., et al. 1992. Determination of bone mineral density by qualitative computed tomography and single photon absorptiometry in subclinical hyperthyroidism: A risk of early osteopaenia in post-menopausal women. *Clin Endocronol* 36: 511–517.

Lemann, J., Jr., Piering, W.F., and Lennon, E.J. 1970. Studies of the acute effects of aldosterone and cortisol on the interrelationship between renal sodium, calcium and magnesium excretion in normal man. *Nephron* 7: 117–130.

Levine, M.A. 2006. Hypoparthyroidism and pseudohypoparathyroidism. In *Endocrinology*, 5th Edition, DeGroot, L., and Jameson, J.L., eds. Elsevier Saunders, Philadelphia, Chapter 82, 1611–1636.

Lindsay, R., Gallagher, J.C., Kleerekoper, M., et al. 2005. Bone response to treatment with lower doses of conjugated estrogens with and without medroxyprogesterone acetate in early postmenopausal women. *Osteoporos Int* 16: 372–379.

Ljunghall, S., Johansson, A.G., Burman, P., et al. 1992. Low plasma levels of insulin-like growth factor-I (IGF-I) in male patients with idiopathic osteoporosis. *J Internal Med* 232: 59–64.

Loffing, J., and Kaissling, B. 2003. Sodium and calcium transport pathways along the mammalian distal nephron: From rabbit to human. *Am J Physiol Renal Fluid Electrolyte Physiol* 284: F628–F643.

Lubahn, D., Joseph, D., Sullivan, P., et al. 1988. Cloning of human androgen receptor complementary DNA and localization to the X chromosome. *Science* 240: 324–326.

Lukert, B.P., and Raisz, L.G. 1990. Glucocorticoid-induced osteoporosis: Pathogenesis and management. *Ann Intern Med* 112: 352–364.

Ma, Y.L., Cain, R.L., Halladay, S., et al. 2001. Catabolic effects of continuous human PTH (1–38) in vivo is associated with sustained stimulation of RANKL and inhibition of osteoprotegerin and gene-associated bone formation. *Endocrinology* 142: 4047–4054.

Manolagos, S.C. 2000. Birth and death of bone cells: Basic regulatory mechanisms and implications for the pathogenesis and treatment of osteoporosis. *Endocrinol Rev* 21: 115–137.

Melmed, S., and Jameson, J.L. 2006. Disorders of the anterior pituitary and hypothalamus. In *Harrison's Endocrinology*, Jameson, J.L., ed. McGraw Hill Companies, New York, Chapter 2, 17–56.

Merriman, H.L., La Tour, D., Linkhart, T.A., et al. 1990. Insulin-like growth factor-I and insulin-like growth factor-II induce c-fos in mouse osteoblastic cells. *Calcif Tissue Int* 46: 258–262.

Mochizuki, H., Hakeda, Y., Wakatsuki, N., et al. 1992. Insulin-like growth factor-I supports formation and activation of osteoclasts. *Endocrinology* 131: 1075–1080.

Mohan, S., and Baylink, D.J. 1991. Bone growth factors. *Clin Orthop Relat Res* 263: 30–48.

Murer, H., Hernando, N., Forster, I., et al. 2000. Proximal tubular phosphate reabsorption: Molecular mechanisms. *Physiol Rev* 80: 1373–1409.

Murray, R.D., Columb, B., Adams, J.E., et al. 2004. Low bone mass is an infrequent feature of the adult growth hormone deficiency syndrome in middle-age adults and the elderly. *J Clin Endocrinol Metab* 89: 1124–1130.

Murray, T.M., Rao, L.G., Divieti, P., et al. 2005. Parathyroid hormone secretion and action: Evidence for discrete receptors for the carboxyl-terminal region and related biological action of carboxyl-terminal ligands. *Endocrinol Rev* 26: 78–113.

Nagano, N. 2006. Pharmacological and clinical properties of calcimimetics: Calcium receptor activators that afford an innovative approach to controlling hyperparathyroidism. *Pharmacol Ther* 109: 339–365.

Naveh-Many, T., Friedlaender, M.M., Mayer, H., et al. 1989. Calcium regulates parathyroid hormone messenger ribonucleic acid (mRNA), but not calcitonin mRNA in vivo in the rat. Dominant role of 1,25-dihydroxyvitamin D. *Endocrinology* 125: 275–280.

Neer, R.M., Arnaud, C.D., Zanchetta, J.R., et al. 2001. Effect of parathyroid hormone (1–34) on fractures and bone mineral density in postmenopausal women with osteoporosis. *New Engl J Med* 344: 1434–1441.

Nielsen, H.A., Mosekilde, L., and Charles, P. 1979. Bone mineral content in hyperthyroid patients after combined medical and surgical treatment. *Acta Radiol Phys Biol* 18: 122–128.

Ontjes, D.A. 2004. The role of estrogens and other steroid hormones in bone metabolism. In *Calcium and Phosphorus in Health*, Anderson, J.J.B., and Garner, S.C., eds. CRC Press, Boca Raton, FL, 207–233.

Peacock, M., Bolognese, M.A., Borofsky, M., et al. 2009. Cinacalcet treatment of primary hyperparathyrodsm: Biochemical and bone densitometric outcomes in a five-year study. *J Clin Endocrinol Metab* 94: 4860–4867.

Pelletier-Morel, L., Fabien, N., Mouhoub, Y., et al. 2008. Hyperparathyroidism in a patient with autoimmune polyglandular syndrome. *Intern Med* 47: 1911–1915.

Pepene, C.E., Kasperk, C.H., Pfeilshifter, J., et al. 2001. Effects of triiodothyronine on the insulin-like growth factor system in primary human osteoblastic cells in vitro. *Bone* 29: 540–546.

Prince, R. Muchmore, D.B., and Siris, E. 2008. Estrogen analogues: Selective estrogen receptor modulators and phytoestrogens. In *Osteoporosis*, 3rd Edition, Marcus, R., Feldman, D., Nelson, D.A., and Rosen, C.J., eds. Elsevier Academic Press, Burlington, MA, Chapter 73, 1705–1723.

Reid, I.R., Wattie, D.J., Evans, M.C., and Stapleton, J.P. 1996. Testosterone therapy in glucocorticoid-treated men. *Arch Intern Med* 156: 1173–1177.

Richy, F., Schacht, E., Bruyere, O., et al. 2005. Vitamin D analogs versus native vitamin D in preventing bone loss and osteoporosis-related fractures: A comparative meta-analysis. *Calcif Tissue Int* 76: 176–186.

Riggs, B.L., Khosla, S., and Melton, L.J. 2002. Sex steroids and the construction and conservation of the adult skeleton. *Endocrinol Rev* 23: 279–302.

Riggs, B.L., Khosla, S., and Melton, L.J. 2008. Estrogen, bone homeostasis and osteoporosis. In *Osteoporosis*, 3rd Edition, Marcus, R., Feldman, D., Nelson, D.A., and Rosen, C.J., eds. Elsevier Academic Press, Burlington, MA, Chapter 40, 1011–1039.

Rosen, C.J., and Adler, R.A. 1992. Longitudinal changes in lumbar bone density among thyrotoxic patients after attainment of euthyroidism. *J Clin Endocrinol Metab* 75: 1531–1534.

Rosen, C.J., and Niu, T. 2008. Growth hormone and insulin-like growth factors: Potential applications and limitation in the management of osteoporosis. In *Osteoporosis*, 3rd Edition, Marcus, R., Feldman, D., Nelson, D.A., and Rosen, C.J., eds. Elsevier Academic Press, Burlington, MA, Chapter 79, 1809–1836.

Ross, D.S., Neer, R.M., Ridgway, E.C., et al. 1987. Subclinical hyperthyroidism and reduced bone density as a possible result of prolonged suppression of the pituitary–thyroid axis with L-thyroxine. *Am J Med* 82: 1167–1170.

Roussouw, J.E., Anderson, G.L., Prentice, R.L., et al. 2002. Risks and benefits of estrogen plus progestin in healthy postmenopausal women: Principal results from the Women's Health Initiative randomized controlled trial. *JAMA* 288: 321–333.

Rubin, J., Ackert-Bickness, C.L., Zhu, L., et al. 2002. IGF-I regulates osteoprotegerin (OPG) and receptor activator of nuclear factor-kappa B ligand (RANKL) in vitro and OPG in vivo. *J Clin Endocrinol Metab* 87: 4273–4279.

Saag, K.G., Zanchetta, J.R., Devogelaer, J.P., et al. 2009. Effects of teriparatide versus alendronate for treating glucocorticoid-induced osteoporosis: Thirty-six month results of a randomized, double-blind, controlled trial. *Arthritis Rheum* 60: 3346–3355.

Saggese, G., Baroncelli, G.I., Bertelloni, S., et al. 1993. Effects of long-term treatment with growth hormone on bone and mineral metabolism in children with growth hormone deficiency. *J Pediatr* 122: 37–45.

Shimada, T., Mizutani, S., Muto, T., et al. 2001. Cloning and characterization of FGF23 as a causative factor of tumor-induced osteomalacia. *Proc Nat Acad Sci (USA)* 98: 6500–6505.

Slatopolsky, E., Finch, J., Denda, M., et al. 1996. Phosphorus restriction prevents parathyroid gland growth. High phosphorus directly stimulates PTH secretion in vitro. *J Clin Invest* 97: 2534–2540.

Smith, E., Boyd, J., Frank, H., et al. 1994. Estrogen resistance caused by a mutation in the estrogen-receptor gene in a man. *New Engl J Med* 331: 1056–1061.

Snyder, P.J., Biller, B.M.K., Zagar, A., et al. 2007. Effect of growth hormone replacement on BMD in adult-onset growth hormone deficiency. *J Bone Miner Res* 22: 762–770.

Snyder, P.J., Peachey, H., Hannoush, P., et al. 1999. Effect of testosterone treatment on bone mineral density in men over 65 year of age. *J Clin Endocrinol Metab* 84: 1966–1972.

Sowers, M.F.-R., Jannausch, M., McConnell, D., et al. 2006. Hormone predictors of bone mineral density changes during the menopausal transition. *J Clin Endocrinol Metab* 91: 1261–1267.

Stewart, A.F. 2005. Hypercalcemia associated with cancer. *New Engl J Med* 352: 373–379.

Stewart, A.F., and Broadus, A.E. 2006. Malignancy-associated hypercalcemia. In *Endocrinology*, 5th Edition, DeGroot, L., and Jameson, J.L., eds. Elsevier Saunders, Philadelphia, Chapter 78, 1555–1564.

Talmage, R.V. 1967. A study of the effect of parathyroid hormone on bone remodeling and calcium homeostasis. *Clin Orthop Rel Res 54*: 163–173.

Talmage, R.V., Doppelt, S.H., and Fondren, F.B. 1976. An interpretation of acute changes in plasma ^{45}Ca following parathyroid hormone administration to thyroparathyroidectomized rats. *Calcif Tissue Res* 22: 117–128.

Tfelt-Hansen, J., and Brown, E.M. 2005. The calcium-sensing receptor in normal physiology and pathophysiology: A review. *Crit Rev Clin Lab Sci* 42: 35–70.

Thakker, R.V., and Juppner, H. 2006. Genetic disorders of calcium homeostasis caused by abnormal regulation of parathyroid hormone secretion or responsiveness. In *Endocrinology*, 5th Edition, DeGroot, L., and Jameson, J.L., eds. Elsevier Saunders, Philadelphia, Chapter 76, 1511–1531.

Tsai, M.J., and O'Malley, B.W. 1994. Molecular mechanisms of action of steroid/thyroid receptor superfamily members. *Annu Rev Biochem* 63: 451–486.

Turner, C.H., Sato, M., and Bryant, H.U. 1994. Raloxifene preserves bone strength and bone mass in ovariectomized rats. *Endocrinology* 135: 2001–2005.

Uzzan, B., Campos, J., Cucherat, M., et al. 1996. Effects on bone mass of long term treatment with thyroid hormones: A meta-analysis. *J Clin Endocrinol Metab* 81: 4278–4289.

van Staa, T.P., Laan, R.F., Barton, I.P., et al. 2003. Bone density threshold and other predictors of vertebral fracture in patients receiving oral glucocorticoid therapy. *Arthritis Rheum* 48: 3224–3229.

van Staa, T.P., Leufkens, H., and Cooper, C. 2007. The epidemiology of corticosteroid-induced osteoporosis: A meta-analysis. *Osteoporos Int* 13: 777–787.

Vidal, O., Lindberg, M.K., Hollberg, K., et al. 2000, Estrogen receptor specificity in the regulation of skeletal growth and maturation in male mice. *Proc Nat Acad Sci (USA)* 97: 5474–5479.

Wang, Y., Nishida, S., Elalieh, H.Z., et al. 2006. Role of IGF-I signaling in regulating osteoclastogenesis. *J Bone Miner Res* 21: 1350–1358.

Weinstein, R.S., Jilka, R.L., Parfitt, A.M., et al. 1998. Inhibition of osteoblastogenesis and promotion of apoptosis of osteoblasts and osteocytes by glucocorticoids. Potential mechanisms of their deleterious effects on bone. *J Clin Invest* 102: 274–282.

Weitzmann, M.N., and Pacifici, R. 2006. Estrogen deficiency and bone loss: An inflammatory tale. *J Clin Invest* 116: 1186–1194.

Wiren, K. 2008. Androgens and skeletal biology: Basic mechanisms. In *Osteoporosis*, 3rd Edition, Marcus, R., Feldman, D., Nelson, D.A., and Rosen, C.J., eds. Elsevier Academic Press, Burlington, MA, Chapter 15, 425–449.

Wood, P.J. 1992. The measurement of parathyroid hormone. *Ann Clin Biochem* 29: 11–21.

Wuster, C., Abs, R., Bengtsson, B.A., et al. 2001. The influence of growth hormone deficiency, growth hormone replacement therapy, and other aspects of hypopituitarism on fracture rate and bone mineral density. *J Bone Miner Res* 16: 398–405.

Wuster, C., Duckeck, G., Ugurel, A., et al. 1992. Bone mass of spine and forearm in osteoporosis and in German normals: Influences of sex, age, and anthropometric parameters. *Eur J Clin Invest* 22: 366–370.

Yeh, J.K., Aloia, J.F., and Semla, H.M. 1984. Interrelation of cortisone and 1,25-dihydroxycholecalciferol on intestinal calcium and phosphate absorption. *Calcif Tissue Int* 36: 608–614.

7 Renal Regulation of Calcium and Phosphate Ions

Philip J. Klemmer and John J.B. Anderson

CONTENTS

INTRODUCTION

An understanding of normal mineral metabolism is essential to understand the classical hormonal endocrine feedback system, which maintains optimal concentrations of calcium and phosphorus in the extracellular fluids while simultaneously serving to regulate external calcium and phosphate balances to facilitate skeletal health. These classical control systems interrelate with each other by means of negative feedback to maintain optimal extracellular concentrations of calcium and inorganic phosphate. Bone not only provides an abundant endogenous source of these minerals to supply extracellular fluids, but it also functions to buffer excess supplies of these minerals entering extracellular fluids from external dietary sources. These same regulatory systems also help maintain skeletal integrity during adult life as well as facilitate skeletal growth during childhood and adolescence. Appropriate mineral balance is maintained across wide ranges of dietary calcium and phosphorus intakes.

The kidney plays a pivotal role in the maintenance of divalent ion homeostasis by virtue of a finely tuned excretory capacity as well as its ability to synthesize the active 1,25-dihydroxycholecalciferol [1,25(OH)$_2$vitamin D], which actively regulates calcium absorption in the small intestine. During fasting periods, the kidneys typically reabsorb about 99% of calcium ions (Ca^{++}) and approximately 95% of the filtered phosphate ions (HPO$_4^=$). The bulk of reabsorption of these ions takes place in the proximal convoluted tubule, where calcium reabsorption is coupled with sodium reabsorption. Following meals, however, these resorptive efficiencies are reduced a few percentage points, and urinary excretions of the two ions are increased to maintain physiological concentrations of these two ions in extracellular fluids. Over a 24-hour period, the external balances of the two elements are maintained while at the same time optimal ionic concentrations of calcium and phosphate are maintained in extracellular fluids. This chapter reviews the renal regulation of calcium and phosphorus in relation to dietary intakes of these two minerals in health.

Renal calcium and phosphate homeostasis are reviewed in this chapter.

CALCIUM

The normal 70-kg adult possesses approximately 1.2 kg of calcium, of which 99% is located within bone and only 1.3 g (0.1%) is located in extracellular fluids. The human kidney is in a unique position to regulate calcium homeostasis. Although by weight the two kidneys represent less than 2% of the total body weight, this organ receives more than 20% of the cardiac output each minute and produces over 180 L of glomerular filtrate each day. The selective reabsorption of greater than 99% of this glomerular filtrate leaves behind approximately 1.4 L of urine each day, which contains not only metabolic waste products but also sufficient calcium and phosphate ions to maintain appropriate balance. The retained divalent ions facilitate growth in childhood and adolescence and steady-state skeletal maintenance in adults. The kidney also helps to regulate optimal concentrations of ionic calcium and phosphorus in extracellular fluids needed for normal neuromuscular and organ function.

Calcium intake from food and supplemental sources varies with race, age, and gender in the United States, but it ranges between 700 and 1000 mg/day for adults. Figure 7.1a and 7.1b depicts calcium and phosphate balance in the normal adult. Using the daily 1,000 mg of calcium intake estimate, it can be seen that the sum of urinary excretion (200 mg) and fecal loss (800 mg) approximates dietary calcium intake (1000 mg/day). Thus, in adult life, until approximately the age of 50 years, zero calcium balance, that is, no net calcium retention, is maintained. The principal site of regulation of calcium balance is the small intestine. The absorption fraction of calcium is approximately 20% to 30% in adults ingesting 1000 mg of calcium in their daily diets. Under conditions

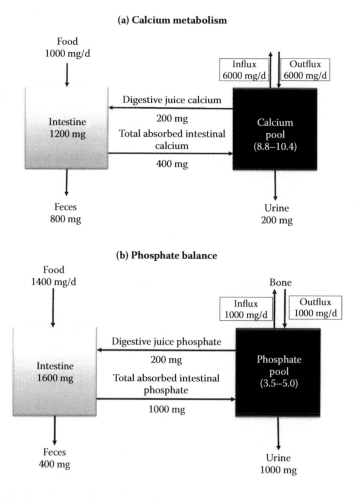

(a) Calcium metabolism

Food
1000 mg/d

Influx
6000 mg/d

Outflux
6000 mg/d

Digestive juice calcium

Intestine
1200 mg

200 mg
Total absorbed intestinal
calcium

Calcium
pool
(8.8–10.4)

400 mg

Feces
800 mg

Urine
200 mg

(b) Phosphate balance

Food
1400 mg/d

Bone

Influx
1000 mg/d

Outflux
1000 mg/d

Digestive juice phosphate

Intestine
1600 mg

200 mg
Total absorbed intestinal
phosphate

Phosphate
pool
(3.5–5.0)

1000 mg

Feces
400 mg

Urine
1000 mg

FIGURE 7.1 (A) Daily calcium balance; (B) daily phosphorus balance. (Adapted from Nordin, B.E.C., ed. 1976. *Calcium, Phosphate and Magnesium Metabolism.* Churchill Livingstone, Edinburgh; modified calcium fluxes based on Talmage, R.V. 1996. Foreword. In *Calcium and Phosphorus in Health and Disease,* Anderson, J.J.B., and Garner, S.C., eds. CRC Press, Boca Raton, FL.)

of low dietary calcium intake, the intestinal absorption fraction of calcium increases to maintain appropriate calcium balance.

Intestinal calcium absorption is primarily regulated by the serum concentration of the active form of vitamin D, that is, $1,25(OH)_2$vitamin D (calcitriol), which becomes critically important during periods of low dietary calcium intakes. The adaptive increase in enteric calcium absorption which occurs during periods of low (<500 mg/day) dietary calcium intake is regulated by increases in the renal synthesis of $1,25(OH)_2$vitamin D derived from 25-hydroxycholecalciferol (calcidiol) in response to increases in parathyroid hormone (PTH) secretion. PTH responds to the ionic concentration of calcium in extracellular fluids by means of the calcium-sensing receptor in cell membranes of the parathyroid gland. During periods of low dietary calcium intake, slight decreases in ionic calcium concentration in extracellular fluid indirectly promote increases in absorption of calcium at the intestinal mucosa by stimulating PTH production, which in turn promotes the formation of increased 1-alpha-hydroxylase activity in the proximal tubule of the kidney. The higher level of active $1,25(OH)_2$vitamin D promotes greater transcellular calcium absorption and helps to maintain zero calcium balance in adults and appropriate positive calcium balance in growing children and adolescents. Reciprocal signaling also occurs during periods of high dietary calcium intake and thus prevents positive calcium balance, which is inappropriate in the adults whose closed epiphyses prevent further skeletal growth. Under conditions of extremely high calcium intake, nonregulated calcium uptake may occur by unregulated paracellular diffusion, that is, absorption between intestinal cells (enterocytes). The kidney is limited in its capacity to compensate for excess enteric calcium absorption (Figure 7.2). In the healthy adult, daily urinary calcium excretion rarely exceeds 4 mg/kg lean body weight. As a consequence of limited urinary calcium excretory capacity, extreme levels of calcium intake, such as exceeding 2300 mg/day, may lead to net positive calcium balance and soft tissue calcification, a condition originally called the milk-alkali syndrome (Hardt and River, 1923), now also referred to as the calcium loading syndrome.

While the kidney regulates intestinal calcium absorption by formation of the active vitamin D hormone, that is, $1,25(OH)_2$vitamin D, it also reclaims most of the massive quantity of calcium within the glomerular filtrate by regulating tubular reabsorption. The kidneys filter about 10 g of calcium each day, and tubular segments reabsorb all but approximately 200 mg of this massive filtered load in men and about 120 mg in women. This level of urinary calcium excretion is maintained across a wide range of calcium intakes by virtue of the tightly regulated calcium absorption in the small intestine. In general, the net amount of calcium absorbed in the small intestine equals the daily urinary calcium excretion (Figure 7.1a).

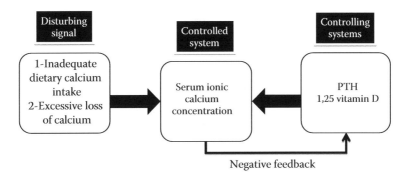

FIGURE 7.2 Serum ionic calcium concentration is maintained within a very narrow range (average 1.1 mM) throughout life by the rapid effects of PTH on calcium flux at the bone envelope and tubular calcium reabsorption in the kidney. Active vitamin D, 1,25 dihydroxycholecalciferol, acts more slowly with respect to maintaining this physiologic set point for ionic calcium concentration in extracellular fluids. (Adapted from Lobaugh, B. 1996. Blood calcium and phosphorus regulation. In *Calcium and Phosphorus in Health and Disease*, Anderson, J.J.B., and Garner, S.C., eds. CRC Press, Boca Raton, FL.)

The regulators of renal calcium excretion include PTH, 1,25(OH)$_2$vitamin D, and other hormones including, but not limited to, insulin, glucagons, and growth hormone. Expansion of the extracellular compartment by high dietary salt intake increases urinary calcium excretion. Sustained excessive intakes of sodium may lead to hypercalciuria and nephrolitiasis. Whether the high dietary sodium contributes to negative external calcium balance, bone loss, and osteoporosis has not been established. Even modest reductions in GFR cause a significant lowering of urinary calcium excretion. Diets rich in animal protein have been shown to cause hypercalciuria, possibly by increasing endogenous acid production which inhibits tubular calcium reabsorption. The ionic calcium concentration in blood and extracellular fluids is tightly regulated at a level between 1.17 and 1.33 mmol/L primarily by the action of PTH on bone. Bone contains greater than 99.5% of the body's calcium reserve, mostly in the form of calcium apatite which forms structural bone. Although bone resorption and formation are normally tightly coupled (1:1), the calcium in apatite crystals is not readily available to buffer minute-to-minute changes in ionic calcium concentration in the extracellular fluid. Rather, the calcium ions in the bone fluid compartment serve to buffer minute-to-minute perturbations in the calcium ion concentration.

A readily available source of exchangeable calcium, however, is found in the bone-lining space (bone envelope or bone compartment) which covers practically all bone surfaces (Talmage, 1996). Ionic calcium held in this reservoir is readily mobilized in response to minute-to-minute changes in the concentration of PTH (Figure 7.3). When ionic serum calcium falls below a physiologic level, the calcium-sensing receptors on the membranes of the parathyroid cells release PTH. This higher level of PTH secretion promotes the release of ionic calcium sequestered in the bone envelope until the serum ionic calcium concentration returns to the physiologic level. Reciprocal changes occur during periods of postprandial calcium absorption, and as the PTH level decreases, the bone

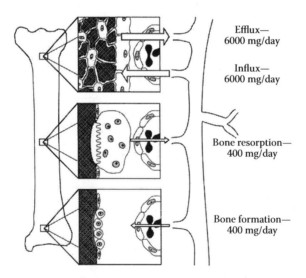

Efflux—
6000 mg/day

Influx—
6000 mg/day

Bone resorption—
400 mg/day

Bone formation—
400 mg/day

FIGURE 7.3 Exchange of calcium between bone and blood. The Ca in blood (and all extracellular fluid) undergoes constant change; both were depleted via Ca ion influx to bone (as Ca and Pi precipitate onto the surface of hydroxyapatite as calcium phosphate crystals) as blood passes through bone and via calcium ion influx from the bone fluid compartment. The tremendous influx of Ca (and Pi) into bone is balanced by an equal amount of Ca (and Pi) ion returned to blood (Ca efflux) by the action of the bone-lining cells and other osteoblast-derived bone cells. The amount of Ca and Pi ions leaving blood through bone formation is at least an order of magnitude less than that of the influx of these ions that results from exceeding the extracellular fluid Ca–Pi solubility product in relation to bone mineral. Similarly, the amount of Ca and Pi ions that can be returned from bone to blood by osteoclastic resorption is quite small, that is, about an order of magnitude lower, and should equal the amount of ions required for bone formation in an individual whose skeleton is undergoing no net change in bone mass, that is, in balance. (Adapted from Talmage, R.V. 1996. Foreword. In *Calcium and Phosphorus in Health and Disease*, Anderson, J.J.B., and Garner, S.C., eds. CRC Press, Boca Raton, FL.)

envelope buffers the rise in ionic calcium concentrations in extracellular fluids by removing calcium ions from the circulation. Thus, in healthy adults, zero calcium balance is maintained over the long term, whereas the set point of ionic calcium concentration in extracellular fluids is tightly regulated between 1.17 and 1.33 mmol/L by the action of PTH at the level of bone and, to a lesser degree, at the level of the renal tubule where PTH acts to increase calcium reabsorption. The major roles of PTH in calcium homeostasis are considered to be increasing the flux of calcium ions from the bone fluid compartment to extracellular fluids and regulating the synthesis of the active form of vitamin D, $1,25(OH)_2$vitamin D. Calcium homeostasis is thus maintained across a wide range of dietary calcium intakes by actions of the kidneys, small intestine, skeleton, and parathyroid glands.

PHOSPHATE

Phosphate homeostasis in the healthy adult differs significantly from that of calcium in that the regulation of serum phosphate concentrations and maintenance of whole-body phosphate balance occur principally at the level of the proximal renal tubule rather than in the small intestine, as is the case for calcium (Anderson et al., 2006). In essence, serum phosphate concentration is regulated through regulated renal excretion rather than by means of regulated intestinal absorption (Lemann et al., 1979).

In recent years, dietary phosphorus intakes have increased as a consequence of phosphate additives in processed foods (Bell et al., 1977). Figure 7.1b depicts phosphate balance in the normal adult with a phosphorus intake of 1400 mg/day, renal excretion of 900 mg/day, and fecal loss of 500 mg/day. Since the total intake and the combined urinary and fecal outputs in health are equal, zero metabolic balance is achieved by adults. Approximately 60% to 70% of dietary phosphorus is absorbed by the small intestine via a sodium/phosphate transporter in the mucosa. Phosphate absorption in the small intestine occurs largely independent of active vitamin D regulation. Instead, regulation of renal phosphate excretion occurs at the level of the proximal tubule in the kidney in response to PTH and FGF-23, a phosphatonin hormone produced by osteocytes in bone. FGF-23 has a phosphaturic effect, and it also reduces the activity of the renal enzyme, 1a-hydroxylase, which, in turn, reduces production of $1,25(OH)_2$vitamin D (Quarles, 2008). After a large phosphate intake from dietary protein sources and/or processed foods containing phosphate additives, PTH and FGF-23 concentrations increase in extracellular fluids. These hormonal increases lead to a reduction in proximal tubular phosphate reabsorption from the glomerular filtrate, thus enhancing urinary phosphate excretion. Thus, these hormonal actions restore balance between dietary phosphate intake and urinary and fecal phosphate excretion.

The set point for ionic phosphate concentration in the extracellular fluids is less tightly defended than that of ionic calcium. Serum phosphate concentrations in adults range between 2.5 and 4.5 mg/dL (0.83–1.5 mmol/L) in fasting adults and demonstrate diurnal and postprandial variations (Calvo et al., 1991). Phosphate flux across the bone envelope contributes to the maintenance of serum phosphate at physiologic concentrations, but this flux has not been adequately investigated.

SUMMARY

Mineral homeostasis, bone metabolism, and kidney function are interrelated by common hormonal control systems. The kidneys tightly regulate the concentrations of calcium and inorganic phosphate ions in the extracellular fluids as well as the total body external balance of these ions across a wide range of dietary calcium and phosphorus intakes. With respect to calcium, these dual roles are achieved by the regulation of calcium flux from the skeleton by PTH and the regulation enteric calcium absorption by the hormonally active form of vitamin D produced in the kidney, $1,25(OH)_2$vitamin D. In contrast, phosphorus homeostasis is regulated almost entirely at the level of the kidney, specifically in the proximal convoluted tubule, which responds to variable levels of PTH and phosphatonins, including FGF-23, to alter tubular absorption of phosphorus from glomerular filtrate. The importance of adequate kidney function in the maintenance of normal mineral homeostasis, cardiovascular health, and skeletal integrity becomes evident when chronic kidney disease develops. These issues, discussed in Chapter 33, make us mindful of the exquisite precision of natural selection in the evolution of these tightly regulated control systems.

REFERENCES

Anderson, J.J.B., Klemmer, P.J., Watts, M.E.S., et al. 2006. Phosphorus. In *Present Knowledge of Nutrition*, vol. I, 9th ed., Bowman, B.A., and Russell, R.M., eds. ILSI Press, Washington, D.C., 383–399.

Bell, R.R., Draper, H.H., Tzeng, D.Y., et al. 1977. Physiological responses of human adults to foods containing phosphate additives. *J Nutr* 107: 42–50.

Calvo, M.S., Eastell, R., Offord, K.P., et al. 1991. Circadian variation in ionized calcium and intact parathyroid hormone: Evidence for sex differences in calcium homeostasis. *J Clin Endocrinol Metab* 72: 69–76.

Hardt, L., and River, A. 1923. Toxic manifestations following the alkali treatment of peptic ulcer. *Arch Intern Med* 31: 171–180.

Lemann, J., Adams, N,D., and Gray, R.W. 1979. Urinary calcium excretion in human beings. *New Engl J Med* 301: 535–541.

Lobaugh, B. 1996. Blood calcium and phosphorus regulation. In *Calcium and Phosphorus in Health and Disease*, Anderson, J.J.B., and Garner, S.C., eds. CRC Press, Boca Raton, FL, 27–43.

Nordin, B.E.C., ed. 1976. *Calcium, Phosphate and Magnesium Metabolism*. Churchill Livingstone, Edinburgh.

Quarles, L.D. 2008. Endocrine functions of bone in mineral metabolism regulation. *J Clin Invest* 118: 3820–3828.

Talmage, R.V. 1996. Foreword. In *Calcium and Phosphorus in Health and Disease*, Anderson, J.J.B., and Garner, S.C., eds. CRC Press, Boca Raton, FL.

Part II

Effects of Specific Nutrients on Bone

8 Calcium and Bone

John J.B. Anderson, Sanford C. Garner, and Philip J. Klemmer

CONTENTS

INTRODUCTION

In addition to fulfilling the needs for calcium ions required in numerous intracellular functions as well as for the regulation of blood clotting (hemostasis), practically all of the remainder of the body's calcium exists in skeletal salts that support the body, enable ambulation, and protect internal organs. A fixed amount of calcium forms the teeth which, after formation, remain static in the oral cavity and which, unlike bone, do not participate in calcium metabolism. In the growing years, dietary calcium contributes greatly to the development of peak bone mass (PBM). Following the achievement of PBM in the second or third decade of life, dietary calcium is needed to replace calcium lost from bone tissue as part of the normal dynamic turnover of the skeleton. Adult bone mineral content (BMC) and bone mineral density (BMD) are better maintained by an adequate amount of calcium in the diet.

Adequate amounts of dietary calcium are necessary for the maintenance of bone mass and calcium metabolic balance, that is, equality between dietary calcium intake and excretion of calcium in the stool and urine. Although dietary intake of calcium, therefore, has a major role in supplying this essential nutrient, hormonal regulation at the intestine and kidneys maintains neutral (zero) calcium balance over a wide range of dietary calcium intakes (Peacock, 2010) (see also Chapter 6).

Low or inadequate consumption of calcium may be partially compensated for by a healthy vitamin D status. Vitamin D enhances intestinal calcium absorption and thereby assists in adaptation to a low calcium intake. Dietary phosphate also interacts with calcium, especially when the phosphorus intake is excessive relative to the calcium intake, and this interaction may be detrimental to bone health. This chapter examines the dietary contributions of calcium and the metabolic and skeletal handling of calcium ions. In addition, the deleterious effects of deficient and excessive intakes of calcium are briefly discussed.

DIETARY SOURCES OF CALCIUM

The amounts of calcium per serving of major calcium-containing foods are given in Table 8.1. A benefit of calcium-rich foods is that they provide good quantities of many additional nutrients besides calcium. Figure 8.1 illustrates the nutrient content of several calcium-rich food sources in comparison with a calcium carbonate supplement and a cola-type of soda drink. Except for dairy foods, few commonly consumed foods in the United States and most other Western nations contain much calcium (Table 8.2). Because of its limited distribution, consuming calcium in sufficient amounts is a challenge for many, and particularly for strict vegetarians or vegans (Havala Hobbs and Anderson, 2009). Based on food consumption surveys, approximately 60% of the calcium consumed by adults in the United States is derived from milk and dairy foods (Looker et al., 1993; Fleming and Heimbach, 1994; Ervin et al., 2004; Anon, 2009). The remainder of calcium is obtained from baked goods, dark green leafy vegetables, and relatively few other foods. For some elderly, who consume little or no dairy products, most of their calcium is obtained from breads and baked goods, which provide some of this mineral but not enough to meet the amount, that is, Dietary Reference Intake (DRI), recommended by the Food and Nutrition Board, Institute of Medicine (IOM) (1997). Fortified food products and beverages, such as orange juice, also provide calcium. The dietary reference intakes (DRIs) for calcium are given in Table 8.3.

A cup (8 oz) of practically any kind of cow's milk provides approximately 300 mg of calcium. This value is the standard to which other foods are compared. Table 8.2 lists the calcium content of selected food items from each food group. The calcium content of vegetarian diets, especially those consumed by vegans, may be sufficient in calcium to maintain good nutritional health if serving sizes are increased to compensate for lower calcium density in these foods (Weaver et al., 1999). Careful selection of calcium-containing plant foods by strict vegetarians is necessary for meeting calcium DRIs (Havala Hobbs and Anderson, 2009).

Low fat dairy products, such as yogurts, are excellent sources of calcium; roughly 30% to 50% more calcium is provided in one serving of yogurt compared with that in a cup of milk. Many young

TABLE 8.1
Approximate Amounts of Calcium per Serving of Major Calcium-Containing Foods

Food	Serving	Calcium, mg
Milk	8 oz	300
Yogurt	1 cup	350
Cheddar cheese	1 oz	200
American cheese	1 slice	175
Cottage cheese	½ cup	65
Tofu, calcium-set	4 oz	145
Salmon, canned, bones	3 oz	165
Kale	½ cup	100
Collards	½ cup	180

Source: USDA National Nutrient Database for Standard Reference, http://www.nal.usda.gov/fnic/foodcomp/search/

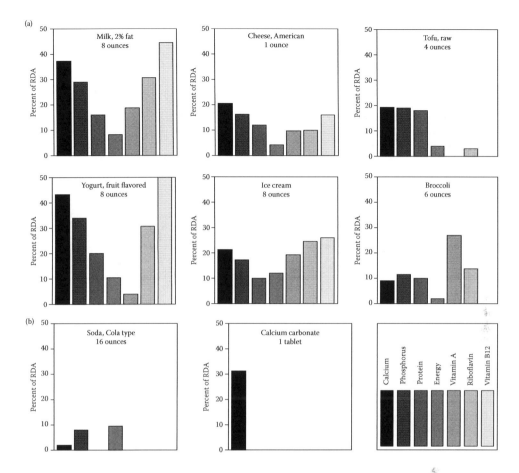

FIGURE 8.1 Nutrient content of selected calcium-rich sources in comparison with a calcium carbonate supplement and a cola-type soft drink. Calcium-rich foods provide more nutrients than calcium. Note the number of other nutrients provided by the food items rich in calcium, but not by a supplement containing calcium alone or by a cola-type soft drink. (Adapted from Anderson, J.J.B., et al. 2005. *Nutrition and Health*, Carolina Academic Press.)

women find yogurt more appealing because they are concerned about dietary fat and its potential contribution to weight gain. Therefore, knowledge of the nutrient composition of various dairy products should help concerned individuals ingest enough calcium while at the same time avoid too much phosphorus or fat.

The actual intakes of calcium and phosphorus, reported in a recent National Health and Nutrition Examination Survey (NHANES) survey based on assessed intakes of a large sample of U.S. adults, have been summarized (see Table 1.2). Compared with the age-specific DRIs, deficits in calcium intakes typically occur beyond 11 years of age, especially in females. Phosphorus intakes, which have been found to be considerably higher than calcium in the NHANES survey, are much higher than their DRIs. Based on NHANES data (Ervin et al., 2004), the adult Ca:P intake ratio of women is approximately 700:1200 (1:1.7 or 0.6:1) (Ervin et al., 2004), compared with the recommended ratio of 1:0.6 (Food and Nutrition Board, IOM, 1997).

DIETARY REFERENCE INTAKES FOR CALCIUM

Calcium is often called a threshold nutrient because intakes need to meet a "threshold" or "window" of intake that satisfies body requirements at all stages of the life cycle. Although age-specific

TABLE 8.2
Calcium Content per Serving of Most Calcium-Containing Foods, According to Food Groups

Milk and Dairy Products	Calcium (mg)	Protein Foods	Calcium (mg)
Milk, whole (8 oz)	276	Tofu, firm, nigari (4 oz)	198
Milk, skim (8 oz)	301	Salmon, canned, bones (3 oz)	212
Yogurt, fruit, low fat (6 oz)	258	Sardines, with bones (3 oz)	325
Ice cream (½ cup)	92	Almonds (2 oz)	141
Ice milk (½ cup)	107	**Fruits and Vegetables**	
Colby cheese (1 oz)	194	Orange (1 medium)	52
American cheese (1 oz)	159	Greens, kale (½ cup)	90
Cheddar cheese (1 oz)	204	Prunes (6)	25
Swiss cheese (1 oz)	224	Green beans (½ cup)	28
Colby cheese (1 oz)	194	Squash, winter (½ cup)	23
Edam cheese (1 oz)	207	**Cereal Grains and Bakery Products**	
Mozzarella cheese (1 oz)	143	White bread, enriched (1 slice)	45
Mozzarella cheese, low fat (1 oz)	222	Whole wheat bread (1 slice)	36
Muenster cheese (1 oz)	203	Cornbread, enriched (2½″ sq)	88
Provolone cheese (1 oz)	214	Pancake, enriched, (4″ diam.)	68
Cottage cheese, creamed (½ cup)	68	Tortilla, corn, enriched (6″ diam.)	19
Ricotta cheese, full milk (½ cup)	255		

Source: USDA National Nutrient Database for Standard Reference, http://www.nal.usda.gov/fnic/foodcomp/search/

TABLE 8.3
Dietary Reference Intakes for Calcium

Age Range	DRI (mg/day)	UL (mg/day)
0 to 6 months	NA	1000
7 to 12 months	NA	1500
1–3 years	700	2500
4–8 years	1000	2500
9–18 years	1300	3000
19–50 years	1000	2500
51–70 years	1000 (M); 1200 (F)	2000
>70 years	1200	2000

Notes: NA = not available. Values for pregnant and lactating women are not included.
Dietary Reference Intakes (DRIs) and tolerable upper intake levels (ULs) are the same for males and females.

Source: Food and Nutrition Board, Institute of Medicine, 2011. *Dietary Reference Intakes for Calcium and Vitamin D.* National Academy Press, Washington, DC.

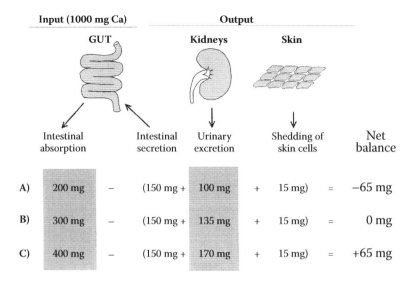

FIGURE 8.2 Three scenarios of calcium balance. Schematic diagrams illustrating three states of calcium balance that occur across the life cycle. In later life (A), 1000 mg of calcium a day may lead to a net negative balance; in early adult life (B), 1000 mg of calcium may be adequate and result in zero balance; and during growth (C), 100 mg of calcium per day may place children and adolescents in positive calcium balance.

calcium requirements cannot easily be determined, even by modern research methods, estimates of the amounts of calcium needed have been established using metabolic balance studies (Matkovic and Heaney, 1992; Hunt and Johnson, 2007) and skeletal calcium accrual analyses based on measurements of total body BMC (Vatanparast et al., 2010). Usual calcium intakes below the threshold or window and those above the threshold or window are considered unhealthy; a schematic diagram (Figure 8.2) illustrates these three conditions of calcium intake.

RECOMMENDED CALCIUM INTAKES IN THE UNITED STATES AND CANADA

The recommended calcium intakes across the life cycle, part of the DRIs, are set forth for the various stages stage of the life cycle. The calcium DRIs and tolerable upper limit intake levels (ULs) are set at estimated daily amounts across the life cycle (Food and Nutrition Board, IOM, 1997) (see Table 8.3). The DRIs for those boys and girls 8 to 19 years of age may be more than enough for optimal skeletal development. Few females in this age range consume 1,300 mg on a regular daily basis, yet most girls achieve reasonable skeletal development and height with lower intakes than their DRI (Bonjour et al., 1997) (see below). Precise requirements for calcium are not known for either males or females, and these recommendations (DRIs) may be set on the high side, especially for females, to optimize PBM development both during adolescent growth and the subsequent skeletal consolidation period of early adulthood, that is, from approximately 19 to 30 years of age (Hunt and Johnson, 2007). Therefore, the calcium DRIs across the life cycle appear to provide a considerable margin of safety, especially for women who typically develop less skeletal mass than do men. Figure 8.3 gives a scenario in which 1000 mg/day may be sufficient for optimal skeletal development from 8 to 19 years of age.

To illustrate the discrepancy between calcium intake data from a U.S. Department of Agriculture survey and DRIs for calcium, the intakes are plotted against age in Figure 8.4. The median calcium intakes of females from 11 years and beyond are much lower than the age-specific DRIs. Males do better, but they still consume less than the DRIs. The typical low intakes of calcium, especially intakes lower than approximately 50% of the DRI, by peripubertal females suggest that PBM accrual may not be optimal in these girls. Similar low calcium intakes are common in similarly

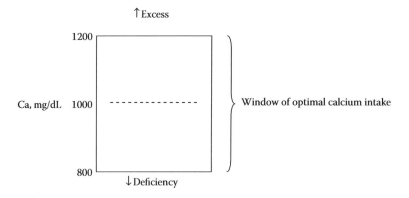

FIGURE 8.3 Optimal range of calcium intake. Scenario in which 1000 mg a day may be sufficient for optimal skeletal development from 8 to 19 years of age, but the current recommendations are 1300 mg/day for boys and girls. Many children and adolescents consume less than 800 mg/day, which implies that these individuals are consuming diets deficient in calcium.

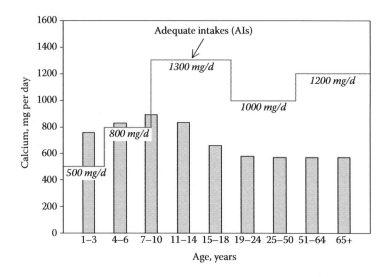

FIGURE 8.4 Discrepancies between calcium intakes (USDA survey) and AIs for calcium across the life cycle. Calcium intakes are plotted against age. AIs or Adequate Intakes were the IOM recommendations for calcium from 1997 to 2011. (Adapted from Anderson, J.J.B., et al. 2005. *Nutrition and Health*, Carolina Academic Press.)

aged females of China and other Asian nations, although Japanese girls have been improving their calcium intakes in recent decades (see Chapter 30).

CALCIUM AND PBM ACCRUAL

Peripubertal calcium intakes have a powerful impact on PBM development, which is typically achieved by approximately the age of 20 years or somewhat later in the third decade, that is, at 30 years or so, when bone consolidation is completed. The World Health Organization recognizes the achievement of PBM and further skeletal mass accrual by the age of 30 years, since the 20- to 29-year-old means of BMC and BMD are used as the healthy adult standards for dual energy x-ray absorptiometry (DXA) measurements (Kanis et al., 1994). DXA scans at later ages are typically compared with those of young healthy adult mean values for BMD. Thus, as part of a healthy diet, calcium intakes during the first two decades of life set the stage for optimal skeletal development, and this optimal PBM accrual is presumed to serve until late in life when declines in bone mass occur (Figure 8.5) (see also Chapter 24).

The concept that a greater PBM may help delay the late-life onset of osteopenia and osteoporosis, and its adverse consequences, has been argued for many years, although direct proof has not been established. Dietary factors, such as calcium, phosphorus, vitamin D, protein, and others, have long been considered as significant determinants of PBM (Heaney et al., 2000; Nieves, 2005; Vatanparast and Whiting, 2006). Results of many research studies have supported the calcium-related skeletal gains in BMC during the peripubertal decade from roughly 8 to 18 years, starting earlier in girls than boys but ending later in boys, depending on pubertal development (Bonjour et al., 1991, 1997; Johnston et al., 1992; Lloyd et al., 1992, 1993; Abrams and Stuff, 1994; Matkovic et al., 1994, 2004; Young et al., 1995; Weaver et al., 1995, 2007 ; Teegarden et al., 1995; Cadogan et al., 1997; Jackman et al., 1997; Martin et al., 2007; Bailey et al., 2000; Abrams, 2005). Also, two studies have found that low calcium intakes during this important period of skeletal growth may contribute [to] fractures in children and adolescents (Goulding et al., 1998; Wyshak and Frisch, 1994).

Studies of dizygotic and monozygotic twin subjects, which benefit from a reduction in genetic variance, have been instrumental in demonstrating the skeletal gains in mass and cross-sectional area or bone size of long bones of the twin receiving the calcium supplement in both the prepubertal and postpubertal periods (Johnston et al., 1992; Young et al., 1995) and in strength parameters (see Chapter 25). Twins, especially monozygotic pairs, have remarkably similar PBM development. This similar development illustrates a strong genetic contribution to PBM, perhaps as high as 80%, but dietary factors and other environmental factors still contribute to this accrual of bone mass (Slemenda et al., 1992).

Gains of bone mass resulting from the addition of calcium supplements, especially during the growth years of early life, may be lost after supplementation ceases. Two reports, one of singleton 12-year-old girls and one of 10- to 12-year-old twins of both genders, have shown that the BMD that was gained by the calcium-supplemented children over 2 to 4 years was subsequently

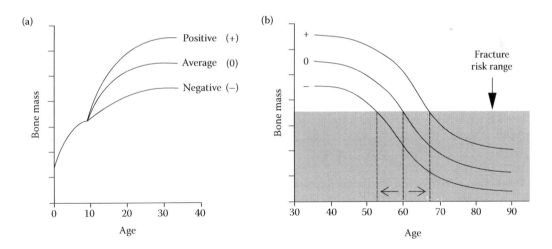

FIGURE 8.5 Early gain and later loss of bone mass across the life cycle. The early gain of bone mass in men and women is shown in the left-hand side of the figure up to about the age of 30 years when peak bone mass is achieved. The peak is higher for men than that for women. The later loss of bone mass is illustrated by the right-hand side of the figure from the age of 50 years and over. After the menopause, at approximately the age of 50 years, in females, and somewhat later in males, the loss of bone mass begins, and it continues at a slow rate of loss after the first postmenopausal decade in women and at about the age of 65 years in men for the rest of an individual's life. Slowing of the bone loss by behavioral factors such as diet and activity retards or delays the onset of osteoporosis. (Adapted from Anderson, J.J.B., et al. 2005. *Nutrition and Health*, Carolina Academic Press.)

lost after cessation of supplements as the treated individuals achieved approximately the same BMD values as their nonsupplemented comparators over the next few years (Lloyd et al., 1994; Slemenda et al., 1997). The conclusion of these short-term dietary studies is that little or no residual benefit continue after calcium supplements stop. Longer periods of calcium intakes that are at least as high as the DRI for growing children have not been examined to assess bone gains that are retained well into adulthood, the presumed benefit of high calcium intakes. In contrast, gains in bone mass related to physical activity during skeletal development are considered to continue into adulthood (see Chapter 23).

Calcium supplementation along with an exercise program has also resulted in improved PBM as measured by BMC (Barr and McKay, 1996; French et al., 2000; Welch and Weaver, 2005; Specker and Vukovich, 2007). BMC is typically chosen because BMD is not as useful a measure in growing children as BMC. A major benefit of regular physical activity is the improvement of bone quality, especially of trabecular or cancellous bone tissue, and dietary calcium availability permissively facilitates this bone consolidation.

Gains of bone size in response to DRIs of calcium occur in most ethnic groups (Weaver et al., 2007). Compared with whites and Asians, African Americans have higher PBM and a lower prevalence of osteoporosis, although gender differences are still evident as fracture rates are greater in black females than those in black males (see Chapter 29). A reason for this high bone mass (and muscle mass) among blacks relates in large part to unknown genetic factors. Because so many blacks are lactose intolerant and refrain from dairy products, they have difficulty obtaining the recommended amounts of calcium for skeletal development during childhood and adolescence. Yet, on average, they exhibit no apparent deleterious effects with respect to the development of PBM. The mechanism or mechanisms that allow blacks to adapt to low calcium intakes and develop superior BMD remain unknown, but a slower action of PTH has been suggested as a reason for increased bone mass. Reasonable calcium intakes, that is, DRI amounts (Food and Nutrition Board, IOM, 1997), however, are still recommended for black adolescents to optimize PBM. A greater "bone" bank may help black women protect against or delay the development of osteoporosis, as their life expectancy is increasing in the United States (Arias, 2010).

Adult Calcium Needs

Adult women and men need adequate amounts of calcium each day to maintain their skeletal mass (BMC) and density (BMD). The calcium recommendations are 1000 mg/day from 19 to 50 years and 1200 beyond the age of 50 years for both genders. Young adult women and men typically continue to gain bone mass via the process of consolidation until approximately 30 years (Halioua and Anderson, 1989). Women, however, begin losing some bone mass during their last decade prior to menopause, that is, during their 40s, as their ovarian estrogen production declines. Men do not lose much bone mass, if any, until a decade or more later when their androgen production decreases. Women who continue reasonably good physical activity during their 30s and 40s may maintain their bone mass for several years longer than others who are less active (Tylavsky et al., 1989).

Beyond 50 years of age, bone loss in women abruptly increases in women as a consequence of the menopausal cessation of ovarian estrogen production. For women, the amount of bone loss from 50 to 80 years has been estimated to be as much as 30% to 50% of their total bone mass (Table 8.4). Women and men beyond 50 years old need to consume sufficient calcium to replace bone loss of calcium, but this zero balance may not occur when bone resorption exceeds bone formation even with additional calcium as supplement (Riis et al., 1987). So, calcium intakes in excess of ~1000 mg/day may not be so well utilized by the skeleton, and neutral (zero) skeletal balance may be impossible to achieve in late life. The DRI of 1200 mg/day for older adults may be reasonably safe, but the excess calcium that is not taken up by the skeleton, may contribute to calcium loading, that is, excessive soft tissue calcification and renal stones (Anderson and Sjoberg, 2001). Some concern exists about excessive intakes of calcium, for example, greater than 1200 to 1500 mg/day, because of arterial

TABLE 8.4
Estimated Relative Gains and Losses of Bone Mass in Females across the Life Cycle

By Age	Gain (%)	Loss (%)
10 years	50–60	
15 years	30–40	
30 years	10	
40 years		
50 years		5–10
60 years		10–20
80 years		15–20
100 years		
Total	100	~30–50

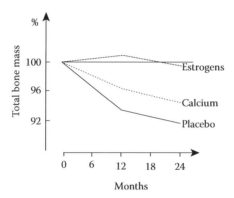

FIGURE 8.6　Relative loss of bone mineral density (BMD) in postmenopausal women. Elderly women receiving a calcium supplement (1000 mg) daily over 2 years in comparison to those receiving estrogen therapy and placebo. (Adapted from Riis, B., et al., *New Engl J Med*, 316, 173–177, 1987.)

calcification and cardiovascular disease (Bolland et al., 2008) and renal stones (Jackson et al., 2006) (see the section "Potential Calcium Toxicity: Arterial Calcification and Renal Stones").

Lactose intolerance from lactase deficiency in a large percentage of the U.S. population, that is, almost 15% of white adults and a higher percentage of African American adults, may also contribute to inadequate calcium and vitamin D intakes and, hence, lower bone density (see the section "Lactose Intolerance and Inadequate Calcium Intake").

ELDERLY CALCIUM NEEDS

Low calcium intakes among the elderly usually result from reductions in milk and cheese consumption. So, meeting the DRI of 1200 mg/day remains almost impossible without the consumption of calcium supplements; 500 mg of calcium supplements per day may be sufficient for most women to achieve the recommended 1000 to 1200 mg/day. Even with consumption above 1500 mg/day from food and supplements, elderly Danish women studied over 3 years still lost BMD (Figure 8.6) (Riis et al., 1987). In older adults, as well as at earlier adult ages, calcium supplements depress PTH secretion and bone resorption; the decrease in bone resorption tends to suppress bone turnover (McKane et al., 1996), making it less dynamic and less able to repair microfractures (Heaney, 2007) (see the section "Potential Calcium Toxicity: Arterial Calcification and Renal Stones").

CALCIUM METABOLISM

This section highlights major aspects of calcium metabolism across the life cycle. Three significant physiological changes occur in the elderly, especially in females, that influence calcium metabolism: intestinal calcium absorption declines, renal calcium reabsorption decreases, and PTH increases. Together, these changes suggest negative calcium balance.

Intestinal Absorption of Calcium

Absorption of calcium ions occurs in the absorbing epithelial cells (enterocytes) via the two-step process common to water-soluble nutrients. Calcium cations, that is, Ca^{2+}, are relatively poorly absorbed compared with inorganic phosphate anions, that is, $HPO_4^=$, also written as P_i. For adults, the net calcium absorption efficiency is approximately 20% to 30%, whereas for phosphate, it is typically about 50% to 70%. Calcium absorption is completed within 2 to 3 hours following a meal, a much slower entry than for phosphate ions (Anderson, 1991). When considering that almost all foods contain phosphorus and only a relatively few contain much calcium, the quantitative absorption of phosphate ions practically always significantly exceeds that of calcium ions from a meal. The absorption of calcium ions may be depressed a percentage point or two, if phosphate is excessive in the diet, because of precipitation of calcium ions by phosphate ions within the gut lumen (see also Chapter 6).

One of the two important interactions that exist for calcium is the enhancement of intestinal calcium absorption, involving the transcellular route, by the hormonal form of vitamin D (see Chapter 10). The vitamin D hormone, derived from prior intake of the vitamin from the diet or from skin biosynthesis, increases the efficiency of calcium ion absorption by stimulating the synthesis of calbindins by the gut absorbing cells. The calbindins carry the calcium ions, four calcium ions per calbindin, across the absorbing cells of the small intestine to the extracellular fluids and blood. At the site of new bone formation in the skeleton, the hormonal form of vitamin D increases the uptake by osteoblasts of calcium ions that are used in making new bone mineral, that is, calcium hydroxyapatite. If both calcium and vitamin D in the diet are low, for example, in a young child who is no longer breast feeding, declines in intestinal calcium absorption and bone mineralization almost certainly occur. Severe deficiencies of each may lead to rickets.

At low intakes of calcium, intestinal absorption percentages of calcium ions typically increase to greater than 30% because of the feedback regulation of the vitamin D hormonal mechanism that improves calcium absorption efficiency. However, when calcium intakes are adequate or high, the vitamin-D-mediated gut absorptive mechanism operates at a much greatly reduced efficiency. Furthermore, it is probable that this mechanism may become totally inactivated to prevent excessive calcium absorption and potential adverse effects of calcium. Thus, the vitamin D adaptation mechanism for calcium absorption depends on a low calcium load (amount) from the diet and increased absorptive efficiency of calcium ions from the diet, as mediated by the vitamin D hormone (see Chapter 10).

At high intakes of calcium, the serum calcium concentration, both total calcium and ionic calcium, increases slightly after a meal. The increase in ionic calcium depresses PTH secretion and, hence, its action on osteoblasts that signal osteoclasts to resorb bone (Martini and Wood, 2002; McKane et al., 1996). A decrease in PTH also reduces proximal tubular calcium reabsorption and thereby increases urinary calcium excretion. Figure 8.7 illustrates the sequence of physiological events following a low intake of calcium from foods or supplements.

To maintain a reasonably constant supply of calcium in blood for tissue functions, a highly regulated serum calcium ion concentration is activated to increase the flow of calcium ions to blood. Although not illustrated here, a calcium-rich meal or supplement reverses this homeostatic regulation by suppressing PTH secretion in this sequence during the first few hours after a calcium-rich meal. The sequence of steps is listed below:

1. Initial positive signal (+) for PTH secretion results from an decrease in serum Ca+2.
2. Parathyroid glands secrete PTH in response to the decrease in the serum Ca+2 concentration.

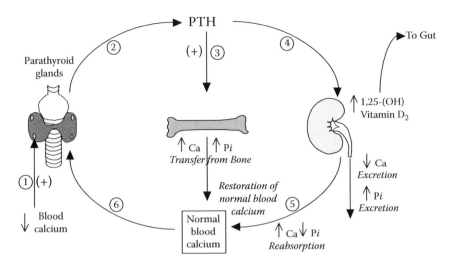

FIGURE 8.7 Regulation of blood calcium (Ca) concentration following intake of a meal low in calcium. The stimulation of parathyroid hormone (PTH) secretion and action on bone and the kidney during fasting. (Adapted from Anderson, J.J.B., et al. 2005. *Nutrition and Health*, Carolina Academic Press.)

3. PTH acts on bone to increase transfer of both Ca and Pi ions to blood.
4. It also acts on the kidneys to increase Ca reabsorption (or decrease Ca excretion). Also, PTH stimulates an increase in renal 1,25(OH)2vitamin D production, which may increase intestinal (gut) Ca absorption over the next 24 hours if calcium intakes are typically low.
5. The net effect of these actions is to return the serum total Ca to normal set level (~10 mg/dL), and the calcium ionic concentration (Ca+2) rises accordingly.
6. A normal serum calcium concentration has little or no influence on PTH secretion by this feedback mechanism until a decline in the Ca ionic concentration triggers PTH secretion. The serum total Ca concentration is highly regulated by this homeostatic mechanism; only small deviations occur under normal conditions.

The absorption of calcium ions is significantly depressed by oxalic acid (oxalate anions) and phytates when they are consumed in the same meal. These binding molecules (anions) carry negative charges that combine with positively charged calcium ions (cations) to reduce the number of calcium ions that are bioavailable and ready for absorption within the gut lumen. Oxalates are high in only a few foods, such as spinach, rhubarb, and beet greens. Factors in spinach other than oxalate may also contribute to the low efficiency of calcium absorption (Heaney et al., 1988). Phytate anions in grains have a similar, but less severe, effect of depressing the absorption of calcium ions. Hence, compared with animal sources, calcium ions from calcium-rich plant sources may be less well absorbed, that is, less bioavailable, depending on the anions or other factors in the plant foods.

Postmenopausal women are generally considered to have a decline in intestinal calcium absorption, which adversely affects calcium balance. This decline may worsen as women enter the decade of their 50s, that is, the post menopause. Because of this reduction in calcium absorption efficiency, the recommendation for dietary calcium was increased for women and men in this stage of the life cycle.

PARATHYROID HORMONE AND THE REGULATION OF SERUM CALCIUM CONCENTRATION

Parathyroid hormone (PTH) is a significant hormone involved in calcium regulation because of its action of removing (pumping) calcium ions from bone to blood during intermeal or fasting periods to maintain blood calcium at its set level, that is, 10 mg/dL (2.5 mmol/L) (Talmage and Talmage, 2006, 2007; Talmage and Mobley, 2008) (see also Chapter 6). Thus, through its major actions on bone and the kidneys, PTH is the major regulator of the blood concentration of calcium, which supplies sufficient amounts of calcium ions for the functional needs of cells. When PTH acts on bone, it stimulates osteoclasts to remove bone mostly from the trabecular surfaces of the vertebrae and the ends of the long bones, and it increases calcium effluxes from the bone extracellular compartment. When PTH acts on the renal tubules, it increases calcium reabsorption and it also blocks phosphate reabsorption, thereby increasing urinary phosphorus losses.

URINARY EXCRETION OF CALCIUM

Several factors contribute to an increase in urinary calcium losses in postmenopausal women after the menopause and older men. Urinary calcium excretion is significantly influenced by several nutrients in the usual diet. The average North American consumes about 15% of food energy from protein, a large portion of which is derived from animal sources, such as meat, fish, poultry, milk, cheese, and eggs. When the individual amino acids are metabolized, they generate acid equivalents, especially sulfuric and phosphoric acids, which must be buffered by serum bicarbonate, cellular proteins, and bone before being excreted by the kidneys.

A modest hypercalciuria (excessive calcium in the urine) may be a normal part of aging, if renal function remains healthy, because of increasing resorption of bone, that is, declining bone mass. In economically advanced societies, however, where a high-meat diet is consumed or where more physical activity is not an everyday phenomenon, the "relative" acid-induced hypercalciuria may be even more significant. For consumers of low amounts of calcium, protein-induced hypercalciuria remains a potentially significant mechanism explaining calcium loss in adults.

A high sodium diet also increases urinary calcium losses because renal calcium excretion is tightly linked to urinary sodium excretion. These minerals are reabsorbed by renal tubules, in part, by a common mechanism that favors sodium reabsorption over calcium (Lemann et al., 1979).

As glomerular filtration rate begins to decline in the later years of the life cycle, lower quantities of the calcium ions are excreted, that is, lower amounts appear in the urine over 24 hours. This decline in urinary calcium reflects lower resulting from a reduction in the formation of the active vitamin D hormonal molecule in urinary calcium by the aging kidney. Under conditions of very high calcium intake, that is, greater than 1400 mg/day, intestinal calcium absorption by older adults may lead to greater retention of calcium, but little in the skeleton. Older adults may risk vascular consequences of a positive calcium balance, that is, arterial calcification (Demer, 1995).

CALCIUM BALANCE

Calcium balance is determined to the extent by which calcium intake from foods and supplements offsets calcium output in urine, feces, and sweat. In calcium balance, the major input is diet, if adequate, and the major outputs are urine and feces. Hormonal control of calcium homeostasis is exerted at the gut, bone, and kidneys, primarily through the actions of PTH. In addition, the major action of the hormonal form of vitamin D is on the absorbing cells of the small intestine when usual calcium intakes are less than adequate. When calcium intakes are not adequate, bone serves as the major source of calcium ions in blood.

During the growth years, this balance is generally positive. In the years from roughly 20 to 40, calcium balance generally remains neutral or zero. In later life, certainly after the age of 50 years, calcium balance is usually negative. During late life, measurements of urinary calcium over a 24-hour period may be needed to assess calcium balance. An increase in urinary calcium in individuals with normal renal function suggests a negative shift in calcium balance and a probable loss of bone mass (see Chapter 7).

In older individuals, calcium balance may seem neutral, but this assessment may be misleading because of ectopic calcification, that is, new bone formation at inappropriate sites, especially in arteries and heart valves (see Chapter 33). In the elderly with normal renal function, the calcification in inappropriate locations contributes to better calcium balance, as a result of reduced or normal urinary calcium losses. If renal function becomes compromised, urinary calcium losses may decline and calcification may substantially increase. Then, calcium balance becomes even better since much less calcium is excreted by the kidneys (see the section "Potential Calcium Toxicity: Arterial Calcification and Renal Stones").

EFFECTS OF DIETARY CALCIUM AND PHOSPHORUS RATIOS ON CALCIUM HOMEOSTASIS

Too much dietary phosphorus may adversely affect bone health by increasing bone resorption (see the section "Parathyroid Hormone and the Regulation of Serum Calcium Concentration"). Bone resorption is the process by which small packets of the bone are degraded, both organic matrix and hard mineral. This process allows calcium and phosphate ions and bone matrix components (biomarkers) to be released into the extracellular fluid and blood. Bone resorption is increased during periods of low calcium and high phosphate intakes, and if it continues for long periods, this diet may adversely affect bone maintenance and reduce BMD (Calvo et al., 1990; Calvo and Park, 1996; Kemi et al., 2009). Therefore, a reasonable intake of calcium in relation to phosphorus is necessary for good bone health. An optimal dietary ratio of calcium to phosphorus for adults ranges between 1:1 and 1:2; a value of 1:1.5 is considered good. Adults who consume too little milk or other dairy products have ratios that are lower than 1:2 and may even approach 1:4.

Figure 8.8 illustrates Ca:P ratios for breast milk; usual dietary intakes during childhood, adolescence, and adulthood; and bone mineral in comparison with the AIs. Constant dietary ratios of 1:2 and less are considered to be potentially detrimental to skeletal health. Recommended daily amounts of calcium and phosphorus are given above (see the section "Dietary Reference Intakes for Calcium").

Increasing the intake of calcium as part of a high phosphate diet does not appear to correct entirely the adverse alterations in calcium metabolism although the Ca:P ratio is improved, as the phosphorus intake still remains too high (Kemi et al., 2010). Over a long period of time, such habitual diets may cause alterations in calcium metabolism that contribute to excessive loss of bone mass and possibly osteoporosis (Calvo et al., 1990; Kemi et al., 2009). It should be noted that these studies were conducted in healthy young women, and they have not been replicated in postmenopausal women.

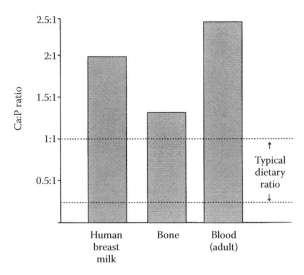

FIGURE 8.8 Ca:P ratios for breast milk; usual dietary intakes during childhood, adolescence, and adulthood; and bone mineral in comparison to the range of ratios of recommended intake amounts (DRIs) of calcium and phosphorus (RDAs).

LACTOSE INTOLERANCE AND INADEQUATE CALCIUM INTAKE

Because many people throughout the world stop synthesizing the enzyme lactase early in life, they become at risk for lactose intolerance, insufficient calcium intake, and poor bone development. If vitamin-D-fortified milk is not consumed, then both calcium and vitamin D, as well as other important nutrients, will not be ingested in adequate amounts to support bone growth. Rickets, either mild or severe, is a likely consequence.

Lactose intolerance almost certainly leads to the avoidance of consuming adequate amounts of calcium by affected individuals. Many African Americans, Asians, and whites who develop lactose intolerance at some time early in life typically avoid milk and often other dairy products. Those who are lactose intolerant may benefit from using lactase-treated milk or from taking calcium supplements beginning as early in life as possible to try to optimize the development of the skeleton, that is, PBM, and then continue supplement use to maintain their bone mass during the adult decades.

Without additional calcium sources in the diet, lactose intolerance may have adverse effects on skeletal mass and density in individuals who inherit the gene controlling the synthesis of the intestinal lactase enzyme. Most ethnic groups throughout the world develop hypolactasia (low state of lactase enzyme) after the first few years of life, which typically leads to a lower efficiency of calcium absorption and to intestinal cramping and other GI symptoms upon milk consumption. Late in life, these lactose intolerants are at increased risk for osteoporotic fractures (Segal et al., 2003).

Despite hypolactasia and low or very low calcium intakes because of low dairy consumption, African American children typically develop bones that are dense and strong. In general, then, African American children have sufficient vitamin D and calcium in their diets during childhood— well after weaning—to absorb the available dietary calcium efficiently and to put it in their skeletons. This pattern differs for white children of Northern European backgrounds and for Asian children who typically consume greater amounts of calcium throughout most of the first two decades. White children obtain most of their calcium from dairy products, whereas Asian children get most from plant sources (see also Chapter 29).

DEFICIENT CALCIUM INTAKES AND THE NEED FOR CALCIUM SUPPLEMENTS

In general, calcium deficiency results from too little ingestion of calcium-rich foods, a fairly common finding in the United States. Such low consumption patterns may contribute to late-life osteopenia and possibly osteoporotic bone fractures, whereas high calcium intakes and regular physical activity will likely help prevent or delay those fractures in later life. Preventive programs for elderly women include recommendations for the consumption of calcium and vitamin D at DRI or greater levels from foods and, typically, supplements. Supplements of these two nutrients have been demonstrated to improve bone measurements in elderly women (Chapuy et al., 1992; Dawson-Hughes et al., 1997), but not in elderly men (Dawson-Hughes et al., 1997). Also, recommendations are made for regular weight-bearing exercises, especially walking at a good pace for 30 minutes four or more days a week, and strength exercises involving upper body muscle groups that help maintain the bone mass and quality of the proximal femur (see later in this chapter).

In modest quantities, calcium supplements may help maintain bone health, that is, bone mass and density, and the reduction of fractures by increasing the Ca:P ratio as well as the amount of calcium in the diet (see Chapter 27). The accumulation of calcium in the body, however, does not necessarily mean that all the additional calcium is put in the skeleton (see below). In older individuals with low calcium intakes, calcium supplements in modest amounts typically improve bone measurements, but an uncertain amount of additional supplemental calcium is now also considered to increase arterial calcification (Persy and D'Haese, 2009; Reid et al., 2010). Therefore, among the elderly, calcium supplements in large amounts (>500 mg/day) may actually exert adverse effects on health and serve as an unintended risk factor for cardiovascular diseases. This effect of extra dietary calcium as a supplement may have a trade-off between the improvement of overall calcium balance of the elderly and the simultaneous adverse effect of increasing calcium updake in coronary and other arteries of the body. A decline in renal function also may contribute to this unhealthy state of arterial calcification. Supplementation with calcium may also improve the effectiveness of bone-conserving drugs during the menopausal transition and in later postmenopausal life, but the usual amount of supplemental calcium recommended per day, 1000 mg, may be higher than necessary without considering typical daily intakes of the individuals.

Adults and elders who obtain 800 to 1000 mg of calcium per day from foods may be doing as well as possible with respect to skeletal maintenance. Yet, most consume less than 800 mg/day, especially the elderly, and they may need a daily supplement of calcium (500 mg or so), along with vitamin D (400 IU/day or more), in an attempt to try to minimize their loss of bone mass and density. The DRIs for calcium remain the best recommendations for the U.S. population, but practically all individuals have difficulty consuming these recommended amounts from foods alone, especially the elderly whose DRI is 1,200 mg/day. Calcium intakes at or above DRIs have relatively little effect on bone compared to antiresorptive drugs (Ontjes and Anderson, 2009).

The concern about excessive calcium loading relates to the higher supplemental amounts that, once absorbed, may not go into bone but rather into arterial walls or other soft tissues. The UL for calcium is 2500 mg/day (Food and Nutrition Board, IOM, 1997), but this high amount may be too much of a risk for health. This issue of excessive supplemental calcium intakes by older adults needs to be more closely monitored in the elderly who have declining renal function.

POTENTIAL CALCIUM TOXICITY: ARTERIAL CALCIFICATION AND RENAL STONES

Toxic effects of calcium may occur with excessive intakes, particularly in cases of overconsumption of calcium supplements. This condition has also recently been referred to as calcium loading (Anderson, 2009). Calcium intakes in excess of needs may contribute to excessive mineralization of soft tissues, that is, calcification of arterial walls in large arteries, such as the aorta; small arteries, such as the coronaries; and the heart valves (Demer, 1995). Calcium salts in arterial walls, as part of rigid bone, limit greatly the elasticity of arteries; the aorta is especially affected. Other than constipation and renal stones, which have been observed in many female calcium supplement users, arterial calcification may be a forthcoming epidemic in older adults, in part because of excessive calcium supplement usage and in part because of reduced renal function. Calcification of coronary arteries, renal arteries, and heart valves may increase the risk of cardiovascular diseases (Bolland et al., 2008) (see also Chapter 33). Despite the fairly liberal UL value of 2,500 mg of calcium a day, adults at risk for these abnormalities may require dietary calcium restriction in an attempt to lessen their condition.

Older adults are often appropriately advised to consume calcium supplements, in amounts of 500 or 1,000 mg/day, to assure that the absorbed calcium will help maintain BMD throughout the skeleton and especially at common sites of fractures. This recommendation, however, may cause adverse effects on calcium balance if renal function has started to decline in older adults. A glomerular filtration rate below 60 is considered the cut point for the beginning of serious renal disease, and it probably also is the point when arterial calcification becomes prominent. In the presence of positive calcium balance, the additional calcium absorbed tends not to be retained by the skeleton, but rather it is retained in soft tissues and the vasculature, that is, new bone at inappropriate sites. Although research has not yet fully established a progression of calcification with age when dietary calcium may be increased (Hsia et al., 2007), evidence suggests that some of the extra calcium from diet and bone resorption is retained in arterial walls (McClelland et al., 2006; Reid et al., 2010). Data from prospective randomized controlled trials are needed to rule in or out this hypothesis.

The tentative conclusion now for older adults is that they must have their renal function checked to obtain their estimated glomerular filtration rate before starting to take calcium supplements—and perhaps before taking vitamin D supplements as well—or even after such supplementation has already been initiated. Calcium from dietary sources may be more preferable than supplemental calcium, but high intakes from foods alone may also contribute to arterial calcification. Calcium loading of the body has long been recognized in the coronaries of the heart, the aorta, the carotid arteries, and heart valves, but the increased risk of death from cardiovascular diseases when this condition exists has only recently become a major concern.

SUMMARY

As an essential nutrient, calcium needs to be consumed in sufficient amounts to meet the body's requirements on a daily basis. Intake amounts need to be within the optimal window that confers health. Although precise estimates of calcium requirements at any stage of the life cycle have not been determined, reasonable estimates of what healthy intakes should actually be have been published by the Institute of Medicine (Food and Nutrition Board, IOM, 1997 and 2011). The calcium recommended DRIs across the life cycle appear to provide a considerable safety factor, especially for women. These DRIs, however, are the same for males and females throughout the life cycle, despite differences in skeletal mass between the genders. Also, they are the same for all ethnic groups, despite differences in bone metabolism. Interactions between calcium and inorganic phosphate and between calcium and vitamin D may potentially have large impacts on the skeleton during growth and young adulthood, and possibly even during bone maintenance in later adulthood. Lactose intolerance also may have adverse effects on calcium and bone metabolism. Finally, calcium supplementation which is generally beneficial in terms of achieving DRIs of calcium may also exert adverse effects on arterial tissue by promoting calcification when total calcium intakes are excessive.

During the period of skeletal growth, physical activity, when regularly performed, has a major positive impact on the accrual of skeletal mass as long as dietary intakes of most nutrients, especially calcium and vitamin D, remain sufficient. Young adult women between 20 and 30 years old may gain an additional 5% to 10% of their skeletal mass over this decade. Optimal nutrient intakes, then, should maximize an individual's PBM by approximately the third decade of life. The growth years may be viewed as a window of opportunity, though short, to obtain dietary calcium in the skeleton and achieve PBM. When epiphyses close, excess calcium from supplements may not improve BMC and BMD appreciably, but it may increase the likelihood of arterial calcification.

Approximately 60% of the calcium consumed by adults in the United States is from milk and dairy products. Deficiencies and more modest insufficiencies of calcium are common in the United States because of insufficient consumption of calcium-rich foods. Women typically have lower calcium intakes than those of men, and many begin taking calcium supplements around the time of the menopause to help delay the adverse effects of low bone mass and density. Such intakes do tend to increase bone mass modestly, especially when consumed with sufficient vitamin D. Excessive calcium intakes, however, may contribute to inappropriate calcification in arterial walls and heart valves, which may be a risk factor for cardiovascular and cerebrovascular diseases.

In conclusion, achieving an adequate calcium intake as part of a healthy diet is often difficult, especially during the growth periods of the lifecycle. Meeting the recommended window of calcium intake, that is, enough but not too much, may be more of a challenge now that calcium supplementation is so widespread, at least in the United States. Future research should generate better understandings of excessive intakes and arterial calcification.

REFERENCES

Abrams, S.A. 2005. Calcium supplementation during childhood: Long-term effects on bone mineralization. *Nutr Rev* 63: 251–255.
Abrams, S.A., and Stuff, J.E. 1994. Calcium metabolism in girls: Current dietary intakes lead to low rates of calcium absorption and retention during puberty. *Am J Clin Nutr* 60: 739–743.

Anderson, J.J.B. 1991. Nutritional biochemistry of calcium and phosphorus. *J Nutr Biochem* 2: 300–307.

Anderson, J.J.B. 2009. Calcium, vitamin D, and bone health: How much do adults need? *Nutr Food Sci* 39: 337–341.

Anderson, J.J.B., and Sjoberg, H.E. 2001. Dietary calcium and bone health in the elderly: Uncertainties about recommendations. *Nutr Res* 21: 263–268.

Anon. 2009. *What We Eat in America, NHANES 2005–2006: Usual Nutrient Intakes from Food and Water Compared to 1997 Dietary Reference Intakes for Vitamin D, Calcium, Phosphorus, and Magnesium.* U.S. Department of Agriculture, Agricultural Research Service, Beltsville Human Nutrition Research Center, Food Surveys Research Group, Washington, D.C. http://www.ars.usda.gov/ba/bhnrc/fsrg

Arias, E. 2010. United States life tables, 2006. *Nat Vital Stat Rep* 58 (21), 40 pp.

Bailey, D.A., Martin, A.D., McKay, H.A., et al. 2000. Calcium accretion in girls and boys during puberty: A longitudinal analysis. *J Bone Miner Res* 15: 2245–2250.

Barr, S.I., and McKay, H.A. 1996. Nutrition, exercise, and bone status in youth. *Int J Sport Nutr* 8: 124–142.

Bolland, M.J., Barber, P.A., Doughty, R.N., et al. 2008. Vascular events in healthy older women receiving calcium supplementation: Randomized controlled trial. *BMJ* 336: 262–265.

Bonjour, J.P., Carrie, A.L., Ferrari, S., et al. 1997. Calcium-enriched foods and bone mass growth in prepubertal girls: A randomized, double-blind, placebo-controlled trial. *J Clin Invest* 99: 1287–1294.

Bonjour, J.P., Theintz, G., Buchs, B., et al. 1991. Critical years and stages of puberty for spinal and femoral bone mass accumulation during adolescence. *J Clin Endocrinol Metab* 73: 555–563.

Cadogan, J., Eastell, R., Jones, N., et al. 1997. Milk intakes and bone mineral acquisition in adolescent girls: Randomized, controlled intervention trial. *BMJ* 315: 1255–1260.

Calvo, M.S., Kumar, R., and Heath, H., III. 1990. Persistently elevated parathyroid hormone secretion and action in young women after four weeks of ingesting high phosphorus, low calcium diets. *J Clin Endocrinol Metab* 70: 1334–1340.

Calvo, M.S., and Park, Y.K. 1996. Changing phosphorus content of the U.S. diet: Potential for adverse effects on bone. *J Nutr* 126: 1168s–1180s.

Chapuy, M.-C., Arlot, M.E., Duboeuf, F., et al. 1992. Vitamin D3 and calcium to prevent hip fractures in elderly women. *New Engl J Med* 327: 1637–1642.

Dawson-Hughes, B., Harris, S.S., Krall, E.A., et al. 1997. Effect of calcium and vitamin D supplementation on bone density in men and women 65 years of age or older. *New Engl J Med* 337: 670–676.

Demer, L. 1995. A skeleton in the atherosclerotic closet. *Circulation* 92: 2029–2032.

Ervin, R.B., Wang, C.-Y., Wright, J.D., et al. 2004. Dietary intake of selected minerals for the United States population: 1999–2000. *Advance Data* No. 341. [CDC, Vital and Health Statistics, U.S. DHHS, Hyattsville, MD, 8 pages]

Fleming, K.H., and Heimbach, J.T. 1994. Consumption of calcium in the US: Food sources and intake levels. *J Nutr* 124: S1426–S1430.

Food and Nutrition Board, Institute of Medicine, 1997. *Dietary Reference Intakes for Calcium, Phosphorus, Magnesium, Vitamin D, and Fluoride.* National Academy Press, Washington, DC.

Food and Nutrition Board, Institute of Medicine, 2011. *Dietary Reference Intakes of Calcium and Vitamin D.* National Academy Press, Washington, DC.

French, S.A., Fulkerson, J.A., and Story, M. 2000. Increasing weight-bearing physical activity and calcium intake for bone mass growth in children and adolescents: A review of intervention trials. *Prev Med* 31: 722–731.

Goulding, A., Cannan, R., Williams, S.M., et al. 1998. Bone mineral density in girls with forearm fractures. *J Bone Miner Res* 13: 143–148.

Halioua, L., and Anderson, J.J.B. 1989. Lifetime calcium intake and physical activity habits: independent and combined effects on bone mass in healthy premenopausal Caucasian women. *Am J Clin Nutr* 49: 534–541.

Heaney, R.P. 2007. Bone health. *Am J Clin Nutr* 85: 300S–303S.

Heaney, R.P., Abrams, S., Dawson-Hughes, B., et al. 2000. Peak bone mass. *Osteoporos Int* 11: 985–1009.

Heaney, R.P., Weaver, C.M., and Recker, R.R. 1988. Calcium absorbability from spinach. *Am J Clin Nutr* 47: 707–709.

Hobbs, S.H., and Anderson, J.J.B. 2009. Calcium and vitamin D. In *The Complete Vegetarian*, Carlson, P., ed. University of Illinois Press, Urbana and Chicago, IL, 78–82.

Hsia, J., Heiss, G., Ren, H., et al. 2007. Calcium/vitamin D supplementation and cardiovascular events. *Circulation* 106: 856–854.

Hunt, C.D., and Johnson, L.K. 2007. Calcium requirements: New estimations for men and women by cross-sectional statistical analyses of calcium balance data from metabolic studies. *Am J Clin Nutr* 86: 1054–1063.

Jackman, L.A., Millane, S.S., Martin, B.R., et al. 1997. Calcium retention in relation to calcium intake and postmenarcheal age in adolescent females. *Am J Clin Nutr* 66: 327–333.

Jackson, R.D., LaCroix, A.Z., Gass, M., et al. for the Women's Health Initiative Investigators. 2006. Calcium plus vitamin D supplementation and the risk of fractures. *New Engl J Med* 354: 669–683.

Johnston, C.C., Jr., Miller, J.Z., Slemenda, C.W., et al. 1992. Calcium supplementation and increases in bone mineral density in children. *New Engl J Med* 327: 82–87.

Kanis, J.A., Melton, L.J., III, Christiansen, C., et al. 1994. The diagnosis of osteoporosis. *J Bone Miner Res* 9: 1137–1141.

Kemi, V.E., Karkkainen, M.U.M., Rita, H.J., et al. 2010. Low calcium:phosphorus ratio in habitual diets affects serum parathyroid hormone concentration and calcium metabolism in healthy women with adequate calcium intake. *Br J Nutr* 103: 561–568.

Kemi, V.E., Rita, H.J., Karkkainen, M.U., et al. 2009. Habitual high phosphorus intakes and foods with phosphate additives negatively affect serum parathyroid concentration: A cross-sectional study on healthy premenopausal women. *Public Health Nutr* 12: 1885–1892.

Lemann, J., Adams, N.D., and Gray, R.W. 1979. Urinary calcium excretion in human beings. *New Engl J Med* 301: 535–541.

Lloyd, T., Andon, M.B., Rollings, N., et al. 1993. Calcium supplementation and bone mineral density in adolescent girls. *JAMA* 270: 841–844.

Lloyd, T., Rollings, N., Andon, M.B., et al. 1992. Determinants of bone density in young women. I. Relationships among pubertal development, total body bone mass, and total body bone density in premenarchal females. *J Clin Endocrinol Metab* 75: 383–387.

Lloyd, T., Rollings, N., Andon, M.B., et al. 1994. Enhanced bone gain in early adolescence due to calcium supplementation does not persist in late adolescence. *J Bone Miner Res* 11: S154. [Abstract]

Looker, A.C., Loria, C.M., Carroll, M.D., et al. 1993. Calcium intakes of Mexican Americans, Cubans, Puerto Ricans, non-Hispanic whites, and non-Hispanic blacks in the United States. *J Am Diet Assoc* 93: 1274–1279.

Martin, B.R., Davis, S., Campbell, W.W., and Weaver, C.M. 2007. Exercise and calcium supplementation: Effects on calcium homeostasis in sportswomen. *Med Sci Sports Exerc* 39: 1481–1486.

Martini, L., and Wood, R.J. 2002. Relative bioavailability of calcium-rich dietary sources in the elderly. *Am J Clin Nutr* 76: 1345–1350.

Matkovic, V., and Heaney, R.P. 1992. Calcium balance during human growth: Evidence for threshold behavior. *Am J Clin Nutr* 55: 992–996.

Matkovic, V., Jelic, T., Wardlaw, G.M., et al. 1994. Timing of peak bone mass in Caucasian females and its implication for the prevention of osteoporosis. *J Clin Invest* 93: 799–808.

Matkovic, V., Landoll, J.D., Badenhop-Stevens, N.E., et al. 2004. Nutrition influences skeletal development from childhood to adulthood: A study of hip, spine, and forearm in adolescent females. *J Nutr* 14: 701S–705S.

McClelland, R.L., Chung, H., Detrano, R., et al. 2006. Distribution of coronary artery calcium by race, gender, and age: Results from the Multi-Ethnic Study of Atherosclerosis (MESA). *Circulation* 113: 30–37.

McKane, W.R., Khosla, S., Egan, K.S., et al. 1996. Role of calcium intake in modulating age-related increases in parathyroid function and bone resorption. *J Clin Endocrinol Metab* 81: 1699–1703.

Nieves, J.W. Osteoporosis: The role of micronutrients. 2005. *Am J Clin Nutr* 81: 1232S–1239S.

Ontjes, D.A., and Anderson, J.J.B. 2009. Nutritional and pharmacologic aspects of osteoporosis. In *Handbook of Clinical Nutrition and Aging*, 2nd ed., Bales, C.W., and Ritchie, C.S., eds. Humana Press, Springer Science, New York, NY.

Peacock, M. 2010. Calcium metabolism in health and disease. *Clin J Am Soc Nephrol* 5: S23–S30.

Persy, V., and D'Haese, P. 2009. Vascular calcification and bone disease: The calcification paradox. *Trends Mol Med* 15: 405–416.

Reid, I., Bolland, M.J., and Grey, A. 2010. Does calcium supplementation increase cardiovascular risk? *Clin Endocrinol* doi:10.1111/j.1365-2265.2010.03792.x

Riis, B., Thomsen, K., and Christiansen, C. 1987. Does calcium supplementation prevent postmenopausal bone loss? A double-blind, controlled clinical trial. *New Engl J Med* 316: 173–177.

Segal, E., Dvorkin, L., Levy, L., et al. 2003. Bone density in axial and appendicular skeleton in patients with lactose intolerance: Influence of calcium intake and vitamin D status. *J Am Coll Nutr* 22: 201–207.

Slemenda, C.W., Christian, J.C., Williams, C.J., et al. 1992. Genetic determinants of bone mass in adult women: A reevaluation of the twin model and the potential importance of gene interaction on heritability estimates. *J Bone Miner Res* 6: 561–567.

Slemenda, C.W., Peacock, M., Hui, S., et al. 1997. Reduced rates of skeletal remodeling are associated with increased bone mineral density during the development of peak skeletal mass. *J Bone Miner Res* 12: 676–682.

Specker, B.L., and Vukovich, M. 2007. Evidence for an interaction between exercise and nutrition for improved bone health during growth. *Med Sport Sci* 51: 50–63.

Talmage, D.W., and Talmage, R.V. 2007. Calcium homeostasis: How bone solubility relates to all aspects of bone physiology. *J Musculoskelet Neuronal Interact* 7: 108–112.

Talmage, R.V., and Mobley, H.T. 2008. Calcium homeostasis: Reassessment of the actions of parathyroid hormone. *Gen Comp Endocrinol* 156: 1–8.

Talmage, R.V., and Talmage, D.W. 2006. Calcium homeostasis: Solving the solubility problem. *J Musculoskelet Neuronal Interact* 6: 402–406.

Teegarden, D., Proulx, W.R., Martin, B.R., et al. 1995. Peak bone mass in young women. *J Bone Miner Res* 10: 711–715.

Tylavsky, F.A., Bortz, A.D., Hancock, R.L., et al. 1989. Familial resemblance of radial bone mass between premenopausal mothers and their college-age daughters. *Calcif Tissue Int* 45: 265–272.

Vatanparast, H., Bailey, D.A., Baxter-Jones, A.D.G., et al. 2010. Calcium requirements for bone growth in Canadian boys and girls during adolescence. *Br J Nutr* 103: 575–580.

Vatanparast, H., and Whiting, S.J. 2006. Calcium supplementation trials and bone mass development in children, adolescents and young adults. *Nutr Rev* 64: 204–209.

Weaver, C.M., Martin, B.R., Plawecki, K.L., et al. 1995. Differences in calcium metabolism between adolescent and adult females. *Am J Clin Nutr* 61: 577–581.

Weaver, C.M., McCabe, L.D., McCabe, G.P., et al. 2007. Bone mineral and predictors of bone mass in white, Hispanic, and Asian early pubertal girls. *Calcif Tissue Int* 81: 352–363.

Weaver, C.M., Proulx, W.R., and Heaney, R. 1999. Choices for achieving adequate dietary calcium with a vegetarian diet. *Am J Clin Nutr* 70 (Suppl): 543S–548S.

Welch, J.M., and Weaver, C.M. 2005. Calcium and exercise affect the growing skeleton. *Nutr Rev* 63: 361–373.

Wyshak, G., and Frisch, R.E. 1994. Carbonated beverages, dietary calcium, the dietary calcium/phosphorus ratio, and bone fractures in girls and boys. *J Adolesc Health* 15: 210–215.

Young, D., Hopper, J.L., Nowson, C.A., et al. 1995. Determinants of bone mass in 10 to 26 year old females: A twin study. *J Bone Miner Res* 10: 558–567.

9 Inorganic Phosphorus
Do Higher Dietary Levels Affect Phosphorus Homeostasis and Bone?[*]

Mona S. Calvo

CONTENTS

INTRODUCTION

The adult body contains approximately 600 g of phosphorus as both inorganic and organic phosphorus (Endres and Rude, 2006). Approximately 510 g or 85% of total body phosphorus is contained in the adult skeleton as organic and inorganic phosphates, and soft tissues contain 15% as both inorganic and organic phosphate, whereas the extracellular fluid contains 0.1% largely as inorganic phosphorus. Cellular phosphates function in many energy-intensive physiologic functions such as muscle contraction, nerve conduction, electrolyte transport, and energy production, in addition to

---

[*] Required Disclaimer: The findings and conclusions presented in this chapter are those of the author and do not necessarily represent the views and opinions of the U.S. Food and Drug Administration. Mention of trade names, product labels, or food manufacturers does not constitute endorsement or recommendations or use by the U.S. Food and Drug Administration.

providing the main structural support of the body as a component of bone mineral. Intracellular phosphates are critical to the regulation of intermediary metabolism of proteins, fats and carbohydrates, gene transcription, and cell growth (Endres and Rude, 2006). These tissue functions are very sensitive to fluxes of inorganic phosphate into soft tissues when blood levels increase due to dietary loading or failing kidney function. To maintain homeostasis of phosphorus, exquisitely sensitive physiologic mechanisms have evolved to tightly regulate the level of inorganic phosphorus in the extracellular fluid (Calvo and Carpenter, 2003).

This chapter focuses on our current understanding of the role of bone and other endocrine organs in the regulation of phosphorus homeostasis. It addresses the question of how the changing inorganic phosphorus content of our food supply influences phosphorus homeostasis and impacts bone health and risk of hypertension and cardiovascular disease.

INORGANIC PHOSPHORUS AND BONE

INORGANIC PHOSPHORUS BALANCE

Extracellular fluid phosphorus is regulated within a very narrow concentration range by hormonal processes that control intestinal absorption and renal excretion (Schiavi and Kumar, 2004). Figure 9.1 shows how balance is maintained between intake and excretion in a normal 70-kg adult consuming approximately 20 mg phosphorus/kg of body weight/day. Phosphorus is absorbed with much greater efficiency than are calcium and other minerals (Lemann, 1993). As much as 80% of ingested phosphorus from highly processed food is absorbed and enters the extracellular fluid pool from which it can be moved in and out of bone as needed (Schiavi and Kumar, 2004). Approximately 70% of the dietary phosphorus is absorbed, but almost 100% of this phosphorus is excreted per day by the kidneys. This excretion enables maintenance of phosphorus homeostasis, which is a balance between the amount absorbed and the amount excreted. Plasma phosphorus levels normally occur within a

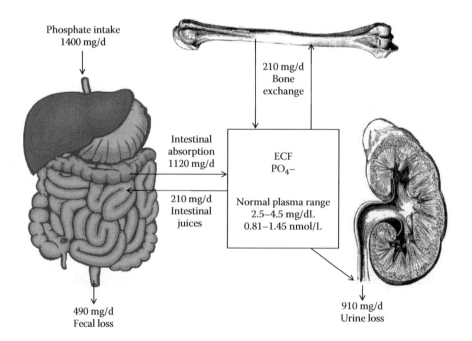

FIGURE 9.1 Maintenance of phosphorus balance in a 70-kg adult consuming 1400 mg of phosphorus daily. Figure was drawn by the author based on schematic presented by Schiavi and Kumar (2004).

very narrow range, 2.5 to 4.5 mg/dL, and maintenance of this set point or narrow range of plasma phosphorus differs from the maintenance of whole body homeostasis. Plasma phosphorus is freely filtered at the glomerulus, and regulation of the amount excreted in the urine occurs at the level of the proximal tubule where it is controlled by a number of factors that either increase or decrease phosphorus reabsorption.

Dietary phosphate loading and depletion are key factors regulating renal phosphate reabsorption. This is achieved by controlling the number of sodium–phosphate cotransporters (NaPiIIa) located on the surface of the renal proximal tubule brush border membrane (Takeda et al., 2004). Phosphorus depletion results in recruitment of existing NaPiIIa cotransporters from intracellular pools, whereas phosphorus loading results in endocytosis of the cotransporters (Takeda et al., 2004). Sabbagh et al. (2009) have recently demonstrated that an intestinal cotransporter (Npt2b) plays a major role in phosphate absorption and overall phosphorus homeostasis. Intestinal phosphate absorption occurs by both passive and active transport, with the active transport controlled by the intestinal cotransporter.

BONE

The skeleton, which comprises most of the inorganic phosphate of the body, serves as a ready reserve of phosphate ions for biological functions, especially cellular uses such as ATP, DNA, RNA, and many other molecules critical for metabolism. Osteocytes, cells embedded in bone, are a source of endocrine factors, such as fibroblast growth factor 23 (FGF23), secreted into the circulation that function in the regulation of phosphorus balance. Bone thus functions in structural support and mineral storage and serves as an endocrine organ.

DIETARY PHOSPHORUS

DIFFERENCES IN ORGANIC AND INORGANIC PHOSPHORUS IN FOOD

Phosphorus in the food supply is either organic, bound to a carbon compound, or inorganic, a phosphate acid or salt not bound to a carbon-containing compound. Examples of organic and inorganic phosphorus commonly found in food are shown in Figure 9.2. Organic forms, such as phytate, the plant storage form of phosphorus in whole grains, and phosphoproteins, such as casein or whey from milk, show a slower rate of phosphorus absorption than that of inorganic phosphate salts (Calvo and Carpenter, 2003; Karp et al., 2007; Uribarri, 2009). Organic phosphorus is generally less bioavailable and must be digested or degraded by enzymatic action such as phytase, which is not produced by the mammalian gastrointestinal tract (Calvo and Carpenter, 2003). Inorganic phosphate salts readily dissociate in the acidic environment of the stomach requiring no enzymatic digestion and therefore are more rapidly and efficiently absorbed and have greater metabolic affects. Evidence of this physiologic difference in the rate of absorption and metabolic affect was recently reported by Karp et al. (2007). They monitored parathyroid hormone (PTH) levels after consumption of high dietary phosphorus from different food sources: meat, whole grain (phytate source), cheese (calcium–phosphoprotein), and a dietary supplement (combination of disodium and trisodium phosphate salt). Inorganic phosphate salts are shown to have metabolic consequences (rise in PTH) in this study, whereas organic phosphorus from foods such as cheese, meat, and whole grains either depressed PTH (cheese affect) or did not differ from the control session where only 500-mg phosphorus was consumed.

PHOSPHORUS ADDITIVES IN FOOD

The phosphorus content of the U.S. diet is increasing as a result of the growing consumption of processed foods containing phosphate additives (Calvo and Park, 1996; Uribarri and Calvo, 2003).

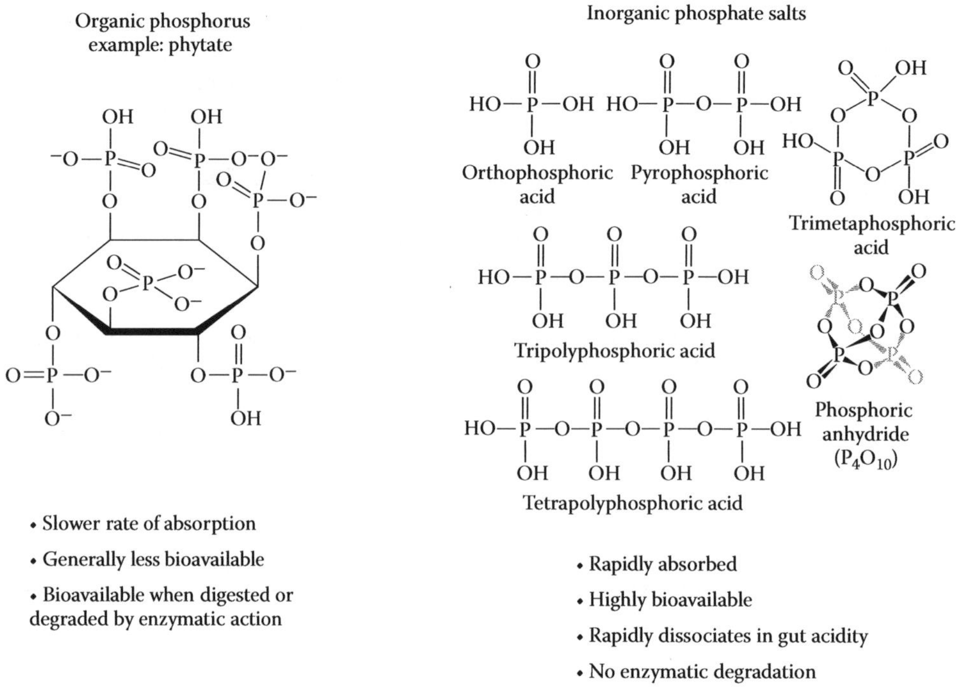
Organic phosphorus
example: phytate
• Slower rate of absorption
• Generally less bioavailable
• Bioavailable when digested or degraded by enzymatic action
Inorganic phosphate salts
Orthophosphoric acid
Pyrophosphoric acid
Trimetaphosphoric acid
Tripolyphosphoric acid
Phosphoric anhydride (P_4O_{10})
Tetrapolyphosphoric acid
• Rapidly absorbed
• Highly bioavailable
• Rapidly dissociates in gut acidity
• No enzymatic degradation

FIGURE 9.2 Structural and physiological differences between organic phosphorus and inorganic phosphate salts.

Almost two decades ago, we reported that the use of phosphorus containing food additives had increased by 17% over the previous report which estimated that phosphorus salts contributed to more than 30% of the adult phosphorus intake (Calvo, 1994). Phosphorus containing additives are inorganic forms of phosphorus widely used in the processing of a broad variety of food categories, ranging from baked goods to restructured meats and cola beverages as shown in Table 9.1 (International Food Additive Council, 2008). Greater use of these very desirable functions of phosphate additives is encouraged by our fast-paced culture's ever-growing consumption of fast food and need for fast-cooking convenience foods (Calvo and Park, 1996; Sarathy et al., 2008). Convenience foods are more highly processed, and the added phosphate salts enable them to cook faster or to be "instant," requiring no or little cooking. An example of such a convenience food product is shown in Table 9.2 which presents the ingredient labels from an "instant" lemon pudding mix, as well as the ingredient label from the "cooked" product made by the same manufacturer. These labels also illustrate that more than one phosphate additive can be found in a product due to their many valued functional properties.

The U.S. Food and Drug Administration (FDA) has considered approved inorganic phosphates to be Generally Recognized as Safe since 1979, and a more recent toxicological review concluded that all four classes of inorganic phosphates exhibit low oral toxicity (Weiner et al., 2001). The toxicology reviewers stated that "humans [with normal renal function] are unlikely to experience adverse effects when the daily phosphorus consumption remains below 70 mg/kg/day." This estimate is equivalent to 4.9 g of phosphorus per day by a 70-kg adult! Current reality is that we have no mechanism to accurately monitor the contributions of these phosphorus additives to total phosphorus intake. Phosphorus intakes from fast foods, convenience foods, or processed food in general are not captured by nutrient composition databases largely because the content changes with the constantly evolving processing techniques and phosphorus content is not required to be listed on the FDA's Nutrition Facts panel (Sullivan et al., 2007; Uribarri, 2009).

TABLE 9.1
Phosphate Use in Foods

Finished Product	Phosphate Ingredient	Phosphate Function
Baked goods		
Baking powder	Sodium acid pyrophosphate 28, monocalcium phosphate	Acid-base reaction with sodium bicarbonate to produce CO_2
Cakes, mixes	Sodium acid pyrophosphate, monocalcium phosphate, salp	Moderate action leavening; double-action leavening
Cake donuts	Sodium acid pyrophosphate 40, sodium acid pyrophosphate 43	Fast-action leavening
Refrigerated dough	Sodium acid pyrophosphate 22	Heat-activated leavening
Beverages		
Colas	Phosphoric acid	Acidulates
Chocolate milk	Tetrasodium pyrophosphate	Suspend cocoa
Dry mixes	Tricalcium phosphate	Prevent caking; clouding agent
Buttermilk	Tetrasodium pyrophosphate, disodium phosphate	Maintain protein dispersion
Orange juice	Tricalcium phosphate	Calcium and phosphorus fortification
Strawberry-flavored milk	Tetrasodium phosphate	Bind iron to maintain pink color
Cereals and pasta		
Cooked cereals	Disodium phosphate, tricalcium phosphate	Decrease cooking time; calcium and phosphorus fortification
Extruded, dry cereals	Disodium phosphate, trisodium phosphate, tricalcium phosphate	Aid in the flow through extruder, calcium and phosphorus fortification
Pasta products	Disodium phosphate	Decrease cooking time
Dairy products		
Instant puddings and cheesecakes	Monocalcium phosphate, disodium phosphate, tetrasodium pyrophosphate	Salts to keep the thickened texture
Hard, soft, and imitation ice cream	Tetrasodium pyrophosphate	Prevent churning or gritty texture development of fat
Imitation dairy products		
Nondairy creamer	Dipotassium phosphate	Buffer for smooth mixing into coffee
Cheese		
Cottage cheese	Phosphoric acid	Direct set by acidification
Dips and sauces	Disodium phosphate, trisodium phosphate, sodium hexametaphosphate	Emulsifying action
Imitation cheese	Disodium phosphate	Emulsifying action
Cheese slices	Disodium phosphate, dipotassium phosphate	Emulsifying action
Starter cultures	Disodium phosphate. Dipotassium phosphate	Inhibit phage growth

continued

TABLE 9.1 (Continued)
Phosphate Use in Foods

Finished Product	Phosphate Ingredient	Phosphate Function
Chips dips	Disodium phosphate, sodium hexametaphosphate, sodium tripolyphosphate	Maintain homogeneity
Baked chips	Monocalcium phosphate	Develop characteristic surface
Meat products		
Ham, corned beef	Sodium tripolyphosphate, and blends with hexametaphosphate	Moisture binding
Sausage franks, bologna	Sodium tripolyphosphate, tetrasodium pyrophosphate, tetrapotassium phosphate, sodium acid pyrophosphate	Emulsion development; reduced sodium; cure color development
Roast beef	Sodium tripolyphosphate	Moisture binding
Seafood		
Shrimp	Sodium tripolyphosphate	Mechanical peeling of shrimp
Canned crab	Sodium acid pyrophosphate	Bind copper from blood to prevent discoloration
Surimi	Sodium tripolyphosphate/tetrasodium pyrophosphate blends	Cryoprotectant to protein
Poultry		
Poultry products	Sodium tripolyphosphate, and blends with sodium hexametaphosphate	Moisture binding
Carcass washes	Trisodium phosphate	Remove salmonella and campylobacter
Egg products		
Whole eggs	Monosodium phosphate, monopotassium phosphate	Color stability
Egg whites	Sodium hexametaphosphate	Improve whipping and foam stability
Fruit and vegetable products		
Tomatoes, berries	Monocalcium phosphate	Maintain firmness when canned
Baked potato chips	Monocalcium phosphate	Create a bubbled surface
French fries, hash browns, potato flakes	Sodium acid pyrophosphate	Bind iron to inhibit iron induced blackening

Source: Data modified from International Food Additive Council. 2008. *Phosphates Use in Foods*. http:www.foodadditives.org/phosphates/phosphate_used_in_food.html (last accessed January 2, 2010).

TABLE 9.2
Example of Convenience Food Product Use of Phosphate Additives

Instant pudding and pie filling

Ingredients: sugar, modified cornstarch, contains less than 2% of natural flavor, disodium phosphate and tetrasodium
pyrophosphate for thickening, monoglycerides and diglycerides (prevent foaming), yellow 5, yellow 6, BHA
(preservative)

Cook and serve pudding and pie filling

Ingredients: cornstarch, sugar, dextrose, modified tapioca starch, fumaric acid (for tartness), contains less than 2% of
natural flavor, salt, hydrogenated soybean oil, yellow 5, yellow 6, BHA (preservative)

Ingredient Label Source: JELL-O brand Lemon Puddings, Product of Kraft Foods Global, In C., Northfield, IL.

Using the available commercial software for estimating nutrient intake, we compared the accuracy
of these indirect methods of estimating phosphorus intake with that of the direct chemical analyses of
the phosphorus content of a variety of diets. We found extreme underestimation of phosphorus intake
(greater than 20%) when software relying on nutrient content databases was used (Oenning et al.,
1988). Phosphorus intake has received little attention in the years since we explored the accuracy of
estimating its intake using these databases. However, recent findings now challenge the safety of high
inorganic phosphorus intake for bone, cardiovascular, and kidney health, all of which underscore the
need for updating the phosphorus content of foods in our national nutrient databases and the need
to require phosphorus content in the Nutrition Facts panel (Alonso et al., 2010; Dhingra et al., 2007;
Foley et al., 2009; Giachelli, 2009; Isakova et al., 2009; Kemi et al., 2009; Uribarri and Calvo, 2003).

Dietary Guidelines for Phosphorus Intake

Table 9.3 shows the U.S. Dietary Guidelines for phosphorus intakes from foods and dietary supplements (Institute of Medicine [IOM], 1997). These guidelines were last reviewed and changed in
1997 when both a Recommended Dietary Allowance (RDA) and an Estimated Average Requirement
(EAR) were established for phosphorus intakes by specific age groups. Relative to the earlier 1989
RDA for phosphorus, changes were made for all age groups, except 9- to 18-year-olds, who require
more of this nutrient during rapid bone accretion. Phosphorus intakes were lowered by 100 mg
from 800 to 700 mg/day in adults. The EAR which is used to evaluate nutrient intake status of a
population was lowered to 580 for adults (IOM, 1997). The Tolerable Upper Intake Level [UL], also
set in 1997, is 4 g of phosphorus per day. As discussed above, this level has come into question,
with the recent evidence linking high serum phosphorus to adverse health outcomes. The RDA and
EAR differ from the labeling guidelines set by the FDA for phosphorus content labeling on food
products. The FDA labeling guidelines are the Reference Daily Intake (RDI) or also termed Daily
Value (DV); however, phosphorus content is not required on the Nutrition Facts panel of food labels.
Listing phosphorus content is optional for food manufacturers and involves only one value, unlike
the RDA. The RDI/DV for phosphorus is 1000 mg, which is usually expressed as a percent of the
DV. When manufacturers opt to list phosphorus content of their product as a percent of the DV, it
often leads to confusion and underestimation of the true phosphorus content. This information is
critical in individuals who must closely monitor their phosphorus intake due to chronic renal failure
(Kalantar-Zadeh et al., 2010; Uribarri, 2009).

Total Dietary Phosphorus Intake

Figure 9.3 shows the median usual intake of phosphorus for various age groups of men and women
taken from the most recent available data from the National Health and Nutrition Education Survey
(NHANES) conducted in 2005 to 2006 (Moshegh et al., 2009). These nationally representative

TABLE 9.3
U.S. Dietary Recommended Intake (DRI) Guidelines for Phosphorus (P) Intake from Foods and Dietary Supplements

1997 DRI, Recommended Dietary Allowance, and Estimated Average Requirement		
Years	mg/d	mg/d
1–3	460	380
4–8	500	405
9–18	1250	1055
19–50	700	580
51–70	700	580
70+	700	580

Tolerable Upper Intake Level (UL) for phosphorus
1997 DRI UL = 4.0 g Pi

Source: Institute of Medicine. 1997. *Dietary Reference Intakes for Calcium, Phosphorus, Magnesium, Vitamin D, and Fluoride.* National Academy Press, Washington, DC.

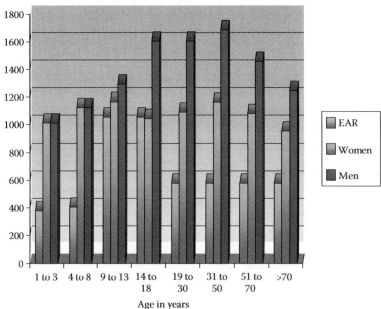

FIGURE 9.3 Median total phosphorus intake (mg/day) of men and women in various age groups compared with the Estimated Average Requirement (EAR) for each age group. Figure drawn by the author from data published for the NHANES 2005–2006 survey. (Moshegh, A., Goldman, J., Ahuja, J., et al. 2009. What we eat in America. NHANES 2005–2006. In *Usual Nutrient Intakes from Food and Water Compared to 1997 Dietary Reference Intakes for Vitamin D, Calcium, Phosphorus, and Magnesium.* U.S. Department of Agriculture Research Service.)

intake estimates are compared with the EAR for each age group. Traditionally, the EAR is used to evaluate intake adequacy of a nutrient at the 50th percentile (median) level of intake. For all ages and genders, except for adolescent girls, the estimated intake of phosphorus greatly exceeds the EAR. Despite the fact that total phosphorus intakes are generally in excess, these values most likely underestimate phosphorus intake in individuals with specific preferences for fast foods or other highly processed foods because the nutrient content databases used for these estimates do not reflect changes in phosphate additive use. Inaccuracy in these estimates presents a critical confounder in studies exploring the relationship between phosphorus intake and disease endpoints.

CURRENT UNDERSTANDING OF THE REGULATION OF PHOSPHORUS HOMEOSTASIS

Our past understanding of phosphorus homeostasis was based on the concept that the body could tolerate wide variations in phosphate intake and plasma levels with little adversity as long as kidney function was maintained. However, current understanding is based on recent research findings indicating that extracellular fluid phosphate levels are tightly regulated within a narrow range and that even slight variations in these levels are associated with chronic disease development. Bergwitz and Juppner (2010), Berndt and Kumar (2009), Isakova et al. (2009), and Quarles (2008) presented valuable reviews of the newfound complexities of the endocrine regulation of phosphorus homeostasis, which is no longer limited to the classic hormones of the parathyroid glands and kidney (active metabolite of vitamin D) but also involves bone and the secretion of FGF23.

REGULATION BY NOVEL INTESTINAL PHOSPHATE SENSOR

A simple overview of our present understanding of the hormonal factors involved in the regulation of phosphorus homeostasis is summarized in Figure 9.4. Phosphorus loading has been shown to immediately trigger an intestinal sensor to release an unidentified endocrine factor that has been shown to stimulate phosphaturia prior to the detection of phosphorus changes in plasma (Kumar, 2009; Berndt et al., 2007). The existence of the proposed phosphate-sensing mechanism within the intestine and the as yet unidentified endocrine factor that signals the kidney to increase phosphate excretion was discovered by administrating phosphate solutions directly into the duodenum of rats (Berndt et al., 2007). Immediate changes in the fractional excretion of phosphate were observed in the phosphate gavaged rats, but not in those rats gavaged with an equivalent amount of sodium chloride or infused with phosphate directly thus bypassing the intestine. Intestinal phosphate sensors offer a rapid response mechanism to maintain phosphorus balance without involving the classic endocrine hormones, PTH and calcitriol, the active form of vitamin D [$1,25(OH)_2D$] (Berndt and Kumar, 2007).

CLASSICAL ENDOCRINE REGULATION

The postulated intestinal phosphaturic factor provides a rapid response mechanism to adapt to changes in dietary phosphorus in contrast to the classical endocrine phosphorus regulating hormones, PTH and the vitamin D endocrine system shown in Figure 9.4 (Kumar, 2009). Classical endocrine feedback loops that function in the long-term adaptation to changes in dietary phosphate are illustrated in Figure 9.5. These classical endocrine changes occur over a longer period of time with chronic changes in the intake of phosphate (Calvo et al., 1988, 1990; Kemi et al., 2009). Oral loads of phosphate salts have been shown to depress ionized calcium and stimulate PTH release, an effect that appears to be dependent on the dose administered (Calvo and Heath, 1988; Kemi et al., 2009). PTH secretion has been shown to remain elevated and plasma calcitriol concentrations unstimulated with chronic consumption of high phosphorus, moderately low calcium diets (Calvo et al., 1990). Portale et al. (1989) demonstrated in humans that the normal stimulation of calcitriol synthesis by PTH is

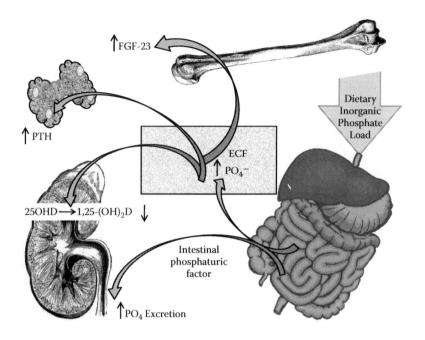

FIGURE 9.4 Factors regulating phosphorus homeostasis in response to dietary loading with inorganic phosphorus. The intestinal phosphaturic factor is thought to be secreted within minutes of ingesting a phosphorus load and acts immediately to increase phosphate excretion. Direct stimulation of fibroblast growth factor 23 (FGF23) release from bone and parathyroid hormone (PTH) from the parathyroid glands requires only a slight elevation of phosphorus in the extracellular fluid which can occur postprandially within less than half an hour. Inhibition of calcitriol [1,25(OH)₂D] occurs after persistent high phosphate loading over several days and results in lower phosphate absorption from the intestine and continued phosphaturia.

attenuated with chronic high dietary phosphorus intake. A decrease in plasma ionized calcium is the major stimulus for PTH release, but direct stimulation of PTH secretion by dietary phosphate loading was recently demonstrated in a rat model (Martin et al., 2005). Phosphate suppression of calcitriol was first observed with the chronic administration of therapeutic treatment (2 g phosphorus per day as inorganic phosphate salts) of patients with idiopathic hypercalciuria. When administered chronically, phosphorus only slightly elevated plasma parathyroid concentrations but significantly reduced plasma calcitriol (Van den Berg et al., 1980). Calcitriol functions to increase intestinal calcium absorption and to a lesser extent to increase phosphorus absorption. Significant reductions in calcitriol concentrations in the face of elevated parathyroid concentrations during chronic oral phosphate loading are puzzling because, until recently, PTH was considered the most potent stimulator of calcitriol synthesis (Calvo and Park, 1996). New factors, the phosphatonins, have recently been determined to also play a major role in the regulation of phosphorus homeostasis (Berndt et al., 2005).

PHOSPHATONIN REGULATION

Emerging evidence suggests that specific factors secreted by osteocytes in bone also participate in maintaining phosphorus homeostasis, notably FGF23, shown in Figures 9.4 and 9.5. FGF23 is one of many factors, loosely termed the "phosphatonins," which were discovered through studies of phosphate-wasting disorders (Schiavi and Kumar, 2004). Through classical endocrine feedback loops, dietary phosphate loading and calcitriol stimulate FGF23 secretion from osteocytes (Nishida et al., 2006; Saito et al., 2005). In turn, elevated FGF23 secretion inhibits renal synthesis of calcitriol

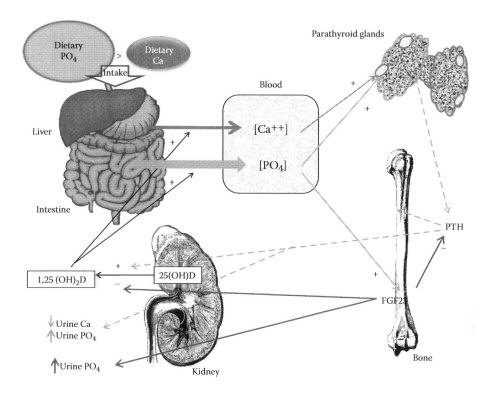

FIGURE 9.5   Schematic representation of the mechanisms regulating phosphorus homeostasis when dietary phosphorus intake exceeds dietary calcium intake. More rapid and more efficient absorption of phosphorus creates an imbalance in the blood, resulting in lower ionized calcium and higher serum phosphate levels, both of which stimulate parathyroid hormone release. Parathyroid hormone (PTH) acts immediately to stimulate renal reabsorption of mineral from bone. The less immediate action of PTH concerns the stimulation of renal alpha-1-hydroxylase increasing the circulating level of calcitriol [1,25(OH)$_2$D] which stimulates the intestinal absorption of both calcium and phosphorus. Slight elevation in blood phosphate concentration will directly stimulate osteocytes in bone to release fibroblast growth factor 23 (FGF23) and other phosphatonins, which inhibit PTH resorptive action in bone and renal synthesis of calcitriol but maintain phosphaturia. These actions can restore the balance between calcium and phosphorus in blood as long as there is sufficient renal function to excrete phosphorus.

from 25-hydroxy vitamin D (Shimada et al., 2004). Short-term phosphate loading in humans stimulates FGF23 secretion, phosphaturia, and suppression of renal calcitriol synthesis (Ferrari et al., 2005; Antoniucci et al., 2006; Burnett et al., 2006; Ito et al., 2007) through apparent parathyroid-independent mechanisms. Ben-Dov et al. (2007) demonstrated that FGF23 inhibits PTH secretion with chronic phosphate loading in rats. These investigators also showed that dietary phosphorus restriction exerts an opposite effect decreasing FGF23, increasing renal phosphate reabsorption, and indirectly increasing renal calcitriol synthesis purportedly by ceasing to inhibit parathyroid secretion. The importance of FGF23 to phosphorus homeostasis is specific to regulation of the wide fluctuations in dietary intake due to the extensive use of phosphate additives. High phosphorus intake is considered the main stimuli of FGF23 secretion as evidenced by the failure of FGF23 levels to increase when serum phosphate levels were raised by nondietary methods (Ito et al., 2007).

PHYSIOLOGIC EFFECTS OF HIGH INORGANIC PHOSPHORUS DIET

EFFECTS ON BONE HEALTH

As world populations increasingly adopt Western culture and diet, such as highly processed convenience foods, we will see growing evidence of a disproportionate increase in phosphorus intake relative to calcium (Calvo and Carpenter, 2003). Few cross-sectional studies in adults relate high phosphorus intake to effects on bone mineral content or bone density, despite a well-established relationship between chronic dietary phosphate loading and adverse skeletal effects in animal models. Experimental studies examining low calcium, high phosphorus consumption have produced hormonal changes that are not conducive to the development or maintenance of peak bone mass, a situation that predisposes women to osteoporosis later in life (Calvo et al., 1990). Both acute and longer exposures to oral phosphorus loading in the presence or absence of adequate calcium intake produce a rise in PTH (Calvo and Carpenter, 2003). Bell et al. (1977) were the first to examine the physiologic effects of diets high in phosphorus containing food additives. Their findings are shown in Table 9.4 that demonstrate a clear effect of phosphorus intake on bone turnover (increased hydroxyproline excretion) and evidence of increased parathyroid activity (increased cyclic adenosine mono phosphate [AMP] excretion). Later, we also examined the effects of chronic high phosphate additive consumption using a more complex study design and direct measures of PTH and calcitriol (Calvo et al., 1988, 1990). In contrast to short-term feeding studies with phosphate salts, our chronic high phosphate additive consumption studies showed a significant reduction or no change in calcitriol levels, despite slight elevations in PTH. We speculate that in these earlier studies, persistent elevation in FGF23 may have inhibited PTH secretion and stimulatory action on calcitriol synthesis. Under conditions of low calcium intake, the dietary phosphate stimulation of FGF23 would impair the body's main adaptive mechanism for adequate calcium absorption and optimal bone accretion, the increased synthesis of calcitriol. The effects of high phosphate additive intake on FGF23 secretion and function in phosphorus homeostasis merit further study.

No prospective dietary studies have been long enough to accurately determine the effect of low calcium, high phosphorus intake on bone mass accretion in young adults. Some more recent cross-sectional studies have shed light on our understanding of the potential adverse effects of some phosphate food additives. Tucker et al. (2006) measured bone mineral density of the spine and hip in older men and women in the Framingham Osteoporosis Study. They regressed bone density data on the frequency of soft drink consumption after multiple adjustment for confounding variables. They found that the intake of cola beverages that contain phosphoric acid but not other carbonated soft drinks, which do not contain phosphoric acid, is significantly associated with low bone mineral density in women but not men. In this study, total calcium intake was lower in women with the highest cola intakes and lowest bone mineral density. Again, we can only speculate that regular consumption of cola beverages with a dose of phosphoric acid may promote lower bone mass by evoking a strong FGF23 response impeding efficiency of calcium absorption by inhibiting calcitriol synthesis, a situation that would exacerbate bone loss if calcium intake was low. More recently, Pinheiro et al.

TABLE 9.4
Physiologic Effects of a Diet High in Foods Containing Phosphate Additives

Biological Measures	Control Diet	High PO$_4$ Diet
Calcium intake	677 mg/day	745
Phosphorus intake	979 mg/day	2125
Urinary calcium	179 mg/day	113 $p < .01$
Urinary phosphorus	427 mg/day	1013 $p < .01$
Urinary hydroxyproline	27.9 mg/day	33.4 $p < .01$
Serum calcium	10.66 mg/100 ml	10.31 $p < .01$
Serum phosphorus	3.76 mg/100 ml	4.43
Urinary cAMP	2.81 nmol/mg creatinine	3.44 $p < .01$

Source: Bell, R.R., et al. *J Nutr*, 107, 42–50, 1977.

(2009) evaluated the association between nutrient intake and osteoporotic fractures in a representative sample of older Brazilian men and women. They demonstrated a relationship between increasing phosphorus intake and bone fractures, showing a 9% increase in risk of fractures for every 100-mg increase in phosphorus intake. Given the rapid rate and high efficiency of absorption and frequency of consumption, specific phosphate additives such as phosphoric acid used in cola beverages merit further study of their influence on bone accretion. These current findings suggest that certain phosphate additives may significantly disrupt phosphorus homeostasis.

EFFECTS ON CARDIOVASCULAR HEALTH

Public health concern is growing over the association between subtle increases in serum phosphate levels within the normal range and increased risk of death and cardiovascular disease (Isakova et al., 2009). Hyperphosphatemia is a significant risk factor for kidney disease progression, vascular calcification, left ventricular hypertrophy, and mortality in chronic kidney disease (CKD) (Block et al., 1998; Giachelli et al., 2001; Jono et al., 2000). Moreover, Shuto et al. (2009) have demonstrated that dietary phosphorus can impair endothelial function. Key strategies to slowing the progression to cardiovascular disease in CKD focus on preventing vascular calcification and damage to the vascular endothelium. These strategies involve restricting phosphorus intake which is difficult given the hidden sources in our foods in the form of phosphorus food additives (Uribarri and Calvo, 2003). Vascular calcification is a major contributor to cardiovascular disease, and a growing body of evidence links small elevations in serum phosphate (high normal range, 3.5–4.5 mg/dl) in young adults with normal renal function with increased coronary artery calcium and increased risk of atherosclerosis (Foley et al., 2009; Giachelli, 2009). Other prospective studies in community-living adults with normal renal function (Dhingra et al., 2007) or patients with previous myocardial infarctions but normal kidney function (Tonelli et al., 2005) showed higher serum phosphorus levels (within normal range) associated with increased cardiovascular disease risk. A recent prospective study of 13,444 participants in the Atherosclerosis Risk in Communities and the Multi-Ethnic Study of Atherosclerosis cohorts reported higher phosphorus intakes associated with lower blood pressure levels when the dietary phosphorus was obtained through the intake of dairy products, but not phosphorus from other dietary sources (Alonso et al., 2010). These findings reinforce the need for better nutrient content data of foods to help distinguish effects of organic phosphorus from those of inorganic phosphorus on critical health measures. Many experts believe that we now have sufficient evidence that higher serum phosphorus within the established normal range promotes cardiovascular calcification, impaired endothelial function, and progression to cardiovascular disease in both normal and CKD patients to justify development of effective strategies to reduce serum phosphorus in the overall population (Tuttle and Short, 2009). Consideration should be given to the development of dietary strategies to reduce phosphorus intake in the overall population by adjusting the use of inorganic phosphorus additives and thus facilitate maintenance of phosphorus homeostasis.

SUMMARY

New knowledge of the role of bone in the endocrine regulation of phosphorus homeostasis has brought new understanding of the mechanisms that could potentially lead to adverse health outcomes resulting from the continued increase in use of inorganic phosphorus in food processing. The phosphorus content of the U.S. diet continues to increase as a result of the growing consumption of highly processed foods such as fast foods and convenience foods. Greater use of phosphate additives in these foods is fueled by our fast-paced culture's need for specific additive functions that allow us to speed the preparation, improve the texture, or restructure food. A growing number of studies are finding that consumption of specific foods or diets rich in phosphorus additives may significantly disrupt phosphorus homeostasis contributing to bone loss, impaired kidney function, and cardiovascular disease. Hyperphosphatemia occurring in chronic renal failure has long been recognized to be a serious risk factor for progression of kidney disease, vascular calcification, left ventricular hypertension, disruption of endothelial function, and mortality, with dietary phosphorus restriction considered to be the best corrective strategy. In both chronic renal failure patients and the general population, vascular calcification is a major contributor to cardiovascular disease. However, growing evidence now links small increases in serum phosphate in individuals with normal renal function to measures of increased coronary artery calcium and increased risk of atherosclerosis. Considering these findings associated with small changes in serum phosphorus, the development of strategies to reduce inorganic phosphorus intake in the general population merits consideration. Adjusting the use of inorganic phosphorus additives in food processing may be a simple approach to reducing phosphorus intake and optimizing the maintenance of phosphorus homeostasis.

REFERENCES

Alonso, A., Nettleton, J.A., Ix, J.H., et al. 2010. Dietary phosphorus, blood pressure, and incidence of hypertension in Atherosclerosis Risk in Communities Study and the Multi-Ethnic Study of Atherosclerosis. *Hypertension* 55: 776–784.

Antoniucci, D.M., Yamashita, T., and Portale, A.A. 2006. Dietary phosphorus regulates serum fibroblast growth factor-23 concentrations in healthy men. *J Clin Endocrinol Metab* 91: 3144–3149.

Bell, R.R., Draper, H.H., Tzeng, D.M., et al. 1977. Physiological responses of human adults to foods containing phosphate additives. *J Nutr* 107: 42–50.

Ben-Dov, I.Z., Gailtzer H., Lavi-Moshayoff, Y., et al. 2007. The parathyroid is a target organ for FG23 in rats. *J Clin Invest* 117: 403–4008.

Bergwitz, C., and Juppner, H. 2010. Regulation of phosphate homeostasis by PTH, vitamin D and FGF-23. *Annu Rev Med* 61: 91–104.

Berndt, T.J., and Kumar, R. 2007. Phosphatonins and the regulation of phosphate homeostasis. *Annu Rev Physiol* 69: 341–359.

Berndt, T.J., and Kumar, R. 2009. Novel mechanisms in the regulation of phosphorus homeostasis. *Physiology (Bethesda)* 24: 17–25.

Berndt, T.J., Schiavi, S., and Kumar, R. 2005. Phosphatonins and the regulation of phosphorus homeostasis. *Am J Physiol (Renal Physiol)* 289: F1170–F1182.

Berndt, T.J., Thomas, L.F., Craig, T.A., et al. 2007. Evidence for a signaling axis by which intestinal phosphate rapidly modulates renal phosphate reabsorption. *PNAS* 104: 11085–11090.

Block, G.A., Hulbert-Shearon, T.E., Levin, N.W., et al. 1998. Association of serum phosphorus and calcium X phosphate product with mortality risk in chronic hemodialysis patients: A national study. *Am J Kidney Dis* 31: 607–617.

Burnett, S.M., Gunawardene, S.C., Bringhurst, F.R., et al. 2006. Regulation of C-terminal and intact FGF-23 by dietary phosphate in men and women. *J Bone Miner Res* 21: 1187–1196.

Calvo, M.S. 1994. The effects of high phosphorus intake on calcium metabolism. In: *Advances in Nutritional Research*, ed. H.H. Draper, 183–207. Plenum Press, New York, NY.

Calvo, M.S., and Carpenter, T.O. 2003. Influence of phosphorus on the skeleton. In: *Nutritional Aspects of Bone Health*, ed. S.I. New and J.-P. Bonjour, 229–265. Royal Chemistry Society, Cambridge, UK.

Calvo, M.S., and Heath, H., III. 1988. Acute effects of oral phosphate–salt ingestion on serum phosphorus, serum ionized calcium and parathyroid hormone in young adults. *Am J Clin Nutr* 47: 1025–1029.

Calvo, M.S., Kumar, R., and Heath, H., III. 1988. Elevated secretion and action of serum parathyroid hormone in young adults consuming high phosphorus, low calcium diets assembled from common foods. *J Clin Endocrinol Metab* 66: 823–829.

Calvo, M.S., Kumar, R., and Heath, H., III. 1990. Persistently elevated parathyroid hormone secretion and action in young women after four weeks of ingesting high phosphorus, low calcium diets. *J Clin Endocrinol Metab* 70: 1334–1340.

Calvo, M.S., and Park, Y.K. 1996. Changing phosphorus content of the U.S. diet: Potential for adverse effects on bone. *J Nutr* 126: 1168s–1180s.

Dhingra, R., Sullivan, L.M., and Fox, C.S. 2007. Relations of serum phosphorus and calcium levels to the incidence of cardiovascular disease in the community. *Arch Intern Med* 167: 879–885.

Endres, D.B., and Rude, R. 2006. Mineral and bone metabolism. In: *Tietz Textbook of Clinical Chemistry and Molecular Diagnostics*, ed. C.A. Burtis, E B. Ashwood, and D.E. Burns, 1891–1965. Elsevier Saunders, St. Louis, MO.

Ferrari, S.L., Bonjour, J.P., and Rizzoli, R. 2005. Fibroblast growth factor-23 relationship to dietary phosphate and renal phosphate handling in healthy young men. *J Clin Endocrinol Metab* 90: 1519–1524.

Foley, R.N., Collins, A.J., Herzog, C.A., et al. 2009. Serum phosphorus levels associate with coronary atherosclerosis in young adults. *J Am Soc Nephrol* 20: 397–404.

Giachelli, C.M. 2009. The emerging role of phosphate in vascular calcification. *Kidney Int* 75: 890–897.

Giachelli, C.M., Jono, S., Shioi, A., et al. 2001. Vascular calcification and inorganic phosphate. *Am J Kidney Dis* 38: S34–S37.

Institute of Medicine. 1997. *Dietary reference intakes for calcium, phosphorus, magnesium, vitamin D, and fluoride*. National Academy Press, Washington, DC.

International Food Additive Council. 2008. *Phosphates Use in Foods*. http:www.foodadditives.org/phosphates/phosphate_used_in_food.html (last accessed January 2, 2010).

Isakova, T., Gutierrez, O.M., and Wolf, M. 2009. A blueprint for randomized trials targeting phosphorus metabolism in chronic disease. *Kidney Int* 76: 705–716.

Ito, N., Fukumoto, S., Takeuchi, Y., et al. 2007. Effect of acute changes of serum phosphate on fibroblast growth factor (FGF)-23 levels in humans. *J Bone Miner Metab* 25: 419–422.

Jono, S., McKee, M.D., Murry, C.E., et al. 2000. Phosphate regulation of vascular smooth muscle cell calcification. *Circul Res* 87: E10–E17.

Kalantar-Zadeh, K., Gutekunst, L., Mehrota, R., et al. 2010. Understanding sources of dietary phosphorus in the treatment of patients with chronic kidney disease. *Clin J Am Soc Nephrol* 5: 519–530.

Karp, H.J., Vaihia, K.P., Kärkkäinen, M.J., et al. 2007. Acute effects of different phosphorus sources on calcium and bone metabolism in young women: A whole-foods approach. *Calcif Tissue Int* 80: 251–258.

Kemi, V., Rita, H.J., Kärkkäinen, M.U.M., et al. 2009. Habitual high phosphorus intakes and foods with phosphate additives negatively affect serum parathyroid concentration: A cross-sectional study on healthy premenopausal women. *Public Health Nutr* 12: 1885–1892.

Kumar, R. 2009. Phosphate sensing. *Curr Opin Nephrol Hypertens* 18: 281–284.

Lemann, J. 1993. Intestinal absorption of calcium, magnesium and phosphorus. In: *Primer on Metabolic Bone Disease and Disorders of Mineral Metabolism*, ed. M.J. Favus, 46–50. Raven Press, New York, NY.

Martin, D.R., Ritter, C.S., Slatopolsky, E., et al. 2005. Acute regulation of parathyroid hormone by dietary phosphate. *Am J Physiol (Endocrinol Metab)* 289: E729–E734.

Moshegh, A., Goldman, J., Ahuja, J, et al. 2009. What we eat in America. NHANES 2005–2006. In: *Usual Nutrient Intakes from Food and Water Compared to 1997 Dietary Reference Intakes for vitamin D, Calcium, Phosphorus, and Magnesium*. U.S. Department of Agriculture Research Service.

Nishida, Y., Taketani, Y., Yammanaka-Okumura, H., et al. 2006. Acute effects of oral phosphate loading on serum fibroblast growth factor 23 levels in healthy men. *Kidney Int* 20: 214–2147.

Oenning, L.J., Vogel, J., and Calvo, M.S. 1988. Accuracy of methods estimating calcium and phosphorus intake in daily diets. *J Am Diet Assoc* 88: 1076–1078.

Pinheiro, M.M., Schuch, N.J., Genaro, P.S., et al. 2009. Nutrient intakes related to osteoporotic fractures in men and women—The Brazilian Osteoporosis Study (Brazos). *Nutr J* 8(6): 1–8.

Portale, A.A., Halloran, B.P., and Morris, R.C., Jr. 1989. Physiologic regulation of the serum concentration of 1,25-dihydroxyvitamin D by phosphorus in normal man. *J Clin Invest* 83: 1494–1499.

Quarles, L.D. 2008. Endocrine functions of bone mineral metabolism regulation. *J Clin Invest* 118: 3820–3828.

Sabbagh, Y., O'Brien, S.P., Song, W., et al. 2009. Intestinal Npt2b plays a major role in phosphate absorption and homeostasis. *J Am Soc Nephrol* 20: 2348–2358.

Saito, H., Maeda, A., Ohtomo, S., et al. 2005. Circulating FGF-23 is regulated by 1 alpha, 25-dihydroxyvitamin D3 and phosphorus in vivo. *J Biol Chem* 280: 2543–2549.

Sarathy, S., Sullivan, C., Leon, J.B., et al. 2008. Fast food phosphorus-containing additives, and the renal diet. *J Renal Nutr* 18: 466–470.

Schiavi, S.C., and Kumar, R. 2004. The phosphatonin pathway: New insights in phosphate homeostasis. *Kidney Int* 65: 1–14.

Shimada, T., Hasegawa, H., Yamazaki, Y., et al. 2004. FGF-a3 is a potent regulator of vitamin D metabolism and phosphate homeostasis. *J Bone Miner Res* 19: 429–435.

Shuto, E., Taketani, Y., Tanaka, R., et al. 2009. Dietary phosphorus acutely impairs endothelial function. *J Am Soc Nephrol* 20: 1504–1512.

Sullivan, C.M., Leon, J.B., and Sehgal, A.R. 2007. Phosphorus-containing food additives and the accuracy of nutrient databases: Implications for renal patients. *J Renal Nutr* 17: 350–354.

Takeda, E., Yamamoto, H. Nashiki, K., et al. 2004. Inorganic phosphate homeostasis and the role of dietary phosphorus. *J Cell Mol Med* 8: 191–200.

Tonelli, M., Sacks, F., Pfeffer, M., et al. 2005. Cholesterol and recurrent events trial investigators relation between serum phosphate levels and cardiovascular event rate in people with coronary disease. *Circulation* 112: 2627–2633.

Tucker, K.L., Morita, K., Qiao, N., et al. 2006. Colas, but not other carbonated beverages, are associated with low mineral density in older women: The Framingham Osteoporosis Study. *Am J Clin Nutr* 84: 936–942.

Tuttle, K., and Short, R. 2009. Longitudinal relationships among coronary artery calcification, serum phosphorus and kidney function. *Clin J Am Soc Nephrol* 4: 1968–1973.

Uribarri, J. 2009. Phosphorus additives in food and their effect in dialysis patients. *Clin J Am Soc Nephrol* 4: 1290–1292.

Uribarri, J., and Calvo, M.S. 2003. Hidden sources of phosphorus in the typical American diet. Does it matter in nephrology? *Semin Dial* 16: 186–188.

Van den Berg, C.J., Kumar, R., Wilson, D.M., et al. 1980. Orthophosphate therapy decreases urinary calcium excretion and serum 1,25-dihydroxyvitamin D concentration in idiopathic hypercalciuria. *J Clin Endocrinol Metab* 51: 998–1001.

Weiner, M.L., Salminen, W.F., Larson, P.R., et al. 2001. Toxicological review of inorganic phosphates. *Food Chem Tox* 39: 759–786.

10 Vitamin D and Bone

Michael F. Holick

CONTENTS

INTRODUCTION

Vitamin D deficiency causes rickets in children and osteomalacia in adults. It also can precipitate and exacerbate osteoporosis including risk of fracture (Holick, 2007). Rickets/osteomalacia by definition means that osteoblasts have laid down a collagen matrix, but a defect exists in its ability to be mineralized. In children, a defect in the mineralization of the osteoid in the long bones and the failure or delay in the mineralization of endochrondal bone formation at the growth plate leads to the classic skeletal deformities of rickets (Holick, 2006) (Figure 10.1). However, in adults, the mineralization defect takes on a different character because of the failure of mineralization of newly formed osteoid at sites of bone turnover of periosteal or endosteal apposition. Several possible causes of poor or absent skeletal mineralization may lead to both rickets and osteomalacia. Although the major cause of rickets/osteomalacia is a deficiency of vitamin D, rare causes include a defect in vitamin D metabolism or in its recognition by calcium-regulating tissues.

VITAMIN D, CALCIUM, AND PHOSPHORUS METABOLISM

The major components of skeletal mineral are calcium and phosphate ions. Thus, any alteration in the calcium–phosphate product in the circulation can result in a mineralization defect of the skeleton. Vitamin D plays a critical role in maintaining both serum calcium and phosphate concentrations (Holick, 2006, 2007; Holick and Garabedian, 2006) (Figure 10.2). Vitamin D is obtained by exposure of the skin to UVB from sunlight, resulting in the biochemical conversion

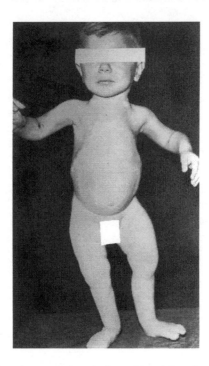

FIGURE 10.1   Child with rickets demonstrating the bowed leg deformity and rachitic rosary. The child is being held up due to severe muscle weakness. (Reproduced from Holick, M.F., *New Engl J Med*, 357, 266–281, 2004. With permission.)

of 7-dehydrocholesterol to previtamin D_3 (Figure 10.2). Previtamin D_3, being thermodynamically unstable, is rapidly converted to vitamin D_3. Once formed, vitamin D is ejected by the epidermal cell into the extracellular space and, by diffusion, enters the circulation bound to the vitamin-D-binding protein (DBP) (Holick, 2006, 2007; Holick and Garabedian, 2006). Vitamin D_3 and vitamin D_2 (D represents D_2 or D_3) in the diet are ingested, and the fat-soluble vitamins are incorporated into chylomicrons and absorbed into the lymphatics. The lymphatic drainage into the thoracic venous system permits the entrance of vitamin D into the circulation where it is bound to the DBP and lipoproteins (Haddad et al., 1993).

Vitamin D is converted in the liver by a vitamin D-25-hydroxylase (25-OHase) to form the major circulating form of vitamin D, 25-hydroxyvitamin D [25(OH)D]. At least four different 25-OHases have been identified in both mitochrondia and in microsomes (Holick, 2006, 2007). 25(OH)D is, however, biologically inert and requires hydroxylation on carbon 1 in the kidneys by the mitochrondial enzyme 25-hydroxyvitamin D-1α-hydroxylase (1-OHase), also known as cyp27B1. This hydroxylation step results in the formation of 1α,25-dihydroxyvitamin D [1,25(OH)$_2$D], which is the biologically active form, that is, hormone, of vitamin D responsible for regulating calcium and phosphorus homeostasis (Holick, 2006, 2007; Holick and Garabedian, 2006). 1,25(OH)$_2$D enters the circulation and is bound to the DBP and travels to its target tissues. In the small intestine, 1,25(OH)$_2$D interacts with its vitamin D nuclear receptor (VDR) that results in the expression of several gene products including the epithelial calcium channel, calbindin$_{9k}$, and a calcium-dependent ATPase (Christakos et al., 2003; Holick, 2006, 2007; Holick and Garabedian, 2006) (Figure 10.2). 1,25(OH)$_2$D increases the efficiency of intestinal calcium absorption. In a vitamin-D-deficient state, the small intestine is able to passively absorb about 10%–15% of dietary calcium. Vitamin D sufficiency enhances the absorption of calcium in the small intestine to about 30%–40% (Holick, 2007).

1,25(OH)$_2$D enhances the efficiency of intestinal calcium absorption principally in the duodenum and to a lesser degree in the jejunum and ileum. 1,25(OH)$_2$D stimulates phosphate absorption

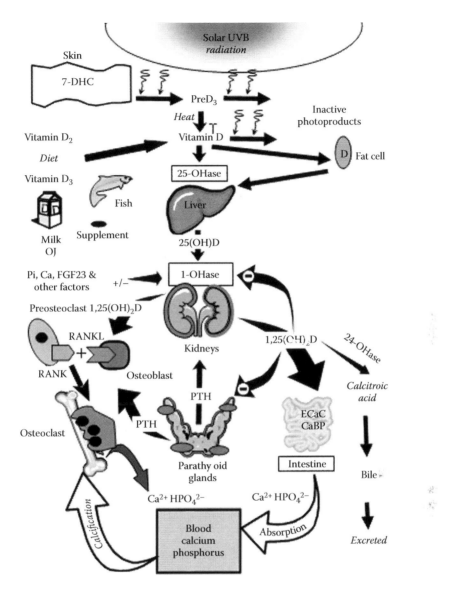

FIGURE 10.2 Schematic representation of the synthesis and metabolism of vitamin D for regulating calcium, phosphorus, and bone metabolism. (Reproduced from Holick, M.F., *New Engl J Med*, AQ9 357, 266–281, 2007. With permission.)

in the jejunum and ileum. The small intestine passively absorbs about 60% of dietary phosphate. $1,25(OH)_2D$ enhances the efficiency of phosphate absorption by an additional 20% to about 80%. When adequate calcium and phosphate are consumed in the diet and vitamin D sufficiency exists, the healthy serum calcium normal range is ~8.6–10.2 mg/dL, and the healthy serum phosphate range is ~2.5–4.5 mg/dL. The calcium–phosphate product (Ca × P) in the circulation and in the extravascular space plays a major role in the normal mineralization of osteoid laid down by osteoblasts.

VITAMIN D'S EFFECT ON BONE METABOLISM

In rodents and humans, vitamin D is not necessary for the mineralization of the osteoid matrix (Balsan et al., 1986; Holick, 2006). This lack of a direct skeletal effect was demonstrated when vitamin-D-deficient rats were either infused with calcium or phosphorus to maintain a normal calcium–phosphate product in the circulation or when they received high-calcium lactose, high-phosphorus diet that maintained a normal serum calcium–phosphate product (Holick, 2006). In both circumstances, bone histology revealed that the mineralization occurred normally without any significant unmineralized osteoid. Vitamin-D-resistant rickets patients have a mutation of their VDR and have severe rickets and osteomalacia. When these patients were infused with calcium and phosphorus to maintain a normal calcium–phosphate product, the unmineralized osteoid became mineralized (Balsan et al., 1986).

1,25(OH)$_2$D interacts with its VDR in osteoblasts to increase the expression of alkaline phosphatase, osteocalcin, and receptor activator of NFκB ligand (RANKL) (Khosla, 2001). Alkaline phosphatase produced by osteoblasts is important in bone mineralization because patients with a decrease in the bone-specific alkaline phosphatase known as hypophosphatasia suffer from a mineralization defect of the osteoid (Parfitt, 1998). Osteocalcin is the major noncollagenous protein in the skeleton. Although its function is not well understood, it appears to have a role in osteoclastic activity (Aubin et al., 2006).

RANKL, once expressed on the surface of an osteoblast, interacts with its receptor RANK on osteoclast precursors. This intimate interaction leads to signal transduction that results in the formation of multinucleated mature osteoclasts (Khosla, 2001; Holick, 2006, 2007; Holick and Garabedian, 2006) (Figure 10.2). The osteoclasts, under the direction of a variety of cytokines (Khosla, 2001; Aubin et al., 2006), increase the destruction of the skeleton by releasing hydrochloric acid to degrade and dissolve the mineral matrix and collagenases and cathepsin K to dissolve the matrix.

During exposure to sunlight, 7-dehydrocholesterol in the skin is converted to previtamin D3. PreD3 immediately converts by a heat dependent process to vitamin D3. Excessive exposure to sunlight degrades previtamin D3 and vitamin D3 into inactive photoproducts. Vitamin D2 and vitamin D3 from dietary sources are incorporated into chylomicrons, transported by the lymphatic system into the venus circulation. Vitamin D (D represents D2 or D3) made in the skin or ingested in the diet can be stored in and then released from fat cells. Vitamin D in the circulation is bound to the vitamin-D-binding protein which transports it to the liver where vitamin D is converted by the vitamin D-25-hydroxylase to 25-hydroxyvitamin D [25(OH)D]. This is the major circulating form of vitamin D that is used by clinicians to measure vitamin D status (although most reference laboratories report the normal range to be 20–100 ng/mL, the preferred healthful range is 30–60 ng/mL). It is biologically inactive and must be converted in the kidneys by the 25-hydroxyvitamin D-1α-hydroxylase (1-OHase) to its biologically active form 1,25-dihydroxyvitamin D [1,25(OH)2D]. Serum phosphorus, calcium fibroblast growth factors (FGF-23), and other factors can either increase (+) or decrease (–) the renal production of 1,25(OH)2D. 1,25(OH)2D feedback regulates its own synthesis and decreases the synthesis and secretion of parathyroid hormone (PTH) in the parathyroid glands. 1,25(OH)2D increases the expression of the 25-hydroxyvitamin D-24-hydroxylase (24-OHase) to catabolize, 1,25(OH)2D to the water-soluble biologically inactive calcitroic acid which is excreted in the bile. 1,25(OH)2D enhances intestinal calcium absorption in the small intestine by stimulating the expression of the epithelial calcium channel (ECaC) and the calbindin 9K (calcium-binding protein; CaBP). 1,25(OH)2D is recognized by its receptor in osteoblasts, causing an increase in the expression of receptor activator of NFκB ligand (RANKL). Its receptor RANK on the preosteoclast binds RANKL, which induces the preosteoclast to become a mature osteoclast. The mature osteoclast removes calcium and phosphorus from the bone to maintain blood calcium and phosphorus levels. Adequate calcium and phosphorus levels promote the mineralization of the skeleton.

Thus, the effect of vitamin D on bone metabolism is to maintain normal serum calcium and phosphate ion concentrations. Vitamin D accomplishes this by increasing intestinal calcium and phosphate absorption and by mobilizing calcium and phosphorus from the skeleton (Holick, 2006, 2007; Holick and Garabedian, 2006).

CAUSES AND CONSEQUENCES OF RICKETS/OSTEOMALACIA

HISTORICAL PERSPECTIVE

Historians have reported bone deformities similar to rickets as early as the second century, but the disease was not considered a significant health problem until the industrialization of northern Europe. Whistler, Glissen, and DeBoot recognized in the mid-1600s that many children who lived in the crowded and polluted cities of northern Europe developed a severe bone-deforming disease (rickety bones) that was characterized by growth retardation, enlargement of the epiphyses of the long bones, deformities of the legs, bending of the spine, knobby projections of the ribcage, and weak and toneless muscles (Rajakumar, 2003; Holick, 2006, 2007) (see Figure 10.1). The incidence of the debilitating bone disease increased dramatically in northern Europe and North America during the industrial revolution, and by the latter part of the 19th century, autopsy studies done in Boston and Leyden, the Netherlands, showed that 80%–90% of children had rickets. In addition, the pelvic bone structure was flattened, and this resulted in a high incidence of infant and maternal morbidity and mortality that led to the widespread use of cesarian sectioning for infant delivery (Rajakumar, 2003; Holick, 2006).

In 1822, Sniadecki (1939) was the first to recognize the importance of sun exposure for the prevention and cure of rickets. Cod liver oil had been intermittently used as a home remedy for rickets, but it often was ineffective. Because of its high prevalence and devastating consequences, many scientists and physicians became interested in finding the cause and cure for rickets. In 1919, Huldschinsky (1919, 1928) found that exposing children to radiation from a sun quartz lamp (mercury arc lamp) or carbon arc lamp was effective in treating rickets as demonstrated by improvement in the children's x-rays (Figure 10.3). He concluded that exposure to ultraviolet radiation was an "infallible remedy" against all forms of rickets in children. Two years later, Hess and Unger (1921) exposed seven rachitic children in New York City to varying periods of sunshine and reported that x-ray examination showed marked improvement in the rickets of each child, as evidenced by calcification of the epiphyses.

Great confusion was expressed as to how either exposure to ultraviolet radiation and sunlight or a dietary factor could prevent and cure rickets. Powers et al. (1921) treated rachitic rats with ultraviolet radiation or cod liver oil and observed the same effect. Hess and Weinstock (1924) and Steenbock and Black (1924) reported that ultraviolet irradiation of various foods and oils imparted antirachitic activity. This discovery led to enhancing the antirachitic activity of milk by exposing milk to ultraviolet radiation or feeding cows ultraviolet-irradiated yeast. This simple fortification practice eradicated rickets (Rajakumar, 2003; Holick, 2006).

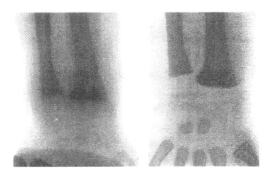

FIGURE 10.3 Florid rickets of the hand and wrist (left panel) and the same wrist and hand radiograph taken after treatment with 1-hour UVR two times a week for 8 weeks. Note the mineralization of the carpel bones and epiphyseal plates (right panel). (Reproduced from Holick, M.F., *New Engl J Med*, 357, 266–281, 2006. With permission.)

Many physicians have assumed that rickets no longer remains a health problem for children in the United States. However, rickets is becoming much more common due to the misconception that breast feeding provides infants with all of their nutritional requirements (Hollis and Wagner, 2004; Holick, 2006). Human breast milk is now known to contain little, if any, vitamin D and, thus, in neonates, especially those of color, are at high risk for vitamin-D-deficiency rickets (Kreiter et al., 2000; Rajakumar, 2003; Holick, 2006). Recently, this high risk of vitamin D deficiency has been recognized by the American Academy of Pediatrics, which now recommends that all infants from the time they are born receive 400 IU of vitamin D a day (Wagner and Greer, 2008).

VITAMIN D DEFICIENCY

Vitamin D deficiency, the most common cause of rickets, prevents the efficient absorption of dietary calcium and phosphorus. In a vitamin-D-deficient state, only 10%–15% of dietary calcium and 50%–60% of dietary phosphorus are absorbed (Holick, 2007). The poor absorption of calcium causes a decrease in serum-ionized calcium. This decline is immediately recognized by the calcium sensor in the parathyroid glands, resulting in an increase in the expression, synthesis, and secretion of parathyroid hormone (PTH) (Brown et al., 1993; Holick, 2006, 2007). PTH conserves calcium by increasing tubular reabsorption of calcium in both the proximal and distal convoluted tubules. PTH, like $1,25(OH)_2D$, enhances the expression of RANKL by osteoblasts to increase the production of mature osteoclasts that mobilize calcium stores from the skeleton. PTH also decreases phosphate reabsorption in the kidney, causing loss of phosphorus into the urine.

The serum calcium is usually normal in a vitamin-D-deficient infant or child. However, the serum phosphate is low, and thus, there is an inadequate calcium × phosphate product that is necessary to mineralize the osteoid laid down by osteoblasts (Figure 10.4). Thus, typically, infants with vitamin-D-deficiency rickets have a normal serum calcium, low normal or low fasting serum phosphorus, elevated alkaline phosphatase, and low 25(OH)D (<15 ng/mL) (Hess and Lundagen, 1922;

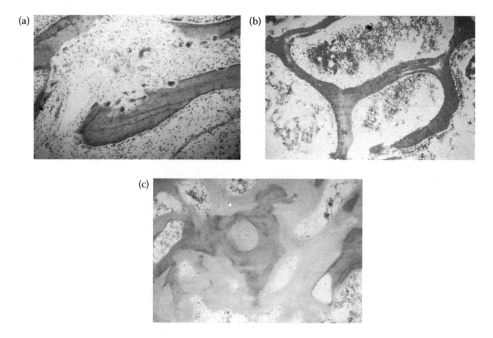

FIGURE 10.4 Bone histology demonstrating (a) increased osteoclastic bone resorption due to secondary hyperparathyroidism, (b) normal mineralized trabecular bone, and (c) osteomalacia with widened unmineralized osteoid (light gray areas). (Reproduced from Holick, M.F., *New Engl J Med*, 357, 266–281, 2004. With permission.)

Hess, 1929; Kreiter et al., 2000; Rajakumar, 2003; Holick, 2006; Wagner et al., 2008). The secondary hyperparathyroidism stimulates the kidneys to produce $1,25(OH)_2D$, and thus $1,25(OH)_2D$ levels are normal or often elevated. Only when the calcium stores in the skeleton are totally depleted will the infant or child become hypocalcemic, which can lead to tetany, tetanic seizures, and death (Hess, 1929; Rajakumar, 2003; Holick, 2006).

INHERITED DISORDERS OF VITAMIN D METABOLISM AND RECOGNITION

Vitamin D–25-Hydroxylase Deficiency

At least four different hepatic enzymes have been found in the mitochondria and microsomes that are capable of metabolizing vitamin D to $25(OH)D$ (Holick, 2006, 2007; Jones, 2007). This is the likely reason there have only been rare reports of a 25-hydroxylase deficiency causing rickets in children (Casella et al., 1994).

Vitamin-D–Dependent Rickets Type I: Pseudovitamin-D–Deficiency Rickets

Before the discovery that vitamin D needed to be metabolized in the liver and kidneys before it could carry out its biologic actions on calcium and phosphorus metabolism, reports were published of children who had rickets but did not respond to physiologic doses of vitamin D. The children had hypocalcemia, hypophosphatemia, elevated alkaline phosphatase, elevated PTH, and severe rachitic changes on x-ray. However, many of these children responded to very large pharmacologic doses of vitamin D. As a result, these children received the diagnosis of vitamin-D-dependent rickets because of their need for much higher amounts of vitamin D to treat your rickets. With the revelation that vitamin D needed to be metabolized in the kidneys to its active form, it was speculated that vitamin-D-dependent rickets was caused by a mutation of the 1-OHase, resulting in either inadequate production of $1,25(OH)_2D$ or the lack of production of $1,25(OH)_2D$ (Figure 10.5). The first insight into the cause of this disorder was when $1,25(OH)_2D_3$ was chemically synthesized and provided to these patients (Fraser et al., 1973). Within several months, there was a dramatic improvement in their serum calcium and phosphorus level with a decrease in alkaline phosphatase and PTH. Thus, vitamin-D-dependent rickets was concluded to be caused by a hereditary defect in the 1-OHase.

The cloning of the 1-OHase gene led to the identification of inactivating mutations that confirmed the hypothesis for the cause of rare genetic disorder (Kitanaka et al., 1998). Patients with pseudovitamin-D-deficiency rickets (PDDR) present in their first year of life with severe hypocalcemia that can cause seizures and carpal pedal spasms, hypophosphatemia, elevated alkaline phosphatase, and PTH. Their blood level of $25(OH)D$ is usually normal, and treating them with physiologic doses of vitamin D had little effect on correcting their abnormal biochemistries (Holick, 2007). The hallmark for making the diagnosis is a low or undetectable blood level of $1,25(OH)_2D$.

If these patients are not appropriately treated with replacement doses of $1,25(OH)_2D_3$, they will have the same skeletal deformities seen in children with severe vitamin D deficiency (Fraser et al., 1973; Holick, 2006, 2007).

These patients respond well to replacement doses of 1–2 mcg of $1,25(OH)_2D_3$ (calcitriol) along with adequate calcium intake. The serum calcium levels begin to rise within 24 hours, and radiologic healing is observed by 3 months (Fraser et al., 1973; Holick, 2006, 2007).

Vitamin-D–Dependent Rickets Type II: Hereditary Vitamin-D–Resistant Rickets

Children who had severe biochemical and skeletal abnormalities associated with vitamin-D-deficiency rickets and who did not respond to physiologic doses of vitamin D and only rarely responded to pharmacologic doses of vitamin D were also considered to have vitamin-D-dependent rickets.

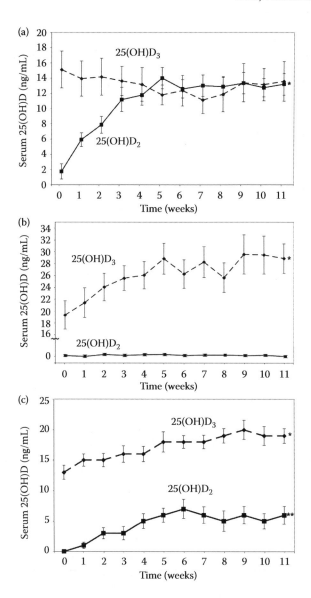

FIGURE 10.5   Effect of vitamin D_2 or vitamin D_3 on serum 25-hydroxyvitamin D_2 [25(OH)D_2] and 25-hydroxyvitamin D_3 [25(OH)D_3] levels. Serum levels of 25(OH)D_2 (-•-)and serum 25(OH)D_3 (-■-) were measured in healthy subjects who received 1000 IU of vitamin D_2 (a), 1000 IU of vitamin D_3 (b), or 500 IU of vitamin D_2 + 500 IU of vitamin D_3 (c) daily for 3 months. Results are presented as means ± SEM over time. In panel A, *$p < .0001$ comparing 25(OH)D_2 from baseline to 3 months. In panel B, *$p < .0001$ comparing 25(OH)D_3 from baseline to 3 months. In panel C, $p = .0014$ comparing 25(OH)D_3 and placebo from baseline to 3 months, **$p = 0.0031$ comparing 25(OH)D_2 and placebo from baseline to 3 months. Note that the serum 25(OH)D_2 levels <4 ng/mL were determined by subtracting the total 25(OH)D_3 from the total 25(OH)D levels. (Reproduced with permission from Holick, M.F., et al. *J Clin Endocrinol Met* 93, 667–668, 2008).

However, unlike children with PDDR who had a low or undetectable blood level of 1,25(OH)$_2$D, these children had a markedly elevated blood level of 1,25(OH)$_2$D (Brooks et al., 1978). It was assumed that these children must have a genetic defect causing a lack of responsiveness to the calcium and bone metabolism to 1,25(OH)$_2$D. The most likely cause was a defective or absent recognition of 1,25(OH)$_2$D due to a mutation of the VDR. These patients had variable responses to replacement doses of $1,25(OH)_2D_3$. A multitude of point mutations of the VDR that cause disruption of hormone-binding or DNA-binding leading to partial resistance to $1,25(OH)_2D_3$ replacement therapy have been identified (Brooks et al., 1978; Holick, 2006, 2007). In some cases, these patients respond to pharmacologic doses of $1,25(OH)_2D_3$. However, other patients do not respond because they have a point mutation that prevents the production of VDR or prevents the VDR from either binding $1,25(OH)_2D$ or permitting the VDR– retinoic acid X receptor (RXR)–$1,25(OH)_2D$ complex from binding to its responsive element within the DNA. Typically, these patients are resistant to both physiologic and pharmacologic doses of $1,25(OH)_2D_3$ (Brooks et al., 1978; Holick, 2006, 2007).

Hereditary vitamin-D-resistant rickets patients have all of the biochemical and clinical manifestations of those with PDDR, with the exception of often having a low blood level of 25(OH)D and a markedly elevated level of $1,25(OH)_2D$. Another clinical manifestation that is not seen in PDDR patients is that some patients develop alopecia beginning the first year of life that progresses to alopecia totalis (Brooks et al., 1978; Holick, 2006).

VITAMIN-D–DEPENDENT RICKETS TYPE III

One case of vitamin-D–resistant rickets has been reported in which an abnormal expression of the hormone-responsive element-binding protein that binds to the vitamin-D-responsive element exists. The abnormal expression prevents the VDR–RXR–$1,25(OH)_2D$ complex from binding to its responsive element. This patient had a normal VDR expression and was completely resistant to $1,25(OH)_2D_3$ (Chen et al., 2003).

STRATEGIES FOR TREATMENT AND PREVENTION OF RICKETS/OSTEOMALACIA

The distinction between vitamin D insufficiency and vitamin D deficiency needs to be kept in mind when recommending supplemental vitamin D, with or without calcium, for the general public to prevent rickets/osteomalacia. Treatment of this disorder typically requires significantly greater doses of vitamin D until the clinical measurements return to the normal ranges.

RESPONSIVENESS TO CALCIUM AND VITAMIN D

The major cause of rickets/osteomalacia is vitamin D deficiency (Hess, 1929; Kreiter et al., 2000; Rajakumar, 2003; Holick, 2007; Wagner and Greer, 2008). Vitamin D deficiency is defined as a serum 25(OH)D < 20 ng/mL. However, to maximize intestinal calcium absorption and to minimize circulating PTH levels, it is desirable to maintain a 25(OH)D > 30 ng/mL (Heaney et al., 2003; Holick, 2007). Thus, vitamin D insufficiency is defined as a 25(OH)D of 21–29 ng/mL (Holick, 2007). To achieve vitamin D sufficiency, at least 1000–2000 IU of vitamin D/day or its equivalent is needed (Heaney et al., 2003; Holick, 2006, 2007; Holick et al., 2008). For every 100 IU of vitamin D_2 or vitamin D_3 ingested, the blood level of 25(OH)D increases by 1 ng/mL (Heaney et al., 2003; Holick et al., 2008). When given daily, vitamin D_2 is equally effective as vitamin D_3 in maintaining serum 25(OH)D levels. However, healthy adults at the end of the winter in Boston receiving 1000 of vitamin D_2 or 1000 IU of vitamin D_3/day or 500 IU vitamin D_2 and 500 IU vitamin D_3/day were unable to achieve a sustained blood level of 25(OH)D > 30 ng/mL (Holick et al., 2008) (Figure 10.5). Most children and adults have a circulating blood level of 25(OH)D of between 15 and 25 ng/mL (Holick, 2006, 2007). Thus, to achieve a blood level of 25(OH)D > 30 ng/mL, it has been recommended that both children and adults take 1000 IU of vitamin D/day along with a multivitamin containing 400 IU of vitamin D. For obese children and adults, the amount of vitamin D ingested should be increased by two- to three-fold because body fat will sequester vitamin D, and obese children and adults need at least two to three times more vitamin D to sustain their blood level of 25(OH)D > 30 ng/mL (Holick, 2006, 2007).

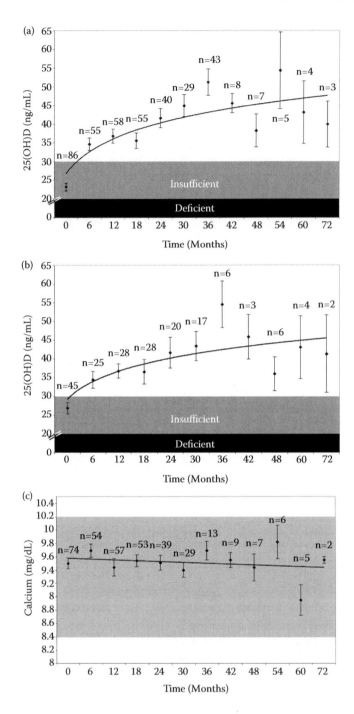

FIGURE 10.6 (a) Mean serum 25-hydroxyvitamin D [25(OH)D] levels in all patients. (b) Mean serum 25(OH)D levels in patients receiving maintenance therapy only. (c) Serum calcium levels: Results for all 86 patients who were treated with 50,000 IU of vitamin D2. (Adapted from Pietras, S.M., et al., *Arch Intern Med*, 169, 1806–1808, 2009 and reproduced from Holick, *M.F., New Engl J Med*, 357, 266–281, 2007. With permission.)

TREATMENT OF VITAMIN D DEFICIENCY

To treat vitamin D deficiency, 50,000 IU of vitamin D_2, which is the only pharmaceutical form of vitamin D available in the United States, once a week for 8 weeks will often fill the empty vitamin D tank and raise the blood level above 30 ng/mL (Malabanan et al., 1998). Patients who are severely vitamin D deficient with a 25(OH)D < 10 ng/mL or patients who are on medications that would enhance vitamin D destruction and obese patients may require an additional 8 weeks of therapy with 50,000 IU of vitamin D_2 (Holick, 2007). Once the blood level of 25(OH)D is above 30 ng/mL, vitamin D sufficiency can be maintained by giving patients 50,000 IU of vitamin D once every 2 weeks. In our clinic, we have found over a 6-year period that the blood levels are sustained between 40 and 50 ng/mL on this regime (Pietras et al., 2009) (Figure 10.6). Alternatively, to treat vitamin D deficiency with vitamin D supplement, 5000 IU of vitamin D/day for 2 months followed by 2000 IU of vitamin D/day will treat vitamin D deficiency and maintain vitamin D sufficiency in most adults.

The graph depicted in Figure 10.6a includes all patients treated with 50,000 IU vitamin D_2 every 2 weeks (maintenance therapy, N = 86). Forty one of the patients were vitamin D insufficient or deficient and first received 50,000 IU vitamin D_2 weekly for 8 weeks before being placed on maintenance therapy of 50,000 IU vitamin D_2 every 2 weeks. Error bars represent the mean ± SEM. Time 0 is the initiation of treatment. Results are shown as mean values averaged for intervals of 6 months. The mean 25(OH)D of each 6-month interval was compared with initial mean 25(OH)D and showed a significant difference of p < .001 for all time points. In patients receiving maintenance therapy, as shown in Figure 10.6b, thirty-eight patients were vitamin D insufficient [25(OH)D levels <21–29 ng/mL] and seven patients were vitamin D sufficient [25(OH)D levels ≥ 30 ng/mL], who were treated only with maintenance therapy of 50,000 IU vitamin D2 every 2 weeks. Error bars represent the mean ± SEM. Time 0 is the initiation of treatment. Results shown are interval mean values averaged for intervals of 6 months. The mean 25(OH)D in each 6-month interval was compared with the mean initial 25(OH)D and showed a significant difference, p < .001, for all time points up to 48 months. The data for interval months 60 and 72 were pooled, and there was a significant difference p < .01 compared with the baseline value. Error bars shown in Figure 10.6c represent standard error of the mean. Time 0 is the initiation of treatment. Results shown are mean values averaged for intervals of 6 months. Normal serum calcium: 8.5–10.2 mg/dL.

The American Academy of Pediatrics recommends that all infants and children receive 400 IU of vitamin D/day (Wagner and Greer, 2008). This daily dose will prevent rickets in infants and children.

Children and adults who have calcium-induced rickets/osteomalacia should be treated with the adequate intake recommendation for calcium, which is 800 mg/day for children under the age of 12 years, 1300 mg/day for teenagers, 1000 mg/day for adults 19–50 years, and 1200 mg/day for adults over the age of 50 years (Institute of Medicine, 1997). Individuals should also be taking an adequate amount of vitamin D, that is, 800–1000 IU per day, for teenagers and adults to maximize the benefit of the calcium on skeletal health.

CONCLUSION

Vitamin D is critically important for bone health. Vitamin D is responsible for regulating intestinal calcium absorption and bone calcium mobilization for the purpose of maintaining serum calcium in a physiologic range to support neuromuscular activity, signal transduction, as well as maintenance of a mineralized skeleton. Rickets/osteomalacia is caused by a defect in the mineralization of osteoid laid down by mature osteoblasts. Once the osteoid is laid down, an adequate calcium–phosphate product in the circulation results in the normal mineralization, with deposition of calcium hydroxyapatite forming mineralized bone. The most common causes of rickets/osteomalacia result from either vitamin D deficiency or calcium deficiency. Any acquired or inherited disorder that alters vitamin D metabolism or its recognition or phosphorus metabolism also causes a mineralization defect of the skeleton. Osteomalacia cannot be distinguished from osteopenia or osteoporosis based either by x-ray examination or by bone mineral density determination. Physicians should be alert to rickets in children and osteomalacia in adults because these disorders are more common than expected. Treatment of vitamin D deficiency and correction of calcium and phosphorus intake inadequacies, that is, nutritional deficiencies, result in complete resolution of rickets/osteomalacia. To maintain maximum skeletal health, all children should ingest at least 400 IU of vitamin D a day and adults should ingest at least 1000 IU of vitamin D a day. However, to take advantage of all of the health benefits of vitamin D, children should be on at least 1000 IU of vitamin D a day and adults should be on 2000 IU of vitamin D a day.

Vitamin D deficiency/insufficiency is now recognized as the most common medical condition worldwide. This deficiency/insufficiency not only has significant consequences for skeletal health of children and adults, but it also has been associated with many chronic diseases. An estimated 50% or more of children and adults in the United States are vitamin D deficient or insufficient. African American children and adults are at especially high risk because of the sun-screening effect of their skin pigment in reducing the efficiency of the sun to produce vitamin D in their skin. Vitamin D deficiency and insufficiency have been linked to increased risk of autoimmune diseases, including type I diabetes; multiple sclerosis and rheumatoid arthritis; cancers of the colon, prostate, and breast; hypertension; heart disease; and stroke, as well as to increased risk of developing infectious diseases including tuberculosis, upper respiratory tract infections, and influenza. To take advantage of the nonskeletal health benefits of vitamin D, children are recommended to receive at least 1000 IU of vitamin D/day, and up to 2000 IU of vitamin D/day is considered safe. Adults need at least 2000 IU of vitamin D/day to maintain a blood concentration of 25(OH)D between 30 and 100 ng/mL.

ACKNOWLEDGMENT

This work was supported in part by a grant from the UV Foundation.

REFERENCES

Aubin, J.E., Lian, J.B., Stein, G.S. 2006. Bone formation: Maturation and functional activities of osteoblast lineage cells. In: *Primer on the Metabolic Bone Diseases and Disorders of Mineral Metabolism*, 6th ed., Favus, M.J., ed. The American Society for Bone and Mineral Research, Washington, DC, 20–29.

Balsan, S., Garabedian, M., Larchet, M., et al. 1986. Long-term nocturnal calcium infusions can cure rickets and promote normal mineralization in hereditary resistance to 1,25-dihydroxyvitamin D. *J Clin Invest* 77: 1661–1667.

Brooks, M.H., Bell, N.H., Love, L., et al. 1978. Vitamin-D-dependent rickets type II: Resistance of target organs to 1,25-dihydroxyvitamin D. *New Engl J Med* 298: 996–999.

Brown, E.M., Gamba, G., Riccardl, D., et al. 1993. Cloning and characterization of an extracellular Ca^{2+}-sensing receptor from bovine parathyroid. *Nature* 366: 575–580.

Casella, S.J., Reiner, B.J., Chen, T.C., et al. 1994. A possible defect in 25-hydroxylation as a cause of rickets. *J Pediatr* 124: 929–932.

Chen, H., Hewison, M. Hu, B., et al. 2003. Heterogeneous nuclear ribonucleoprotein (hnRNP) binding to hormone response elements: A cause of vitamin D resistance. *PNAS (USA)* 100: 6109–6114.

Christakos, S., Dhawan, P., Liu, Y., et al. 2003. New insights into the mechanisms of vitamin D action. *J Cell Biochem* 88: 695–705.

Fraser, D., Kooh, S.W., Kind, H.P., et al. 1973. Pathogenesis of hereditary vitamin-D-dependent rickets. An inborn error of vitamin D metabolism involving defective conversion of 25 hydroxyvitamin D to 1 alpha,25-dihydroxyvitamin D. *New Engl J Med* 289: 817–822.

Haddad, J.G., Matsuoka, L.Y., Hollis, B.W., et al. 1993. Human plasma transport of vitamin D after its endogenous synthesis. *J Clin Invest* 91: 2552–2555.

Heaney, R.P., Davies, K.M., Chen, T.C., et al. 2003. Human serum 25-hydroxycholecalciferol response to extended oral dosing with cholecalciferol. *Am J Clin Nutr* 77: 204–210.

Hess, A.F. 1929. *Rickets Including Osteomalacia and Tetany*. Lea J. Febiger, Philadelphia, PA, 401–429.

Hess, A.F., and Lundagen, M.A. 1922. A seasonal tide of blood phosphate in infants. *J Am Med Assoc* 79: 2210–2212.

Hess, A.F., and Unger, L.J. 1921. The cure of infantile rickets by sunlight. *J Am Med Assoc* 77: 39–41.

Hess, A.F., and Weinstock, M. 1924. Antirachitic properties imparted to inert fluids and to green vegetables by ultraviolet irradiation. *J Biol Chem* 62: 301–313.

Holick, M.F. 2006. Resurrection of vitamin D deficiency and rickets. *J Clin Invest* 116: 2062–2072.

Holick, M.F. 2007. Vitamin D deficiency. *New Engl J Med* 357: 266–281.

Holick, M.F., Biancuzzo, R.M., Chen, T.C., et al. 2008. Vitamin D$_2$ is as effective as vitamin D$_3$ in maintaining circulating concentrations of 25-hydroxyvitamin D. *J Clin Endocrinol Metab* 93: 677–681.

Holick, M.F., and Garabedian, M. 2006. Vitamin D: Photobiology, metabolism, mechanism of action, and clinical applications. In: *Primer on the Metabolic Bone Diseases and Disorders of Mineral Metabolism*, 6th ed., Favus, M.J., ed. American Society for Bone and Mineral Research: Washington, DC, 129–137.

Hollis, B.W., and Wagner, C.L. 2004. Assessment of dietary vitamin D requirements during pregnancy and lactation. *Am J Clin Nutr* 79: 717–726.

Huldschinsky, K. 1919. Heilung von Rachitis durch Kunstliche Hohensonne. *Deutsche Med Wochenschr* 45: 712–713.

Huldschinsky, K. 1928. *The Ultra-violet Light Treatment of Rickets*. Alpine Press, NJ, 3–19.

Jones, G. 2007. Expanding role for Vitamin D in chronic kidney disease: Importance of blood 25-OH-D levels and extra-renal 1α-hydroxylase in the classical and nonclassical actions of 1α,25-dihydroxyvitamin D$_3$. *Semin Dialysis* 20: 316–324.

Khosla, S. 2001. The OPG/RANKL/RANK system. *Endocrinology* 142: 5050–5055.

Kitanaka, S., Takeyama, K.I., Murayama, A., et al. 1998. Inactivating mutations in the human 25-hydroxyvitamin D$_3$ 1α-hydroxylase gene in patients with pseudovitamin D-deficient rickets. *New Eng J Med* 338: 653–661.

Kreiter, S.R., Schwartz, R.P., Kirkman, H.N., et al. 2000. Nutritional rickets in African American breast-fed infants. *J Pediatr* 137: 2–6.

Malabanan, A., Veronikis, I.E., Holick, M.F. 1998. Redefining vitamin D insufficiency. *Lancet* 351: 805–806.

Parfitt, A.M. 1998. Osteomalacia and related disorders. In: *Metabolic Bone Disease and Clinically Related Disorders*, 3rd ed., Avioli, L.V., and Krane, S.M., eds. Academic Press, San Diego, CA, 327–386.

Pietras, S.M., Obayan, B.K., Cai, M.H., et al. 2009. Vitamin D$_2$ treatment for vitamin D deficiency and insufficiency for up to 6 years. *Arch Intern Med* 169: 1806–1808.

Powers, G.F., Park, E.A., Shipley, P.G., et al. 1921. The prevention of rickets in the rat by means of radiation with the mercury vapor quartz lamp. *Proc Soc Exp Biol Med* 19: 120–121.

Rajakumar, K. 2003. Vitamin D, cod-liver oil, sunlight, and rickets: A historical perspective. *Pediatrics* 112: 132–135.

Sniadecki, J. 1939. (1768–1838) On the cure of rickets. (1840) Cited by Mozolowski, W. *Nature* 143: 121–124.

Steenbock, H., and Black, A. 1924. The reduction of growth-promoting and calcifying properties in a ration by exposure to ultraviolet light. *J Biol Chem* 61: 408–422.

Wagner, C.L., and Greer, F.R., and the Section on Breastfeeeding and Committee on Nutrition. (2008). Prevention of rickets and Vitamin D deficiency in infants, children, and adolescents. *Pediatrics* 122:1142–1152.

11 Vitamin A and Bone

Håkan Melhus

CONTENTS

INTRODUCTION

In 1998, we reported that intake of vitamin A at levels only slightly greater than the recommended daily intake was associated with reduced bone density and increased risk of hip fractures (Melhus et al., 1998). The study was prompted by consistent animal and *in vitro* data, reports on osteoporosis as a toxic effect of long-term therapy with synthetic retinoids, and the observation that Sweden and Norway, for unknown reasons, have the world's highest incidence of osteoporotic fractures and that the vitamin A intake in these countries is unusually high due to a high consumption of fortified milk products, cod liver oil, and multivitamins (Melhus et al., 1998).

The results of the observational studies published 1998–2002, together with the recognition that the large increase in vitamin A intake from fortified foods and supplements during the preceding decades had resulted in an oversupplementation especially among the elderly (Anderson, 2002), led to a reassessment of the levels of vitamin A supplementation and food fortification both in the United States and in Europe. Retinol levels have generally been reduced in multivitamins. In addition, in Sweden, AD-vitamins given to all children have been replaced by D-vitamin, and the retinol levels in low-fat dairy products have been reduced. In Norway, the retinol level in cod liver oil has been reduced by 75%.

For ethical reasons, no randomized clinical trials evaluating the effects of vitamin A on bone have been undertaken, but since 1998, over 20 observational human studies have been published, and they are the focus of this chapter. Together, they can be said to illustrate the spectrum of difficulties in performing and interpreting the results of this kind of study.

In this chapter, vitamin A, its structure, and food sources are described. Recommended intakes are given, and the effects of vitamin A on bone are summarized. Before describing the different observational studies, methods and difficulties in assessing vitamin A exposure and the outcome bone health are reviewed.

TERMINOLOGY

The term *vitamin A* refers to a family of essential, fat-soluble dietary compounds that play an important role in vision, bone growth, reproduction, cell differentiation, and regulation of the immune system. The alcohol form of vitamin A, (all-*trans-*) retinol, and its fatty acid ester derivatives, retinyl esters (most commonly, retinyl palmitate), are referred to as *preformed vitamin A* (Figure 11.1). In published literature, the terms *vitamin A*, *retinol*, and *preformed vitamin A* are often used interchangeably. Whereas retinyl esters are the storage form of vitamin A, retinol functions as a prehormone, which is transported to target tissues where it is converted to the active forms of vitamin A (Figure 11.2). In the eye, the active metabolite is 11-*cis* retinal. In all other target organs, retinol is converted to all-*trans*-retinoic acid and possibly also to 9-*cis* retinoic acid. The term *retinoids* refers to retinol, its metabolites, and synthetic analogues that have a similar structure. Beta-carotene is a precursor for vitamin A (Figure 11.1). It is a tail-joined retinal dimer and is more efficiently converted to retinol than are other compounds of the class of plant pigments called *carotenoids*, owing to their relation to the carotenes. Beta-carotene and other carotenoids, such as β-carotene and β-cryptoxanthin, that the body can transform to active forms of vitamin A are referred to as *provitamin A* (McDowell, 2000).

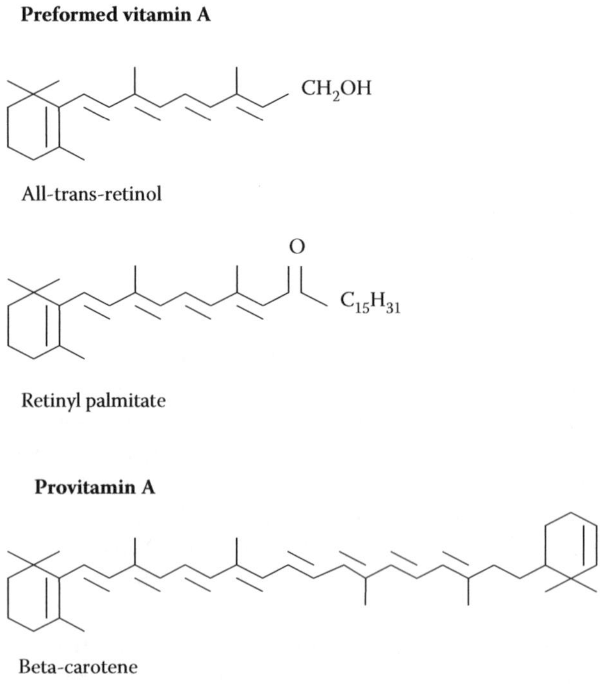

FIGURE 11.1 Vitamin A overview.

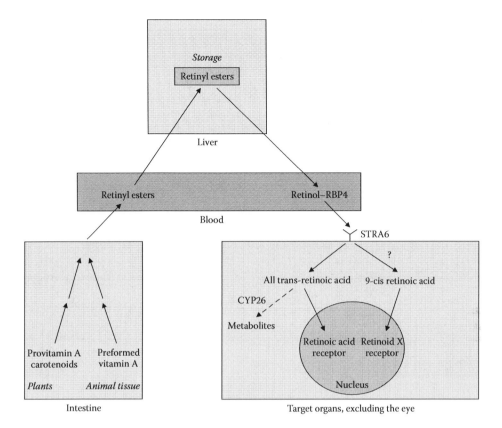

FIGURE 11.2   Vitamin A overview. Vitamin A is obtained as provitamin A carotenoids in plant foods or as preformed vitamin A in the form of retinyl esters from animal sources. In the intestine, provitamin A carotenoids are cleaved to retinal and converted to retinol. Retinyl esters are hydrolyzed to retinol. Retinol is then reesterified and incorporated to chylomicrons, which circulate in the intestinal lymph before entering the general circulation. Chylomicron remnants are cleared by the liver, where the retinyl esters are stored. After hydrolysis of retinyl esters to retinol, retinol binds to retinol-binding protein (RBP) 4 and the vitamin is transported from the liver to target organs. Retinol is taken up by a specific RBP4 receptor, STRA6, and converted to all-*trans* retinoic acid (ATRA), and possibly also 9-*cis* RA. In the eye, retinol is converted to 11-*cis* retinal which binds to opsin. In other target organs, retinol is oxidized to ATRA, which binds to its specific nuclear RA receptor. The enzyme CYP26 converts ATRA to polar metabolites, which can be conjugated and eliminated.

SOURCES OF VITAMIN A

Preformed vitamin A is found in foods of animal origin, such as liver, meats, milk products, eggs, and fatty fish. Because retinyl esters are stored in the liver of both fish and mammals, cod liver oil and other liver products contain very high levels. Common sources are also fortified foods (such as margarine and breakfast cereals) and dietary supplements. Many orange fruits and green vegetables are sources of provitamin A carotenoids, for example, carrots, spinach, sweet potatoes, cantaloupes, broccoli, squash, mango, apricots, peas, and papaya (Sporn et al., 1994; McDowell, 2000).

RECOMMENDED DIETARY INTAKES OF VITAMIN A

In the United States, recommendations for vitamin A are provided in the Dietary Reference Intakes (DRI) developed by the Institute of Medicine (IOM) (Food and Nutrition Board, IOM, 2001). Three important types of reference values included in the DRIs are Recommended Dietary Allowances (RDA), Adequate Intakes (AI), and Tolerable Upper Intake Levels (UL). The RDA recommends the average daily dietary intake level that is sufficient to meet the nutrient requirements of nearly all (97%–98%) healthy individuals in each age and gender group (Table 11.1A). An AI is set when there are insufficient scientific data to establish an RDA. AIs meet or exceed the amount needed to maintain nutritional adequacy in nearly all people (Table 11.1B). The UL is the highest level of daily vitamin A intake that is likely to pose no risk of adverse health effects in almost all individuals (Table 11.2) (Food and Nutrition Board, IOM, 2001).

SKELETAL EFFECTS OF PROVITAMIN A CAROTENOIDS

There is no evidence of bone toxicity from provitamin A carotenoids in laboratory animals or humans (Armstrong et al., 1994; Sahni et al., 2009a, 2009b). Beta-carotene produces no bone

TABLE 11.1A
Recommended Dietary Allowances (RDAs) for Vitamin A

Children	
1–3 years	300
4–8 years	400
Males	
9–13 years	600
14 years and older	900
Females	
9–13 years	600
14 years and older	700
Pregnancy	
14–18 years	750
19 years and older	770
Lactation	
14–18 years	1200
19 years and older	1300

TABLE 11.1B
Adequate Intakes (AIs) of Vitamin A for Infants (Males and Females)

0–6 months	400
7–12 months	500

Note: RDAs and AIs are listed as micrograms of retinol activity equivalents/day. 1 RAE = 3.3 IU.

Source: Food and Nutrition Board, Institute of Medicine. 2001. *Dietary Reference Intakes for Vitamin A, Vitamin K, Arsenic, Boron, Chromium, Copper, Iodine, Iron, Manganese, Molybdenum, Nickel, Silicon, Vanadium, and Zinc.* National Academy Press, Washington, DC.

resorption or other significant change in bone *in vitro* (Kamm et al., 1984). Moreover, these compounds do not cause skeletal malformations (Armstrong et al., 1994). Important reasons are that the cleavage of provitamin A carotenoids to retinal in the intestine is a highly regulated step (Bachmann et al., 2002; Takitani et al., 2006) and that an excess of carotenoids can be stored in the skin, resulting in a yellow to yellow-orange discoloration, or carotenodermia.

SKELETAL EFFECTS OF PREFORMED VITAMIN A AND RETINOIDS IN ANIMALS

Evidence from animal studies has clearly shown that high doses of retinol can have adverse skeletal effects (Binkley and Krueger, 2000). This research on vitamin A toxicity was primarily carried out between 1925 and 1950. Nieman and Obbink (1954) provided an extensive review of these studies. Skeletal lesions were reported in 31 different studies, and laboratory animals included rat, mouse, guinea pig, rabbit, chicken, duck, and dog. The most prominent features of toxic doses of retinol were a thinning of the long bones and spontaneous fractures (Table 11.3). These findings have been confirmed in more recent studies (Frankel et al., 1986; Hough et al., 1988; Wu et al., 1996). The active form of vitamin A, retinoic acid, and synthetic retinoids induce the same characteristic bone thinning (Teelmann, 1981; Kneissel et al., 2005). The available data suggest that these adverse

TABLE 11.2
Tolerable Upper Intake Levels (ULs)
for Preformed Vitamin A

Age (Years)	ULs for Preformed Vitamin A (µg/day)
0–1	600
1–3	600
4–8	900
9–13	1700
14–18	2800
Adults	3000

Source: Food and Nutrition Board, Institute of Medicine. 2001. *Dietary Reference Intakes for Vitamin A, Vitamin K, Arsenic, Boron, Chromium, Copper, Iodine, Iron, Manganese, Molybdenum, Nickel, Silicon, Vanadium, and Zinc.* National Academy Press, Washington, DC.

TABLE 11.3
Major Findings Related to Bone in Animals with
Hypervitaminosis A

Spontaneous fractures
Thinning of long bones
Premature closure of epiphyses
Retardation of growth
No or little effect on mineralization, except when vitamin D is low.
Toxicity is cumulative and reversible.

effects occur as a result of increased bone resorption and decreased bone formation. It has been pointed out that most studies on laboratory animals have used very high doses administered to young growing animals and that results from such studies may not be directly relevant to human osteoporosis (Binkley and Krueger, 2000). However, subclinical hypervitaminosis A in mature rats leads to reduced bone diameter (Johansson et al., 2002), and the same changes, although smaller in magnitude, also occur in aged rats (Kneissel et al., 2005).

There are several important observations in animal studies that may help us to interpret human studies. First, retinol has no or little effect on mineralization, except when vitamin D is present at a marginal level (Aburto and Britton, 1998a, 1998b). When there is sufficient vitamin D, retinol increases the risk of fracture by a mechanism that reduces the diameter of the bone but not the bone mineral density (BMD) (Lind et al., 2006). This is in contrast to vitamin D. If this is true also in humans, BMD measurements (which are used to diagnose osteoporosis) will not detect the adverse effects caused by an excessive intake of retinol. Second, vitamin A toxicity is cumulative. The duration of onset and frequency of fractures are dose related. This has been most clearly shown for the retinoid etretinate (Teelmann, 1981). Fractures occurred as early as 10–14 days at doses of 10–15 mg/kg/day. In contrast, with 3 mg/kg/day, fractures were not observed earlier than after 5–6 months. The fractures were preceded by a markedly intensified remodeling of the bones with deformations, increased periosteal osteoclastic activity, thickening of the periosteum, and accelerated ossification of the epiphyseal line. In addition, an augmented endosteal osteoblastic activity resulting in marked reduction of bone diameter and increasing porosity, particularly of the long bones, was noted. All side effects were reversible after cessation of treatment (Teelmann, 1981; Melhus, 2003).

CASE REPORTS IN HUMANS

Case reports of children and adults who have ingested massive doses of vitamin A describe most of the findings that have been found in animals (Table 11.4) (Kamm et al., 1984; Armstrong et al., 1994). However, only one case of fracture due to hypervitaminosis A has been reported in man (Ruby and Mital, 1974). A girl 1 year and 3 months old had been given a daily dose of 15 mg in a water-soluble preparation for 7 months. Roentgenograms showed a fracture of the right humerus. Only remnants of the distal femoral epiphyses were visible, and both were seemingly impressed into the metaphyses, which were irregular. The serum vitamin A was elevated by a factor of five.

Vitamin A has an effect on bone turnover also in humans (Jowsey and Riggs, 1968). The micro-radiographic appearance of bone taken during and after a period of high vitamin A intake revealed that there was an increase in the size of the osteocyte lacunae, resorption surfaces were a factor of six above the normal, and there was an absence of a comparative increase in bone formation. Similar findings with numerous resorptive lacunae and no index of bone formation have been described in a French patient (Baglin et al., 1986).

The lowest dose inducing chronic hypervitaminosis A has not been defined. In some cases, doses as low as about 0.1–0.3 mg/kg/day (Schurr et al., 1983; Carpenter et al., 1987) have been suggested to cause toxicity in children.

TABLE 11.4
Major Findings Related to Bone in Human Subjects with Hypervitaminosis A

Bone and joint pain
Thinning of bone cortex
Premature closure of epiphyses
Retardation of growth
Hyperostosis
Calcification of tendons and ligaments

As described above, preclinical studies demonstrated that synthetic retinoids have effects on bones that mimic the effects of hypervitaminosis A. When these retinoids were introduced in clinical dermatology in the late 1970s, relatively high doses were used, and premature closure of epiphyses (Milstone et al., 1982), hyperostosis (Pittsley and Yoder, 1983), calcification of ligaments and tendons (DiGiovanna et al., 1986), and thinning of long bones and traumatic fractures (Prendiville et al., 1986) were all reported within a few years.

HUMAN STUDIES

Results from observational studies of the effect of retinol on bone health are inconsistent. This may be due, in part, to differences in population studied, study designs, assessment of retinol intake or vitamin A status, and method used to measure bone health. Some aspects of these will therefore be discussed.

POPULATION STUDIES

About half of all studies on vitamin A and bone health have been conducted in the United States and one third in the Nordic countries. The reason for this is that the highest incidence of osteoporotic fracture is found in these countries, especially Norway and Sweden (Johnell et al., 1992; EPOS Group, 2002; Kanis et al., 2002). The dietary intake of retinol is higher in Nordic countries than that in southern Europe and the United States (Cruz et al., 1991; Scientific Advisory Committee on Nutrition, 2005). One important reason for this is that the milk consumption is higher in Nordic countries (International Dairy and Federation, 1995). This is possibly due to lactose tolerance (Sahi, 1994), which is a genetic adaptation to vitamin D deficiency; at northern latitudes, the cutaneous synthesis of previtamin D during the long winter season is undetectable (Burgaz et al., 2007). Historically, the intake of dairy products, fatty fish, cod liver oil, and AD-vitamins has therefore been important in these countries. Low-fat milk products are not fortified with vitamin A in Sweden anymore, so the United States and Canada are now the only countries in which these products are fortified with AD-vitamins.

STUDY DESIGN

The majority of the studies on bone mineral are cross-sectional, whereas prospective studies dominate when fracture is the endpoint. For reasons discussed below, a cohort study with multiple assessments of retinol intake or vitamin A status, a good follow-up, and fracture as endpoint is important to obtain reliable results. Case–control studies have a lower quality grade on a standard scale of medical evidence (Phillips et al., 2001), and it is interesting to note that the results from these (Table 11.5) often show that vitamin A has positive effects on BMD. A problem with case–control studies is that of confounding. Cases with osteoporosis are more likely to be older, have lower BMI, and have poorer health compared with those of controls. If serum retinol is found to be lower in cases than in controls, it is impossible to separate whether this is the cause or a consequence of other factors. Differences in age and BMI can be adjusted for in the statistical analysis, but to control for differences in general health will require very detailed information about comorbidities and intricate statistical modeling.

DIETARY ASSESSMENT OF VITAMIN A

Multiple methods have been used to ascertain retinol intake, with the Food Frequency Questionnaire (FFQ) being the instrument of choice in large nutritional epidemiological studies. Two other dietary instruments that have been commonly used are the 24-h dietary recall and the dietary record (DR). It is generally accepted that all these methods have advantages and limitations, and none of them is

---

TABLE 11.5

Studies Examining the Association between Vitamin A Intake and Bone Mineral

Year	Country	Study Design	Study Sample	Dietary Assessment	Bone Measurement	Nutrient/Biomarker	Association	Reference
1985	United States	Cross-sectional	912 ♀, 1208 ♂ 43–81 years	24-hour recall + previous week	SPA	Total vitamin A	0 (+)	Yano et al., 1985
1985	United States	Cross-sectional	324 ♀, 55–80 years	24-hour recall	SPA	Total vitamin A	0	Sowers et al., 1985
1986	United States	Four-year calcium trial	99 ♀, 35–65 years	Multiple 24-hour records	SPA	Total vitamin A	0 (+ and –)	Freudenheim et al., 1986
1990	United States	Cross-sectional	246 ♀, 55–80 years	Not assessed	SPA	Serum retinol	0	Sowers and Wallace, 1990
1993	United States	Cross-sectional	281 ♀, 50–60 years	FFQ	SPA	Retinol	0 (+)	Hernandez-Avila et al., 1993
1995	United States	Physical exercise trial	66 ♀, 28–39 years	Three 4-day records	DXA	Total vitamin A	0 (+)	Houtkooper et al., 1995
1997	United Kingdom	Cross-sectional	426 ♀, 45–59 years	Three-day record	DXA	Total vitamin A	0	Earnshaw et al., 1997
1998	Sweden	Cross-sectional	175 ♀, 28–74 years	Four 1-week records	DXA	Retinol	–	Melhus et al., 1998
2001	United States	Cross-sectional	2888 ♀, 2902 ♂, 20–80+ years	Not assessed	DXA	Serum retinyl esters	0	Ballew et al., 2001a, 2001b
2001	Iceland	Cross-sectional	408 ♀, 70 years	FFQ	DXA	Retinol	0	Sigurdsson et al., 2001
2002	United States	Four-year longitudinal	570 ♀, 388 ♂, 55–92 years	FFQ	DXA	Retinol	Inverse U-shaped	Promislow et al., 2002

Year	Country	Study Type	Subjects	Dietary Assessment	Bone Measure	Vitamin A Measure	Association	Reference
2003	Italy	Case–Control	♀ ≥ 60y, 75 with osteoporosis, 75 controls	Not assessed	DXA	Plasma retinol	+	Maggio et al., 2003
2003	England	Longitudinal	470 ♂, 474 ♀, 67–79y	Seven-day records at baseline	DXA × 2 (2–5y apart)	Vitamin A, beta-carotene	0	Kaptoge et al., 2003
2003	Canada	Cross-sectional	58 ♀, 45–75y	Retrospective questionnaires	DXA	Retinol	0	Suzuki et al., 2003
2004	Scotland	Longitudinal	891 ♀, 45–55y	FFQ × 2 (5–7y apart)	DXA × 2 (5–7y apart)	Vitamin A/Retinol	0 (–)	Macdonald et al., 2004
2004	Denmark	Cross-sectional + longitudinal	2016 ♀, median 50y	Four-day or 7-day food records (5y apart)	DXA × 2 (5y apart)	Retinol, beta-carotene	0	Rejnmark et al., 2004
2005	United States	Cross-sectional	11,068 ♀, 50–79y	FFQ	DXA	Vitamin A, retinol, beta-carotene	0 (–)	Wolf et al., 2005
2005	United Kingdom	Nested case–control	312 cases, 934 controls from 2606 ♀, >75y	Not assessed	DXA	Serum retinol, RE, beta-carotene	+	Barker et al., 2005
2006	United States	Case–Control	27 ♀ with osteoporosis, 24 ♀ without osteoporosis, 48–83y	Three-day food records	DXA	Vitamin A	0	Penniston et al., 2006
2008	Sweden	Longitudinal	78 ♂, 21–25y at baseline	Not assessed	DXA × 2 (2y apart)	Serum retinol	0	Hogstrom et al., 2008
2008	Norway	Retrospective	3052 ♀, 50–70y	Questionnaire	SXA	Childhood cod liver oil intake	–	Forsmo et al., 2008

Notes: SPA = singe-photon absorptiometry, FFQ = Food Frequency Questionnaire, DXA = dual-energy X-ray absorptiometry. 0 = no significant association, + = positive association, – = negative association, (+) = weak positive or partly positive association (e.g., in subgroups), (–) = weak negative or partly negative association, DXA = dual-energy X-ray absorptiometry, SXA = single energy X-ray absorptiometry, FFQ = Food Frequency Questionnaire, RE = retinyl esters, y = years.

entirely satisfactory (Henriquez-Sanchez et al., 2009). Because retinol is found in very high concentrations in a limited number of foods (liver, liver products, fortified foods, and supplements), some of which may be consumed infrequently, it is difficult to obtain reliable estimates of average consumption (especially with the 24-hour recall method) and to identify consumers of high levels of retinol (Scientific Advisory Committee on Nutrition, 2005). The intraindividual variation can cause random error when classifying persons by intake of retinol and produce a bias that systematically underestimates the strength of associations to bone health. It has been estimated that three to nine independent measurements may be required to distinguish reliably even large differences (Tangney et al., 1987). Osteoporosis develops over many years, and repeated measurements are also required to identify changes in diet over time. It is important to recognize that the majority of published studies are based on one single dietary assessment and find no association with bone health. In fact, there are only four studies with three or more independent measurements of retinol intake (Tables 11.5 and 11.6). One study used multiple 24-hour records; one study, three 4-day records; one study, four 7-day records; and the best designed study performed five independent measurements of retinol intake by FFQs over 18 years. In this latter study with five FFQs, the association with hip fracture was not significant when only the baseline measurement was used for analyses (Feskanich et al., 2002), emphasizing the importance of repeated measurements.

Another problem in correctly assessing the vitamin A intake is the bioconversion of carotenoids. For more than 30 years, it was generally accepted that 6 μg of beta-carotene and 12 μg of other provitamin A carotenoids had the same vitamin activity as 1 μg of retinol (FAO/WHO, 1967). However, several studies published in the 1990s showed that the bioefficacy of beta-carotene in plant foods was considerably less. Therefore, the U.S. Food and Nutrition Board, IOM (2001) introduced the term *retinol activity equivalent* (RAE), where 1 μg RAE = 1 μg retinol = 12 μg beta-carotene = 24 μg other provitamin A carotenoids. The development of techniques using isotope-labeled beta-carotene and retinol has advanced our knowledge further and shown that this bioconversion is quite variable; 1 mol beta-carotene can provide anything between 0 and 0.27 mol retinol (Lin et al., 2000; van Lieshout et al., 2001; Hickenbottom et al., 2002).

The activity of the enzyme responsible for the conversion of beta-carotene to retinal in the intestine, the β,β-carotene 15,15′-monooxygenase (βCMOOX), is upregulated in vitamin A deficiency and downregulated by an increased intake of retinyl esters or beta-carotene (van Vliet et al., 1996). It has been shown that retinoic acid reduces, and a retinoic acid receptor alpha antagonist significantly increases the intestinal enzyme activity. Moreover, a retinoic-acid-responsive element has been identified in the promoter of the μCMOOX gene. These results are consistent with a transcriptional feedback regulation of the enzyme by RA via the specific nuclear receptors (Bachmann et al., 2002; Takitani et al., 2006). Thus, the bioconversion of beta-carotene seems to be determined by the body's needs for the vitamin. This inefficiency of bioconversion explains why provitamin A carotenoids do not cause hypervitaminosis A even when ingested in large amounts.

ASSESSMENT OF VITAMIN A STATUS

Serum Retinol

Serum retinol levels reflect the liver stores of vitamin A, but not in a linear fashion. The levels are homeostatically controlled (usually around 2 μmol/L) over the physiologic range of liver vitamin A concentrations and are therefore generally unaffected by normal retinol intakes (Willett et al., 1983; Krasinski et al., 1989). When liver stores are exhausted (<20 μg/g liver), serum retinol values tend to fall, and when the capacity for storage in the liver is exceeded (>300 μg/g liver) or the rate of intake is greater than the rate it can be removed by the liver, serum values tend to increase. Thus, except in cases of deficiency or excess, retinol levels in the serum are not good indicators of vitamin A status (Olson, 1984). This may, in part, explain why serum retinol does not correlate with normal dietary intakes (Garry et al., 1987; Roidt et al., 1988; Booth et al., 1997), but it does with supplement use (Garry et al., 1987; Roidt et al., 1988; Sowers and Wallace, 1990; Opotowsky and Bilezikian, 2004; Barker et al., 2005).

An advantage of serum retinol as a measure of retinol exposure is that it tends to be stable for many months. In one study, serum retinol measurements taken 4 months apart correlated highly ($r = 0.79$), while estimates of vitamin A intake among the same group correlated less well ($r = 0.47$) (Kardinaal et al., 1995).

A number of other factors may also influence the levels. Serum retinol has, for example, been positively associated with age, weight, serum lipids, socioeconomic status, and renal failure and negatively associated with smoking, alcohol consumption, infections, and chronic liver diseases. With the exception of serum lipids and infections, all the other confounding factors also influence the risk of fracture (Michaelsson et al., 2003) and need to be considered in the statistical analysis.

Serum Retinyl Esters

Retinyl esters from animal food sources are transported from the intestine via the lymph to the liver, where they are stored. In contrast to retinol, which is homeostatically controlled, the serum levels of retinyl esters will increase markedly after each vitamin-A-rich meal. In fasting serum, most of the circulating vitamin A is found in the form of retinol, and only a small proportion is retinyl esters. This may explain why total intake of vitamin has not been found to correlate with serum retinyl esters (Scientific Advisory Committee on Nutrition, 2005). By contrast, in some cases of vitamin A intoxication, the retinyl ester to retinol ratio was found to exceed 10% (Smith and Goodman, 1976), and long-term use of retinol supplements has been associated with higher serum retinyl esters in elderly subjects (Krasinski et al., 1989). Serum retinyl esters have therefore been used as a marker of retinol toxicity in two studies on BMD (Table 11.5) and two on fractures (Table 11.6). However, serum retinyl esters may more reflect a temporary excess in vitamin A intake rather than long-term vitamin A intake and storage. In patients with vitamin A toxicity, serum retinyl esters decrease faster than serum retinol after discontinuation of vitamin A supplements (Smith and Goodman, 1976). Studies of plasma kinetics have shown that the clearance of serum retinyl esters varies substantially from one person to another (Bitzen et al., 1994; Reinersdorff et al., 1996; Johansson and Melhus, 2001), with an average increase in clearance of more than 50% over a 12-hour period after an intake of vitamin A of 1.0 to 1.5 mg (Krasinski et al., 1990).

ASSESSMENT OF BONE HEALTH

In studies of factors influencing bone health, the most clearly defined outcome of interest is bone fracture following minimal trauma. Most studies, however, use the intermediate outcome measure of BMD (Scientific Advisory Committee on Nutrition, 2005). Techniques to measure BMD, such as single-photon absorptiometry (SPA) and dual-energy X-ray absorptiometry (DXA), determine the amount of mineral per unit area and not volume. This means that BMD measurements are influenced by the size, shape, and orientation of the bone and therefore are more useful in prospective studies, where changes can be assessed over time. There are six such prospective studies (Table 11.5). If retinol reduces the size rather than the BMD in humans in the same way as in animals, peripheral quantitative computer tomography and other methods that can provide a measure of volumetric density may be necessary to more accurately assess the adverse skeletal effects of retinol.

The most serious and important consequence of osteoporosis is hip fractures. In studies that use fracture as outcome, hip fractures are therefore of special relevance. They have generally been identified via hospital discharge records or are self-reported. Some studies have confirmed medical record data with radiographic records or home visits. A problem with self-reported fractures is selection bias. Fracture patients have a substantially increased risk of death that persists several years post fracture (Bliuc et al., 2009). This risk of death is most pronounced for hip

TABLE 11.6
Studies Examining the Association between Vitamin A and Fracture Risk

Year	Country	Study Design	Study Sample	Vitamin A Assessment	Identification of Fractures	Mean Intake/ Level	Results	Reference
1990	United States	Retrospective	246 ♀, 56 cases (31 fx in the last 10y) 55–80y	Serum retinol, 24-h food recall, interview for suppl	Self-reported by interview	Total vit A food + suppl 0.9 mg RE	No association	Sowers and Wallace, 1990
1998	Sweden	Nested case–control, 2–64 months follow-up (SMC)	66,651 ♀, 247 hip fx cases, 873 controls, 40–76y	FFQ of usual intake of 60 foods during previous 6 months	Hospital discharge records	Retinol from food: cases 0.96 mg, controls 0.8 mg RE	OR = 2.05, ≥1.5 mg vs. <0.5 mg	Melhus et al., 1998
1998	Sweden	Prospective, 2.4y follow-up (MDCS)	6576♂, 160 any fx cases, 51 fragility fx, 46–68y	Seven-day menu book, + FFQ	Local hospital registry + X-ray examinations	Cases, 1.96 mg; controls, 1.82 mg	No association	Elmstahl et al., 1998
2002	United States	Prospective, 18y follow-up (NHS)	72,337 ♀, 603 hip fx, 34–77y	FFQs every 4y, mean intake determined from 5 FFQs	Self-reported by questionnaire	Retinol from food + suppl, 1.2 mg	RR = 1.89, ≥2 mg vs. <0.5 mg	Feskanich et al., 2002
2003	Sweden	Prospective, 30y follow-up (ULSAM)	Cohort 2322 ♂, 266 any fx, 84 hip fx, 49–51y	Serum retinol, serum beta-carotene, 7-day food record in 1138 men 20y after entry	Hospital discharge, orthopedic + radiographic records	Retinol from food 1.1 mg	Rate ratio =2.5 for hip fx; >2.64 μM (5th) vs. 2.17–2.36 μM (3rd quintile)	Michaelsson et al., 2003
2004	United States	Prospective, 9.5y follow-up (IWHS)	34,703 ♂ + ♀, 6502 any fx, 525 hip, 55–69y	FFQ 127 items + suppl question	Self-reported	Tot vit A 4.33 mg RE, retinol food + suppl 1.16 mg	No association (RR hip fx for suppl users 1.18 (0.99–1.41)	Lim et al., 2004

Year	Country	Study design/follow-up	Cohort	Assessment	Records	Retinol/vitamin A	Result	Reference
2004	Denmark	Nested case–control, 5y follow-up (DOPS)	Cohort 2016 ♀, 163 fx cases (extremities or spine), 978 controls, 45–58y	Four- or 7-day record	Hospital discharge records	Retinol food 0.53 mg, food + suppl 1.21 mg	No association	Rejnmark et al., 2004
2004	United States	Prospective, 22y follow-up (NHANES I)	2799 ♂, 172 hip fx, 50–74y	Serum vit A (retinol + retinyl esters)	Self-reported, confirmed by hospital records	Serum retinol 2.0 μM	HR = 2.1 for ≥2.56 μM (5th) and 1.9 for ≤1.61 μM (1st) vs. 1.90–2.13 μM (3rd quintile)	Opotowsky and Bilezikian, 2004
2005	United Kingdom	Nested case–control, 3.7y follow-up	2606 ♀, 312 any fx cases, 92 hip fx, 934 controls, >75y	Serum retinol, retinyl esters, beta-carotene	Medical records, home visits	1.95 μM any fx, 2.00 μM controls. 1.91 μM hip fx, 1.94 μM controls	No association, supplement use HR = 0.76	Barker et al., 2005
2006	United States	Prospective, 17y follow-up (LWCS)	8877 ♀, 5101 ♂, mean 73.7 + 74.9y, 1227 hip fx, 445 wrist fx, 729 spine fx	Questionnaire about suppl	Self-reported + hospital discharge records	68% of ♀ and 61% ♂ took vit A containing suppl	♀ suppl users wrist fx HR = 1.15 hip HR 1.07(1.00–1.15)	White et al., 2006
2009	United States	Prospective, 6.6y follow-up (WHI)	75,747 ♀, 10,405 total fx, 588 hip fx, mean age 63y	FFQ × 2	Questionnaire, medical records	Retinol from food + suppl, 0.98 mg	No association, RR = 1.15 in low vit D + high vit A	Caire-Juvera et al., 2009

Notes: RE = retinol equivalents, fx = fracture(s), y = years, vit = vitamin, suppl = supplement, FFQ = Food Frequency Questionnaire, OR = odds ratio, RR = relative risk, HR = hazard ratio, SMC = Swedish Mammography Cohort, MDCS = Malmö Diet and Cancer Study, NHS = Nurses' Health Study, ULSAM = Uppsala Longitudinal Study of Adult Men, IWHS = Iowa Women's Health Study, DOPS = Danish Osteoporosis Prevention Study, NHANES = National Health and Nutrition Examination Survey, LWCS = Leisure World Cohort in Southern California, WHI = Women's Health Initiative.

fractures, which have the highest mortality risks in the first 6 months post fracture (Farahmand et al., 2005).

STUDIES WITH BONE MINERAL AS ENDPOINT

Before 1990, no human studies were reported that explicitly examined the relationship between vitamin A and bone health. Three studies in the 1980s had included vitamin A in investigations of diet, especially calcium, and bone health (Table 11.5).

The association between diet and bone mineral content (BMC) was investigated in a population of elderly Japanese residents (1368 men and 1098 women) living in Hawaii (Yano et al., 1985). Dietary intake was obtained by the 24-hour recall method, and BMC was measured by SPA. In the analysis of data, all subjects who reported atypical dietary intakes during the previous 24 h were excluded, leaving 1208 men and 912 women for the analyses. If all subjects who consumed liver in the previous 24 h were excluded is unclear. Participants were also asked to estimate the frequency of eating selected food containing relatively large amounts of calcium during the previous week, and they received a mailed questionnaire in which they were asked to list the brand names and amounts of supplementary minerals and vitamins consumed in the past week. There were no correlations between vitamin A intake and BMC in men. Of the five examined sites, dietary plus supplementary vitamin A was very modestly associated with BMC at the distal radius and ulna in women. Covariables included age, weight, height, history of nonviolent fracture, current use of estrogen (women), and current use of thiazides. No difference in BMC was found between users and nonusers of supplements.

With similar methods and only one single 24-h recall, it was found that "vitamin A intake was negatively correlated with bone density values at a level which approached significance" in 324 postmenopausal women in Iowa (Sowers et al., 1985).

As part of a 4-year clinical trial of 99 women randomly assigned to placebo or calcium supplements, the effect of energy and 14 nutrients on BMC of the radius, humerus, and ulna was examined (Freudenheim et al., 1986). Up to seventy-two 24-h recall records were collected for each woman in this study from Wisconsin. A positive association between vitamin A and rate of humeral bone loss was found among the nine premenopausal women in the placebo group. In contrast, in the postmenopausal women of the calcium supplemented group, there was an inverse correlation between vitamin A intake and the rate of change in ulna BMC. In a single patient receiving a high supplemental dose (average intake 14,624 IU/day), bone loss was very rapid with no other reason apparent.

Sowers and Wallace (1990) extended their initial study by evaluating vitamin A intake, serum retinol concentrations, and radial bone mass in 246 postmenopausal women. The correlation between serum retinol and dietary food intake estimated from 24-hour food recall was only 0.02, but serum retinol levels were higher among vitamin A supplement users (1.69 ± 0.52 μmol/L) compared with those among nonusers (1.55 ± 0.52 μmol/L, $p < .03$). After controlling for age, current estrogen replacement, and current thiazide use, they observed no association between vitamin A supplement use or serum retinol with radial bone mass (Sowers and Wallace, 1990).

In a study from Massachusetts (Hernandez-Avila et al., 1993), the influence of dietary, anthropomorphic, and hormonal factors on bone density in a cross-sectional sample of 281 premenopausal and perimenopausal women was investigated. Dietary information was obtained using an FFQ (Willett et al., 1987). Bone density was measured using SPA in the midshaft and the ultradistal radius. The investigators observed no associations between dietary variables and midshaft bone density, but retinol, vitamin D, and vitamin C were all positively but weakly associated with ultradistal radius density. Women who used multivitamins had higher values than the values of those who did not. It was not possible to distinguish which nutrients were responsible for this association.

Houtkooper et al. (1995) assessed the relationship between total energy intake, nutrient intake, body composition, exercise group status, and annual rates of change in BMD measured by DXA in

66 premenopausal women living in Arizona and taking calcium supplements. Neither calcium nor other nutrients were significant variables in regression models predicting BMD slopes at the spine or at any femur site, but vitamin A or carotene was associated with slowing the annual rate of total body bone loss. Intakes from supplements were not included in the analyses.

In the British Early Postmenopausal Intervention Cohort (EPIC) study (Earnshaw et al., 1997), BMD was measured with DXA. Dietary assessment was performed with a 3-day unweighed DR. No correlation between any dietary variable, including calcium, and BMD was found in 426 women.

In the first study that distinguished between retinol and beta-carotene (Melhus et al., 1998), the association between dietary retinol or beta-carotene and BMD in 175 Swedish women was investigated. Diet was assessed from four 1-week DRs. In a multivariable analysis, retinol intake was negatively associated with BMD. When subjects with intakes >1.5 mg/day were compared with those with intakes <0.5 mg/day, BMD was significantly reduced at all five examined sites. Dietary intake of beta-carotene was not associated with BMD.

In a cross-sectional analysis of the Third National Health and Nutrition Examination Survey (NHANES III) (Ballew et al., 2001a), the association between fasting serum retinyl esters and BMD was analyzed in 5790 adults. Although about one third of the participants had fasting serum retinyl esters ≥10% of total serum vitamin A and one quarter or more had osteopenia/osteoporosis at one or more sites, the study showed no significant association between fasting serum retinyl ester concentration, or fasting serum retinyl esters as percent of total vitamin A, and BMD at any site.

In a book chapter, a study of 70-year-old Icelandic women (n = 232) was published (Sigurdsson et al., 2001). Dietary intake was assessed using an FFQ, with 130 food items reflecting intake from the past 3 months. More than half of the retinol was obtained from cod liver oil and multivitamins. No association of retinol intake and BMD was observed.

In the Rancho Bernardo Study (Promislow et al., 2002), the association between BMD and bone loss, and total and supplemental retinol intake was studied in a cohort of 570 elderly women and 388 men who were followed for 4 years. Dietary intake of vitamin A was assessed by a dietary questionnaire at baseline. Half of the women and more than a third of the men were taking retinol-containing supplements. After stratification by supplement use, regression analyses showed an inverse U-shaped association of retinol intake with baseline BMD and BMD change.

In a case–control study of Italian women (Maggio et al., 2003), 75 subjects with osteoporosis (BMD T-score ≤ −3.5 at the femoral neck) and 75 controls were examined. Plasma retinol was found to be decreased in osteoporotic women (2.14 vs. 2.37 μM). In a subsequent analysis of 45 of these women with osteoporosis and 45 of the controls, plasma retinol, but not carotenoids, was positively correlated with femoral neck BMD (Maggio et al., 2006).

In a study from England (Kaptoge et al., 2003), 470 men and 474 women that were recruited from a diet and cancer study (EPIC-Norfolk) were studied. Seven-day food diaries were used to calculate dietary intake of some 31 nutrients and 22 food groups. BMD loss was measured using DXA on two occasions about 3 years apart. In men, there was no evidence of an effect of any of the nutrients evaluated. In women, only low intake of vitamin C was associated with faster rate of BMD loss.

In a small study from Canada (Suzuki et al., 2003), 58 postmenopausal women not taking estrogen were examined. Dietary intakes were assessed by retrospective questionnaires. Increased retinol intake from supplements had no adverse effect on BMD.

In a longitudinal study of mainly premenopausal women (45–55 years at baseline and 50–60 years at follow-up 5–7 years later) in the Aberdeen Prospective Osteoporosis Screening Study (Macdonald et al., 2004), it was found that greater femoral neck BMD loss was associated with increased dietary intake of retinol, but this negative association was no longer significant when retinol from supplements was included.

The relations between vitamin A intake and BMD and fracture risk were investigated in the Danish Osteoporosis Prevention Study—a prospective study on the effect of hormone replacement therapy (Rejnmark et al., 2004). Cross-sectional analysis at baseline and after 5 years showed no association between intake of retinol and BMD at any site.

In a cross-sectional analysis of 11,068 women, who were participants in the Women's Health Initiative (WHI) (Wolf et al., 2005), a negative association between total beta-carotene intake and femoral neck BMD was unexpectedly found. The finding was not consistent in that it was not significant for dietary intake alone, serum beta-carotene, or for other BMD sites. Retinol and other antioxidants were unrelated to BMD.

In a case–control study of 312 incident osteoporotic fracture cases (92 hip fractures) and 934 controls, nested in a prospective study of 2606 British women over the age of 75 years (Barker et al., 2005), a tendency for increased serum retinol to predict benefit rather than harm in terms of BMD ($r = 0.09$, $p = .002$) was noted. Comorbidities or socioeconomic variables were not adjusted for in the analyses of this study.

In a case–control study of 30 postmenopausal women with osteoporosis and 29 women with normal BMD from Wisconsin (Penniston et al., 2006), it was observed that serum retinyl esters were not elevated in either group, but serum retinol, total vitamin A (retinol + retinyl esters), use of supplements containing preformed vitamin A, and BMI were lower in women with osteoporosis. A trend existed for the association of serum retinyl esters as percentage of total vitamin A with osteoporosis ($p = .07$). Adjustment was only made for BMI and triacylglycerols.

In a longitudinal study of 78 healthy young Swedish males (Hogstrom et al., 2008), the influence of retinol on peak bone mass was investigated. The mean serum retinol concentration was high (2.43 μM), but serum retinol was not associated with peak BMD or BMD changes during the 2-year follow-up.

Finally, 3052 Norwegian women aged 50–70 years had forearm BMD measured with single X-ray absorptiometry in a substudy of the population-based Nord-Trøndelag Health Study (Forsmo et al., 2008). Women reporting childhood cod liver oil intake had significantly lower BMD than that of women with ingestion of cod liver oil. The authors described this result as unexpected and paradoxical, considering the good bone health intentions behind the long-standing cod liver oil recommendations in Norway.

Thus, although methodological limitations exist in many of these studies, which may explain discrepancies and produce a bias that will systematically underestimate the strength of associations, the effect of vitamin A on bone mineral appears to be similar to that in animals, that is, no or little effect is observed.

STUDIES WITH FRACTURES AS ENDPOINT

Eleven published studies have examined the most important endpoint, fracture (Table 11.6). In the first study by Sowers and Wallace (1990) described above, fracture history was also examined. Fracture history was self-reported and obtained by interview. Only 56 women reported an atraumatic fracture, 31 in the past 10 years, among these women. No linear association was found between serum retinol and fracture risk. (Nonlinear associations were not investigated.)

The Swedish BMD study (Melhus et al., 1998) also included a nested case–control study of 247 women with a first hip fracture and 873 age-matched controls. Dietary vitamin A intake was estimated from a semiquantitative FFQ, and hip fracture was identified by using hospital discharge records and confirmed by record review. For every 1-mg increase in daily intake of retinol, the risk for hip fracture increased by 68%. For intakes >1.5 mg/day compared with intakes <0.5 mg/day, the risk for hip fracture was doubled. Dietary intake of beta-carotene was not associated with BMD or hip fracture risk.

In another study from Sweden (Elmstahl et al., 1998), dietary risk factors for fracture in men aged 46–68 years were studied. The diet was assessed using a combined 7-day menu book for hot meals, beverages, and dietary supplements and a quantitative FFQ. The incident fractures that occurred during the mean observation time of 2.4 years were retrieved from the local hospital registry and registry of X-ray examinations. The study showed that the retinol intake in Sweden was high also in men, but there was no association between retinol, calcium, or vitamin D intake and fracture risk. A serious limitation of this study is that of the 160 men who had at least one fracture; only 51 of these had fragility fractures. This may explain why physical activity paradoxically was positively associated with fractures.

The study with the best estimate of vitamin A intake is the Nurses' Health Study (Feskanich et al., 2002). The intake was assessed every 4 years using an FFQ. Mean cumulative intake data from five FFQs were obtained. There were 603 incident hip fractures resulting from low or moderate trauma. Women in the highest quintile of total vitamin A intake from food and supplements ($\geq$3 mg retinol equivalents/day) had a significantly elevated relative risk of hip fracture (1.48 [95% confidence interval [CI] 1.05–2.07]) compared with that of women in the lowest quintile of intake (<1.25 mg retinol equivalents/day). This increased risk was attributable primarily to retinol (relative risk 1.89 [95% CI 1.33–2.68] comparing $\geq$2 mg/day vs. <0.5 mg/day). Beta-carotene did not contribute significantly to fracture risk. A retinol intake $\geq$1.5 mg/day as compared with an intake of <0.5 mg/day was associated with a relative risk of 1.64 for hip fracture similar to the odds ratio of 1.54 reported from Sweden (Melhus et al., 1998). Multivitamins were the primary contributors to total retinol (35%–43% of intake). Liver was the primary food source of retinol (22% in 1980 and 15% in 1994). Multivitamins were used by 34% of the cohort in 1980 and 53% by 1996.

Only three prospective studies have used a biological marker of vitamin A status to assess the risk of fractures. The first was published in the *New England Journal of Medicine* (Michaelsson et al., 2003). In a population-based study of 2322 men, serum retinol and beta-carotene levels were measured at baseline. Fractures were documented in 266 men during 30 years of follow-up. In multivariable analysis, the relative risk was 1.64 for any fracture and 2.47 for hip fracture among men in the highest quintile for serum retinol (>2.64 μmol/L), as compared with the middle quintile (2.17–2.36 μmol/L). Because serum retinol levels do not increase until the capacity for storage in the liver is exceeded, it is interesting that there was an exponential rise in the rate–ratio curve for men with serum levels above approximately 3 μmol/L. Men with >3.6 μmol/L had an overall risk of fracture that was seven-fold greater than that in those with lower concentrations. The serum beta-carotene level was not associated with risk of fracture.

The relationship between fracture risk and total vitamin A and retinol intake in a prospective study of 34,703 postmenopausal women from the Iowa Women's Health Study (Lim et al., 2004) was examined. Intake at baseline was assessed using a semiquantitative FFQ. Fractures were self-reported. Thirty-five percent of participants reported using supplements containing retinol or beta-carotene. These users of supplements had a 1.18-fold increased risk of incident hip fracture compared with that of nonusers (95% CI 0.99–1.41), but there was no evidence of a dose–response relationship or of an increased risk for total fractures. Limitations of this study include the single FFQ, that fractures were self-reported, and that no distinction was made between fractures due to high trauma events and those due to low/moderate events.

In the Danish study (Rejnmark et al., 2004) described above, a case–control study of fractures was included. During the 5 years of follow-up, 163 women sustained a fracture of the appendicular skeleton and/or the vertebrae. The number of hip fractures was not reported. Each case was matched to six controls. Average dietary intake was lower (0.53 mg/day) than that in Sweden and the United States, but not associated with fracture risk.

The second study that used a biological marker of vitamin A status was the prospective analysis of the NHANES I follow-up study (Opotowsky and Bilezikian, 2004) on 2799 women aged 50–74 years at baseline. There were 172 incident hip fractures during the 22-year follow-up period. A U-shaped relationship between serum vitamin A (retinol + retinyl esters) and hip fracture risk. Fracture risk was significantly higher among subjects in the lowest ($\leq$1.61 μmol/L) and highest quintile ($\geq$2.56 μmol/L) compared to the risk among those in the middle quintile (1.90–2.13 μmol/L).

The third study using a biomarker of vitamin A status was a nested case–control study conducted in the United Kingdom (Barker et al., 2005). The results differ from those in the Swedish and American studies. Within the placebo arm of a cohort of elderly women participating in a prospective study of hip fracture, they examined serum retinol, retinyl palmitate, and beta-carotene as predictors of incident hip and other fractures. After a mean follow-up of 3.7 years, 312 osteoporotic fracture cases, of which 92 had sustained a hip fracture, were identified and matched to 934 controls. Risk of any osteoporotic fracture was slightly less in the highest quartile (>2.42 μmol/L) of serum retinol compared with that in the lowest quartile (<1.66 μmol/L) (hazard ratio [HR] 0.85; 95% CI 0.69–1.05). The composition of the multivitamins was not recorded, but multivitamin or cod liver oil supplement users had higher serum retinol levels (mean 2.07 μmol/L) than those of nonusers (mean 1.95 μmol/L) and they had a lower risk of any fracture (HR 0.76; 95% CI 0.60–0.96). Comorbidities or socioeconomic variables were not adjusted for in the analyses of this study. Also, mean retinol intakes are higher in Sweden than in the United States and United Kingdom (Scientific Advisory Committee on Nutrition, 2005). This is also reflected in the serum retinol levels (mean levels among cases were 1.91 μmol/L and 1.94 μmol/L among controls in the U.K. study, 2.02 μmol/L in the U.S. study, and in the Swedish study, the median was 2.26 μmol/L). These differences may actually be even more pronounced because the women in this British study were about 15 years older than the women in NHANES I, and serum retinol has been shown to increase with age (McLaren, 1981; Sowers and Wallace, 1990; Ballew et al., 2001b). The lowest quartile (<1.66 μmol/L) was used as reference in the U.K. study. This level is close to the lowest quintile in the U.S. study (≤1.61 μmol/L), which was associated with an increased risk of hip fracture. This could, in part, be an explanation to why risk of any osteoporotic fracture was slightly less in the highest quartile compared with the lowest quartile in the U.K. study.

In the Leisure World Cohort Study in southern California (White et al., 2006), incident fractures of the hip (n = 1227), wrist (n = 445), and spine (n = 729) were identified in 13,978 residents surveyed over the course of two decades. Mean age at entry was 74.9 years for men and 73.7 years for women. Information about supplement use was collected via a questionnaire, and fractures were identified from four follow-up surveys, hospital discharge records, and death certificates. Women, but not men, who used vitamin A supplements had modestly increased rates of hip fracture (HR 1.07; 95% CI 1.00–1.15) and wrist fracture (HR 1.15; 95 CI 1.07–1.23).

Finally, the relation between total vitamin A and retinol intakes and the risk of incident total and hip fracture was also examined in the WHI Observational Study (Caire-Juvera et al., 2009). Fractures were self-reported or reported by proxy respondents, and 78% of self-reported hip fractures and 71% of self-reported single-site fractures could be confirmed by medical records. Dietary intake was assessed at baseline and at year 3 of follow-up with the WHI FFQ. There were 10,405 total fractures and 588 hip fractures among the 75,747 participants during 6.6 years of follow-up. There was no association between total vitamin A or retinol and fracture risk, but women with vitamin D intake below the mean (11 μg/day) in the highest quintile of intake of both vitamin A (HR 1.19; 95% CI 1.04–1.37) and retinol (HR 1.15; 95% CI 1.03–1.29) had a modest increased risk of total fracture. The total average of vitamin D intake (from food and supplements) was 2.5–4 μg higher in this and the Iowa Women's Health Study compared with that in the Nurses' Health Study (Caire-Juvera et al., 2009).

SUMMARY

In animals, beta-carotene and other provitamin A carotenoids had no adverse effects on bone, whereas high doses of retinol and other retinoids induced spontaneous fractures by a mechanism that reduces the bone diameter. No or little effect on mineralization has been observed, except when vitamin D was low.

Consistent with animal studies, no negative effects of provitamin A carotenoids have been found in man, and most human observational studies of the relationship between retinol intake and BMD find no association. The methods that have been used to measure BMD determine the amount of mineral per unit area, but not volume, and it is therefore unknown if retinol reduces the bone diameter. Results from studies with fracture as endpoint show some heterogeneity, but the majority of prospective studies found that an excessive intake of vitamin A is associated with increased risk of fracture. Currently, insufficient evidence exists to determine at what level of intake the risk increases. Prospective studies with more reliable and long-term assessments of retinol intake are necessary to clarify this. High levels of retinol are only found in liver and dietary supplements containing retinol, including cod liver oil. Because the intake of liver has decreased over the last 30 years and the retinol levels in supplements recently have been reduced, the negative effects of retinol on bone health should diminish in the future.

Vitamin A and bone is perhaps best summarized with the classical words of Paracelsus (1493–1541): *Alle Ding' sind Gift, und nichts ohn' Gift; allein die Dosis macht, daß ein Ding kein Gift ist.* "All things are poison and nothing is without poison, only the dose permits something not to be poisonous."

REFERENCES

Aburto, A., and Britton, W.M. 1998a. Effects and interactions of dietary levels of vitamins A and E and chole-calciferol in broiler chickens. *Poult Sci* 77: 666–673.

Aburto, A., and Britton, W.M. 1998b. Effects of different levels of vitamins A and E on the utilization of chole-calciferol by broiler chickens. *Poult Sci* 77: 570–577.

Anderson, J.J. 2002. Oversupplementation of vitamin A and osteoporotic fractures in the elderly: To supplement or not to supplement with vitamin A. *J Bone Miner Res* 17: 1359–1362.

Armstrong, R., Ashenfelter, K., Eckoff, C., et al. 1994. General and reproductive toxicology of retinoids. In *The Retinoids*. 2nd ed., Sporn, M., Roberts, A., and Goodman, D., eds. Raven Press, New York, NY.

Bachmann, H., Desbarats, A., Pattison, P., et al. 2002. Feedback regulation of beta,beta-carotene 15,15′-monooxygenase by retinoic acid in rats and chickens. *J Nutr* 132: 3616–3622.

Baglin, A., Hagege, C., Franc, B., et al. 1986. A systemic-like disease: Chronic vitamin A poisoning. *Ann Med Interne (Paris)* 137: 142–146.

Ballew, C., Bowman, B.A., Russell, R.M., et al. 2001a. Serum retinyl esters are not associated with biochemical markers of liver dysfunction in adult participants in the third National Health and Nutrition Examination Survey (NHANES III), 1988–1994. *Am J Clin Nutr* 73: 934–940.

Ballew, C., Bowman, B.A., Sowell, A.L., et al. 2001b. Serum retinol distributions in residents of the United States: Third National Health and Nutrition Examination Survey, 1988–1994. *Am J Clin Nutr* 73: 586–593.

Barker, M.E., Mccloskey, E., Saha, S., et al. 2005. Serum retinoids and beta-carotene as predictors of hip and other fractures in elderly women. *J Bone Miner Res* 20: 913–920.

Binkley, N., and Krueger, D. 2000. Hypervitaminosis A and bone. *Nutr Rev* 58: 138–144.

Bitzen, U., Winqvist, M., Nilsson-Ehle, P., et al. 1994. Retinyl palmitate is a reproducible marker for chylomicron elimination from blood. *Scand J Clin Lab Invest* 54: 611–613.

Bliuc, D., Nguyen, N.D., Milch, V.E., et al. 2009. Mortality risk associated with low-trauma osteoporotic fracture and subsequent fracture in men and women. *JAMA* 301: 513–521.

Booth, S.L., Tucker, K.L., Mckeown, N.M., et al. 1997. Relationships between dietary intakes and fasting plasma concentrations of fat-soluble vitamins in humans. *J Nutr* 127: 587–592.

Burgaz, A., Akesson, A., Oster, A., et al. 2007. Associations of diet, supplement use, and ultraviolet B radiation exposure with vitamin D status in Swedish women during winter. *Am J Clin Nutr* 86: 1399–1404.

Caire-Juvera, G., Ritenbaugh, C., Wactawski-Wende, J., et al. 2009. Vitamin A and retinol intakes and the risk of fractures among participants of the Women's Health Initiative Observational Study. *Am J Clin Nutr* 89: 323–330.

Carpenter, T.O., Pettifor, J.M., Russell, R.M., et al. 1987. Severe hypervitaminosis A in siblings: Evidence of variable tolerance to retinol intake. *J Pediatr* 111: 507–512.

Cruz, J. A., Moreiras-Varela, O., Van Staveren, W.A., et al. 1991. Intake of vitamins and minerals. Euronut SENECA investigators. *Eur J Clin Nutr* 45(Suppl 3): 121–138.

Digiovanna, J.J., Helfgott, R.K., Gerber, L.H., et al. 1986. Extraspinal tendon and ligament calcification associated with long-term therapy with etretinate. *New Engl J Med* 315: 1177–1182.

Earnshaw, S.A., Worley, A. and Hosking, D.J. 1997. Current diet does not relate to bone mineral density after the menopause. The Nottingham Early Postmenopausal Intervention Cohort (EPIC) Study Group. *Br J Nutr* 78: 65–72.

Elmstahl, S., Gullberg, B., Janzon, L., et al. 1998. Increased incidence of fractures in middle-aged and elderly men with low intakes of phosphorus and zinc. *Osteoporos Int* 8: 333–340.

EPOS Group. 2002. Incidence of vertebral fracture in Europe: Results from the European Prospective Osteoporosis Study (EPOS). *J Bone Miner Res* 17: 716–724.

FAO/WHO. 1967. Requirements of vitamin A, thiamine, riboflavin and niacin. *Report of a Joint FAO/WHO Expert Group*. WHO Technical Report Series, Rome, Italy.

Farahmand, B.Y., Michaelsson, K., Ahlbom, A., et al. 2005. Survival after hip fracture. *Osteoporos Int* 16: 1583–1590.

Feskanich, D., Singh, V., Willett, W.C., et al. 2002. Vitamin A intake and hip fractures among postmenopausal women. *JAMA* 287: 47–54.

Food and Nutrition Board, Institute of Medicine. 2001 *Dietary Reference Intakes for Vitamin A, Vitamin K, Arsenic, Boron, Chromium, Copper, Iodine, Iron, Manganese, Molybdenum, Nickel, Silicon, Vanadium, and Zinc*. National Academy Press, Washington, DC.

Forsmo, S., Fjeldbo, S.K., and Langhammer, A. 2008. Childhood cod liver oil consumption and bone mineral density in a population-based cohort of peri- and postmenopausal women: The Nord-Trondelag Health Study. *Am J Epidemiol* 167: 406–411.

Frankel, T.L., Seshadri, M.S., Mcdowall, D.B., et al. 1986. Hypervitaminosis A and calcium-regulating hormones in the rat. *J Nutr* 116: 578–587.

Freudenheim, J.L., Johnson, N.E., and Smith, E.L. 1986. Relationships between usual nutrient intake and bone-mineral content of women 35–65 years of age: Longitudinal and cross-sectional analysis. *Am J Clin Nutr* 44: 863–876.

Garry, P.J., Hunt, W.C., Bandrofchak, J.L., et al. 1987. Vitamin A intake and plasma retinol levels in healthy elderly men and women. *Am J Clin Nutr* 46: 989–994.

Henriquez-Sanchez, P., Sanchez-Villegas, A., Doreste-Alonso, J., et al. 2009. Dietary assessment methods for micronutrient intake: A systematic review on vitamins. *Br J Nutr* 102(Suppl 1): S10–S37.

Hernandez-Avila, M., Stampfer, M. J., Ravnikar, V. A., et al. 1993. Caffeine and other predictors of bone density among pre- and perimenopausal women. *Epidemiology* 4: 128–134.

Hickenbottom, S.J., Follett, J.R., Lin, Y., et al. 2002. Variability in conversion of beta-carotene to vitamin A in men as measured by using a double-tracer study design. *Am J Clin Nutr* 75: 900–907.

Hogstrom, M., Nordstrom, A. and Nordstrom, P. 2008. Retinol, retinol-binding protein 4, abdominal fat mass, peak bone mineral density, and markers of bone metabolism in men: The Northern Osteoporosis and Obesity (NO2) Study. *Eur J Endocrinol* 158: 765–770.

Hough, S., Avioli, L.V., Muir, H., et al. 1988. Effects of hypervitaminosis A on the bone and mineral metabolism of the rat. *Endocrinology* 122: 2933–2939.

Houtkooper, L.B., Ritenbaugh, C., Aickin, M., et al. 1995. Nutrients, body composition and exercise are related to change in bone mineral density in premenopausal women. *J Nutr* 125: 1229–1237.

International Dairy and Federation. 1995. Consumption statistics for milk and milk products. *Bull Int Dairy Fed* 301: 14–16.

Johansson, S., Lind, P.M., Hakansson, H., et al. 2002. Subclinical hypervitaminosis A causes fragile bones in rats. *Bone* 31: 685–689.

Johansson, S., and Melhus, H. 2001. Vitamin A antagonizes calcium response to vitamin D in man. *J Bone Miner Res* 16: 1899–1905.

Johnell, O., Gullberg, B., Allander, E., et al. 1992. The apparent incidence of hip fracture in Europe: A study of national register sources. *Osteoporos Int* 2: 298–302.

Jowsey, J. and Riggs, B. 1968. Bone changes in a patient with hypervitaminosis A. *J Clin Endocrinol Metab* 28: 1833–1835.

Kamm, J., Ashenfelter, K., and Ehmann, C. 1984. Preclinical and clinical toxicology of selected retinoids. In *The Retinoids*. 1st ed., Sporn, M., Roberts, A., and Goodman, D., eds. Academic Press, London.

Kanis, J.A., Johnell, O., De Laet, C., et al. 2002. International variations in hip fracture probabilities: Implications for risk assessment. *J Bone Miner Res* 17: 1237–1244.

Kaptoge, S., Welch, A., Mctaggart, A., et al. 2003. Effects of dietary nutrients and food groups on bone loss from the proximal femur in men and women in the 7th and 8th decades of age. *Osteoporos Int* 14: 418–428.

Kardinaal, A.F., Van 't Veer, P., Brants, H.A., et al. 1995. Relations between antioxidant vitamins in adipose tissue, plasma, and diet. *Am J Epidemiol* 141: 440–450.

Kneissel, M., Studer, A., Cortesi, R., et al. 2005. Retinoid-induced bone thinning is caused by subperiosteal osteoclast activity in adult rodents. *Bone* 36: 202–214.

Krasinski, S.D., Cohn, J.S., Schaefer, E.J., et al. 1990. Postprandial plasma retinyl ester response is greater in older subjects compared with younger subjects. Evidence for delayed plasma clearance of intestinal lipoproteins. *J Clin Invest* 85: 883–892.

Krasinski, S.D., Russell, R.M., Otradovec, C.L., et al. 1989. Relationship of vitamin A and vitamin E intake to fasting plasma retinol, retinol-binding protein, retinyl esters, carotene, alpha-tocopherol, and cholesterol among elderly people and young adults: Increased plasma retinyl esters among vitamin A-supplement users. *Am J Clin Nutr* 49: 112–120.

Lim, L.S., Harnack, L.J., Lazovich, D., et al. 2004. Vitamin A intake and the risk of hip fracture in postmenopausal women: The Iowa Women's Health Study. *Osteoporos Int* 15: 522–529.

Lin, Y., Dueker, S.R., Burri, B.J., et al. 2000. Variability of the conversion of beta-carotene to vitamin A in women measured by using a double-tracer study design. *Am J Clin Nutr* 71: 1545–1554.

Lind, P. M., Johansson, S., Ronn, M., et al. 2006. Subclinical hypervitaminosis A in rat: Measurements of bone mineral density (BMD) do not reveal adverse skeletal changes. *Chem Biol Interact* 159: 73–80.

Macdonald, H.M., New, S.A., Golden, M.H., et al. 2004. Nutritional associations with bone loss during the menopausal transition: Evidence of a beneficial effect of calcium, alcohol, and fruit and vegetable nutrients and of a detrimental effect of fatty acids. *Am J Clin Nutr* 79: 155–165.

Maggio, D., Barabani, M., Pierandrei, M., et al. 2003. Marked decrease in plasma antioxidants in aged osteoporotic women: Resuits of a cross-sectional study. *J Clin Endocrinol Metab* 88: 1523–1527.

Maggio, D., Polidori, M.C., Barabani, M., et al. 2006. Low levels of carotenoids and retinol in involutional osteoporosis. *Bone* 38: 244–248.

McDowell, L. 2000. *Vitamins in Animal and Human Nutrition.* Iowa State University Press, Ames, Iowa.

McLaren, D.S. 1981. The luxus vitamins—A and B12. *Am J Clin Nutr* 34: 1611–1616.

Melhus, H. 2003. Vitamin A and fracture risk. In *Nutritional Aspects of Bone Health.* J.-P. Bonjour, and New, S., eds. The Royal Society of Chemistry, Cambridge, UK, 369–372.

Melhus, H., Michaëlsson, K., Kindmark, A., et al. 1998. Excessive dietary intake of vitamin A is associated with reduced bone mineral density and increased risk for hip fracture. *Ann Intern Med* 129: 770–778.

Michaelsson, K., Lithell, H., Vessby, B., et al. 2003. Serum retinol levels and the risk of fracture. *New Engl J Med.* 348: 287–294.

Milstone, L.M., Mcguire, J., and Ablow, R.C. 1982. Premature epiphyseal closure in a child receiving oral 13-cis-retinoic acid. *J Am Acad Dermatol* 7: 663–666.

Nieman, C., and Obbink, H. 1954. The biochemistry and pathology of hypervitaminosis A. *Vitam Horm* 12: 69–99.

Olson, J.A. 1984. Serum levels of vitamin A and carotenoids as reflectors of nutritional status. *J Natl Cancer Inst* 73: 1439–1444.

Opotowsky, A.R., and Bilezikian, J.P. 2004. Serum vitamin A concentration and the risk of hip fracture among women 50 to 74 years old in the United States: A prospective analysis of the NHANES I follow-up study. *Am J Med* 117: 169–174.

Penniston, K.L., Weng, N., Binkley, N., et al. 2006. Serum retinyl esters are not elevated in postmenopausal women with and without osteoporosis whose preformed vitamin A intakes are high. *Am J Clin Nutr* 84: 1350–1356.

Phillips, B., Ball, C., Sackett, D., et al. 2001. Levels of evidence. Oxford Centre for Evidence-Based Medicine. www.cebm.net/index.aspx?o+1047. Accessed March 10, 2010.

Pittsley, R.A., and Yoder, F.W. 1983. Retinoid hyperostosis. Skeletal toxicity associated with long-term administration of 13-cis-retinoic acid for refractory ichthyosis. *New Engl J Med.* 308: 1012–1014.

Prendiville, J., Bingham, E.A., and Burrows, D. 1986. Premature epiphyseal closure—A complication of etretinate therapy in children. *J Am Acad Dermatol* 15: 1259–1262.

Promislow, J.H., Goodman-Gruen, D., Slymen, D.J., et al. 2002. Retinol intake and bone mineral density in the elderly: The Rancho Bernardo Study. *J Bone Miner Res* 17: 1349–1358.

Reinersdorff, D.V., Bush, E. and Liberato, D.J. 1996. Plasma kinetics of vitamin A in humans after a single oral dose of [8,9,19–13C]retinyl palmitate. *J Lipid Res* 37: 1875–1885.

Rejnmark, L., Vestergaard, P., Charles, P., et al. 2004. No effect of vitamin A intake on bone mineral density and fracture risk in perimenopausal women. *Osteoporos Int* 15: 872–880.

Roidt, L., White, E., Goodman, G.E., et al. 1988. Association of Food Frequency Questionnaire estimates of vitamin A intake with serum vitamin A levels. *Am J Epidemiol* 128: 645–654.

Ruby, L.K., and Mital, M.A. 1974. Skeletal deformities following chronic hypervitaminosis A: A case report. *J Bone Joint Surg Am* 56: 1283–1287.

Sahi, T. 1994. Genetics and epidemiology of adult-type hypolactasia. *Scand J Gastroenterol* Supplement 202: 7–20.

Sahni, S., Hannan, M.T., Blumberg, J., et al. 2009a. Inverse association of carotenoid intakes with 4-y change in bone mineral density in elderly men and women: The Framingham Osteoporosis Study. *Am J Clin Nutr* 89: 416–424.

Sahni, S., Hannan, M.T., Blumberg, J., et al. 2009b. Protective effect of total carotenoid and lycopene intake on the risk of hip fracture: A 17-year follow-up from the Framingham Osteoporosis Study. *J Bone Miner Res* 24: 1086–1094.

Schurr, D., Herbert, J., Habibi, E., et al. 1983. Unusual presentation of vitamin A intoxication. *J Pediatr Gastroenterol Nutr* 2: 705–707.

Scientific Advisory Committee on Nutrition. 2005. Review of dietary advice on vitamin A. The Stationary Office, London.

Sigurdsson, G., Franzon, L., Thorgeirsdottir, H., et al. 2001. A lack of association between excessive dietary intake of vitamin A and bone mineral density in seventy-year old Icelandic women. In *Nutritional Aspects of Osteoporosis*. Burckhardt, P., Dawson-Hughes, B., and Heaney, R.P., eds. Academic Press, San Diego, CA.

Smith, F., and Goodman, D. 1976. Vitamin A transport in human vitamin A toxicity. *New Engl J Med* 294: 805–808.

Sowers, M.F., and Wallace, R.B. 1990. Retinol, supplemental vitamin A and bone status. *J Clin Epidemiol* 43: 693–699.

Sowers, M.R., Wallace, R.B. and Lemke, J.H. 1985. Correlates of mid-radius bone density among postmenopausal women: A community study. *Am J Clin Nutr* 41: 1045–1053.

Sporn, M., Roberts, A., and Goodman, D. 1994. *The Retinoids: Biology, Chemistry and Medicine*. Raven Press, New York, NY.

Suzuki, Y., Whiting, S.J., Davison, K.S., et al. 2003. Total calcium intake is associated with cortical bone mineral density in a cohort of postmenopausal women not taking estrogen. *J Nutr Health Aging* 7: 296–299.

Takitani, K., Zhu, C.L., Inoue, A., et al. 2006. Molecular cloning of the rat beta-carotene 15,15′-monooxygenase gene and its regulation by retinoic acid. *Eur J Nutr* 45: 320–326.

Tangney, C.C., Shekelle, R.B., Raynor, W., et al. 1987. Intra- and interindividual variation in measurements of beta-carotene, retinol, and tocopherols in diet and plasma. *Am J Clin Nutr* 45: 764–769.

Teelmann, K. 1981. Experimental toxicology of the aromatic retinoid Ro 10–9359 (etretinate). In *Retinoids: Advances in Basic Research and Therapy*. Orfanos, C., Braun-Falco, O., Farber, E., Grupper, C., Polano, M., and Schuppli, R., eds. Springer-Verlag, Berlin and Heidelberg.

van Lieshout, M., West, C.E., Muhilal, et al. 2001. Bioefficacy of beta-carotene dissolved in oil studied in children in Indonesia. *Am J Clin Nutr* 73: 949–958.

van Vliet, T., Van Vlissingen, M.F., Van Schaik, F., et al. 1996. Beta-carotene absorption and cleavage in rats is affected by the vitamin A concentration of the diet. *J Nutr* 126: 499–508.

White, S.C., Atchison, K.A., Gornbein, J.A., et al. 2006. Risk factors for fractures in older men and women: The Leisure World Cohort Study. *Gend Med* 3: 110–123.

Willett, W.C., Reynolds, R.D., Cottrell-Hoehner, S., et al. 1987. Validation of a semi-quantitative Food Frequency Questionnaire: Comparison with a 1-year diet record. *J Am Diet Assoc* 87: 43–47.

Willett, W.C., Stampfer, M.J., Underwood, B.A., et al. 1983. Vitamins A, E, and carotene: Effects of supplementation on their plasma levels. *Am J Clin Nutr* 38: 559–566.

Wolf, R.L., Cauley, J.A., Pettinger, M., et al. 2005. Lack of a relation between vitamin and mineral antioxidants and bone mineral density: Results from the Women's Health Initiative. *Am J Clin Nutr* 82: 581–588.

Wu, B., Xu, B., Huang, T.Y., et al. 1996. [A model of osteoporosis induced by retinoic acid in male Wistar rats]. *Yao Hsueh Hsueh Pao* 31: 241–245.

Yano, K., Heilbrun, L.K., Wasnich, R.D., et al. 1985. The relationship between diet and bone mineral content of multiple skeletal sites in elderly Japanese-American men and women living in Hawaii. *Am J Clin Nutr* 42: 877–888.

12 Vitamin K and Bone

Cees Vermeer and Marjo H.J. Knapen

CONTENTS

INTRODUCTION

The human diet contains different forms of vitamin K. Green vegetables, notably spinach, kale, broccoli, and sprouts, are the main sources of phylloquinone (vitamin K_1); menaquinones (vitamin K_2) form a family of closely related compounds produced by a number of microorganisms including lactic acid and propionic acid bacteria, as well as by *Bacillus subtilis natto*. In Europe and Northern America, cheese and curd cheese are the main dietary sources of vitamin K_2, whereas in Japan, natto (fermented soy beans), a popular food, is extremely rich in menaquinone-7, one of the long-chain menaquinones (Booth et al., 1993; Shearer and Bolton-Smith, 2000; Schurgers and Vermeer, 2000). Also, bacteria in the gut produce large amounts of vitamin K_2, but hardly any of it is absorbed because of the lack of bile salts at the site of production. Dietary vitamin K_2 accounts for approximately 10% of the total vitamin K intake, but its better absorption and much longer half-life than K_1 make it an important contributor to total human vitamin K status.

CHARACTERISTICS OF VITAMIN K

A common characteristic of all forms of vitamin K is the methylated naphthoquinone ring system substituted with a variable aliphatic side chain at the 3-position. In K_1, this side chain is constituted of four isoprenoid residues, the last three of which are saturated. In K_2, the number of isoprenyl residues is variable, but all are unsaturated. The nomenclature is MK-n, where n stands for the number of isoprenyl residues in the side chain. Obviously, the lipophilic character of the menaquinones increases at increasing side-chain length. The most common menaquinones in the human diet are MK-4 through MK-6 (classified as the short-chain menaquinones) and MK-7 through MK-9 (the long-chain menaquinones).

The function of all forms of vitamin K is to serve as a cofactor for the endoplasmic reticulum (ER) enzyme gammaglutamate carboxylase (GGCX), which converts certain polypeptide-bound glutamate residues into gammacarboxyglutamate (Gla). This vitamin-K-dependent carboxylation is a posttranslational modification accomplished during the maturation of secretory proteins that are equipped with a GGCX recognition sequence. Presently, 15 Gla-containing proteins have been identified, including four blood coagulation factors (all synthesized in the liver), the bone Gla-protein osteocalcin (exclusively synthesized by osteoblasts) and matrix Gla-protein (MGP). MGP is mainly synthesized by chondrocytes in cartilage and by smooth muscle cells in the arterial vessel wall. In these proteins, the Gla residues form strong calcium-binding groups which are essential for their biological function. During vitamin K deficiency or after intake of vitamin K antagonists, for example, warfarin (coumadin), uncarboxylated Gla-proteins devoid of biological activity, is formed (Berkner, 2005; Shearer and Newman, 2008).

Following intestinal absorption, the K vitamins are taken up in triglycerides to be transported to the liver, where they can be utilized for the synthesis of the clotting factors. Notably, the long-chain menaquinones, however, are subsequently incorporated into low-density lipoproteins which are transported to extrahepatic tissues such as bone and vessel wall (Schurgers and Vermeer, 2002). During the last decade, experiments in vitamin-K-deficient animals and in coumarin-treated subjects have unfolded a general principle in the pharmacokinetics of K vitamins: the liver takes what it needs and the excess (mainly K_2) is redistributed to other tissues. In coumarin-treated volunteers treated with increasing doses of vitamin K, this principle is exemplified by the preferential carboxylation of the clotting factors (hepatic) well before the first sign of osteocalcin (extrahepatic) carboxylation was observed (Schurgers et al., 2004). These data were found for both K_1 and K_2 and are consistent with the recently published triage theory, which holds that during episodes of dietary vitamin K insufficiency, the body selectively transports vitamins to tissues carrying out functions that are vital for immediate survival (McCann and Ames, 2009). Obviously, prevention of bleeding is more important for survival than bone loss or vascular calcification in old age. In this way, it can be understood why in the healthy population having undercarboxylation of the clotting factors does not exist, whereas 20%–30% of the osteocalcin and MGP circulate in their uncarboxylated, inactive forms.

Although high vitamin K intake was shown to be associated with low risk for osteoporosis (Feskanich et al., 1999), cardiovascular disease (Gast et al., 2009), and cancer (Nimptsch et al., 2008), research has not examined whether long-term subclinical vitamin K deficiencies contribute to age-related diseases. This concept of chronic vitamin K deficiency also raises the question of how to define human vitamin K requirement. Dietary reference intakes (DRIs) for vitamin K in various countries range between 1 and 1.5 µg/kg body weight/day or between 80 and 120 µg/day (for adults). These figures are based on the doses required to ensure complete carboxylation of the clotting factors; many studies have shown that these amounts are insufficient to support full carboxylation of the extrahepatic Gla-proteins. Here, we define *vitamin K deficiency* as a state in which the hepatic vitamin K status is too low to allow complete carboxylation of all clotting factors, whereas *vitamin K insufficiency* is defined as a state in which more than 5% of an extrahepatic Gla-protein occurs in its uncarboxylated form. According to this definition, nearly all nonsupplemented healthy adults are vitamin K insufficient. Before addressing the question of whether increased vitamin K intake—for instance, by using nutrient supplements or functional foods—may have benefits for bone health, we describe the various Gla-proteins reported to reside in bone.

VITAMIN-K–DEPENDENT PROTEINS IN BONE

Thus far, five Gla-proteins have been identified in or associated with bone: osteocalcin (Hauschka and Reid, 1978), MGP (Price et al., 1983), growth-arrest-specific gene 6 protein (Gas6) (Katagiri et al., 2001), protein S (Maillard et al., 1992), and periostin, a protein abundantly found in the periosteum which was recently found to contain four widely separated Gla domains (Coutu et al., 2008). MGP is the most potent inhibitor of soft tissue calcification presently known, and it is synthesized in chondrocytes and, under certain conditions, also in osteoblasts. Gas6 is a cell growth regulator also involved in bone differentiation and resorption (Katagiri et al., 2001). One of the functions of protein S is to serve as a cofactor for protein C in the inhibition of the blood coagulation cascade; in the circulation, a large fraction of serum proteins is bound to the C4-binding protein of the complement system, but the function for the C4BP/PS complex remains unclear. No specific role for protein S in bone has been reported, but it is synthesized in various cells including osteoblasts (Maillard et al., 1992). Hereditary protein S deficiency has been associated with osteopenia (Pan et al., 1990). Periostin has primarily been studied as a recombinant protein produced in the absence of the vitamin-K-dependent carboxylase system. In this form, *in vitro* studies have demonstrated a potential role in extracellular matrix mineralization, whereas the role of carboxylated periostin remains to be elucidated. The most recently discovered Gla-protein is the Gla-rich protein (GRP), which is expressed in many vertebrate tissues, but most abundantly in cartilage. GRP has been suggested to play a role in calcium regulation in the extracellular environment (Viegas et al., 2008).

Remarkably, no clear function has been described for osteocalcin, the most abundant noncollagenous protein in bone. Transgenic mice showed that it is a negative regulator of bone growth and that it may have a role in the appropriate deposition of hydroxyapatite crystals in bone and that it most likely functions as a regulator of bone mineral maturation (Ducy et al., 1996). Other researchers have found that osteocalcin has chemoattractant activity for osteoclasts. Recently, osteocalcin has also been postulated to act as a hormone that stimulates fat metabolism in adipose tissue (Lee et al., 2007). At this time, however, the precise function of osteocalcin is unclear, and its main practical importance is gained from its use as a circulating biomarker for osteoblast activity (total osteocalcin antigen) and for the vitamin K status of bone tissue (fraction of osteocalcin that is uncarboxylated). Since so many vitamin-K-dependent proteins have been identified in bone, and because at least two of them (osteocalcin and MGP) occur in a partly uncarboxylated form in the majority of the adult population, vitamin K intake is likely associated with bone health. Cell culture experiments in primary osteoblasts showed a marked stimulation of calcification by all forms of vitamin K, and these studies suggest that vitamin K promotes the transition of osteoblasts into osteocytes while at the same time decreasing the osteolytic potential of these osteocytes. The mechanisms by which vitamin K optimizes calcification, as part of the process of bone formation, and integrity *in vivo* may help explain the net positive effect of vitamin K on bone formation (Atkins et al., 2009).

VITAMIN K STATUS AND BONE HEALTH

Many observational studies have demonstrated that poor vitamin K status is associated with low bone mineral density (BMD) and increased fracture risk. In these studies, vitamin K status was assessed in one of three ways: by dietary intake (food frequency questionnaires), by circulating vitamin K concentrations (only vitamin K_1 was measured), or by the degree to which circulating osteocalcin had been carboxylated (reflecting vitamin K status of bone tissue). Pioneers in this fields were Hart and colleagues, who observed unusually low circulating vitamin K levels in patients with bone fractures and in osteoporotic patients (Hart et al., 1984). Feskanich and colleagues and Booth and coworkers first associated dietary K intake with bone health (Feskanich et al., 1999; Booth et al., 2003). Szulc and coinvestigators and Luukinen and coresearchers found strong correlations between the circulating levels of uncarboxylated osteocalcin (ucOC) and bone health (Szulc et al., 1996; Luukinen et al., 2000). These studies have been confirmed by other researchers. Remarkably, all the investigators mentioned above first found the relation of vitamin K deficiency with fracture risk, and only years later with low BMD. This paradox may be related to the role of vitamin K in regulating the synthesis of bone matrix proteins, especially collagen which contributes to bone strength independently of BMD.

An important question is what is the most reliable method to establish vitamin K status. Circulating vitamin K species mostly reflect the diet of the day prior to blood sampling, but analytical procedures are insufficiently sensitive to detect the low levels of circulating long-chain menaquinones, which also have K activity and which are especially important for extrahepatic tissues. Food frequency questionnaires give an overall picture of dietary intakes and a fair estimate of dietary preferences, but they are not highly accurate and do not correct for food matrix. K_1 from green vegetables, for instance, is absorbed at efficiencies of only 5% to 15% (depending on concomitant fat intake), whereas the absorption of K_2 from cheese is almost complete, that is, ~100%. It seems, therefore, that tissue-specific Gla-proteins, like osteocalcin of bone, form the most reliable markers for vitamin K status of the tissue in which they were produced, especially if the noncarboxylated protein is expressed as a fraction of the total protein antigen or as a ratio between uncarboxylated and carboxylated protein.

INTERVENTION TRIALS

The effect of vitamin K on bone strength remains a matter of controversy, mainly because many of the studies showing a beneficial effect were underpowered or too short in duration. Only a limited number of clinical intervention trials published today meet the criteria of more than 2 years of treatment and more than 100 subjects investigated. These trials are summarized in Table 12.1. The study reported by Shiraki et al. (2000) included 241 osteoporotic women receiving either calcium (150 mg/day) or calcium plus vitamin K_2 (45 mg/day) over a period of 2 years. Lumbar BMD decreased in the control group (calcium alone), but it remained constant in the vitamin-K_2-treated group. Also, the incidence of clinical fractures was significantly higher in the control group than that in K_2-treated group.

Braam et al. (2003) included 180 nonosteoporotic postmenopausal women randomized into three groups of 60 each. They were treated for 2 years with placebo, calcium + vitamin D, or calcium + vitamin D + vitamin K_1 (1 mg/day). Vitamin K_1 decreased the rate of bone loss, that is, BMD, as measured by dual-energy x-ray absorptiometry, by about 30% as compared with the calcium + vitamin D group. Knapen et al. (2007) included 325 nonosteoporotic postmenopausal women randomized to receive either placebo or vitamin K_2 (45 mg/day) for 3 years. No effect on BMD was observed, but it was shown that vitamin K_2 induced a beneficial change in the geometry of the hip. The calculated bone strength of the hip remained constant during the entire study period in the K_2 group, whereas a significant decrease of the calculated bone strength was observed in the placebo group. Similar to the results of Braam et al. (2003), Bolton-Smith et al. (2007) showed a synergetic

---

TABLE 12.1
Overview of Randomized Clinical Intervention Studies Testing Effects of K Vitamins on Bone Quality and Bone Strength

Investigator (Year of Publication)	Bone Quality (BMD/BMC)	Bone Strength (Fractures, Geometry)
Shiraki et al. (2000)	Positive effect on lumbar BMD	Fracture incidence decreased
Braam et al. (2003)	Positive effect on hip BMD	Not measured
	Rate of bone loss decreased	
Knapen et al. (2007)	No effect on BMD	Femoral neck width increased
	Positive effect on hip BMC	Positive effect on indices for hip bone strength
Bolton-Smith et al. (2007)	Positive effect on BMC and BMD	Not measured
	Only seen at ultradistal radius	
Cheung et al. (2008)	No effect on BMD or BMC	Decreased fracture incidence
		Study not designed for fracture risk monitoring
Booth et al. (2008)	No effect on BMD or BMC	Not measured
Inoue et al. (2009)	Not measured	Fracture risk decreased
		Only found in patients with >4 vertebral fractures

Notes: The references listed in this table describe all vitamin K intervention trials published until December 2009 meeting the criteria of a treatment period of at least 2 years and at least 100 subjects included in the trial. Conclusions in this paper are based on these seven trials.

effect of 200 μg/day of vitamin K and calcium + vitamin D on bone metabolism in a 2-year study among 244 postmenopausal women, This study, however, was hampered by the fact that in the placebo group no bone loss was observed at the most critical site, that is, the hip.

Cheung et al. (2008) reported a study among 440 osteopenic women receiving either placebo or vitamin K_1 (5 mg/day) for 2 years. These researchers did not find an effect of vitamin K on BMD, but—although the study was not powered to examine fractures or cancers—significant decreases of the incidence of both fractures and cancers in the vitamin-K-treated group were found. The reduced cancer incidence is remarkable, because recently a large population-based study also showed an inverse correlation between vitamin K intake and prostate cancer incidence (Nimptsch et al., 2008).

Booth et al. (2008) enrolled 452 elderly men and women in a 3-year study who received either a multivitamin containing calcium and vitamin D or the same multivitamin plus 500 μg/day of vitamin K_1. No effect of vitamin K treatment was found. Finally, Inoue et al. (2009) reported a study among over 4000 postmenopausal women receiving either calcium or calcium plus vitamin K_2 (45 mg/day) for 3 years. Although the cumulative 48-month incidence rate of new clinical fractures was lower in the combined therapy group, the difference was only significant in the subgroup with at least five baseline fractures. Also, the loss of height was less with the combined therapy than with monotherapy among patients 75 years of age or older at enrollment and those with at least five vertebral fractures at enrollment. The authors concluded that vitamin K_2 may especially prevent vertebral fractures in patients with more advanced osteoporosis.

Throughout the literature, the effects of vitamin K status on the reduction of fracture incidence are remarkably more evident than improvements of BMD or bone mineral content (BMC), even in trials not designed to monitor fractures (Cheung et al., 2008). One explanation for this persistent observation of a lowered fracture incidence is that BMD and BMC are not appropriate endpoints to monitor the effect of vitamin K on bone strength or fracture risk. Another explanation for the lack of effect in some epidemiologic studies is that only poor vitamin K status is associated with increased fracture risk. It would be logical to investigate the effect of vitamin K on bone health in subjects preselected for poor dietary vitamin K status, but none of the published reports have included subjects with poor vitamin K intakes. We recommend that a placebo-controlled study be performed in early postmenopausal women, who are at great risk of rapid bone loss and who have established poor dietary vitamin K status as a prerequisite risk factor.

VITAMIN K IN CHILDHOOD

Children's bone is different from adult bone in that it continues to grow in length, and it rapidly accumulates mass up to late adolescence. These characteristics are demonstrated by the high activity of the osteoblasts that generate the high concentrations of circulating bone formation markers including osteocalcin. Serum concentrations of both inactive ucOC and the active form, carboxylated osteocalcin (cOC), are high, as is the ratio ucOC/cOC, suggesting a relative excess of ucOC which is characteristic of poor vitamin K status during bone growth (Van Summeren et al., 2007). Apparently, vitamin K is depleted from bone tissue because of the 10-fold higher osteocalcin synthesis rate of children compared with adult bone, resulting in a 10-fold higher vitamin K requirement for the growth of bone compared with the maintenance needs of vitamin K by adult bone. The increased requirement is compensated for neither by a higher dietary vitamin K intake nor by increased vitamin K uptake by osteoblasts from the blood circulation, resulting in a marked vitamin K insufficiency of the bone tissue. Recent studies have demonstrated that vitamin K insufficiency is more pronounced during childhood than in any other stage of life and that an inverse relationship exists between serum ucOC levels and both the rate of bone turnover (Kalkwarf et al., 2004) and BMD (Van Summeren et al., 2008).

Before answering the question of whether children will benefit from increasing their intakes of vitamin K, it is important to learn if we can correct the apparent vitamin K insufficiency of children's bone by giving them vitamin K supplements in doses not exceeding the DRIs. The first placebo-controlled vitamin K_2 intervention study in healthy children between 6 and 10 years of age was published by Van Summeren et al. (2009). The children received either vitamin K_2 (45 µg/day of menaquinone-7 as MenaQ7 capsules) or placebo during 8 weeks, and it was demonstrated that after the 8-week period the ucOC/cOC ratio rapidly declined in the vitamin K-treated group. The dose of 45 µg/day is comparable with the DRI for children of that age. Now that it has been established that the vitamin K status in children's bone is extremely low and that it can be corrected by vitamin K supplements, the question arises whether higher vitamin K intakes should be recommended for children. Although no obvious dangers or disadvantages exist, it is not known whether children would benefit from vitamin K supplements given during their entire growth period. Vitamin K intake by children has declined substantially during the past half century (Prynne et al., 2005). Present strategies of bone health promotion and osteoporosis prevention include aiming to achieve a high peak bone mass in the young adults so that they are optimally prepared to withstand bone loss during the later stages of life without fracture. Whether or not vitamin K should be included in this strategy is not clear at this time.

SAFETY OF HIGH VITAMIN K INTAKE

The best known function of vitamin K is its requirement for the synthesis of functional blood clotting factors and therefore normalization of hemostasis in vitamin-K-deficiency bleeding. During hepatic vitamin K deficiency or when vitamin K antagonists are used, uncarboxylated species of the clotting factors are produced, which lack procoagulant activity. Experimental animals receiving vitamin-K-deficient diets develop severe vitamin K deficiency and exsanguinate within 3 weeks. Under these conditions, administration of vitamin K quickly normalizes hemostasis and prevents death (Groenen-van Dooren et al., 1993). A widespread misperception is that, in subjects with a normal hemostasis, extra vitamin K intake would lead to a hypercoaguble state and hence to an increased risk of thrombosis and thromboembolism. No scientific support for this notion, however, exists.

This scenario is evidently not true. The most sensitive technique presently available to assess thrombosis risk is the endogenous thrombin potential (ETP) in which platelet-free plasma is activated to form thrombin; the amount of thrombin formed during a 30-minute period is then monitored using a chromogenic method (Hemker et al., 2006). Adverse effects monitoring in several of our intervention trials included ETP measurement, and in this way, several hundreds of participants treated with 10 mg/day of vitamin K_1 or even 45 mg/day of vitamin K_2 were evaluated for increased thrombosis tendency during intervention periods of 2 to 3 years. Neither increased thrombosis risk nor other adverse effects were found in these studies. These results are consistent with the statement of the Institute of Medicine (2001) that vitamin K has a very wide safety range and that no evidence of toxicity has been associated with the intake of either phylloquinone (vitamin K_1) or menaquinone (vitamin K_2).

Although no upper tolerable levels for vitamin K have been defined, it is well known that subjects using oral anticoagulants, such as warfarin, acenocoumarol, or phenprocoumon, should avoid taking high doses of vitamin K (either by diet or as supplements), especially if the intake fluctuates from day to day. Oral anticoagulant drugs act as vitamin K antagonists and are prescribed during episodes of high thrombosis risk. Obviously, such drugs should not be combined with high doses of vitamin K. In a study among anticoagulated volunteers, low-dose vitamin K intake (100 µg/day of K_1 or 50 µg/day of K_2) was demonstrated not to affect the level of anticoagulation (international normalized ratio) in a clinically relevant way (Schurgers et al., 2007).

CONCLUSIONS

Although the results remain inconclusive, the majority of published studies have shown a mild positive effect of high vitamin K intake, that is, an adequate vitamin K status, on bone strength, especially if taken in combination with calcium and vitamin D (Cockayne et al., 2006; Iwamoto et al., 2009). Most negative outcomes were found in trials of 1 year or shorter, whereas long-term intervention trials and retrospective studies of life-long dietary habits almost invariably showed a positive correlation between high vitamin K intake and bone health. Many indications suggest that BMD, BMC, or circulating biomarkers for bone metabolism are not suitable endpoints to establish an effect of vitamin K on bone health. Since the molecular functions of vitamin K–dependent proteins in bone are largely unknown, it is difficult to determine the appropriate surrogate markers indicative of bone health in intervention studies. Therefore, large trials in which fracture risk or calculated bone strength are used as endpoints may be the one way to demonstrate unequivocally the importance of vitamin K for bone health. Moreover, such trials should be performed using selected subjects with poor bone vitamin K status, based on their assessment of low osteocalcin carboxylation.

Vitamin K supplements may also be important in another way. Women at risk of rapid bone loss or with high fracture risk often receive supplements containing calcium, vitamin D, or both. Recently, it was suggested that either of these regimens induces coronary artery calcification and cardiovascular mortality (Bolland et al., 2008). MGP is the only known calcification inhibitor in the arterial vessel wall; hence, it is the major tool for the vessel wall to prevent local arterial calcification. Like other extrahepatic Gla-proteins, however, MGP is not fully carboxylated in the majority of the people examined (Schurgers et al., 2008), which means that a substantial fraction of MGP produced in the vessel wall remains inactive. Hence, the calcification-inhibitory potential of the vasculature can be improved by increased vitamin K intake, which is especially important during periods of increased calcium loading, to increase carboxylation of the GRPs. Therefore, we recommend that extra vitamin K should always accompany calcium supplements or calcium plus vitamin D supplements.

REFERENCES

Atkins, G.J., Welldon, K.J., Wijenayaka, A.R., et al. 2009. Vitamin K promotes mineralization, osteoblast to osteocyte transition and an anti-catabolic phenotype by {gamma}-carboxylation dependent and independent mechanisms. *Am J Physiol Cell Physiol* 297: C1358–C1367.

Berkner, K.L. 2005. The vitamin K-dependent carboxylase. *Annu Rev Nutr* 25: 127–149.

Bolland, M.J., Barber, P.A., Doughty, R.N., et al. 2008. Vascular events in healthy older women receiving calcium supplementation: Randomised controlled trial. *Brit Med J* 336: 262–266.

Bolton-Smith, C., McMurdo, M.E.T., Paterson, C.R., et al. 2007. Two-year randomized controlled trial of vitamin K_1 (phylloquinone) and vitamin D_3 plus calcium on the bone health of older women. *J Bone Miner Res* 22: 509–519.

Booth, D.L., Dallal, G., Shea, M.K., et al. 2008. Effect of vitamin K supplementation on bone loss in elderly men and women. *J Clin Endocrinol Metab* 93: 1217–1223.

Booth, S.L., Broe, K.E., Gagnon, D.R., et al. 2003. Vitamin K intake and bone mineral density in women and men. *Am J Clin Nutr* 77: 512–516.

Booth, S.L., Sadowski, J.A., Weihrauch, J.L., et al. 1993. Vitamin K1 (phylloquinone) content of foods: A provisional table. *J Food Comp Anal* 6: 109–120.

Braam, L.A.J.L.M., Knapen, M.H.J., Geusens, P., et al. 2003. Vitamin K_1 supplementation retards bone loss in postmenopausal women between 50 and 60 years of age. *Calcif Tissue Int* 73: 21–26.

Cheung, A.M., Tile, L., Lee, Y., et al. 2008. Vitamin K supplementation in postmenopausal women with osteopenia (ECKO trial): A randomized controlled trial. *PLoS Med* 5: 1461–1472.

Cockayne, S., Adamson, J., Lanham-New, S., et al. 2006. Vitamin K and the prevention of fractures: Systematic review and meta-analysis of randomized controlled trials. *Arch Intern Med* 166: 1256–1261.

Coutu, D.L., Wu, J.H., Monette, A., et al. 2008. Periostin, a member of a novel family of vitamin K-dependent proteins, is expressed by mesenchymal stromal cells. *J Biol Chem* 283: 17991–18001.

Ducy, P., Desbois, C., Boyce, B., et al. 1996. Increased bone formation in osteocalcin-deficient mice. *Nature* 382: 448–452.

Feskanich, D., Weber, P., Willett, W.C., et al. 1999. Vitamin K intake and hip fractures in women: A prospective study. *Am J Clin Nutr* 69: 74–79.

Gast, G.C.M., de Roos, N.M., Sluijs, I, et al. 2009. A high menaquinone intake reduces the incidence of coronary heart disease. *Nutr Metab Cardiovasc Dis* 19: 504–510.

Groenen-van Dooren, M.M.C.L., Soute, B.A.M., Jie, K.-S.G., et al. 1993. The relative effects of phylloquinone and menaquinone-4 on the blood coagulation factor synthesis in vitamin K-deficient rats. *Biochem Pharmacol* 46: 433–437.

Hart, J.P., Catterall, A., Dodds, R.A., et al. 1984. Circulating vitamin K_1 levels in fractured neck of femur. *Lancet* 324 (8397): 283.

Hauschka, P.V., and Reid, M.L. 1978. Vitamin K dependence of a calcium-binding protein containing gammacarboxyglutamic acid in chicken bone. *J Biol Chem* 253: 9063–9068.

Hemker, H.C., Al Dieri, R., De Smedt, E., et al. 2006. Thrombin generation, a function test of the haemostatic–thrombotic system. *Thromb Haemost* 96: 553–561.

Inoue, T., Fujita, K., Kishimoto, H., et al. 2009. Randomized controlled study on the prevention of osteoporotic fractures (OF study): A phase IV clinical study of 15-mg menatetrenone capsules. *J Bone Miner Metab* 27: 66–75.

Institute of Medicine. 2001. Vitamin K. In: *Dietary Reference Intakes for Vitamin A, Vitamin K, Arsenic, Boron, Chromium, Copper, Iodine, Iron, Manganese, Molybdenum, Nickel, Silicon, Vanadium, and Zinc.* National Academy Press, Washington, DC.

Iwamoto, J., Sato, Y., Takeda, T., et al. 2009. High-dose vitamin K supplementation reduces fracture incidence in postmenopausal women: A review of the literature. *Nutr Res* 29: 221–228.

Kalkwarf, H.J., Khoury, J.C., Bean, J., et al. 2004. Vitamin K, bone turnover, and bone mass in girls. *Am J Clin Nutr* 80: 1075–1080.

Katagiri, M., Hakeda, Y., Chikazu, D., et al. 2001. Mechanism of stimulation of osteoclastic bone resorption through Gas6/Tyro 3, a receptor tyrosine kinase signaling, in mouse osteoclasts. *J Biol Chem* 276: 7376–7382.

Knapen, M.H.J., Schurgers, L.J., and Vermeer, C. 2007. Vitamin K_2 supplementation improves bone geometry and bone strength indices in postmenopausal women. *Osteoporos Int* 18: 963–972.

Lee, N.K., Sowa, H., Hinoi, E., et al. 2007. Endocrine regulation of energy metabolism by the skeleton. *Cell* 130: 456–469.

Luukinen, H., Käkönen, S.-M., Petterson, K., et al. 2000. Strong prediction of fractures among older adults by the ratio of carboxylated to total serum osteocalcin. *J Bone Miner Res* 15: 2473–2478.

Maillard, C., Berruyer, M., Serre, C.M., et al. 1992. Protein S, a vitamin K-dependent protein, is a bone matrix component synthesized and secreted by osteoblasts. *Endocrinology* 130: 1599–1604.

McCann, J.C., and Ames, B.N. 2009. Vitamin K, an example of triage theory: Is micronutrient inadequacy linked to diseases of aging? *Am J Clin Nutr* 90: 889–907.

Nimptsch, K., Rohrmann, S., and Linseisen, J. 2008. Dietary intake of vitamin K and risk of prostate cancer in the Heidelberg cohort of the European Prospective Investigation into Cancer and Nutrition (EPIC-Heidelberg). *Am J Clin Nutr* 87: 985–992.

Pan, E.Y., Gomperts, E.D., Millen, R., et al. 1990. Bone mineral density and its association with inherited protein S deficiency. *Thromb Res* 58: 221–231.

Price, P.A., Urist, M.R., and Otawara, Y. 1983. Matrix Gla-protein, a new gammacarboxyglutamic acid-containing protein which is associated with the organic matrix of bone. *Biochem Biophys Res Commun* 117: 765–771.

Prynne, C.J., Thane, C.W., Prentice, A., et al. 2005. Intake and sources of phylloquinone (vitamin K(1)) in 4-year-old British children: Comparison between 1950 and the 1990s. *Publ Health Nutr* 8: 171–180.

Schurgers, L.J., Cranenburg, E.C., and Vermeer, C. 2008. Matrix Gla-protein: The calcification inhibitor in need of vitamin K. *Thromb Haemost* 100: 593–603.

Schurgers, L.J., Shearer, M.J., Hamulyák, K., et al. 2004. Effect of vitamin K on the stability of oral anticoagulant treatment: Dose response relationship in healthy subjects. *Blood* 104: 2682–2689.

Schurgers, L.J., Teunissen, K.J., Hamulyák, K., et al. 2007. Vitamin K-containing dietary supplements: Comparison of synthetic vitamin K1 and natto-derived menaquinone-7. *Blood* 109: 3279–3283.

Schurgers, L.J., and Vermeer, C. 2000. Determination of phylloquinone and menaquinones in food: Effect of food matrix on circulating vitamin K concentrations. *Haemostasis* 30: 298–307.

Schurgers, L.J., and Vermeer, C. 2002. Differential lipoprotein transport pathways of K-vitamins in healthy subjects. *Biochim Biophys Acta* 1570: 27–32.

Shearer, M.J., and Bolton-Smith, C. 2000. The U.K. food data-base for vitamin K and why we need it. *Food Chem* 68: 213–218.

Shearer, M.J., and Newman, P. 2008. Metabolism and cell biology of vitamin K. *Thromb Haemost* 100: 530–547.

Shiraki, M., Shiraki, Y., Aoki, C., et al. 2000. Vitamin K_2 (menatetrenone) effectively prevents fractures and sustains lumbar bone mineral density in osteoporosis. *J Bone Miner Res* 15: 515–521.

Szulc, P., Chapuy, M.-C., Meunier, P.J., et al. 1996. Serum undercarboxylated osteocalcin is a marker of the risk of hip fracture: A three year follow-up study. *Bone* 18: 487–488.

Van Summeren, M.J.H., Braam, L.A.J.L.M., Lilien, M.R., et al. 2009. The effect of menaquinone-7 (vitamin K_2) supplementation on osteocalcin carboxylation in healthy prepubertal children. *Br J Nutr* 102: 1171–1178.

Van Summeren, M.J.H., Braam, L.A.J.L.M., Noirt, F., et al. 2007. Pronounced elevation of undercarboxylated osteocalcin in healthy children. *Pediatr Res* 61: 366–370.

Van Summeren, M.J.H., van Coeverden, S.C.C.M., Schurgers, L.J., et al. 2008. Vitamin K status is associated with childhood bone mineral content. *Br J Nutr* 100: 852–858.

Viegas, C.S., Simes, D.C., Laizé, V., et al. 2008. Gla-rich protein (GRP), a new vitamin K-dependent protein identified from sturgeon cartilage and highly conserved in vertebrates. *J Biol Chem* 283: 36655–36664.

13 The Iron Factor in Bone Development

Denis M. Medeiros and Erika Bono

CONTENTS

INTRODUCTION

Osteoporosis is a major public health threat for an estimated 44 million Americans or 55% of the people 50 years of age and older. In the United States today, 10 million individuals are estimated to already have the disease, and almost 34 million more are estimated to have low bone mass, placing them at increased risk for osteoporosis. In 2005, osteoporosis-related fractures were responsible for an estimated $19 billion in costs. By 2025, experts predict that these costs will rise to approximately $25.3 billion (National Osteoporosis Foundation, 2008).

Calcium and vitamin D are crucial for maintaining bone health and preventing diseases of aging such as osteoporosis. Deficiency of these nutrients increases the risk for developing this disease. These two nutrients are critical in promoting bone growth and development in the formative years. Other nutrients have also received attention because of their roles in bone health. For instance, the balance between dietary phosphorus and calcium is important for bone. Also, excess dietary intakes of protein and sodium may also have negative effects upon bone. Other micronutrients, such as magnesium, ascorbic acid, selenium, copper, vitamin A, boron, zinc, and vitamin K, also impact upon bone, as has been demonstrated when one of these nutrients is either lacking or deficient in a diet (Anderson et al., 1998; Ilich and Kerstetter, 2000; Palacios, 2006). For instance, in animals, magnesium deficiency results in decreased bone strength and volume, poor bone development, and uncoupling of bone formation and resorption (Ilich and Kerstetter, 2000). Manganese supplementation along with calcium, copper, and zinc resulted in a greater gain in bone compared with supplementation with calcium alone (Ilich and Kerstetter, 2000).

Another nutrient, iron, has been demonstrated to play a role in bone strength primarily because of experimental animal research. A few human studies also suggest an association between iron and bone health. Although iron itself is not as important as are calcium and vitamin D in promoting bone health, nevertheless, iron has an essential role in collagen formation, which directly impacts on bone integrity. Because iron deficiency is the second most common public health nutrition problem in the United States, it may have relevance to suboptimal bone development. Insufficient iron intake may foster the detrimental effects on bone health that result from suboptimal calcium and/ or vitamin D intakes.

THEORETICAL UNDERPINNINGS

COLLAGEN CROSS-LINKING

Our group has investigated trace elements, such as copper and iron, as they relate to bone health. We initially observed that copper deficiency led to increased fragility in bone, an observation also reported by others (Rucker et al., 1969a, 1969b, 1975; Rucker, 1972; Opsahl et al., 1982; Jonas et al., 1993). A key role for copper exists as a component in a cupro-enzyme, lysyl oxidase, which is a rate-limiting enzyme in collagen strengthening. This enzyme catalyzes the production of aldehydes from lysine. Specifically, the epsilon amino group of lysine and hydroxylysine residues is converted to the reactive aldehydes, allysine and hydroxyallysine, respectively (Figure 13.1). These products then form an aldol cross-link, as shown in Figure 13.2. Collagen and elastin cross-linking are dependent upon this reaction, an important reaction from a biological perspective because it gives these connective tissue proteins their strength. Without active lysyl oxidase, tissues rich in collagen and elastin decline in strength, that is, reduced response to physical stress. The weakened connective tissues are one reason aneurysms and cardiac valve abnormalities occur in copper deficiency (Medeiros et al., 1991). With respect to bone, type I collagen is likely compromised in copper deficiency, and this leads to more fragile bones.

ROLE OF IRON IN COLLAGEN CROSS-LINKING

A major reason to investigate iron in bone tissue is that iron is required for lysine to be hydroxylated prior to reacting with lysyl oxidase. This hydroxylation step requires a unique reaction and enzyme, in this case, lysyl hydroxylase. Another similar enzyme also involved with collagen metabolism and thereby bone is prolyl hydroxylase, which catalyzes the formation of hydroxyproline from proline. In both reactions, ascorbate, molecular oxygen, α-ketoglutarate, and ferrous iron are required for this reaction (Figure 13.3). Both iron and ascorbate are required for several hydroxylase reactions (Switzer and Summer, 1972, 1973; Anderson et al., 1998).

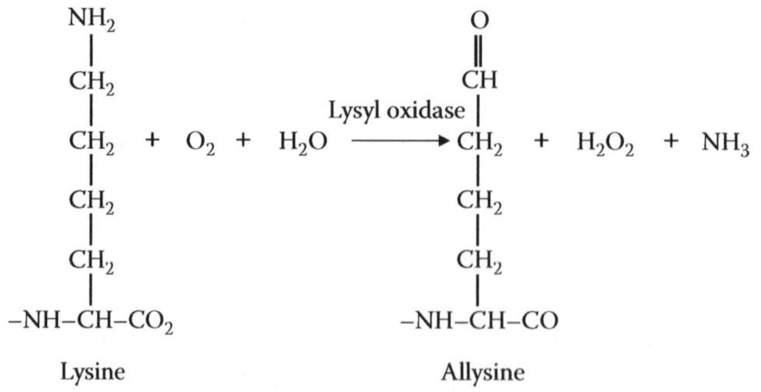

$$
\begin{array}{ccc}
\text{NH}_2 & & \text{O} \\
| & & \| \\
\text{CH}_2 & & \text{CH} \\
| & \text{Lysyl oxidase} & | \\
\text{CH}_2 + \text{O}_2 + \text{H}_2\text{O} \longrightarrow & \text{CH}_2 + \text{H}_2\text{O}_2 + \text{NH}_3 \\
| & & | \\
\text{CH}_2 & & \text{CH}_2 \\
| & & | \\
\text{CH}_2 & & \text{CH}_2 \\
| & & | \\
-\text{NH}-\text{CH}-\text{CO}_2 & & -\text{NH}-\text{CH}-\text{CO} \\
\text{Lysine} & & \text{Allysine}
\end{array}
$$

FIGURE 13.1 Reaction of lysine and the copper containing enzyme lysyl oxidase in producing allysine prior to cross-linking reaction in collagen synthesis.

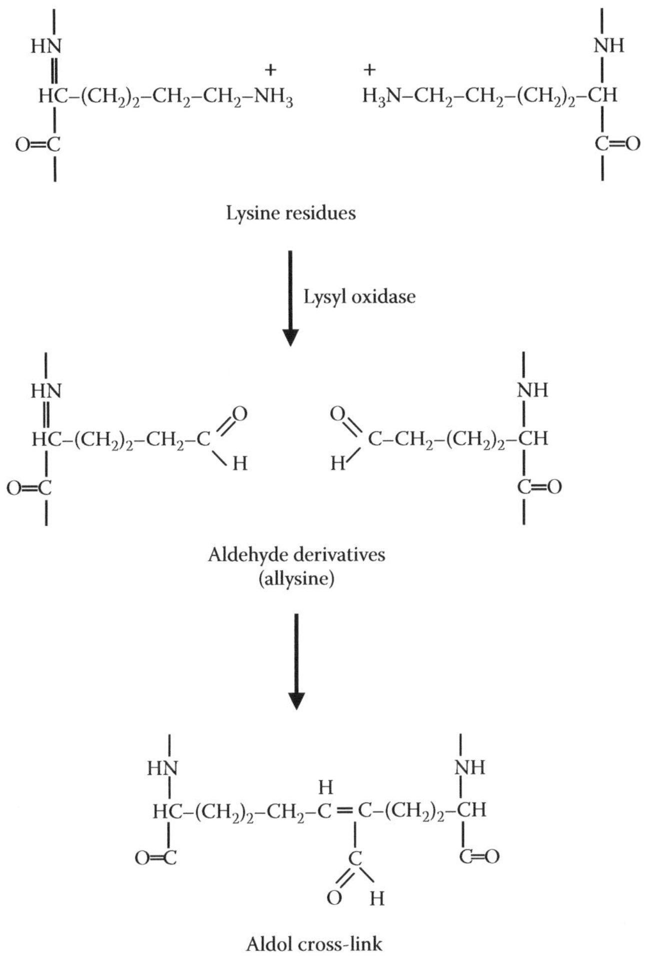

FIGURE 13.2 Complete cross-linking reactions mediated by lysyl oxides for collagen development.

COPPER DEFICIENCY AND BONE

To provide background for understanding the role of iron in bone development and remodeling, a review of our knowledge of copper and bone provides comparison to the role of iron. Much of our understanding of copper as it relates to bone comes from the studies of Rucker (1972), Rucker et al. (1969a, 1969b, 1975), Opsahl et al. (1982), and Jonas et al. (1993). In these studies, elastin- and collagen-containing tissues, such as blood vessels, tendon, and bone, demonstrated decreased mechanical strength in copper deficiency that was associated with deficient collagen and elastin cross-linking. Torsional strength of bone in copper deficiency was noted to be decreased in chick tibia (Opsahl et al., 1982). Decreased activity of lysyl oxidase was also reported in this study. Jonas et al. (1993), who reported decreased torsional loading in femurs from copper-deficient rats, suggested that because the calcium content of the femurs did not differ by copper treatment, the difference in torsional strength was likely due to a decrease in collagen cross-linking. However, the issue of decreased bone mineralization in copper deficiency was reported earlier by Smith and colleagues (2002) who demonstrated lower bone mineral density (BMD), as measured by dual-energy x-ray absorptiometry (DXA) in the fifth lumbar vertebra and the proximal femur in copper-deficient rats. Furthermore, biochemical markers of bone formation, such as changes in blood alkaline

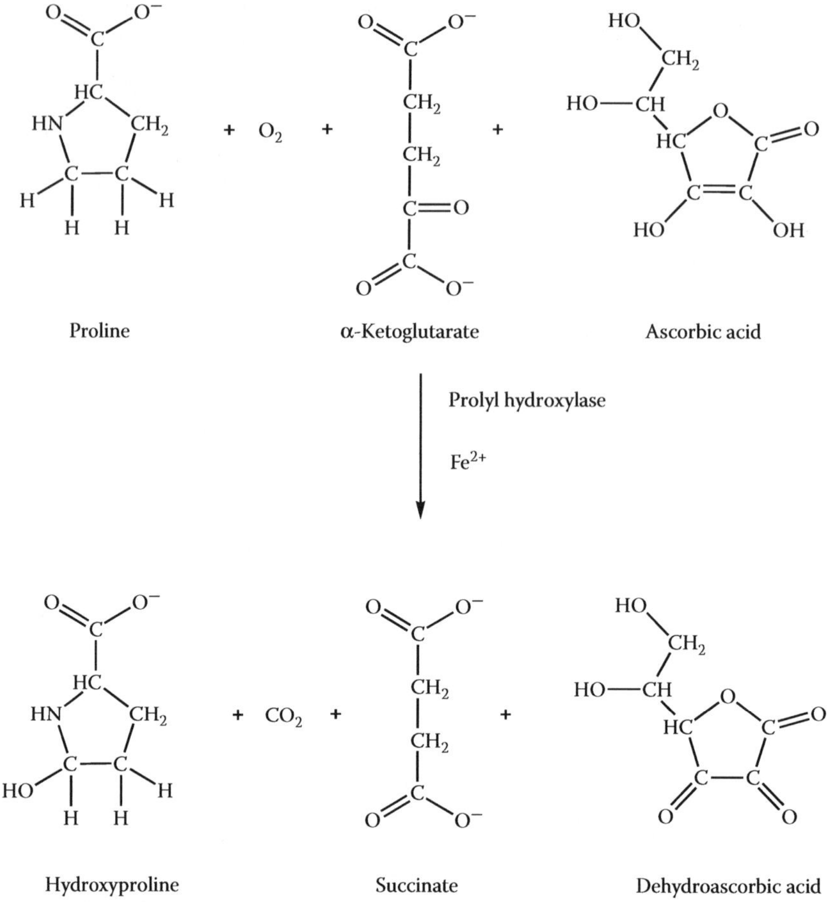

FIGURE 13.3 A role for iron in collagen. Here proline is hydroxylated to hydroxyproline in the presence of an iron-dependent enzyme, prolyl hydroxylase, and ascorbic acid. α-Ketoglutarate is used as a substrate in the reaction with a succinate product, both of which are tricarboxylic acid cycle (TCA) intermediates.

phosphatase activity, were not noted, which indirectly suggested an accelerated bone resorption as the reason for decreased BMD in the bones of copper-deficient rats.

IRON DEFICIENCY AND BONE

ANIMAL STUDIES

We were the first laboratory to report a possible role for iron in bone integrity. Initially, our laboratory had been studying the role of copper and iron deficiency upon cardiac metabolism and cardiac hypertrophy. In the course of a usual study, we noted that the bones from iron-deficient rats appeared to be more fragile upon dissection of the carcass. A review of the literature suggested that iron could play a role in bone via hydroxylase coenzyme partner, as reviewed above. In our first study, we compared rats fed either control diets, iron-deficient diets, or copper-deficient diets from weaning until 5 weeks thereafter. Animals were sacrificed and assessed for iron stores and had their femurs removed and x-rays developed for morphometric analysis and then submitted to a three-point bending test for strength analysis (Medeiros et al., 1997). We reported that in iron-deficient and copper-deficient rats, the breaking strength decreased in femurs. Iron and copper deficiency both resulted in smaller cortical and larger medullary areas in a part of the femur.

With this new information, more defined studies were planned to confirm and explain in greater detail the changes that occur in bone of rats that were fed iron-deficient diets. One issue that needed to be addressed appeared to be the relative perturbation of iron deficiency upon bone as compared with that of calcium restriction; the latter, of course, is a commonly accepted culprit in the genesis of osteoporosis. We conducted a study in which four groups of weanling male rats were fed diets either deficient in iron (5 to 8 mg Fe/kg diet), low in calcium (1.0 g calcium/kg diet), or deficient in both minerals as compared with a control diet that contained adequate amounts of both nutrients (Medeiros et al., 2002). Extra care was taken in preparing the diets as we wanted to rigorously control the dietary intake levels of both calcium and iron. Because of our concern about avoiding any iron contamination in this and other studies, we used 5% avicel as a source of fiber rather than cellulose, as cellulose has a rather high iron background content. For the low-calcium diets, we used chemically pure calcium phosphate dibasic and magnesium carbonate. Also, because of concern about the phosphate components of the diet, we elected to control the phosphorus level in the diet at 0.56%. This diet was very low in iron content (5 to 8 mg Fe/kg diet). Rats were fed the control or iron-deficient diets for 5 weeks. Results revealed that cortical widths were reduced in all experimental groups, with the calcium-restricted and the calcium/iron-deficient groups having the greatest reductions in cortical width. Total femur and tibia widths were decreased in all experimental groups. The iron-deficient group had an increase in the medullary width. Calcium restriction and iron deficiency either alone or in combination resulted in reduced BMD and cortical bone area. In this animal model, iron deficiency clearly had a negative impact upon bone health, and in combination with calcium restriction, even greater negative effects were observed.

A fundamental issue in the study previously cited (Medeiros et al., 2002) was that the low iron content of the diet resulted in severe iron deficiency and multiple adverse skeletal and nonosseous effects. The animals had greatly reduced body weight, and thus the issue of food intake during iron deficiency had to be taken into consideration. Another study was designed with similar diets, and rats were allocated to one of four groups: control (ad libitum), calcium-restricted, iron-deficient, or a control group pair fed to the iron-deficient group (Medeiros et al., 2004). The pair-fed control group simply meant that the amount of food consumed by the iron-deficient group was determined daily and an equal amount of control diet was provided to the pair-fed rats. The results revealed that while the pair-fed rats did have small but greater decreases in whole body and femur BMD and bone mineral content (BMC) than those of the control group, both the calcium-restricted and the iron-deficient groups had much greater reductions in BMD and BMC at the same measurement sites than the pair-fed group (Table 13.1).

These results suggested that the impact of iron deficiency was independent of low caloric intake and a reduced body weight resulting from iron deficiency. In this same study, we examined the lumbar region of the animals as well as the microarchitecture of lumbar vertebrae. The third lumbar vertebra (L_3) revealed decreases in bone volume and total bone volume, decreased trabecular number

TABLE 13.1

Whole Body and Femur BMD of Rats That Were Fed Control, Calcium-Deficient, Iron-Deficient, or Pair-Fed Diets[1,2] (Mean ± SEM)

Variable	Control	Ca−	Fe−	Pair-Fed
Whole-body BMD, g/cm²				
3 weeks	0.122 ± 0.0025[a]	0.093 ± 0.0023[b]	0.119 ± 0.0034[a]	0.117 ± 0.0031[a]
5 weeks	0.142 ± 0.0018[a]	0.091 ± 0.0014[d]	0.129 ± 0.0019[c]	0.135 ± 0.0012[b]
Femur BMD, g/cm²	0.183 ±.0042[a]	0.096 ± 0.0015[d]	0.161 ± 0.0030[c]	0.173 ± 0.0021[b]

[1] Pair-fed group was fed the control diet in an amount consumed by the iron-deficient group (Fe−).

[2] Means in a row without a common superscript differ, $p \leq .05$.

and thickness, a lower structural model index, and increased trabecular separation in each of the nutrient-deficient groups compared with the control and pair-fed groups. Finite element analysis was used to further analyze the data. This analytic method uses a computer simulation technique, often employed in engineering and other physical sciences, to predict how materials and structures will respond when loads are placed upon them. Finite element analysis revealed that a lower force was needed to compress the vertebrae that had lower stiffness, but that a greater von Mises stress was needed in the calcium-restricted and iron-deficient groups compared with both the control and pair-fed groups. Von Mises stress is the internal stress in the bone when a constant force is applied. These findings mean that greater internal stresses existed in the lumbar vertebrae of the calcium-restricted and iron-deficient groups. Urine concentrations of deoxypyridinium cross-links, serum osteocalcin, and 1, 25-dihydroxycholecalciferol were increased in calcium-restricted rats compared with the other three groups. Iron deficiency apparently did not affect these measures. The lack of change in serum 1,25-dihydroxycholecalciferol concentrations were unexpected because it had been reported that 1α-hydroxylase involves a reaction that is dependent upon a flavoprotein, that is, an iron-sulfur protein, and cytochrome P-450, also iron containing (DeLuca, 1976). Regardless, this study provided further evidence that iron deficiency had a detrimental impact upon the microarchitecture of L_3 and other vertebrae and that the bone effects were independent of the amount of food ingested.

The final study from our laboratory sought to answer the question as to whether marginal iron intake, as opposed to a very severe iron deficiency (as used in the above studies), would produce similar adverse effects on bone (Parelman et al., 2006). Our goal was to address more specifically the likelihood of iron deficiency in humans might be a factor affecting bone health. This investigation, therefore, evaluated marginal iron and calcium intakes upon the same bone parameters as in our previous study (Medeiros et al., 2004). We assigned 32 male weanling rats to one of four diets: control (ad libitum), marginal calcium in the amount of 2.5 g Ca/kg diet (compared with 1.0 g Ca/kg diet in previous studies), marginal iron in the amount of 12 mg Fe/kg diet (compared with 5 to 8 mg Fe/kg diet in previous studies), or a diet marginal in both calcium and iron. Because the diets were higher in calcium and iron, we elected to feed these diets to animals for 10 weeks instead of the usual 5 weeks. As would be expected, rats fed the marginal iron diet did have lower hematocrit readings compared with those of iron-adequate rats. Using similar measures as reported above, the whole-body BMD was lower in the marginal calcium group, and whole-body BMC was lower in the marginal iron group when compared with the controls (Medeiros et al., 2004). Marginal calcium or marginal iron intake resulted in decreased BMD of the femur. There was a trend (p = .06) for the doubly deficient group to have lower BMD than those of the other three treatment groups. Furthermore, the most revealing findings concerned the L_4 vertebrae, in that BMD was lower in all three experimental groups compared with the control group. The overall BMC was lower in both the marginal iron and the marginal calcium groups than in the groups with adequate iron and the control rats. Microcomputed tomography analysis revealed that marginal iron L_4 and marginal calcium L_4 had reduced connectivity of the trabeculae. Moreover, in the marginal iron rats, trabecular number was decreased and trabecular separation was increased, which results in enhanced porosity (Figure 13.4). Finite element analysis suggested that the marginal iron group was less likely to withstand compression force and could break at lower external stress than was the control group.

Control   Iron-restricted

FIGURE 13.4 Example of trabecular bone of L_4 in rats fed either a control diet containing adequate levels of iron or a diet marginal in iron (12 mg Fe/kg diet). The arrow denotes increased porosity in the vertebrae for a rat fed an iron-restricted diet.

A follow-up study of iron chelation in hFOB osteoblast cells, that is, iron deficiency induced by an iron chelator, was designed to test whether iron deficiency in bone-forming cells influences type I collagen formation (Parelman et al., 2006). No differences in type I collagen levels were found between iron-deficient cells and control cells. Interestingly, we did observe decreased mineralization associated with iron chelation treatment. These *in vitro* results supported, at least in part, the *in vivo* studies, which demonstrated decreased mineralization in rats consuming an iron-restricted diet.

McClung et al. (2008) did not report any differences in bone-breaking threshold as a result of marginal iron intake. However, a major difference in their study compared with ours (Parelman et al., 2006) was that their rats began the iron-deficient diets at 10 weeks of age. Although they were fed these diets for 12 weeks, this was an insufficient period of time for animals to develop iron-deficiency anemia. Presumably, the animals in this report had stored up sufficient iron reserves by the time the study started. In contrast, our study provided an iron-deficient diet starting at weaning (when limited iron accretion by the liver occurs in comparison with an older rat), and all the rats developed iron-deficiency anemia.

Another critical issue may be the specific period in the life cycle that the limited intake of iron is fed. Dietary iron deficiency might be more detrimental to the bones of rapidly growing rats after weaning than later in life. Other laboratories have been able to corroborate our finding of the negative impact of a postweaning iron-deficient diet upon bone development (Katsumata et al., 2006, 2009). For example, Katsumata et al. (2009) investigated whether iron deficiency would decrease BMD in weanling male rats. Two groups of six rats each were fed a control (ad libitum) or an iron-deficient diet, and a third group, similar to our previous study (Medeiros et al., 2004), was pair-fed a control diet in an amount consumed by the iron-deficient rats. The diet was the AIN-93G diet, a modification of the AIN-77 diet previously used by our laboratory. The rats were allowed to consume their respective diets for 4 weeks. BMC and BMD were measured, and bone histomorphometry was assessed. The iron-deficient rats did develop both anemia and greater heart weights, common signs of severe dietary iron deficiency. Supporting our previous studies, BMC and BMD measurements were significantly lower in the femurs of the iron-deficient groups compared with the control and pair-fed groups. Lower bone-volume-to-total-bone-volume ratio in the iron-deficient group was also demonstrated. Whereas trabecular thickness did not differ among the three groups, trabecular number was significantly decreased in both iron-deficient groups, and trabecular separation was higher as well.

These findings are consistent with increased porosity in iron-deficient rats and are in agreement with our previous studies (Medeiros et al., 2004; Parelman et al., 2006). These investigators also assessed osteoid volume, osteoid surface, and osteoid thickness. All of these parameters were reduced in the iron-deficient groups compared with those of controls. Mineralizing surface, mineral apposition rate, bone formation rate, and adjusted apposition rate were also significantly lower in the iron-deficient group. The percentage of bone surface occupied by osteoclasts was decreased in the iron-deficient group as was osteoclast number. Biochemical measures, such as blood osteocalcin concentrations and urinary deoxypyridinoline levels, were lower in the iron-deficient group, whereas the C-terminal telopeptide of type I collagen was higher in the iron-deficient group. The lower osteocalcin levels suggested lower bone formation in the iron-deficient group. The reductions of deoxypyridinoline and C-terminal telopeptide of type I collagen suggested that bone resorption is decreased in iron deficiency. We did not find changes of osteocalcin and urinary deoxypyridinoline in our study, nor did we report differences in 1,25-dihydroxycholecalciferol, as these authors did (Medeiros et al., 2004). McClung and coinvestigators (2008) pointed out that the degree of anemia, a major determinant of the results, in their study was much greater than in ours.

HUMAN STUDIES

No conclusive data exist that dietary iron or adequate iron status may be beneficial in humans as it relates to bone integrity and BMD, but a few studies suggest the benefit of sufficient iron intake for skeletal health. The first study published by Harris and colleagues (2003) assessed 242 women 40 to 66 years of age for a variety of bone-related variables as part of the Bone, Estrogen, and Strength Training (BEST) Study. This randomized clinical trial examined the impact of exercise on BMD in early postmenopausal women. As part of this study, the investigators had access to 3-day dietary records and BMD measurements of the lumbar spine at L_2 to L_4, greater trochanter, femur neck, Ward's triangle, and whole body (Figure 13.5). Using multiple regression techniques and adjustments for pertinent confounding variables, dietary iron intake was associated with greater BMD at all skeletal sites. This relationship was significant even after adjustment for dietary calcium and protein. Specifically, subjects who consumed greater than 20 mg of dietary iron per day and had a calcium intake between 800 and 1200 mg per day had the most significant increases in BMD.

A second investigation by the same group using subjects from the BEST study (Maurer et al., 2005) provided additional support to the idea that iron may be related to bone mass and density. Here, hormone replacement therapy was considered in a 1-year longitudinal study of 116 women who received hormone replacement and 112 women who did not receive replacement therapy. This study used 8-day dietary records and had the same BMD measurements as in the previous report (Harris et al., 2003). Iron intake was shown to be positively related to BMD in the greater trochanter and Ward's triangle only in women receiving hormone replacement therapy. For those women in the lowest tertile of calcium intake, femur neck BMD increased as iron intake increased.

A study of a British group of 32 women aged 46 to 55 years who were not on hormone replacement therapy suggested an independent positive association between dietary iron and BMD (Abraham et al., 2006). The women were followed for a period of 11 to 14 years and had periodic weighed-food intakes and BMD measurements at L_2 to L_4 of the vertebral column. Again, dietary iron intake was positively related to BMD, even after adjusting for calcium and protein intakes. A larger cross-sectional study of the same subjects enrolled in this study revealed that, among 244 females within the same age range, a positive association between dietary iron and BMD was found at all bone sites (Farrell et al., 2009).

Perhaps the ultimate test short of a randomized clinical trial with iron supplementation is illustrated by a study conducted by Moran et al. (2008), in which young Israeli soldiers in basic training were evaluated for risk factors that might predict stress fractures. The study included 227 females and 83 males. None of the males developed stress fractures during basic training, but 27 females did develop stress fractures during the 4-month period of basic training. Females with iron deficiency

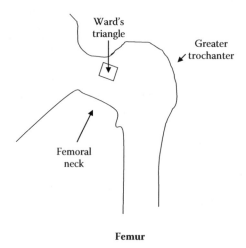

Femur

FIGURE 13.5 Diagram of a femur in which DXA measures are often made for bone mineral density measurements. Note that the greater trochanter and an area on the femur neck called Ward's triangle are often measured in bone studies.

had a greater risk of developing stress fractures. These results are intriguing and should be further investigated because of relevance to other military units as well as to athletes who may be consuming an iron-poor diet.

SUMMARY

Experimental studies have revealed that dietary factors other than protein, calcium, and vitamin D, that is, other micronutrients, may have a role in skeletal development and maintenance. Magnesium, ascorbic acid, selenium, vitamin A, boron, zinc, and vitamin K are some of the most common nutrients known to have roles in bone growth and maintenance. Also, copper is known to promote bone integrity as a cofactor for the enzyme lysyl oxidase, which promotes cross-linking among collagen fibrils, thereby enhancing strength in bone as well as in other collagen-containing tissue. Iron has been shown to play a role in supporting bone strength in both animal and human studies. From a theoretical perspective, two iron-dependent enzymes act in support of collagen cross-linking: lysyl hydroxylase and prolyl hydroxylase. Experimentally, data from animal models indicate that bone mineralization appears to be compromised as a result of either severe iron deficiency or marginal iron deficiency.

Human and animal studies are consistent in finding that bone mineral density and content, as measured by DXA, are decreased with lower iron intake. Stress fractures may occur in young women athletes and military recruits with iron deficiency. One important study revealed an increased incidence of stress fractures among iron-deficient female military recruits compared with none in iron-replete female military recruits in basic training. These findings have implications from a practical perspective because iron insufficiency, and less commonly, iron-deficiency anemia, is a common U.S. and worldwide problem. A precise mechanism regarding the linkage between iron deficiency and poor bone development and bone loss in young adults has not yet been determined. Randomized clinically controlled trials of BMD in females of various ages, with or without iron supplementation, appear to be warranted.

ACKNOWLEDGMENTS

This was supported in part by K-State Research and Extension Multistate project number W2002; "Nutrient Bioavailabilty—Phytonutrients and Beyond."

REFERENCES

Abraham, R., Walton, J., Russell, L., et al. 2006. Dietary determinants of post-menopausal bone loss at the lumbar spine: A possible beneficial effect of iron. *Osteoporos Int* 17: 1165–1173.

Anderson, J.J.B., Stender, M., Rondano, P., et al. 1998. In *Nutrition in Exercise and Sport*, I. Wolinsky, ed., 219–244. CRC Press, Boca Raton, FL.

DeLuca, H.F. 1976. Metabolism of vitamin D: Current status. *Am J Clin Nutr* 29: 1258–1270.

Farrell, V., Harris, M., Lohman, T.G., et al. 2009. Comparison between dietary assessment methods for determining associations between nutrient intakes and bone mineral density in postmenopausal women. *J Am Diet Assoc* 109: 899–904.

Harris, M.M., Houtkooper, L.B., Stanford, V.A., et al. 2003. Dietary iron is associated with bone mineral density in healthy postmenopausal women. *J Nutr* 133: 3598–3602.

Ilich, J.Z., and Kerstetter, J.E. 2000. Nutrition in bone health revisited: A story beyond calcium. *J Am Coll Nutr* 19: 715–737.

Jonas, J., Burns, J., Abel, E.W., et al. 1993. Impaired mechanical strength of bone in experimental copper deficiency. *Ann Nutr Metab* 37: 245–252.

Katsumata, S., Katsumata-Tsuboi, R., Uehara, M., et al. 2009. Severe iron deficiency decreases both bone formation and bone resorption in rats. *J Nutr* 139: 238–243.

Katsumata, S., Tsuboi, R., Uehara, M., et al. 2006. Dietary iron deficiency decreases serum osteocalcin concentration and bone mineral density in rats. *Biosci Biotechnol Biochem* 70: 2547–2550.

Maurer, J., Harris, M.M., Stanford, V.A., et al. 2005. Dietary iron positively influences bone mineral density in postmenopausal women on hormone replacement therapy. *J Nutr* 135: 863–869.

McClung, J.P., Andersen, N.E., Tarr, T.N., et al. 2008. Physical activity prevents augmented body fat accretion in moderately iron-deficient rats. *J Nutr* 138: 1293–1297.

Medeiros, D.M., Bagby, D., and Ovecka, G. 1991. Myofibrillar, mitochondrial and valvular morphological alterations in cardiac hypertrophy among copper deficient rats. *J Nutr* 121: 815–824.

Medeiros, D.M., Ilich, J., Ireton, J., et al. 1997. Femur from rats fed diets deficient in copper or iron have decreased mechanical strength and altered mineral composition. *J Trace Elem Exp Med* 10: 197–203.

Medeiros, D.M., Plattner, A., Jennings, D., et al. 2002. Bone morphology, strength and density are compromised in iron-deficient rats and exacerbated by calcium restriction. *J Nutr* 132: 3135–3141.

Medeiros, D.M., Stoecker, B., Plattner, A., et al. 2004. Iron deficiency negatively affects vertebrae and femurs of rats independently of energy intake and body weight. *J Nutr* 134: 3061–3067.

Moran, D.S., Israeli, E., Evans, R.K., et al. 2008. Prediction model for stress fracture in young female recruits during basic training. *Med Sci Sports Exerc* 40: S636–S644.

National Osteoporosis Foundation. 2008. *Fast Facts on Osteoporosis.* http://www.nof.org/osteoporosis/diseasefacts.htm (accessed October 29, 2009).

Opsahl, W., Zeronian, H., Ellison, M., et al. 1982. Role of copper in collagen cross-linking and its influence on selected mechanical properties of chick bone and tendon. *J Nutr* 112: 708–716.

Palacios, C. 2006. The role of nutrients in bone health, from A to Z. *Crit Rev Food Sci Nutr* 46: 621–628.

Parelman, M., Stoecker, B., Baker, A., et al. 2006. Iron restriction negatively affects bone in female rats and mineralization of hFOB osteoblast cells. *Exp Biol Med* 231: 378–386.

Rucker, R.B. 1972. The effect of copper deficiency on bone strength and the metabolism of aortic elastin. In *Trace Substances in Environmental Health VI.* R.S. Riggins ed., 153–157. University of Missouri Press, Columbia, MO.

Rucker, R.B., Parker, H.E., and Rogler, J.C. 1969a. Effect of copper deficiency on chick bone collagen and selected bone enzymes. *J Nutr* 98: 57–63.

Rucker, R.B., Parker, H.E., and Rogler, J.C. 1969b. The effects of copper on collagen cross-linking. *Biochem Biophys Res Comm* 34: 28–32.

Rucker, R.B., Riggins, R.S., Laughlin, R., et al. 1975. Effects of nutritional copper deficiency on the biomechanical properties of bone and arterial elastin metabolism in the chick. *J Nutr* 105: 1062–1070.

Smith, B.J., King, J.B., Lucas, E.A., et al. 2002. Skeletal unloading and dietary copper depletion are detrimental to bone quality of mature rats. *J Nutr* 132: 190–196.

Switzer, B.R., and Summer, G.K. 1972. Collagen synthesis in human fibroblasts: Effects of ascorbate, α-ketoglutarate and ferrous ion on proline hydroxylation. *J Nutr* 102: 721–728.

Switzer, B.R., and Summer, G.K. 1973. Inhibition of collagen synthesis by α, α'-dipyridyl in human skin fibroblasts in culture. *In Vitro* 9: 160–166.

14 Micronutrients and Bone

Elizabeth Grubert and Jeri W. Nieves

CONTENTS

INTRODUCTION

The most recent definition of osteoporosis is a disease characterized by loss of bone mass, accompanied by microarchitectural deterioration of bone tissue, that leads to an unacceptable increase in the risk of skeletal failure (fracture). Osteoporosis and low bone mass are currently estimated to be a major public health threat for almost 44 million U.S. men and women aged 50 years and older, or 55% of the population in that age range (America's Bone Health: The State of Osteoporosis and Low Bone Mass in Our Nation, 2002). In fact, one in two women and one in four men over the age of 50 years will fracture at some point in their lifetime. The costs to the healthcare system associated with osteoporotic fracture are approximately 17 billion dollars annually (Gabriel et al., 2002; Ray et al., 1997; Tosteson et al., 2001), with each hip fracture having total medical costs of $40,000.

Adequate nutrition plays a major role in the prevention and treatment of osteoporosis; the nutrients of greatest importance are calcium and vitamin D, and this will be discussed in Chapters 8 and 10. In this chapter, we cover various micronutrients including sodium, vitamin C, magnesium, fluoride, boron, silicon, copper, zinc, and the B vitamins.

It is increasingly clear that exposures to a complex of nutrients and food constituents interact to affect bone status. In addition to identifying the role of individual components, a great need exists to understand the interactions of these factors within diets to make effective recommendations for prevention of bone loss and osteoporosis in the aging population (Tucker, 2003).

SODIUM

Sodium may lead to an increase in renal calcium excretion. The mean urinary calcium loss is 1 mmol/100 mmol sodium for males and females at all ages (Teucher and Fairweather-Tait, 2003).

If the amount of calcium consumed and absorbed is less than the amount needed to offset these obligatory urinary calcium losses associated with sodium intake, then bone mass will be negatively impacted. In observational studies, higher salt intakes can lead to higher levels of circulating parathyroid hormone and greater rates of bone resorption in postmenopausal women and men (Harrington and Cashman, 2003; Jones et al., 1997). Furthermore, those with low-calcium and high-salt diets may have lower bone mineral density (BMD), although this is not always the case (Devine et al., 1995; Harrington and Cashman, 2003; Massey and Whiting, 1996; Mizushima et al., 1999).

The effect of dietary sodium on calcium retention and the influence of race were studied in 35 adolescent girls (22 black and 13 white) who participated in two 20-day metabolic summer camps. At the end of the intervention, both race and sodium intake significantly correlated with calcium retention ($p < .01$). The high-sodium diet (3.96 g/day) significantly reduced calcium retention in both whites and blacks ($p < .01$), primarily through a decrease in net calcium absorption. However, black girls excreted significantly less calcium in the urine than did white girls, regardless of diet ($p < .05$) (Wigertz et al., 2005).

The relationship between sodium intake, sodium and calcium excretion, and BMD of the total hip was measured in 50 Caucasian and 39 African American postmenopausal women. Sodium excretion was found to be a significant predictor of calcium excretion in both postmenopausal African American and Caucasian postmenopausal women. The relationship between sodium and calcium excretion is modulated by calcium intake, and the relationship is strongest at low calcium intakes (≤1000 mg/day). However, sodium excretion was not a significant predictor of total hip BMD in elderly African American and Caucasian postmenopausal women (Carbone et al., 2003).

In postmenopausal women who had baseline sodium excretions equal to or greater than the average sodium intake in the United States (≥3.4 g/day), a low-sodium diet (2 g/day) for 6 months resulted in significant decreases in sodium excretion ($p = .01$), in calcium excretion ($p = .01$), and in bone turnover ($p = .04$). However, no significant changes were found in intact PTH ($p = .97$) or 1,25 dihydroxyvitamin D ($p = .49$) with the low-sodium diet. These findings suggest that in postmenopausal women with sodium intakes 3.4 g/day or more, a low sodium diet may have benefits for skeletal health (Carbone et al., 2005). In a study of 1098 men and women over the age of 65 years, sodium intake, reflected by urinary-sodium-to-creatinine ratio (Na/Cr), was the major factor linking blood pressure and osteoporosis, as shown by the inverse relationship with BMD. These findings lend further emphasis to the health benefits of salt reduction in our population both in terms of hypertension and osteoporosis (Woo et al., 2009). Further support of the role of salt in bone health comes from the finding that the Dietary Approaches to Stop Hypertension diet was shown to reduce bone turnover (Lin et al., 2003).

Results of cross-sectional and prospective investigations on high salt intake and long-term bone health are inconclusive. In general, markers of bone resorption do relate to sodium intake, but BMD does not typically relate to sodium intake. Clearly, increased sodium intake will lead to increased renal calcium excretion. This relationship may be modified by protein or potassium intake as well as by genotype or salt sensitivity (Harrington and Cashman, 2003; Harrington et al., 2004a, 2004b). In addition, adequate intake of calcium may allow a more liberal use of sodium in the diet. The anion is also important, with sodium chloride increasing urinary calcium more than other salts such as sodium bicarbonate or sodium acetate (Carbone et al., 2003; Frassetto et al., 2001). In general, sodium intake will not be a problem in the face of adequate calcium intake (Carbone et al., 2003) or potassium intake (Harrington and Cashman, 2003). Furthermore, if American Heart Association guidelines are followed (1500 mg sodium/day), there should be no negative impact of sodium on bone health. However, further study of the impact of sodium consumption on peak bone mass is warranted.

VITAMIN C

Vitamin C is an essential cofactor for collagen formation and synthesis of hydroxyproline and hydroxylysine (see Chapter 13). Vitamin C may also reduce oxidative stress. Rich dietary sources of vitamin C include citrus fruit and juices, peppers, broccoli and tomato products, and green leafy vegetables. The dietary reference intakes for vitamin C are 75 mg/day for adult women and 90 mg/day for adult men.

In an observational study of 533 women, results suggest that antioxidant vitamin E or C supplements may suppress bone resorption in nonsmoking postmenopausal women (Pasco et al., 2006). Other epidemiological studies have shown a positive association between vitamin C and bone mass, although the results are not always significant. In these studies, low intakes of vitamin C are associated with a faster rate of bone loss in women of varying ages, and one study found that higher vitamin C was associated with fewer fractures; however, randomized clinical trials are lacking (Freudenheim et al., 1986; Hall & Greendale, 1998; Hernandez-Avila et al., 1993; Kaptoge et al., 2003; Leveille et al., 1997; Macdonald et al., 2004; New et al., 1997; Odland et al., 1972; Prynne et al., 2006; Sowers et al., 1985; Weber, 1999). After adjustment for important BMD-related covariates, increasing intakes of antioxidants (including vitamin C) were not independently associated with BMD, but a significant interaction between intake of vitamin C and hormone therapy on BMD was found in a cohort from the Women's Health Initiative Observational Study and Clinical Trial (Wolf et al., 2005).

Tucker et al. (2002) evaluated the bone density of 213 men and 393 women, with the average age among them of 75 years, at the start in the Framingham Osteoporosis study, over a 4-year period to determine if any association existed between vitamin C intake and bone health. Using a diet questionnaire given to participants at baseline and again 4 years later, the researchers evaluated the change in bone density in the hip, spine, and arm over the follow-up period. Vitamin C and vitamin E intake were of primary interest, but whether participants smoked or were on hormone replacement therapy was taken into account. Men in the highest vitamin C intake (>300 mg/day; >3 times the recommended intake in men) had less bone loss than that of men in the lowest group of vitamin C intake (106 mg). A similar finding in women was not significant, and it was shown that vitamin C may interact with estrogen use, calcium, and vitamin E (Sahni et al., 2008). Because it is not possible to separate the effects of vitamin C supplements from vitamin C in fruits and vegetables in some studies (Macdonald et al., 2004; Sahni et al., 2008), the recommendation is to obtain the needed amounts of vitamin C only from fruits and vegetables for skeletal health rather than from supplements. In fact, higher fruit and vegetable intakes may have positive effects on bone mineral status in both younger and older age groups so that this recommendation should cover the lifespan (Prynne et al., 2006). Recommended intakes of five or more servings of fruits and vegetables per day should supply enough vitamin C for bone health. Future studies of vitamin C and bone health need to take into account gender, estrogen use, and intake of other nutrients to assess any potential interactions.

MAGNESIUM

Magnesium, when complexed with adenosine-5'-triphosphate, takes part in many intracellular enzyme reactions, including the synthesis of proteins and nucleic acid. Magnesium is an electrolyte mineral that contributes to alkalinity and is important in acid base balance. The current intakes recommended for healthy adult males are 420 mg and those for women are 320 mg/day. Because magnesium is present in most foods, particularly legumes, vegetables, nuts, seeds, fruits, grains, fish, and dairy, severe magnesium deficiency is, therefore, rarely seen in healthy people. However, many intakes in the United States fall below the recommended intake levels, as the mean magnesium intakes for males and females are 323 and 228 mg/day, respectively. Magnesium deficiency can also occur if concomitant disorders exist and/or medications place individuals at further risk for magnesium depletion (Rude and Gruber, 2004; Rude et al., 2004). Magnesium deficiency can be detected with biochemical measurements, that is, low serum magnesium, low serum calcium, and resistance to vitamin D, or via clinical symptoms, that is, muscle twitching, muscle cramps, high blood pressure, and irregular heartbeat. A small metabolic study showed that consuming a diet deficient in magnesium, which resulted in negative magnesium balance, may affect calcium, potassium, and cholesterol metabolism (Nielsen, 2004).

In preadolescent girls, a positive relationship between ultrasound determination of bone mass of the calcaneus and dietary magnesium intake was found (Wang et al., 1999), suggesting that this mineral was important in skeletal growth and development. Magnesium in serum and hair was associated with greater BMD in premenopausal women, and the ratio of serum calcium to magnesium was a significant indicator of BMD (Song et al., 2007). The intake of fruits and vegetables, containing vitamin C, magnesium, and potassium, may protect against premenopausal bone loss, but magnesium alone may not be protective against declines in BMC and BMD (Macdonald et al., 2004). In other studies of premenopausal women, magnesium intake was related to lumbar spine BMD in a cross-sectional evaluation (New et al., 2000), and a significant relationship was found over a 1-year period between dietary magnesium intake and rate of change of BMD of the lumbar spine and total body calcium (Houtkooper et al., 1995). A study of postmenopausal women showed a positive correlation between BMD of the forearm and magnesium intake (Tranquilli et al., 1994). Several small epidemiological studies have found that higher magnesium intakes are associated with higher BMD in elderly men and women, although rates of bone loss over 4 years were only related to magnesium intake in men (Tucker et al., 1999). In 2038 older black and white men and women (aged 70 to 79 years) enrolled in the Health, Aging and Body Composition Study, a greater magnesium intake was significantly related to higher BMD in white women and men, but not in black women and men, which may have been related to differences in dietary assessment (Ryder et al., 2005).

Only a few small controlled clinical trials of magnesium supplementation on bone have been conducted (Nielsen, 1990; Stendig-Lindberg et al., 1993), and they were primarily effective in magnesium-depleted subjects. Overall, observational and clinical trial data concerning magnesium and BMD or fractures are inconclusive, and in fact, one recent study from the Women's Health Initiative surprisingly reported that higher intakes of magnesium were associated with a higher risk of wrist fracture (Durlach et al., 1998; Jackson et al., 2003; Nielsen, 1990; Rude and Olerich, 1996; Stendig-Lindberg et al., 1993; Tucker et al., 1999).

Little evidence has been reported that magnesium is needed to prevent osteoporosis in the general population. Results relating magnesium to BMD are often confounded by coexisting limited intakes of other nutrients that are important for skeletal health. Clearly, a magnesium supplement may be required in frail elderly with poor diets (Durlach et al., 1998) and in persons with intestinal disease, alcoholics, or persons on treatment with diuretics or chemotherapy that depletes magnesium. In addition, as calcium supplements sometimes result in constipation, a supplement with magnesium might be useful in helping to keep bowel habits regular.

FLUORIDE

Fluoride is an essential trace element that is required for skeletal and dental development. The adequate daily adult intake is 4 mg for males and 3 mg for females. The concentration of fluoride in the soil, water, and many foods varies by geographic region. Major dietary sources include drinking water, tea, coffee, rice, soybeans, spinach, onions, and lettuce.

Fluoride interacts with mineralized tissues in a number of ways. At low doses, the fluoride may be passively incorporated into the mineral, stabilizing mineral surfaces against dissolution. At higher doses, such as those used previously for treatment of osteoporosis, the fluoride may alter the amount and structure of tissue present, including altering the interface between the collagen and mineral and causing a painful condition associated with extraosseous calcification and brittle bones. At very high doses, skeletal fluorosis may occur, characterized by debilitating changes in the skeleton; this can even occur in communities where the local drinking water has naturally high fluoride levels, much greater than 1 ppm in fluoridated waters (Chachra et al., 2008). High doses of fluoride can stimulate osteoblasts; however, the quality of bone that is formed may be abnormal and the effect on fracture rates is unclear (Riggs, 1993).

The impact of more typical intakes of fluoride on the skeleton was evaluated in the Iowa Fluoride Study/Iowa Bone Development Study. Longitudinal fluoride intake at levels of intake typical in the United States (mean 0.68 mg per day) is only weakly associated with BMC or BMD in boys and girls at age 11 years. Additional research is warranted to better understand possible gender- and age-specific effects of fluoride intake on bone development (Levy et al., 2009).

No benefit of adding fluoride supplements to an adult diet exists for skeletal health. The lower doses of fluoride typically found in drinking water have no effect on bone density or on reducing fractures (Cauley et al., 1995; Kurttio et al., 1999; Suarez-Almazor et al., 1993).

B VITAMINS

The role of B vitamins in skeletal health has been the subject of many recent research studies. Elevated serum homocysteine levels may be caused by deficiencies of folate (folic acid), vitamin B_{12}, or vitamin B_6. Homocysteine has recently been linked to fragility fractures, including hip fractures in older men and women (Gjesdal et al., 2006; van Meurs et al., 2004). Incident osteoporosis-related fractures were assessed in 702 Italian participants aged 65–94 years, with a mean follow-up of 4 years, and it was found that low serum folate was responsible for the association between homocysteine and risk of osteoporosis-related fractures in elderly persons (Ravaglia et al., 2005).

In two recent studies, poor vitamin B_{12} status was associated with low BMD in men and women and osteoporosis in elderly women but not men (Dhonukshe-Rutten et al., 2003; Tucker et al., 2005). It is unclear whether associations such as this are only a result of B_{12} deficiency or an indication of overall poor nutrition and frailty. Based on data collected on older men and women, that is, aged >55 years, who underwent dual-energy x-ray absorptiometry (DXA) scans of the hip as participants in phase 2 of the third U.S. National Health and Nutrition Examination Survey (n = 1550), the prevalence of osteoporosis in those with serum B_{12} in the lowest quartile was two times greater than that in individuals with serum B_{12} in the highest quartile (Morris et al., 2005). Homocysteine and vitamin B_{12} status indicators were negatively associated with BMD in older Americans (Stone et al., 2004). Whether this association reflects a causal relation remains unclear.

In 1002 men and women (mean age 75 years) in the Framingham Osteoporosis study, low serum B vitamin concentrations were noted to be a risk factor for decreased bone health, although these low concentrations did not fully explain the relationship between elevated homocysteine and hip fracture (McLean et al., 2008). In fact, controlled trials are clearly needed to determine whether treatment with B vitamins would reduce fracture rates among community-dwelling cohorts (McLean and Hannan, 2007). The Hordaland Homocysteine Study is a population-based study of more than 18,000 men and women in Western Norway, and among women in this study, raised homocysteine levels were associated with decreased BMD and increased risk of osteoporosis (Refsum et al., 2006). Low folate concentrations were related to more than a two-fold elevation in hip fracture risk versus higher folate concentrations (McLean et al., 2008).

In some studies, folate is more strongly related to BMD than any other B vitamin (Baines et al., 2007; Cagnacci et al., 2003, 2008; Rejnmark et al., 2008). However, in a 2-month study of folic acid supplementation in 61 healthy individuals, short-term folic acid supplementation did not affect biochemical bone markers in subjects without osteoporosis but who had a low folate status (Herrmann et al., 2006), and combined administration of folic acid, B_6, and B_{12} over 1 year had no effect on bone turnover (Herrmann et al., 2007). However, in older Japanese, folic acid and [me]cobalamin reduced hip fracture as compared with placebo (Sato et al., 2005). In the Rotterdam study, those with the highest quartile of B_6 intake had a lower risk of fracture than that of individuals with low B_6 intakes (Yazdanpanah et al., 2007). Clearly, a need exists for long-term clinical trial data to determine the role of each B vitamin in skeletal health.

OTHER NUTRIENTS

BORON

Boron is not an essential nutrient, so no recommended intakes have been published. Boron is present in several foods, such as fruits, vegetable, nuts, eggs, wine, and dried foods (Nielsen, 2008). A significant number of people, however, do not consistently consume more than 1 mg a day of boron (Nielsen, 1998), and whether such a low intake is of clinical concern is unknown. A small study noted that urinary boron excretion changes rapidly with changes in boron intake, indicating that the kidney is the site of homeostatic regulation (Sutherland et al., 1998). Although a few studies have found that 3 mg daily of boron may have a positive effect on bone (Nielsen, 1990; Nielsen et al., 1987), controlled trials are lacking.

COPPER

Copper is an essential element required by many enzymes including lysyl oxidase, which is required for cross-linking of collagen. Severe deficiency does have profound effects on bone (see also Chapter 13). A small study of 25 females with low bone mass found a correlation between the plasma copper concentrations and BMD of the lumbar spine as measured using DXA and quantitative computerized tomography (Chaudhri et al., 2009). Clearly, further study is needed regarding the role of copper in bone health.

ZINC

A few intervention trials using zinc supplements have generated variable results on bone turnover and BMD (Gur et al., 2002; Strause et al., 1994); in one study, a mixture of trace elements on bone was investigated (Strause et al., 1994). Profound zinc deficiency leads to reduced bone growth and maturation, but little evidence has been reported showing that dietary zinc levels have an effect on bone mass or fractures related to osteoporosis. In a metabolic study of 21 women, low dietary zinc (3 mg/day) resulted in undesirable changes in circulating calcitonin and osteocalcin. However, a high intake of zinc may be a health concern for individuals consuming less than the recommended amounts of magnesium because of a zinc–magnesium interaction (Nielsen and Milne, 2004).

SILICON

Cereals provide the greatest amount of silicon in the U.S. diet (about 30%), followed by fruit, beverages (hot, cold, and alcoholic beverages combined), and vegetables; together, these foods provided over 75% of the silicon intake. Silicon intakes may be suboptimal (McNaughton et al., 2005); a reported decrease of silicon concentrations occurs with age, especially in women (Bisse et al., 2005). Dietary silicon may be beneficial to bone and connective tissue health on the basis of recently reported strong positive associations between dietary silicon intake and BMD in U.S. and U.K. cohorts (Jugdaohsingh, 2007). The biological role of silicon in bone health remains unclear, although a number of possible mechanisms, including effects on the synthesis of collagen and/or its stabilization and on matrix mineralization, have been suggested.

In a cross-sectional study of a sample of 2847 participants in the Framingham Offspring cohort (aged 30–87 years), dietary silicon correlated positively and significantly with BMD at all hip sites in men and premenopausal women, but not in postmenopausal women (Jugdaohsingh et al., 2004). Silicon appears to mediate the positive association between beer and BMD, but not of wine or liquor, in the Framingham Offspring cohort (aged 29–86 years) (Tucker et al., 2009). Results associating silicon to skeletal health require further follow-up.

COMBINATIONS OF TRACE MINERALS

Subclinical zinc and/or copper deficiency, resulting from a reduced dietary intake of micronutrients and reduced absorption (Thomson and Keelan, 1986), may result in bone loss. Both zinc and copper are essential cofactors for enzymes involved in the synthesis of various bone matrix constituents. Calcium supplementation may accentuate the problem of reduced serum zinc and copper levels by impairing the absorption and retention of these nutrients (Snedeker et al., 1982). The relationships among BMD and zinc, copper, and calcium in the meal and hair of 470 urban and rural elderly people were studied, and the amount of zinc, copper, and calcium in the meal was positively correlated with BMD (Li et al., 2005).

Although significant correlations were found between serum elements, such as calcium, sodium, potassium, magnesium, zinc, iron, copper, and selenium, no significant differences in the concentrations of these elements were found in 290 women assigned to groups with osteoporosis, low bone mass, or normal bone mass (Liu et al., 2009). Two studies have shown that a combination of several minerals (zinc, manganese, and copper) with calcium was able to reduce spinal bone loss in postmenopausal women (Gur et al., 2002; Strause et al., 1994). These data indicate that individual or combinations of trace elements do not have a clear impact on skeletal health; hence, the effects of trace minerals on bone remain unknown. Therefore, the best advice is for individuals to consume a varied diet with adequate intakes of fruits, vegetables, cereals, and proteins to obtain enough of all the trace elements.

CONCLUSIONS

The known benefits of calcium and vitamin D on bone cannot be considered in isolation from the other components of the diet, especially vitamins and the trace minerals. However, the needs of the other micronutrients for optimizing bone health can be easily met by a healthy varied diet that is high in fruits, vegetables, legumes, cereals, and adequate amounts of animal protein. In elderly individuals, greater attention should be placed on B vitamin status and homocysteine levels.

REFERENCES

National Osteoporosis Foundation, *America's Bone Health: The State of Osteoporosis and Low Bone Mass in Our Nation.* Report of the National Osteoporosis Foundation, Washington, DC, 2002.

Baines, M., Kredan, M.B., Davison, A., et al. 2007. The association between cysteine, bone turnover, and low bone mass. *Calcif Tissue Int* 81: 450–454.

Bisse, E., Epting, T., Beil, A., et al. 2005. Reference values for serum silicon in adults. *Anal Biochem* 337: 130–135.

Cagnacci, A., Bagni, B., Zini, A., et al. 2008. Relation of folate, vitamin B12 and homocysteine to vertebral bone mineral density change in postmenopausal women. A five-year longitudinal evaluation. *Bone* 42: 314–320.

Cagnacci, A., Baldassari, F., Rivolta, G., et al. 2003. Relation of homocysteine, folate, and vitamin B12 to bone mineral density of postmenopausal women. *Bone* 33: 956–959.

Carbone, L.D., Barrow, K.D., Bush, A.J., et al. 2005. Effects of a low sodium diet on bone metabolism. *J Bone Miner Metab* 23: 506–513.

Carbone, L.D., Bush, A.J., Barrow, K.D., et al. 2003. The relationship of sodium intake to calcium and sodium excretion and bone mineral density of the hip in postmenopausal African-American and Caucasian women. *J Bone Miner Metab* 21: 415–420.

Cauley, J.A., Murphy, P.A., Riley, T.J., et al. 1995. Effects of fluoridated drinking water on bone mass and fractures: The study of osteoporotic fractures. *J Bone Miner Res* 10: 1076–1086.

Chachra, D., Vieira, A.P., and Grynpas, M.D. 2008. Fluoride and mineralized tissues. *Crit Rev Biomed Eng* 36: 183–233.

Chaudhri, M.A., Kemmler, W., Harsch, I., et al. 2009. Plasma copper and bone mineral density in osteopenia: An indicator of bone mineral density in osteopenic females. *Biol Trace Elem Res* 129: 94–98.

Devine, A., Criddle, R.A., Dick, I.M., et al. 1995. A longitudinal study of the effect of sodium and calcium intakes on regional bone density in postmenopausal women. *Am J Clin Nutr* 62: 740–745.

Dhonukshe-Rutten, R.A., Lips, M., de Jong, N., et al. 2003. Vitamin B-12 status is associated with bone mineral content and bone mineral density in frail elderly women but not in men. *J Nutr* 133: 801–807.

Durlach, J., Bac, P., Durlach, V., et al. 1998. Magnesium status and ageing: An update. *Magnes Res* 11: 25–42.

Frassetto, L., Morris, R.C., Jr., Sellmeyer, D.E., et al. 2001 Diet, evolution and aging—The pathophysiologic effects of the post-agricultural inversion of the potassium-to-sodium and base-to-chloride ratios in the human diet. *Eur J Nutr* 40: 200–213.

Freudenheim, J.L., Johnson, N.E., and Smith, E.L. 1986. Relationships between usual nutrient intake and bone-mineral content of women 35–65 years of age: Longitudinal and cross-sectional analysis. *Am J Clin Nutr* 44: 863–876.

Gabriel, S.E., Tosteson, A.N., Leibson, C.L., et al. 2002. Direct medical costs attributable to osteoporotic fractures. *Osteoporos Int* 13: 323–330.

Gjesdal, C.G., Vollset, S.E., Ueland, P.M., et al. 2006. Plasma total homocysteine level and bone mineral density: The Hordaland Homocysteine Study. *Arch Intern Med* 166: 88–94.

Gur, A., Colpan, L., Nas, K., et al. 2002. The role of trace minerals in the pathogenesis of postmenopausal osteoporosis and a new effect of calcitonin. *J Bone Miner Metab* 20: 39–43.

Hall, S.L., and Greendale, G.A. 1998. The relation of dietary vitamin C intake to bone mineral density: Results from the PEPI study. *Calcif Tissue Int* 63: 183–189.

Harrington, M., Bennett, T., Jakobsen, J., et al. 2004a. Effect of a high-protein, high-salt diet on calcium and bone metabolism in postmenopausal women stratified by hormone replacement therapy use. *Eur J Clin Nutr* 58: 1436–1439.

Harrington, M., Bennett, T., Jakobsen, J., et al. 2004b. The effect of a high-protein, high-sodium diet on calcium and bone metabolism in postmenopausal women and its interaction with vitamin D receptor genotype. *Br J Nutr* 91: 41–51.

Harrington, M., and Cashman, K.D. 2003. High salt intake appears to increase bone resorption in postmenopausal women but high potassium intake ameliorates this adverse effect. *Nutr Rev* 61: 179–183.

Hernandez-Avila, M., Stampfer, M.J., Ravnikar, V.A., et al. 1993. Caffeine and other predictors of bone density among pre- and perimenopausal women. *Epidemiology* 4: 128–134.

Herrmann, M., Stanger, O., Paulweber, B., et al. 2006. Folate supplementation does not affect biochemical markers of bone turnover. *Clin Lab* 52: 131–136.

Herrmann, M., Umanskaya, N., Traber, L., et al. 2007. The effect of B-vitamins on biochemical bone turnover markers and bone mineral density in osteoporotic patients: A 1-year double blind placebo controlled trial. *Clin Chem Lab Med* 45: 1785–1792.

Houtkooper, L.B., Ritenbaugh, C., Aickin, M., et al. 1995. Nutrients, body composition and exercise are related to change in bone mineral density in premenopausal women. *J Nutr* 125: 1229–1237.

Jackson, R., Bassford, T., Cauley, J., et al. 2003. The impact of magnesium intake on fractures: Results from the Women's Health Initiative Observational Study (WHI-OS). Abstract presented at Annual Meeting of American Society for Bon and Mineral Research.

Jones, G., Beard, T., Parameswaran, V., et al. 1997. A population-based study of the relationship between salt intake, bone resorption and bone mass. *Eur J Clin Nutr* 51: 561–565.

Jugdaohsingh, R. 2007. Silicon and bone health. *J Nutr Health Aging* 11: 99–110.

Jugdaohsingh, R., Tucker, K.L., Qiao, N., et al. 2004. Dietary silicon intake is positively associated with bone mineral density in men and premenopausal women of the Framingham Offspring cohort. *J Bone Miner Res* 19: 297–307.

Kaptoge, S., Welch, A., McTaggart, A., et al. 2003. Effects of dietary nutrients and food groups on bone loss from the proximal femur in men and women in the 7th and 8th decades of age. *Osteoporos Int* 14: 418–428.

Kurttio P., Gustavsson N., Vartiainen T., et al. 1999. Exposure to natural fluoride in well water and hip fracture: A cohort analysis in Finland. *Am J Epidemiol* 150: 817–824.

Leveille, S.G., LaCroix, A.Z., Koepsell, T.D., et al. 1997. Dietary vitamin C and bone mineral density in postmenopausal women in Washington State, USA. *J Epidemiol Community Health* 51: 479–485.

Levy, S.M., Eichenberger-Gilmore, J., Warren, J.J., et al. 2009. Associations of fluoride intake with children's bone measures at age 11. *Community Dent Oral Epidemiol* 37: 416–426.

Li, W., Tian, Y., Song, X., et al. 2005. Relationship between BMD and Zn, Cu, Ca levels in the hair and meal in elderly people. *J Huazhong Univ Sci Technolog Med Sci* 25: 97–99.

Lin, P.H., Ginty, F., Appel, L.J., et al. 2003. The DASH diet and sodium reduction improve markers of bone turnover and calcium metabolism in adults. *J Nutr* 133: 3130–3136.

Liu, S.Z., Yan, H., Xu, P., et al. 2009. Correlation analysis between bone mineral density and serum element contents of postmenopausal women in Xi'an urban area. *Biol Trace Elem Res* 131: 205–214.

Massey, L.K., and Whiting, S.J. 1996. Dietary salt, urinary calcium, and bone loss. *J Bone Miner Res* 11: 731–736.

McLean, R.R., and Hannan, M.T. 2007. B vitamins, homocysteine, and bone disease: Epidemiology and pathophysiology. *Curr Osteoporos Rep* 5: 112–119.

McLean, R.R., Jacques, P.F., Selhub, J., et al. 2008. Plasma B vitamins, homocysteine, and their relation with bone loss and hip fracture in elderly men and women. *J Clin Endocrinol Metab* 93: 2206–2212.

McNaughton, S.A., Bolton-Smith, C., Mishra, G.D., et al. 2005. Dietary silicon intake in post-menopausal women. *Br J Nutr* 94: 813–817.

Mizushima, S., Tsuchida, K., and Yamori, Y. 1999. Preventive nutritional factors in epidemiology: Interaction between sodium and calcium. *Clin Exp Pharmacol Physiol* 26: 573–575.

Morris, M.S., Jacques, P.F., and Selhub, J. 2005. Relation between homocysteine and B-vitamin status indicators and bone mineral density in older Americans. *Bone* 37: 234–242.

New, S.A., Bolton-Smith, C., Grubb D.A., et al. 1997. Nutritional influences on bone mineral density: A cross-sectional study in premenopausal women. *Am J Clin Nutr* 65: 1831–1839.

New, S.A., Robins, S.P., Campbell, M.K., et al. 2000. Dietary influences on bone mass and bone metabolism: Further evidence of a positive link between fruit and vegetable consumption and bone health? *Am J Clin Nutr* 71: 142–151.

Nielsen, F.H. 1990. Studies on the relationship between boron and magnesium which possibly affects the formation and maintenance of bones. *Magnes Trace Elem* 9: 61–69.

Nielsen, F.H. 1998. The justification for providing dietary guidance for the nutritional intake of boron. *Biol Trace Elem Res* 66: 319–330.

Nielsen, F.H. 2004. The alteration of magnesium, calcium and phosphorus metabolism by dietary magnesium deprivation in postmenopausal women is not affected by dietary boron deprivation. *Magnes Res* 17: 197–210.

Nielsen, F.H. 2008. Is boron nutritionally relevant? *Nutr Rev* 66: 183–191.

Nielsen, F.H., Hunt, C.D., Mullen, L.M., et al. 1987. Effect of dietary boron on mineral, estrogen, and testosterone metabolism in postmenopausal women. *Faseb J* 1: 394–397.

Nielsen, F.H., and Milne, D.B. 2004. A moderately high intake compared to a low intake of zinc depresses magnesium balance and alters indices of bone turnover in postmenopausal women. *Eur J Clin Nutr* 58: 703–710.

Odland, L.M., Mason, R.L., and Alexeff, A.I. 1972. Bone density and dietary findings of 409 Tennessee subjects. 1. Bone density considerations. *Am J Clin Nutr* 25: 905–907.

Pasco, J.A., Henry, M.J., Wilkinson, L.K., et al. 2006. Antioxidant vitamin supplements and markers of bone turnover in a community sample of nonsmoking women. *J Womens Health (Larchmt)* 15: 295–300.

Prynne, C.J., Mishra, G.D., O'Connell, M.A., et al. 2006. Fruit and vegetable intakes and bone mineral status: A cross sectional study in 5 age and sex cohorts. *Am J Clin Nutr* 83: 1420–1428.

Ravaglia, G., Forti, P., Maioli, F., et al. 2005. Folate, but not homocysteine, predicts the risk of fracture in elderly persons. *J Gerontol A Biol Sci Med Sci* 60: 1458–1462.

Ray, N.F., Chan, J.K., Thamer, M., et al. 1997. Medical expenditures for the treatment of osteoporotic fractures in the United States in 1995: Report from the National Osteoporosis Foundation. *J Bone Miner Res* 12: 24–35.

Refsum, H., Nurk, E., Smith, A.D., et al. 2006. The Hordaland Homocysteine Study: A community-based study of homocysteine, its determinants, and associations with disease. *J Nutr* 136: 1731S–1740S.

Rejnmark, L., Vestergaard, P., Hermann, A.P., et al. 2008. Dietary intake of folate, but not vitamin B2 or B12, is associated with increased bone mineral density 5 years after the menopause: Results from a 10-year follow-up study in early postmenopausal women. *Calcif Tissue Int* 82: 1–11.

Riggs, B.L. 1993. Formation-stimulating regimens other than sodium fluoride. *Am J Med* 95: 62S–68S.

Rude, R.K., and Gruber, H.E. 2004. Magnesium deficiency and osteoporosis: Animal and human observations. *J Nutr Biochem* 15: 710–716.

Rude, R.K., Gruber, H.E., Norton, H.J., et al. 2004. Bone loss induced by dietary magnesium reduction to 10% of the nutrient requirement in rats is associated with increased release of substance P and tumor necrosis factor-alpha. *J Nutr* 134: 79–85.

Rude, R.K., and Olerich, M. 1996. Magnesium deficiency: Possible role in osteoporosis associated with gluten-sensitive enteropathy. *Osteoporos Int* 6: 453–461.

Ryder, K.M., Shorr, R.I., Bush, A.J., et al. 2005. Magnesium intake from food and supplements is associated with bone mineral density in healthy older white subjects. *J Am Geriatr Soc* 53: 1875–1880.

Sahni, S., Hannan, M.T., Gagnon, D., et al. 2008. High vitamin C intake is associated with lower 4-year bone loss in elderly men. *J Nutr* 138: 1931–1938.

Sato, Y., Honda, Y., Iwamoto, J., et al. 2005. Effect of folate and mecobalamin on hip fractures in patients with stroke: A randomized controlled trial. *JAMA* 293: 1082–1088.

Snedeker, S.M., Smith, S.A., and Greger, J.L. 1982. Effect of dietary calcium and phosphorus levels on the utilization of iron, copper, and zinc by adult males. *J Nutr* 112:136–143.

Song, C.H., Barrett-Connor, E., Chung, J.H., et al. 2007. Associations of calcium and magnesium in serum and hair with bone mineral density in premenopausal women. *Biol Trace Elem Res* 118: 1–9.

Sowers, M.R., Wallace, R.B., and Lemke, J.H. 1985. Correlates of mid-radius bone density among postmenopausal women: A community study. *Am J Clin Nutr* 41: 1045–1053.

Stendig-Lindberg, G., Tepper, R., and Leichter, I. 1993. Trabecular bone density in a two year controlled trial of peroral magnesium in osteoporosis. *Magnes Res* 6: 155–163.

Stone, K.L., Bauer, D.C., Sellmeyer, D., et al. 2004. Low serum vitamin B-12 levels are associated with increased hip bone loss in older women: A prospective study. *J Clin Endocrinol Metab* 89: 1217–1221.

Strause, L., Saltman, P., Smith, K.T., et al. 1994. Spinal bone loss in postmenopausal women supplemented with calcium and trace minerals. *J Nutr* 124: 1060–1064.

Suarez-Almazor, M.E., Flowerdew, G., Saunders, L.D., et al. 1993. The fluoridation of drinking water and hip fracture hospitalization rates in two Canadian communities. *Am J Public Health* 83: 689–693.

Sutherland, B., Strong, P., and King, J.C. 1998. Determining human dietary requirements for boron. *Biol Trace Elem Res* 66: 193–204.

Teucher, B., and Fairweather-Tait, S. 2003. Dietary sodium as a risk factor for osteoporosis: Where is the evidence? *Proc Nutr Soc* 62: 859–866.

Thomson, A.B., and Keelan, M. 1986. The aging gut. *Can J Physiol Pharmacol* 64: 30–38.

Tosteson, A.N., Gabriel, S.E., Grove, M.R., et al. 2001. Impact of hip and vertebral fractures on quality-adjusted life years. *Osteoporos Int* 12: 1042–1049.

Tranquilli, A.L., Lucino, E., Garzetti, G.G., et al. 1994. Calcium, phosphorus and magnesium intakes correlate with bone mineral content in postmenopausal women. *Gynecol Endocrinol* 8: 55–58.

Tucker, K.L. 2003. Dietary intake and bone status with aging. *Curr Pharm Des* 9: 2687–2704.

Tucker, K.L., Chen, H., Hannan, M.T., et al. 2002. Bone mineral density and dietary patterns in older adults: The Framingham Osteoporosis Study. *Am J Clin Nutr* 76: 245–252.

Tucker, K.L., Hannan, M.T., Chen, H., et al. 1999. Potassium, magnesium, and fruit and vegetable intakes are associated with greater bone mineral density in elderly men and women. *Am J Clin Nutr* 69: 727–736.

Tucker, K.L., Hannan, M.T., Qiao, N., et al. 2005. Low plasma vitamin B12 is associated with lower BMD: The Framingham Osteoporosis Study. *J Bone Miner Res* 20: 152–158.

Tucker, K.L., Jugdaohsingh, R., Powell, J.J., et al. 2009. Effects of beer, wine, and liquor intakes on bone mineral density in older men and women. *Am J Clin Nutr* 89: 1188–1196.

van Meurs, J.B., Dhonukshe-Rutten, R.A., Pluijm, S.M., et al. 2004. Homocysteine levels and the risk of osteoporotic fracture. *New Engl J Med* 350: 2033–2041.

Wang, M.C., Moore, E.C., Crawford, P.B., et al. 1999. Influence of pre-adolescent diet on quantitative ultrasound measurements of the calcaneus in young adult women. *Osteoporos Int* 9: 532–535.

Weber, P. 1999. The role of vitamins in the prevention of osteoporosis—A brief status report. *Int J Vitam Nutr Res* 69: 194–197.

Wigertz, K., Palacios, C., Jackman, L.A., et al. 2005. Racial differences in calcium retention in response to dietary salt in adolescent girls. *Am J Clin Nutr* 81: 845–850.

Wolf, R.L., Cauley, J.A., Pettinger, M., et al. 2005. Lack of a relation between vitamin and mineral antioxidants and bone mineral density: Results from the Women's Health Initiative. *Am J Clin Nutr* 82: 581–588.

Woo, J., Kwok, T., Leung, J., et al. 2009. Dietary intake, blood pressure and osteoporosis. *J Hum Hypertens* 23: 451–455.

Yazdanpanah, N., Zillikens, M.C., Rivadeneira, F., et al. 2007. Effect of dietary B vitamins on BMD and risk of fracture in elderly men and women: The Rotterdam study. *Bone* 41: 987–994.

15 Dietary Protein's Impact on Skeletal Health

Anna K. Surdykowski, Anne M. Kenney,
Karl L. Insogna, and Jane E. Kerstetter

CONTENTS

INTRODUCTION

Both dietary calcium and vitamin D are undoubtedly beneficial to skeletal health. In contrast, despite intense investigation, the impact of dietary protein on calcium metabolism and bone balance remains controversial. Further complicating this debate is the potential difference that animal and vegetable protein sources may have on skeletal health. One previously held view is that diets high in protein were considered to be detrimental to bone, because the inorganic acids generated from the metabolism of amino acids increase urinary calcium excretion. According to this hypothesis, continued loss of calcium in the urine eventually results in negative calcium balance and loss of calcium from skeletal stores, including osteopenia if systemic acidosis is chronic. An alternative hypothesis is that a higher intake of protein increases circulating levels of insulin-like growth factor-1 (IGF-1), increases intestinal calcium absorption and improves muscle strength and mass, all of which may potentially benefit skeletal health.

This review provides the scientific evidence supporting the latter hypothesis that dietary protein works synergistically to support both calcium retention and bone metabolism.

PROTEIN REQUIREMENTS AND INTAKES

The Food and Nutrition Board, Institute of Medicine, the National Academies and Health Canada set dietary reference intakes (DRIs) for all of the macronutrients and micronutrients in our diet (Institute of Medicine, Standing Committee on the Scientific Evaluation of Dietary Reference Intakes, Food and Nutrition Board, 2002). The recommended dietary allowance (RDA) is defined as the intake that is sufficient to meet the needs of nearly all of the population (97.5%) and is perhaps the most commonly used reference value for protein. The RDA for protein in individuals aged 14 years and higher is 0.8 g/kg body weight. The acceptable macronutrient distribution range (AMDR) is defined as "a range of intakes that is associated with reduced risk of chronic diseases

223

TABLE 15.1

Dietary Protein Intake (g/kg) in the United States from the NHANES 2003–2004 Database (Usual Intakes from Food Compared to Estimated Average Requirement [EAR])[a]

	Mean ± SD	Percentiles							EAR	Percentage less than EAR
		5	10	25	50	75	90	95		
Males										
19–30 (n = 470)	1.5 ± 0.4	0.9	1.0	1.2	1.4	1.7	2.0	2.2	0.7	<3
31–50 (n = 624)	1.4 ± 0.3	0.9	1.0	1.2	1.4	1.6	1.8	1.9	0.7	<3
51–70 (n = 555)	1.2 ± 0.3	0.8	0.8	1.0	1.1	1.3	1.5	1.7	1.7	<3
71 + (n = 391)	1.0 ± 0.3	0.7	0.7	0.9	1.0	1.2	1.4	1.5	0.7	<3
Females										
19–30 (n = 393)	1.2 ± 0.3	0.7	0.8	1.0	1.2	1.4	1.6	1.8	0.7	<3
31–50 (n = 612)	1.1 ± 0.3	0.7	0.8	0.9	1.1	1.3	1.5	1.6	0.7	4.0
51–70 (n = 606)	1.1 ± 0.3	0.6	0.7	0.9	1.0	1.2	1.5	1.6	0.7	7.2
71 + (n = 406)	1.0 ± 0.3	0.6	0.7	0.8	0.9	1.1	1.3	1.4	0.7	8.6

[a] Data from individuals with two days of reliable intake from NHANES 2003–2004. Body weights adjusted to nearest ideal body weight for children and adults. Results generated using SIDE program.

Source: Adapted from Fulgoni, V.L., 3rd, *Am J Clin Nutr*, 87, 1554S–1557S, 2008.

while providing adequate intakes of essential nutrients." The protein AMDR for adults is 10%–35% of total caloric intake.

Although Americans are typically considered to consume a high-protein diet, the 2003–2004 National Health and Nutrition Examination Survey (NHANES) dietary data do not support this notion for everyone. Fulgoni (2008) analyzed the latest NHANES data to characterize mean protein intakes according to age and sex categories (Table 15.1). These data show a trend toward decreased protein intake with age. Men, on average, consume more protein than women at all stages of life. Whereas 10% of women between the ages of 19 and 50 years had a protein intake at or below the RDA, 25% of the women over the age of 70 years were eating 0.8 or fewer g/kg (body weight) of protein each day. Overall, 10% of the entire population over 70 years did not meet the RDA for protein. In addition, 50% of adults aged 71 years and older consumed less than 1 g/kg protein, an amount slightly above the RDA (Fulgoni, 2008). Therefore, not all adults consume a high-protein diet, and individuals that consume the lowest protein diets, that is, the elderly, are at the highest risk of bone loss.

PROTEIN-INDUCED METABOLIC ACIDOSIS AND BONE LOSS

An increase in dietary protein results in greater calcium excretion in the urine (Kerstetter and Allen, 1994). The source of this urinary calcium is not completely clear. Early research, up to the mid-1970s, suggested that intestinal calcium absorption was modulated by dietary protein (Wapnir, 1990). However, subsequent calcium balance studies failed to duplicate the original findings. Because the skeleton contains approximately 99% of the body's calcium, the increased losses of urinary calcium (in excess of absorption) would support the notion that the skeleton was the most likely source of the extra urinary calcium.

Therefore, the traditional hypothesis held that a high intake of protein, particularly from animal sources, generates a high fixed metabolic acid load, because the animal proteins contain higher amounts of sulfur- and phosphorus-containing amino acids. Dietary protein is the major contributor to endogenous acid production; the U.S. diet can generate 100 mEq of acid daily, primarily phosphate and sulfate anions (Barzel and Massey, 1998). Should the kidneys and lungs be unable to completely handle this diet-induced acid load, a source of additional buffer would be necessary via osteoclast-activated bone resorption. The large bicarbonate reservoir of the skeleton would provide this buffer, and calcium would consequently be released with the carbonate (Kerstetter et al., 2003). This hypothesis is supported by both cellular and animal studies (Arnett, 2003). Several human intervention trials demonstrate that the addition of a base, such as bicarbonate or citrate, suppresses bone resorption (Sebastian et al., 1994; Jehle et al., 2006), further supporting the hypothesis.

The central question becomes, does this endogenous acid production from a high-protein diet have a sufficient magnitude to adversely impact bone? In the healthy individual, the lungs work to regulate pH by immediately expiring carbon dioxide, a metabolic by-product, while the kidney helps with buffering by excreting excess hydrogen ions primarily as ammonium ions and secondarily as phosphates, the so-called titratable acidity. The tandem actions of the kidneys and lungs very tightly and effectively regulate the pH of arterial blood. This tightly regulated homeostatic mechanism defends normal blood pH at 7.40 (constant) within a narrow pH range of 7.38 to 7.42, even in the face of variable day-to-day acid loads from dietary sources (Bonjour, 2005). Because food proteins are typically consumed throughout the daytime hours, acid generation occurs during the postprandial periods, thus providing ample time for neutralization during the fasting periods. The mechanism by which acidosis induces bone loss is through activation of osteoclasts via a slight decline in extracellular pH. However, the pH of extracellular fluid bathing cells deviates little from 7.40, and the initial activation of osteoclastic resorption requires a decline in the systemic pH of only approximately 0.2 units (Arnett, 2003). Small pH changes between 7.25 and 7.15 showed the greatest changes in osteoclast-mediated bone resorption (Arnett, 2003).

It is not known if the extracellular pH in bone tissue is within this range or whether it changes following an animal-protein–containing meal. Given that the induced acid load from food is distributed over the course of a day, and in view of the robust buffering capacity of the renal and respiratory systems, it seems unlikely that increasing dietary (animal) protein would lead in healthy patients to osteoclast-dependent bone resorption, a conclusion also reached by Bonjour (2005).

A recent meta-analysis by Fenton et al. (2009) evaluated the relationship between the acid-generating capacity of the diet and urinary calcium, calcium balance, and markers of bone resorption. Five studies were selected based on preset methodological criteria. Although a significant positive relationship between net acid excretion (NAE) and urinary calcium did exist, NAE was not associated with calcium balance or markers of bone resorption. The findings of this meta-analysis suggest that the increased acid-generating capacity of a high-protein diet may lead to increased urinary calcium loss, but this loss does not necessarily translate to negative calcium balance or bone loss.

EPIDEMIOLOGICAL STUDIES

Epidemiological data largely support a positive association between protein intake and bone health. A few studies conducted in premenopausal adult women and adolescents have found a positive linkage between high dietary protein and bone (Beasley et al., 2010; Zhang et al., 2010). The vast majority of studies, however, have examined older adults. For example, Hannan et al. (2000) evaluated the relationship between baseline protein intake and 4-year change in bone mineral density (BMD) in 615 subjects with a mean age of 75 years. When percent protein intake was divided into quartiles, the group with the lowest protein intake (ranging from 0.21 to 0.71 g protein/kg) demonstrated the greatest loss in BMD. The highest quartile consumed 1.24 to 2.78 g/kg protein and demonstrated the least loss in BMD over the 4-year period (Hannan et al., 2000).

Promislow et al. (2002) investigated the association between protein intake and BMD in a community-dwelling cohort of 572 women and 388 men aged 55–92 years living in Rancho Bernardo, California. For each increment of 15 g of animal protein daily, small but significant increases were found in women only over a 4-year period in BMD at the hip, femoral neck, spine, and total body. Interestingly, this association did not hold for consumers of vegetable protein nor was it observed in men. Nonetheless, the authors concluded that animal protein improved the skeletal health of elderly women!

In a 5-year cohort study of 862 elderly women, food frequency questionnaires and dual-energy x-ray absorptiometry scans were used to examine the relationship between dietary protein at baseline and body composition 5 years later (Meng et al., 2009). After 5 years, there was greater bone mineral content (BMC) in those consuming the highest amount of protein (>87g/day) than in those consuming a moderate-protein (66–87g/day) or low-protein (<66g/day) diet. Whole-body BMC and appendicular BMC were 5.3% and 6.0% greater in the highest versus lowest tertile of protein intake, respectively. Subjects consuming the highest amount of protein also had significantly higher whole body lean muscle mass than that of subjects consuming the moderate or low levels of protein. These data support the hypothesis that protein intake positively impacts bone and muscle while also suggesting that the greater BMC may be due in part to an interaction between muscle and bone (Meng et al., 2009).

A systematic review and meta-analysis of protein intake and bone health were recently reported by Darling et al. (2009). These investigators initially collected over 2000 potential studies, of which 61 met the inclusion criteria for the systematic review in that they measured both dietary protein and bone parameters (BMD or BMC, bone turnover, or fracture) in healthy adults. Overall, the authors could find little support for a negative relationship between dietary protein and bone. In fact, from the cross-sectional surveys, the pooled r values did not identify any negative association between protein intake and BMD/BMC at the clinically important skeletal sites. If anything, a slight positive association showed that protein was able to account for 1% to 2% of BMD measurements. Darling's group further studied 19 randomized, placebo-controlled trials and found an overall slightly positive impact of protein supplementation (from all different sources) on lumbar BMD. These small changes in bone, however, did not translate to a beneficial association between dietary protein and fracture rates. In other words, no significant association (either positive or negative) of protein intake with fracture incidence was found in either the qualitative review or the meta-analysis. This meta-analysis does not support the contention that higher dietary protein is detrimental to bone, but it does suggest that a small yet potentially important positive effect may result from a higher protein intake. Although these epidemiological findings of positive protein-bone associations are important, they cannot establish a causal relationship between protein and bone.

ISOTOPIC STUDIES

Several recent short-term feeding studies used calcium isotopes (generally considered the most sensitive and specific method) to evaluated calcium metabolism with different levels of dietary protein in humans. In a randomized crossover study of 15 healthy postmenopausal women, Roughead et al. (2003) assigned participants to low-meat-protein (12% of energy) and high–meat-protein (20% of energy) diets, each containing 600-mg calcium for 8-week periods. After a 4-week adjustment period on each diet, 2-day diets were labeled with ^{47}Ca, and whole-body scintillation counting was performed over the subsequent 28 days. If the traditional hypothesis were correct, one would expect to see lower calcium retention among the group consuming the higher protein level. However, no significant difference was seen in calcium retention between the groups. Rather, a trend toward better calcium retention was observed on the higher protein diet. The high– and low–meat-protein diet also did not adversely affect biochemical markers of bone turnover (Roughead et al., 2003).

In a follow-up randomized, controlled feeding study conducted by this same team of investigators, 27 postmenopausal women were assigned to either a low-calcium (675 mg Ca/day) or high-calcium (1510 mg Ca/day) diet. Subjects consumed low-protein (10% of energy) and high-protein (20% of energy) diets containing their assigned calcium level for 7 weeks each, with a 3-week washout period in between. After 3 weeks on each diet, 2-day diets were labeled with ^{47}Ca isotopes, and whole-body scintillation counting followed. On the lower calcium diet, fractional calcium absorption increased with the higher protein diet (in comparison with the low-protein diet); however, on the higher calcium diet, this effect was not seen. Of further importance, the higher protein diet significantly increased serum IGF-1, an anabolic hormone that may be beneficial to bone. The higher protein diet also reduced urinary deoxypyridinoline, a marker of bone collagen breakdown (Hunt et al., 2009).

In a final study, dual stable isotopes were used to evaluate the effect of a 10-day dietary intervention containing a moderate-protein (1.0g/kg) or high-protein (2.1g/kg) diet and a low intake of calcium (800 mg) in healthy women (Kerstetter et al., 2005). The high-protein diet resulted in a significant, 42% relative increase (7.7% raw) in intestinal calcium absorption and a significant increase in calcium excretion. No statistically significant differences were seen in kinetic measures of bone turnover between the moderate- and high-protein diets. However, the higher protein diet caused a significantly lower urinary fraction of calcium from bone origin. These data suggest that, at least acutely, hypercalciuria secondary to increased dietary protein is, in fact, the result of increased intestinal calcium absorption. Further, although not significant, there was a trend toward lower bone turnover in the high protein group, which may positively impact bone (Kerstetter et al., 2005). In all of the above isotopic studies (Roughead et al., 2003; Kerstetter et al., 2005; Hunt et al., 2009) where dietary protein had a positive effect on calcium and bone, dietary calcium was limited to 600–800 mg. At higher calcium intakes, the impact is less evident.

However, in a recent pilot feeding study, Ceglia et al. (2009) observed no increase in intestinal calcium absorption on a high-protein (1.5g/kg) versus low-protein (0.5g/kg) diet using dual-tracer stable isotopes. This intervention did not keep phosphorous constant. The high-dietary-phosphorus load that naturally accompanies a high–dietary-protein diet may blunt any change in intestinal calcium absorption (Ceglia et al., 2009). In addition, these subjects also received 1200-mg elemental calcium, which could have masked any effect of a change in dietary protein, as it did in the study by Hunt et al. (2009).

The strength of the design of the feeding studies, with each subject serving as his or her own control, and the methods used to measure calcium metabolism make these findings an important addition to the epidemiological data supporting a positive relationship between long-term higher protein intake and bone health. However, the dietary feeding studies are limited by their short-term nature and small sample sizes.

If experimental diets contain high levels of calcium, the impact of protein on absorption may not be evident (Ceglia et al., 2009; Hunt et al., 2009). On the other hand, when dietary calcium is limited (Kerstetter et al., 1998, 2005; Hunt et al., 2009), the effect of protein on calcium absorption becomes apparent. Because dietary calcium is inadequate in many older individuals, inadequate dietary protein may compound the problem of calcium bioavailability, whereas increasing protein may help to rectify it. The age of subjects may be important as older adults often have modest declines in glomerular filtration rate, which means that they retain more acid and calcium.

POTENTIAL PROTEIN-INDUCED MECHANISMS OPERATING TO IMPROVE CALCIUM BALANCE

Several potential mechanisms might explain how increasing the amount of protein in the diet could potentially benefit calcium retention and bone homeostasis, including improved calcium absorption, increased production of IGF-1, and gain in lean body mass (Figure 15.1). These potential mechanisms probably overlap and are not necessarily exclusive.

Experimental feeding studies demonstrate that increases in dietary protein enhance intestinal calcium absorption beginning at 1 week and at least to 7 weeks (Kerstetter et al., 2005; Hunt et al., 2009). If more calcium is absorbed from the intestine on a higher protein diet, parathyroid hormone (PTH) would be expected to decrease, resulting in reduced rates of bone resorption and bone loss. A significantly lower level of PTH observed in the trial with 10 individuals on a 10-day high-protein (1.5g/kg) versus low-protein (0.5g/kg) diet supports this hypothesis (Ceglia et al., 2009). In another

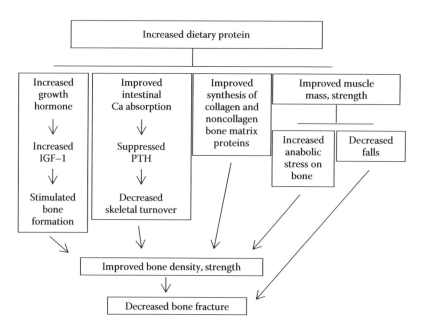

FIGURE 15.1 Potential mechanisms by which increased dietary protein positively impacts bone health. (Adapted from Gaffney-Stomberg, E., et al., *J Am Geriatr Soc*, 57, 1073–1079, 2009.)

short-term study, serum PTH was 1.6 to 2.7 times higher in women consuming low-protein (0.7g/kg) versus moderate-protein (1.0g/kg) diets for 14 days (Kerstetter et al., 1997).

One mechanism by which dietary protein may increase intestinal calcium absorption is by an effect on gastric acid secretion. Calcium is absorbed in the ionized form by the small intestines. When ingested, calcium is in a food matrix or it is complexed with an anion, but not in an ionized form or readily available. Adequate gastric acid must be secreted to facilitate the release of calcium from these complexes and matrices, which allows for ionic calcium absorption. (Older adults may not have optimal gastric acid secretion.) However, the clinical intervention trials addressing this question, which usually used a proton pump inhibiting (PPI) drug to increase gastric pH, did not generate consistent conclusions. For example, Recker (1985) was the first to observe that fasting patients with achlorhydria absorbed less calcium (from a calcium carbonate supplement) than did control subjects with normal gastric acid production. In agreement with this finding are the results of a randomized crossover trial in which a significant decrease in fasting calcium absorption (from calcium carbonate) was observed when elderly women were given a PPI drug which blocked gastric acid production (O'Connell et al., 2005). On the other hand, during fed conditions, the blockage of gastric acid excretion by a PPI drug did not impact calcium absorption (Serfaty-Lacrosniere et al., 1995). Therefore, the influence of gastric acid on intestinal calcium absorption may be dependent on whether subjects are fed or fasted.

To explore further the mechanisms underlying the effect of dietary protein on intestinal calcium absorption, we developed a rat model that simulates the acute response in humans (Gaffney-Stomberg et al., 2010). Female Sprague-Dawley rats were fed a control (20%), low-protein (5%), or high-protein (40%) diet for 1 week at which point duodenal mucosa was harvested and brush border membrane vesicles (BBMV) were prepared to evaluate calcium uptake. By day 7, urinary calcium was more than two-fold higher in the 40% protein group compared with that in the control group (4.2 mg/day vs. 1.7 mg/day, p < .05). Rats consuming the 40% protein diet both absorbed and retained more Ca compared with the 5% protein group in which absorption was 48.5% vs. 34.1% and retention was 45.8% vs. 33.7%, respectively (p < .01). The BBMV calcium uptake results suggest that a higher protein intake improves Ca absorption, at least in part, by increasing cellular calcium uptake.

Another potential mechanism involves IGF-1, a key mediator of bone growth (Geusens and Boonen, 2002), that is regulated by dietary protein (Bonjour et al., 1997, 2001). In two studies employing high protein intakes, significantly greater levels of IGF-1 were found in subjects consuming the higher protein diets (Dawson-Hughes et al., 2004; Hunt et al., 2009). The anabolic effect of IGF-1 on muscle, rather than bone, may help further explain the positive relationship, though indirect, between dietary protein and bone. Thus, protein-induced increases in IGF-1 may indirectly benefit bone because of a direct enhancing action on muscle tissue and strength, which also increases bone strength.

A frequently overlooked fact is that changes in bone mass and muscle strength tend to track together over the life span (Wolfe, 2006). The maintenance of bone strength is dependent upon maintenance of muscle mass, and a trophic effect of muscle contraction has a direct anabolic effect on bone (Wolfe, 2006). Like bone, muscle mass decreases with age; after the age of 40 years, skeletal muscle loss occurs at a rate of approximately 0.5%–1.0% per year (Paddon-Jones et al., 2008). Houston et al. (2008) evaluated the association between protein intake and lean body mass, largely skeletal muscle, over a 3-year period in 2066 black and white individuals between the ages of 70 and 79 years. Subjects with protein consumption in the highest quintile (median intake 1.1 g/kg/day) had significantly lower rates of loss of muscle mass ($p < .05$) than those in subjects in the lowest quintile of protein intake (median intake 0.7 g/kg/day) (Houston et al., 2008).

The relationship between protein intake and muscle mass in the aging population may be modulated by timing of food consumption, frequency of intake, quality of protein, presence or absence of other macronutrients, and physical activity. A recent hypothesis suggests that the consumption of high-quality protein at each meal (25–30 g) may combat sarcopenia by slowing or preventing muscle loss in the aging elderly population (Paddon-Jones and Rasmussen, 2009). The maintenance of good skeletal health in late life, including the avoidance of falls associated with aging, may be highly dependent on the maintenance of adequate muscle mass and function, which is in turn dependent to some extent on an adequate daily intake of dietary protein. The relationships among dietary protein, muscle mass, muscle strength and function, risk of falls and fracture, and bone density and bone health are complex and not yet well delineated.

Because 50% of bone volume represents protein in the organic matrix, especially collagen, and continuous bone remodeling occurs, a higher intake of protein may positively impact bone formation and help maintain a greater bone mass (Heaney and Layman, 2008). Clearly, further findings from cross-sectional population trials and well-designed, long-term protein interventions are needed to define the relationships among dietary protein, bone health, and fractures.

SUMMARY

The current RDA for protein of 0.8 g/kg for adults was designed to provide the minimum amount of protein necessary to prevent a deficiency. The amount of protein that is required in the diet to optimize bone and muscle health is quite different and likely to be higher. Some groups of individuals in the United States consume inadequate protein diets; for example, 25% of women over the age of 70 years consume 0.8 g/kg protein or less per day, and overall, 10% of the population over 70 years does not meet the RDA for protein. Many epidemiological studies have found a significant positive relationship between protein intake and bone mass or density. Similarly, isotopic studies have also demonstrated greater calcium retention and absorption by individuals consuming high-protein diets, particularly when the calcium content of the diet was limiting. High-protein intake may positively impact bone health by several mechanisms, including calcium absorption, stimulation of the secretion of IGF-1, and enhancement of lean body mass. Clearly, long-term clinical intervention trials in which dietary protein is increased to 1.0–1.5 g/kg in healthy and well-nourished older individuals should be conducted to assess the effect of the level of dietary protein on muscle, bone, and fracture risk. Meanwhile, a limitation of protein in the diets of older individuals to improve bone health does not appear to be scientifically warranted.

A widely held view is that high intakes of animal protein result in increased bone resorption, reduced BMD, and increased fractures because of its ability to generate a high fixed metabolic acid load. The hypothesis is supported by cellular and animal studies and human trials showing the addition of a base such as potassium bicarbonate or citrate which suppresses bone resorption (see review by Arnett, 2003 and Pizzorno et al., 2010). However, the consistency of the controlled isotopic studies as well as the recent epidemiological meta-analyses calls into question this conventional view. Clearly, further protein controlled human intervention trials are needed to establish causality and more clearly define the role of dietary protein and skeletal health.

REFERENCES

Arnett, T. 2003. Regulation of bone cell function by acid-base balance. *Proc Nutr Soc* 62: 511–520.

Barzel, U.S., and Massey, L.K. 1998. Excess dietary protein can adversely affect bone. *J Nutr* 128: 1051–1053.

Beasley, J.M., Ichikawa, L.E., Ange, B.A., et al. 2010. Is protein intake associated with bone mineral density in young women? *Am J Clin Nutr* 91: 1311–1316.

Bonjour, J.P. 2005. Dietary protein: An essential nutrient for bone health. *J Am Coll Nutr* 24: 526S–536S.

Bonjour, J.P., Ammann, P., Chevalley, T., et al. 2001. Protein intake and bone growth. *Can J Appl Physiol* 26 Suppl: S153–S166.

Bonjour, J.P., Schurch, M.A., Chevalley, T., et al. 1997. Protein intake, IGF-1 and osteoporosis. *Osteoporos Int* 7 Suppl 3: S36–S42.

Ceglia, L., Harris, S.S., Abrams, S.A., et al. 2009. Potassium bicarbonate attenuates the urinary nitrogen excretion that accompanies an increase in dietary protein and may promote calcium absorption. *J Clin Endocrinol Metab* 94: 645–653.

Darling, A.L., Millward, D.J., Torgerson, D.J., et al. 2009. Dietary protein and bone health: A systematic review and meta-analysis. *Am J Clin Nutr* 90: 1674–1692.

Dawson-Hughes, B., Harris, S.S., Rasmussen, H., et al. 2004. Effect of dietary protein supplements on calcium excretion in healthy older men and women. *J Clin Endocrinol Metab* 89: 1169–1173.

Fenton, T.R., Lyon, A.W., Eliasziw, M., et al. 2009. Meta-analysis of the effect of the acid-ash hypothesis of osteoporosis on calcium balance. *J Bone Miner Res* 24: 1835–1840.

Fulgoni, V.L., III. 2008. Current protein intake in America: Analysis of the National Health and Nutrition Examination Survey, 2003–2004. *Am J Clin Nutr* 87: 1554S–1557S.

Gaffney-Stomberg, E., Insogna, K.L., Rodriguez, N.R., et al. 2009. Increasing dietary protein requirements in elderly people for optimal muscle and bone health. *J Am Geriatr Soc* 57: 1073–1079.

Gaffney-Stomberg, E., Sun, B., Cucchi, C., et al. 2010. The effect of dietary protein on intestinal calcium absorption in rats. *Endocrinology* 151: 1071–1078.

Geusens, P.P., and Boonen, S. 2002. Osteoporosis and the growth hormone-insulin-like growth factor axis. *Horm Res* 58 Suppl 3: 49–55.

Hannan, M.T., Tucker, K.L., Dawson-Hughes, B., et al. 2000. Effect of dietary protein on bone loss in elderly men and women: The Framingham Osteoporosis Study. *J Bone Miner Res* 15: 2504–2512.

Heaney, R.P., and Layman, D.K. 2008. Amount and type of protein influences bone health. *Am J Clin Nutr* 87: 1567S–1570S.

Houston, D.K., Nicklas, B.J., Ding, J., et al. 2008. Dietary protein intake is associated with lean mass change in older, community-dwelling adults: The Health, Aging, and Body Composition (Health ABC) Study. *Am J Clin Nutr* 87: 150–155.

Hunt, J.R., Johnson, L.K., and Fariba Roughead, Z.K. 2009. Dietary protein and calcium interact to influence calcium retention: A controlled feeding study. *Am J Clin Nutr* 89: 1357–1365.

Institute of Medicine, Standing Committee on the Scientific Evaluation of Dietary Reference Intakes, Food and Nutrition Board. 2002. *Dietary Reference Intakes for Energy, Carbohydrates, Fiber, Fat, Protein and Amino Acids (Macronutrients)*. National Academy Press, Washington, DC.

Jehle, S., Zanetti, A., Muser, J., et al. 2006. Partial neutralization of the acidogenic Western diet with potassium citrate increases bone mass in postmenopausal women with osteopenia. *J Am Soc Nephrol* 17: 3213–3222.

Kerstetter, J.E., and Allen, L.H. 1994. Protein intake and calcium homeostasis. *Adv Nutr Res* 9: 167–181.

Kerstetter, J.E., Caseria, D.M., Mitnick, M.E., et al. 1997. Increased circulating concentrations of parathyroid hormone in healthy, young women consuming a protein-restricted diet. *Am J Clin Nutr* 66: 1188–1196.

Kerstetter, J.E., O'Brien, K.O., Caseria, D.M., et al. 2005. The impact of dietary protein on calcium absorption and kinetic measures of bone turnover in women. *J Clin Endocrinol Metab* 90: 26–31.

Kerstetter, J.E., O'Brien, K.O., and Insogna, K.L. 1998. Dietary protein affects intestinal calcium absorption. *Am J Clin Nutr* 68: 859–865.

Kerstetter, J.E., O'Brien, K.O., and Insogna, K.L. 2003. Dietary protein, calcium metabolism, and skeletal homeostasis revisited. *Am J Clin Nutr* 78: 584S–592S.

Meng, X., Zhu, K., Devine, A., et al. 2009. A 5-year cohort study of the effects of high protein intake on lean mass and BMC in elderly postmenopausal women. *J Bone Miner Res* 24: 1827–1834.

O'Connell, M.B., Madden, D.M., Murray, A.M., et al. 2005. Effects of proton pump inhibitors on calcium carbonate absorption in women: A randomized crossover trial. *Am J Med* 118: 778–781.

Paddon-Jones, D., and Rasmussen, B.B. 2009. Dietary protein recommendations and the prevention of sarcopenia. *Curr Opin Clin Nutr Metab Care* 12: 86–90.

Paddon-Jones, D., Short, K.R., Campbell, W.W., et al. 2008. Role of dietary protein in the sarcopenia of aging. *Am J Clin Nutr* 87: 1562S–1566S.

Pizzorno, J., Frassetto, L.A., and Katzinger, J. 2010. Diet-induced acidosis: Is it real and clinically relevant? *Br J Nutr* 103:1185–1194.

Promislow, J.H., Goodman-Gruen, D., Slymen, D.J., et al. 2002. Protein consumption and bone mineral density in the elderly: The Rancho Bernardo Study. *Am J Epidemiol* 155: 636–644.

Recker, R.R. 1985. Calcium absorption and achlorhydria. *N Engl J Med* 313: 70–73.

Roughead, Z.K., Johnson, L.K., Lykken, G.I., et al. 2003. Controlled high meat diets do not affect calcium retention or indices of bone status in healthy postmenopausal women. *J Nutr* 133: 1020–1026.

Sebastian, A., Harris, S.T., Ottaway, J.H., et al. 1994. Improved mineral balance and skeletal metabolism in postmenopausal women treated with potassium bicarbonate. *N Engl J Med* 330: 1776–1781.

Serfaty-Lacrosniere, C., Wood, R.J., Voytko, D., et al. 1995. Hypochlorhydria from short-term omeprazole treatment does not inhibit intestinal absorption of calcium, phosphorus, magnesium or zinc from food in humans. *J Am Coll Nutr* 14: 364–368.

Wapnir, R. 1990. Calcium, magnesium and phosphorus absorption, nutritional status and effect of proteins. In Wapnir, R., ed. *Protein Nutrition and Mineral Absorption*. CRC Press, Boca Raton, FL.

Wolfe, R.R. 2006. The underappreciated role of muscle in health and disease. *Am J Clin Nutr* 84: 475–482.

Zhang, Q., Ma, G., Greenfield, H., et al. 2010. The association between dietary protein intake and bone mass accretion in pubertal girls with low calcium intakes. *Br J Nutr* 103: 714–723.

16 Omega-3 Fatty Acids and Bone Metabolism

Bruce A. Watkins, Kevin Hannon, Mark F. Seifert, and Yong Li

CONTENTS

INTRODUCTION

The purpose of this chapter is to review the literature on omega-3 fatty acids and bone biology based on *in vivo* investigations and bone cell cultures. A recent search for publications indexed from January 1, 1999, to the present in PubMed using specific key words, resulted in the following number of refereed publications. The following key words were searched: *PUFA and bone*, 57 publications; *omega-3 and bone*, 89 publications; *fatty acids and bone*, 315 publications; and *lipids and bone*, 7891 publications. Publications for this review were selected based on human and animal studies that used or investigated the actions of omega-3 fatty acids or utilized bone cell cultures to understand their actions on bone formation.

Herein, we explain the actions of omega-3 fatty acids on (1) the relationships between muscle and bone, (2) bone formation and bone mineral status *in vivo*, (3) recent findings in human and animal models, and (4) arthritis. The current findings of omega-3 fatty acids and their effects on bone modeling and remodeling are summarized and presented in table format (Tables 16.1 and 16.2). A major limitation of the research on omega-3 fatty acids and bone is the lack of consistent test mixtures and protocols to evaluate bone formation and resorption in modeling and remodeling bone. However, the future is promising because of the positive association between docosahexaenoic acid (DHA) and bone mineral density (BMD) in children and, in some studies, in adults.

Fundamental knowledge on the differences between the actions of eicosapentaenoic acid (EPA) and DHA in bone cell cultures and animal models is now developing. The research is also testing various mechanisms

TABLE 16.1
Reported Observations of n-3 PUFA on Bone in Human Subjects

References	Type of n-3 PUFA	Human Subject	Bone Modeling or Remodeling	Observations
Eriksson et al., 2009	Analyzed for DHA, ALA	85 healthy Caucasian 8-yr-olds (50 boys and 35 girls)	Modeling	• LA, total n-6 PUFA, and the high ratio of n-6:n-3 PUFA were negatively associated with BMD. • AA was positively correlated with BMC and BMD of total body.
Gronowitz et al., 2008	Analyzed for ALA, EPA, and DHA	14 men with cystic fibrosis (aged 21.6 ± 2.2 yr), 42 healthy men as control (19.5 ± 0.2 yr)	Modeling	• The endosteal circumference of radius was positively associated with serum PL DHA, while it was negatively associated with the ratio of n-6:n-3 PUFA in the patient group. • No such association was found in the control group.
Hogstrom et al., 2007	Analyzed for DHA and total n-3	78 healthy young men with a mean age of 16.7 yr at baseline	Modeling	• Concentrations of DHA and total n-3 PUFA were positively associated with total and spine BMD at 22 yr of age.
Gronowitz et al., 2006	Analyzed for DHA	54 patients (25 males and 29 females, 35 children and 19 adults) with cystic fibrosis (6–33 yr, median 16 yr)	Modeling	• The lumbar spine BMD Z-score correlated negatively with the ratio of AA:DHA. • Fatty acid status influenced BMD in cystic fibrosis children, but not in adults.
Weiler et al., 2005	Analyzed for EPA and DHA	Healthy infants at birth (16 females and 14 males) and at 15 days	Modeling	• Cord RBC AA was positively correlated with infant whole-body BMC. • AA:EPA positively correlated with lumbar spine 1–4 BMC and femur BMC. • Maternal RBC AA was positively correlated with whole-body BMC. • Femur BMC was negatively predicted by maternal DHA.
Dawczynski et al., 2009	Treated with ALA, EPA, DPA(n-3), and DHA	45 RA patients (43 females and 2 males) Age 57.9 ± 10.8 yr (for the 39 subjects who completed the study)	N/A	• The n-3 PUFA (ALA, EPA, and DHA) suppressed COX-2 expression. • n-3 PUFA did suppress the immune response as lymphocytes and monocytes were found to be significantly decreased. • Supplementing increased total plasma levels of EPA and DHA. • No improvement in the duration of morning stiffness, number of tender joints, and number of swollen joints was seen by dietary n-3 supplementation.
Griffith et al., 2009	Analyzed for ALA, EPA, and DHA	126 subjects (94 females, 32 males, mean age 69.7 ± 10.5 yr)	Remodeling	• Research was done in patients undergoing orthopedic surgery with various underlying conditions. • No correlation was detected between marrow fatty acid concentrations (AA, EPA, and DHA) and bone mineral status in patients with normal, low, or osteoporotic BMD. • No dietary intake information was obtained from these patents. • Mixing postmenopausal women with similar aged men confounds the result.

Study	Treatment/Analysis	Subjects	Type	Findings
Griel et al., 2007	Treated with ALA (walnuts and flaxseed oil)	23 human subjects (20 males of 48.6 ± 1.6 yr and 3 females of 58.3 ± 2.7 yr)	Remodeling	• Serum NTx levels were significantly lower following the ALA diet. • There was no change in levels of bone-specific alkaline phosphatase activity across the three dietary treatments.
Martinez-Ramirez et al., 2007	Analyzed for n-3	167 patients aged 65 yr or more (mean age 73.2 yr, 80% women) with a low-energy fracture + matched controls at 1:1	Remodeling	• A higher ratio of MUFA to PUFA was associated with a reduced risk of fracture. • The intake of n-6 PUFA was associated with an elevated risk of fracture.
Hamazaki et al., 2006	Analyzed for EPA	256 men (22–59 yr of age) and 95 women (22–66 yr)	Remodeling	• The beta coefficient of the numbers of remaining teeth and EPA concentrations in the fraction was 0.89 (per 1% EPA, p = .007).
Baggio et al., 2005	Analyzed for EPA, DHA, and total n-3	30 renal transplant patients (19 males; mean age 44 yr, range 22–65 years)	Remodeling	• The ratio of n-3 PUFA:AA was positively correlated to BMD. • BMD improvement was positively related to EPA but negatively related to plasma phospholipid AA modification.
Rousseau et al., 2009	Analyzed for total n-3	247 men (118) and women (129) aged 60 yr and older (overall 78.9 ± 6.8 yr)	Remodeling	• There was an association between greater reported n-3 PUFA intake and higher BMD.
Zwart et al., 2009	Treated with fish	Bed rest study: 16 healthy subjects Short-duration spaceflight: (7 male and 3 female astronauts, aged 36–54 yr) Long-duration spaceflight: 24 crew members	Remodeling	• A higher intake of n-3 PUFA was associated with less N-telopeptide excretion during bed rest. • Higher fish consumption was associated with reduced BMD loss after space flight.
Wang et al., 2008	Reported total n-3	293 healthy subjects (63% female, 58.0 ± 5.5 yr)	Remodeling	• Intake of n-6 PUFA was associated with an increased risk of bone marrow lesions.
Weiss et al., 2005	Analyzed for ALA, EPA, and total n-3	Community-dwelling men (n = 642, 72.9 ± 9.3 yr) and women (n = 564, 74.0 ± 9.2 yr for those without hormone therapy, n = 326, 69.4 ± 8.6 yr for those with hormone therapy)	Remodeling	• There was a significant inverse association between the ratio of dietary LA:ALA and BMD at the hip. • An increasing ratio of total dietary n-6:n-3 PUFA was significantly and independently associated with lower BMD at the hip in all women.

Notes: AA = arachidonic acid; ALA = alpha-linolenic acid; BMC = bone mineral content; BMD = bone mineral density; COX = cyclooxygenase; DHA = docosahexaenoic acid; DPA = docosapentaenoic acid; EPA = eicosapentaenoic acid; LA = linoleic acid; PL = phospholipids; PUFA = polyunsaturated fatty acids; MUFA = monounsaturated fatty acids; N/A = not applicable; NTx = cross-linked N-telopeptides of type I collagen; RBC = red blood cell; yr = year.

TABLE 16.2
Reported Observations of n-3 PUFA on Bone in Animal Models

Reference	Type of n-3 PUFA	Animal Model	Bone Modeling or Remodeling	Observations
Kohut et al., 2009	Treated with DHA	Male low-birth-weight (3-day-old) and very-low-birth-weight Cotswold piglets (5-day-old)	Modeling	• Higher intake of AA and DHA lowered bone resorption relative to controls. • Dietary treatments did not change the bone formation rate.
Lobo et al., 2009	Treated with ALA (soybean oil) and fish oil	Male Wistar rats (6-wk-old)	Modeling	• Feeding fish oil to rats significantly increased BMC.
Korotkova et al., 2004	Treated with ALA (linseed oil and soybean oil)	Rat dams (day 7 of gestation) and 3-wk-old female pups Modeling	Modeling	• Femur length and cortical cross-sectional bone area and bone mineral content were significantly higher in the n-6 + n-3 PUFA group than in the other groups. • Cortical bone thickness in the n-6 + n-3 PUFA group was increased compared with the n-3 PUFA group. • Regulatory mechanisms were influenced by the ratio of n-6:n-3 PUFA early in life and not compensated for by the introduction of an ordinary diet after weaning.
Reinwald et al., 2004	Treated with ALA and DHA	Weaning 21-day-old Long-Evans rats	Modeling	• n-3 PUFA deficiency diminished structural integrity in rat tibia. • Rats repleted with n-3 PUFA demonstrated accelerated bone modeling (cross-sectional geometry) and an improved second moment in tibiae compared with those of control n-3-adequate rats.
Watkins et al., 2000	Treated with menhaden oil	Weanling Sprague-Dawley rats	Modeling	• Bone PGE_2 was positively correlated with the ratio of AA:EPA. • The ratio of AA:EPA or PGE_2 in bone was negatively correlated to bone formation rate. • Serum bone-specific alkaline phosphatase activity was greater in rats fed a diet high in n-3.
Lau et al., 2009a, 2009b	Analyzed for ALA, EPA, and DHA	Male and female fat-1 and wild type mice (3-wk-old)	Modeling and remodeling	• The ratio of n-6:n-3 PUFA in the femur and vertebra was negatively correlated with BMC and peak load. • ALA, EPA, and DHA were positively correlated with BMC (or BMD) and peak load.
Nielsen and Stoecker, 2009	Treated with menhaden oil	Female rats (dams and pups to 21 wk)	Modeling and remodeling	• Fish oil instead of safflower oil increased the maximum force to break and the bending moment of the femur, especially in rats fed adequate boron.
Bendyk et al., 2009	Treated with tuna fish oil	6- to 8-wk-old female BALB/c mice	Remodeling	• Tuna fish treatment reduced alveolar bone loss in induced periodontitis. • Alveolar bone loss was inversely related to n-3 PUFA tissue levels.

Reference	Treatment	Model	Category	Findings
Sacco et al., 2009	Treated with ALA (flaxseed)	3-month-old female Sprague-Dawley OVX rats	Remodeling	• Flaxseed + low-dose estrogen therapy resulted in the highest bone mineral density and peak load at the lumbar vertebrae, with no effect on bone mineral density or strength in the tibia and femur.
Poulsen et al., 2008a	DHA	7-month-old female Sprague-Dawley OVX rats	Remodeling	• Combined treatment with 17beta-estradiol + DHA was more effective than was either treatment alone at preserving femur BMC and lowering circulating concentrations of proinflammatory IL-6.
Vardar-Sengul et al., 2008	Treated with EPA and DHA	Adult male Sprague-Dawley (205 ± 29.3 g) rats	Remodeling	• Selective cyclooxygenase-2 inhibitor, prophylactic n-3 PUFA, and a combination of these two agents can inhibit gingival tissue MMP-8 expression.
Poulsen et al., 2007	Treated with EPA and DHA	7-month-old female Sprague-Dawley OVX rats	Remodeling	• The OVX-induced decrease in lumbar spine BMC was significantly attenuated by DHA but not by EPA or GLA supplementation or supplementation with a mixture of all three long-chain PUFA. • Endosteal circumferences of tibiae were significantly greater in DHA and EPA compared with OVX.
Shen et al., 2007	Treated with menhaden oil	Male F344 BNF1 rats (12-months-old)	Remodeling	• Rats fed the n-3 PUFA diet had the highest values for peak load, ultimate stiffness, and Young's modulus. • Rats fed the n-3 PUFA diet had lower values for formation rate, osteoclast number, and eroded surface in proximal tibia but higher values for periosteal mineral apposition and formation rates in tibia shaft.
Ward and Fonseca, 2007	Treated with menhaden oil	Sham or OVX CD-1 mice (6-months-old)	Remodeling	• Fish oil, either alone or combined with isoflavone, resulted in a higher BMD of LV. • Fish oil + isoflavone resulted in a higher peak load of LV4.
Shen et al., 2006	Treated with menhaden oil	Male F344 × BNF1 rats (12-months-old)	Remodeling	• Rats fed the n-3 PUFA diet had the highest bone mineral content and cortical + subcortical BMD. • Rats fed the n-3 PUFA diet had higher values for serum insulin-like growth factor-I, parathyroid hormone, 1,25-(OH)$_2$ vitamin D$_3$, and bone-specific alkaline phosphatase activity but lower bone NO production and urinary Ca.
Watkins et al., 2006	Treated with DHA	3-month-old female OVX rats	Remodeling	• DHA-rich diets resulted in a significantly lower bone loss among the OVX rats. • DHA in the diet preserved rat femur BMC in the absence of estrogen.
Watkins et al., 2005	Treated with menhaden oil	3-month-old female OVX rats	Remodeling	• Among the OVX rats, those fed the n-3 PUFA + isoflavone diet had a significantly higher value for tibial BMC. • The concentration of serum pyridinoline cross-links was significantly lower in the n-3 PUFA+ isoflavone group.

Notes: AA = arachidonic acid; ALA = alpha-linolenic acid; BMC = bone mineral content; BMD = bone mineral density; DHA = docosahexaenoic acid; EPA = eicosapentaenoic acid; GLA = γ-linolenic acid; IL = interleukin; LV = lumbar vertebra; MMP = matrix metallopeptidase; NO = nitric oxide; OVX = ovariectomized; PGE$_2$ = prostaglandin E$_2$; PUFA = polyunsaturated fatty acids; wk = week.

of omega-3 fatty acid actions on gene expression. One evolving area of research in bone that has great potential to improve bone health is identifying how omega-3 fatty acids may alter receptor functions of the endocannabinoid signaling system. These aspects of omega-3 fatty acids and bone are also described.

MUSCLE AND BONE RELATIONSHIPS AND OMEGA-3 FATTY ACIDS

Healthy and optimally functioning muscle and bone are vital for normal musculoskeletal growth,
beginning at birth, and proceeding into adolescence and adulthood, and muscles are also necessary for maintaining the integrity of the skeletal system in the adult. Muscles exert biomechanical
force-generated signals of the muscle/bone unit described by Schoenau and Frost (2002) for bone
growth in children up to adults and in remodeling the skeletal system of the adult to minimize
risk of osteoporosis and bone fractures (Figure 16.1). The mechanostat theory best describes how
the biomechanical signals that emanate from muscle affect bone, that is, as part of the muscle/
bone unit. Substantial clinical and epidemiological evidence supports the premise that osteoporosis
prevention must incorporate strategies to enhance peak bone mass early in life and to limit bone
loss with aging. To understand the current science of the biomechanical and biochemical factors
controlling bone growth in the young and which support musculoskeletal health throughout life, the
fundamental principles of muscle and bone growth are examined along with environmental agents,
mainly polyunsaturated fatty acids (PUFA), that influence this process. The relatively new nutrient
candidates that are intimately involved in this process are the omega-3 (or n-3) PUFA. Specifically,
DHA (22:6n-3) has been shown to support bone growth (Hogstrom et al., 2007), minimize muscle
and bone loss (Poulsen et al., 2008a; Watkins et al., 2006, 2007), and improve bone architecture
(mechanical properties testing) to resist long-bone fractures (Reinwald et al., 2004).

Our research, and that of others, demonstrates important actions for n-3 PUFA in supporting
optimal bone modeling and osteoblast functions, normalizing muscle insulin response to reduce the
risk of obesity and diabetes, and minimizing chronic inflammation in the musculoskeletal system
with estrogen decline and aging. The principle n-3 PUFA involved in this aspect of nutrition and

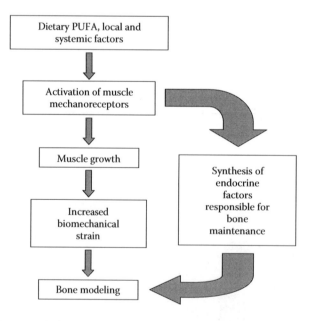

FIGURE 16.1 Muscles cause the largest loads and strains on bone to model and remodel bone tissue throughout life. These strains help control the biological mechanisms that determine whole bone strength and architecture, as explained by the mechanostat theory. Several dietary factors including essential fatty acids and the
amounts of PUFA of the n-6 and n-3 families can influence muscle health. See text for details.

health appears to be DHA, an essential fatty acid for neural growth and retinal development in the infant (Uauy et al., 2001).

DHA has been associated with elevated bone mass (Watkins et al., 2006) and enhanced intestinal calcium absorption and retention (Haag et al., 2003; Poulsen et al., 2007), as well as reduced prostaglandin biosynthesis and bone resorption (Kang and Weylandt, 2008; Rahman et al., 2008). DHA improved bone mass in young rats with diabetes (a risk factor for low bone mass) (Yamada et al., 1995). Ovariectomized (OVX) rats fed either fish oil or DHA experienced attenuated loss of bone mineral, and in some cases, this observation was associated with increased bone formation and decreased bone resorption biomarkers (Watkins et al., 2005, 2006). In advanced aging, n-3 PUFA found in menhaden oil (which includes DHA) also attenuated bone loss in intact male rodents (Shen et al., 2006, 2007). Thus, in several studies, dietary sources of DHA benefit the musculoskeletal system by enhancing peak bone mass during growth and preserving bone mass during estrogen loss, as well as supporting muscle mass during advanced aging to prevent muscle atrophy and osteopenia.

Healthy muscle is crucial in providing proper biomechanical signals needed to facilitate bone growth, proper architecture, and maintenance of mineral throughout life (Fricke and Schoenau, 2007). Muscle loss is followed by osteopenia at all ages (Carmeli et al., 2002; Giangregorio and McCartney, 2006). Moreover, substantial research has demonstrated that n-3 PUFA, including DHA, reduces muscle loss during cachexia (defined as the massive loss of up to 80% of both adipose tissue and skeletal muscle in cancer patients) (Khal and Tisdale, 2008; Smith et al., 2004; Tisdale, 1996, 2002). Thus, dietary approaches to attenuate age-associated muscle loss or losses of muscle and bone because of disuse may result in numerous health benefits beyond improvement of bone mineral content (BMC).

Other aspects of the actions of n-3 PUFA include observations from studies conducted with DHA on bone modeling in rats. DHA supplemented to n-3-PUFA-deficient growing rats restored the n-3 PUFA content (including DHA) of bone tissue compartments including femoral marrow and cortical bone (Li et al., 2003a) and resulted in compensatory bone modeling and improvements in femur and tibia bone architecture (Reinwald et al., 2004). Moreover, Watkins et al. (2000) found that DHA was more efficiently incorporated into femoral marrow polar lipids than was EPA in growing rats and that the periosteum of the femur was highly enriched with DHA (10%–14%) compared with EPA (0.4%–0.3%). Hence, DHA appears to be more important than EPA for the periosteum, which supports osteoblastic activity, and enriching or restoring DHA concentrations in the periosteum, which has an abundance of osteoblasts, is rich with blood and lymph vessels and has a complex nerve supply.

In a lipopolysaccharide (LPS)-induced experimental periodontitis model using adult male Sprague-Dawley rats (205 ± 29.3 g), feeding n-3 PUFA (40 mg/kg/day, 60% EPA + 40% DHA) for 14 days inhibited gingival matrix metallopeptidase (MMP)-8 (a collagenase regulated by proinflammatory cytokines) expression and increased tissue inhibitor of MMP (TIMP)-1 (endogenous downregulators of MMPs) expression, but the DHA-rich diet did not affect alveolar bone loss (Vardar-Sengul et al., 2008).

OVX rats supplemented with DHA (expressed as a low ratio of n-6:n-3 PUFA of 5:1) had higher femur BMC compared with that of rats receiving a lower amount of DHA, that is, a ratio of n-6:n-3 PUFA of 10:1 (Watkins et al., 2006). DHA supplementation in OVX rats correlated with higher bone-specific alkaline phosphatase and lower pyridinoline (Pyd) cross-links, a marker of bone resorption. The diet containing DHA moderated the actions of linoleic acid (LA, the essential dietary n-6 PUFA) to support a bone biomarker profile that is associated with greater BMC in the femur of estrogen-deficient rats (Watkins et al., 2006). A lower total dietary PUFA content (both n-6 and n-3 PUFA and their ratio) led to a significantly higher osteocalcin level but lower values for Pyd and deoxypyridinoline in OVX rats compared with that of rats given a higher dietary PUFA content. With respect to the ratio of n-6:n-3 PUFA in this study, an excess of n-6, typical of the American diet, may exceed the capacity of n-3 PUFA to moderate the potential negative effect of n-6 PUFA.

This research supports the concept that n-3 PUFA, specifically DHA in this case, maintains higher BMC in estrogen deficiency that correlates with higher biomarkers of bone formation and lower bio-markers of bone resorption compared with n-6 PUFA. Further, the actions of n-3 PUFA and lower total dietary n-6 PUFA both diminish the negative impact of excess n-6 PUFA on bone.

In OVX rats (female Sprague-Dawley, 7-month-old) fed DHA (DHA in ethyl ester form, 0.5 g/kg/day), BMC was conserved in lumbar spine, femur, and tibial trabeculae, whereas feeding EPA had no such effect on these bone sites (Poulsen et al., 2007). Feeding OVX rats (female Sprague-Dawley, 7-month-old) DHA (DHA in ethyl ester form, 0.5 g/kg/day) combined with 17β-estradiol conserved femur BMC and lowered circulating proinflammatory interleukin (IL)-6 better than did individual treatment of either DHA or 17β-estradiol (Poulsen et al., 2008a). However, combining DHA with a phytoestrogen, either genistein or daidzein, did not show any beneficial effect on bone mineral conservation in this animal model.

Rather interesting relationships between dietary n-3 PUFA and cyclooxygenase-2 (COX-2) expression in human subjects have been reported. An n-3 PUFA supplement (1.1 g alpha-linolenic acid (ALA), 0.7 g EPA, 0.1 g docosapentaenoic acid, and 0.4 g DHA) in yogurt significantly decreased LPS-stimulated COX-2 expression in a randomized double-blind placebo-controlled crossover study (Dawczynski et al., 2009).

In children, serum fatty acid profiles were found associated with bone mineralization in healthy 8-year-old boys and girls (Eriksson et al., 2009). Consistent with the findings in rats in our labora-tory (Watkins et al., 2000), serum phospholipid LA was found to be negatively associated with BMD of the total body and lumbar spine, and this same pattern was found for both the total serum n-6 PUFA concentration and the ratio of n-6:n-3 PUFA. The correlations between serum phospholipid EPA, DHA, the ratio of arachidonic acid (AA) to EPA (AA:EPA) or ratio of AA:DHA, and bone parameters were not statistically significant in this subject group (Eriksson et al., 2009). In human infants, whole-body BMC was positively predicted by cord red blood cell (RBC) AA content, and lumbar vertebrae (L1–4) and femur BMC were positively associated with cord ratio of AA:EPA but negatively related to maternal DHA (Weiler et al., 2005). Clearly, blood and other tissue analyses of PUFA need to be considered as potential markers of bone status, and as the research advances in this area, a clearer relationship will be found for specific fatty acids, their ratios, and bone status.

RESEARCH FINDINGS OF N-3 PUFA AND BONE

PUFA ACTIONS ON BONE CELL FUNCTIONS AND BONE MODELING

PGE_2 is a robust modulator of biochemical activity in bone and has been reported to influence osteo-blast function (Watkins et al., 2001). At moderate levels, PGE_2 supports bone formation, but at high concentrations, it promotes bone resorption (Watkins et al., 2000). In growing rats, a high dietary ratio of n-6:n-3 PUFA was positively correlated with lower bone formation rates and higher capacity for *ex vivo* PGE_2 production in bone (Figure 16.2) (Watkins et al., 2000). Our laboratory confirmed that n-3 PUFA not only reduced the production of PGE_2 *in vivo* but also affected the expression of COX-2, a key enzyme that catalyzes the biosynthesis of PGE_2 from AA, in osteoblastic bone cell cultures (Watkins et al., 2003). Furthermore, n-3 PUFA feeding helped maintain BMC in OVX rats (Watkins et al., 2005, 2006) and mice (Fernandes et al., 2003). Moreover, n-3 PUFA levels in bone and osteoblastic cell cultures have been shown to coincide with the elevated levels of bone formation markers that are indicative of enhanced bone formation activity (Watkins et al., 2000, 2001, 2003).

Generally, DHA can function to attenuate AA conversion to prostanoids, and although DHA is not an eicosanoid precursor, it would provide an important means for modulating AA prostanoid-mediated physiological and pathological processes (Mori and Beilin, 2001; Raisz et al., 1989). The need for understanding the role of n-3 PUFA in musculoskeletal health is further justified by the most recent dietary reference intakes published by the Institute of Medicine of the National Academies for these fatty acids (Institute of Medicine, 2002).

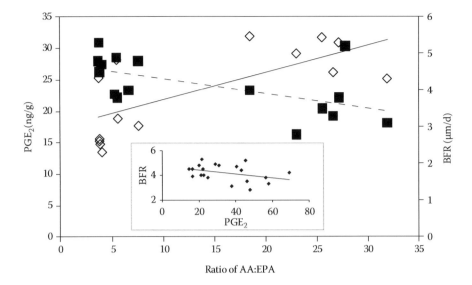

FIGURE 16.2 Relationships between the ratio of AA:EPA in bone and *ex vivo* bone PGE$_2$ production and bone formation in the rat. A positive correlation (shown as solid linear trend line that can be expressed as y = 0.439x + 17.389) was observed between *ex vivo* bone PGE$_2$ (y) and the ratio of AA:EPA (x) in bone (■). A negative correlation (shown as dotted linear trend line that can be expressed as y = 20.0396x + 4.705) was found between bone formation rate (BFR) (y) and the ratio of AA:EPA (x) (◊). The panel insert shows a negative correlation (shown as solid linear trend line that can be expressed as y = 20.0194x + 4.819) between BFR (y) and *ex vivo* PGE$_2$ (x) production in bone. Bone alkaline phosphatase activity (bone formation marker) was greater in rats fed a diet high in n-3 PUFA or a low dietary ratio of n-6:n-3 PUFA. (Adapted from Watkins, B. A., Li, Y., Allen, K. G. D., et al., *J Nutr* 130, 2274–84, 2000.)

The evidence suggests that the n-3 PUFA (EPA and DHA) increase bone formation rates in growing rodents, and the response is associated with lowering PGE$_2$ *ex vivo* in bone (Watkins et al., 2000) (see Figure 16.2). Furthermore, consistent with elevating n-3 PUFA in bone tissues by feeding dietary sources of EPA and DHA to rodents, a reduction of COX-2 protein but higher bone alkaline phosphatase (ALP) activity was observed in osteoblast-like cells (Watkins et al., 2003). What is not clear is how n-3 PUFA may influence genes and transcription factors associated with osteoblasts and osteoclasts. The core binding factor α1 (Cbfa1), a transcription factor of osteoblast differentiation, was higher in MC3T3-E1 cells after 7 days of exposure to EPA at different doses (1 and 10 μM) compared with AA treatment but lower compared with AA treatment (10 and 100 μM) at 14 days (Watkins et al., 2003). The expression values for Cbfa1 were normalized to the vehicle control (VC), and generally all fatty acid treatments except conjugated LA increased expression compared with the VC. Hence, these data suggest that fatty acids may be stimulatory or inhibitory to osteoblast expression of Cbfa1.

A way in which n-3 PUFA may be beneficial to bone formation, related to the relationships demonstrated in Figure 16.2, is to reduce bone tissue concentrations of AA for PGE$_2$ production as a means to control osteoclastic activity and bone loss. For example, PGE$_2$ has been implicated in osteoclastogenesis in that this prostanoid promotes osteoclast formation by increasing the expression of receptor activator of nuclear factor kappa B ligand (RANKL) (Li et al., 2002), and Suda et al. (2004) reported that PGE$_2$ decreases osteoblastic expression of osteoprotegerin (OPG), which is a decoy receptor for RANKL. In addition, PGE$_2$, a proposed receptor agonist to bone morphogenetic protein-2 (BMP-2), may potentiate the effects of BMP-2 on osteoclastogenesis (Blackwell et al., 2009). Therefore, a major action of n-3 PUFA on bone can be the direct effects on reducing AA concentrations as well as decreasing the production of PGE$_2$ and attenuating its downstream actions (cytokines and transcription factors) to influence both osteoblasts and osteoclasts, as shown in Figure 16.3.

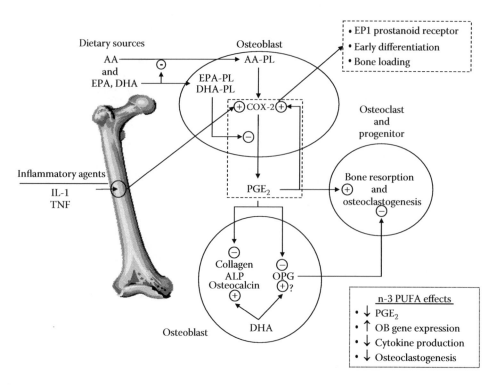

FIGURE 16.3 In bone, some actions of EPA and DHA are reducing the production of PGE_2 either by lowering the substrate levels (AA in phospholipids) or effects on the activity or expression of COX in osteoblasts. In addition, substitution of EPA for AA in phospholipids can result in the production of PGE_3. These actions are, in part, how n-3 PUFA influences the activity of osteoblasts and osteoclasts. EPA was reported to upregulate Cbfa1 (osteoblast differentiation); however, the responses appear to be related to both the concentration of fatty acids in and duration of culture time in osteoblast-like cells. In addition, reducing PGE_2 has direct effects on osteoblasts that appear related to their functions in bone formation and to the downregulation of genes of pathways inducing osteoclastogenesis (osteoprotegerin [OPG] and receptor activator of nuclear-κB ligand [RANKL]). Some evidence in osteoblast-like cell cultures indicates that EPA and DHA decrease PGE_2-induced RANKL expression. Thus, the current findings suggest that with respect to osteoclastogenesis, n-6 PUFA via PGE_2 and n-3 PUFA (EPA and DHA) may exert their actions through different genes and proteins. We have shown that elevated PGE_2 production in bone (resulting from a diet rich in n-6 PUFA and low in n-3 PUFA) is associated with decreased *in vivo* bone formation in rodents (as shown in Figure 16.1). The beneficial actions of DHA in bone appear to be similar in muscle to prevent its atrophy in rodent models of hindlimb suspension and its association with higher BMD in growing individuals as described in the text.

During growth and development, the collective behavior of skeletal elements is organized to facilitate the bone modeling process in children. In long bones, surface drifts (the net loss [net resorption] or gain [net formation] of bone) resulting from physical strain on bone (Epker and Frost, 1965) occur during appositional growth that influences the bone modeling process in the young. Other long bone dimensions including cortical thickness, marrow cavity diameter, external diaphyseal and metaphyseal diameters, longitudinal curvatures, total cortical mass, and cross-sectional geometries can also be attributed to bone modeling activity. Bones of equal material quality but of differing geometries can vary in their degree of stiffness and potential to withstand stress or fracture (Ehrlich and Lanyon, 2002). Hence, bone modeling is a physiological activity significant to skeletal competency, whereas remodeling processes throughout adult life determine fracture risk commensurate with skeletal disease (Ehrlich and Lanyon, 2002).

Until skeletal maturity is attained, over 90% of the periosteal and endosteal bone surfaces are continuously involved in bone appositional and resorptional activities that result in morphological changes pertinent to growth and reshaping (Ehrlich and Lanyon, 2002; Frost, 2003b). During bone modeling (e.g., long bone appositional growth), surface drifts occur, which alter bone cortical thickness, marrow cavity diameter, external diaphyseal and metaphyseal diameters, longitudinal curvatures, total cortical mass, and cross-sectional geometries (Frost, 2003b). These changes in the geometrical character of bone tissue govern the quality of bone, which is determined not only by its material properties but also by architectural, physical, and biological factors that influence its mechanical properties (Ehrlich and Lanyon, 2002; Frost, 2003b; Judex et al., 2003). Investigators have demonstrated that dietary factors including lipids can impact bone morphology and mechanical properties (Mori and Beilin, 2001; Wohl et al., 1998). Evaluation of bone mechanical properties, both structural and material, can be instrumental in elucidating the quality of bone architecture during bone modeling, as demonstrated with n-3 repletion in rats by our laboratory (Reinwald et al., 2004).

BONE AND MUSCLE DEVELOPMENT AND THEIR INTERDEPENDENCE: THE MUSCLE–BONE UNIT

Muscle and bone form an operational unit that controls the growth, maintenance, and operation of these organs. Muscles generate the largest loads and strains on the modeling and remodeling of bone throughout life (see Figure 16.1). These strains help control the biological mechanisms that determine whole bone strength (Schoenau and Frost, 2002). This relationship between muscle and bone is best described by the mechanostat theory, as previously explained, which states that increasing muscle mass and force during development creates the stimulus for the increase in bone mass and strength. Most hormones and other nonmechanical agents can modify the relationship between bone strength and muscle strength but cannot replace it (Schoenau and Frost, 2002). This codependence of muscle and bone means that the study of these two organ systems must be done as a unit and cannot be achieved practically as independent entities. As stated by Rauch and colleagues, "if muscle forces drive bone development, then analyses of muscle function should be added to the armamentarium of clinicians diagnosing bone disorders" (Rauch et al., 2004).

Postnatally, the mechanostat theory is supported by a large volume of work that correlates muscle strength with bone density and strength. For example, peak velocity in lean body mass accretion precedes that of peak velocity of BMC accretion by a few months (Rauch et al., 2004). Very active humans without exceptionally strong muscles, such as marathon runners, lack the whole bone strength that weight lifters obtain (Frost, 2003a; Schoenau and Frost, 2002). Forearm muscle strength is significantly correlated with BMD (Ozdurak et al., 2003). Also supporting the theory is the observation that when muscle mass is decreased in children, such as those with cerebral palsy or muscular dystrophy, in comparison with their normal peers, BMD is significantly reduced (Gray et al., 1992; Lingam and Joester, 1994).

According to Frost, the mechanostat theory (see Figure 16.1) is a result of muscle-derived flexural loads that are symmetrically oriented around the cross-sectional circumference of bone, causing a uniform increase in bone diameter (Frost, 1973). However, repetitive, similar dynamic flexural straining asymmetrically around the bone activates the flexure-drift feedback system and causes drifts of lamellar bone surfaces in tissue space. Bone surfaces will move toward the flexural concavity that arises when the flexural loads are applied, with convex-tending surfaces activating an osteoclastic drift (osteoclasts solubilize the basic organic and inorganic constituents of the bone and return them to the blood, thus facilitating bone resorption) and concave-tending ones activating osteoblastic drift (bone deposition by osteoblasts). Therefore, muscle forces have the capacity to control the shape and density of long bones and, hence, their architecture to resist fracture.

As an example of diet effects on postnatal bone development, our laboratory examined repletion of n-3 PUFA in n-3-PUFA-deficient rats. In this investigation, three groups of rats were studied, second-generation n-3-deficient, n-3-repleted, and a control n-3-adequate rats (Reinwald et al., 2004). The n-3-adequate diet contained ALA (2.6% of total fatty acids) and DHA (1.3% of total fatty acids). Fatty acid composition of the hindlimb tissues (bone and muscle) of chronically n-3-deficient rats revealed a marked increase in n-6 PUFA (20:4n-6 or AA, 22:4n-6, and 22:5n-6) and a corresponding decrease in n-3 PUFA (18:3n-3, EPA, 22:5n-3, and DHA). Measurement of bone mechanical properties (energy to peak load) of tibiae showed that n-3 deficiency diminished structural integrity (Reinwald et al., 2004). Rats repleted with n-3 PUFA demonstrated accelerated bone modeling (cross-sectional geometry) and an improved second moment in tibiae compared with control n-3-adequate rats after 28 days of dietary treatment. This study showed that repletion with dietary n-3 PUFA restored the ratio of n-6:n-3 PUFA in bone compartments (compared with the adequate n-3 PUFA group) and reversed the compromised bone modeling in n-3-deficient rats (Reinwald et al., 2004). Although this study showed the important relationship between bone modeling and improved bone architecture in rats, it is consistent with the concept that bone strength and BMD are related, and in our study, bone strength (based on mechanical property testing) was higher with n-3 PUFA repletion in rats. Thus, indirectly, because muscle-derived loads model bone and determine bone strength or BMD (Ozdurak et al., 2003), repleting n-3 PUFA to n-3-deficient rats in our study is suggestive that n-3 PUFA would improve this muscle–bone relationship to model bone and increase bone strength. In support of the role n-3 PUFA plays in muscle–bone relationship, it is reported that feeding fish oil (containing EPA and DHA) prevented lean body mass loss during a state of cachexia in a mouse model (Tisdale and Dhesi, 1990).

Increased circulating cytokines such as tumor necrosis factor-alpha (TNFα), IL-6, and IL-1β occur in chronic disease states (Levine et al., 1990; Valdez and Lederman, 1997). However, local expression of proinflammatory cytokines could exert a more significant effect on muscle atrophy than could systemically derived cytokines, as skeletal muscle can synthesize TNFα (De Bleecker et al., 1999), IL-1 (Belec et al., 1997), and IL-6 (Bartoccioni et al., 1994; Li et al., 2003b; Saghizadeh et al., 1996; Schulze et al., 2003). Recently, Spate and Schulze reported that the cytokines IL-1β and TNFα activate the ATP-dependent proteolytic pathway and increase proteolysis in muscle (Spate and Schulze, 2004).

TNFα is thought to activate proteolysis through a pathway that involves stimulation of reactive oxygen species (ROS) production and ROS signaling in muscle (Garg and Aggarwal, 2002; Goossens et al., 1995; Li et al., 2000). This activated ROS system then stimulates ATP-dependent proteolysis (Gomes-Marcondes and Tisdale, 2002; Li et al., 2005). Increases in ROS activity and oxidative stress to levels greater than that can be normally neutralized by intracellular antioxidant defenses (which remain unchanged) (Barreiro et al., 2005) are associated with muscle mass loss in catabolic states such as cancer (Tisdale, 2001), sarcopenia (Spiers et al., 2000), and immobilization (Kondo et al., 1993). Similar to the prostaglandin story, the effects of cytokines on muscle protein synthesis and degradation depend on the specific cytokine. Although the above-mentioned cytokines are deleterious for muscle health, IL-15 positively affects parameters associated with skeletal muscle fiber hypertrophy (Quinn et al., 1995). In a tumor-bearing rat model (AH-130 ascites hepatoma), IL-15 treatment significantly slowed the rates of protein degradation to spare skeletal muscle mass from cancer-induced wasting (Carbo et al., 2000). The underlying mechanism on these alterations was reported to be linked to the inhibition of the ATP–ubiquitin-dependent proteolytic pathway (Carbo et al., 2000).

Dietary sources of n-3 PUFA have been found to inhibit the negative effects of cytokines in muscle but may have a significant role in this capacity by moderating PGE_2 production in bone (Figure 16.3). In contrast, dietary lipids rich in n-6 PUFA enhance IL-1 production and tissue responsiveness to cytokines, whereas those rich in n-3 PUFA have the opposite effect (Grimble and Tappia, 1998). The exact mechanism behind this selective effect of n-3 PUFA is not clear. In addition, it is not known what effects n-3 PUFA exert on the synthesis and activity of the positive-acting cytokines, such as IL-15. Clearly though, n-3 PUFA have the ability to control muscle protein synthesis and degradation by regulating the action of muscle-degrading prostanoids and cytokines.

DHA is likely vital to normal bone physiology as a physical constituent of bone compartments, periosteum (nerve abundant tissue), and cortical bone (Li et al., 2003a) for biological maintenance in muscle (in preventing muscle atrophy) and muscle–bone interdependence in modeling bone

(Reinwald et al., 2004). We hypothesize that the endocannabinoid (EC) system, which is fundamentally involved in bone cell differentiation and mature functioning of the skeletal system (Bab et al., 2008), provides some aspect of muscle-to-bone communications yet identified but highly likely because this system influences obesity and insulin sensitivity in muscle and bone cell functions. The EC system, through activation of its receptors, is responsible for differentiation of osteoblasts and osteoclastogenesis (Idris et al., 2008; Ofek et al., 2006) and is a target for modulation by dietary n-3 PUFA that would decrease the AA-derived agonists and may also influence the receptors in muscle and bone.

ROLE OF MATERNAL N-3 PUFA STATUS ON FETAL AND POSTNATAL DEVELOPMENT

Barker and his colleagues postulated that some chronic diseases associated with aging may be programmed in very early life (Godfrey and Barker, 2001). This supposition was initially termed "the fetal origins of adult disease hypothesis." One of the major ideas of this hypothesis is that the effects of early programming are most pronounced when there is a mismatch between early nutritional deprivation and later nutritional affluence. Many examples of metabolic programming exist. For example, premature infants who consumed breast milk (generally higher in DHA content than formula) had lower mean arterial blood pressure at 13 to 16 years of age than that of age-matched, previously premature individuals given standard infant formula (Singhal et al., 2001). The influence of infant growth on long-term muscle strength appears to continue into adult age. Sarcopenia, considered an age-related loss in muscle mass and strength, has its origins in early life (Sayer et al., 2004), as does compromised BMC (Sayer and Cooper, 2005). Muscle metabolism appears to be programmed early in development (Taylor et al., 1995), and nutrition during neonatal life can alter muscle metabolic properties (Harrison et al., 1996).

It has become clear that n-3 PUFA are important for optimal fetal development, and these fatty acids appear to be involved in metabolic programming. This programming is relevant for industrialized countries where consumption of n-6 PUFA has greatly eclipsed the intake of n-3 PUFA from plants and marine food products. The dietary ratio of n-6:n-3 PUFA has now risen to more than 10:1 (Kris-Etherton et al., 2000), and because the ratio of n-6:n-3 PUFA in the milk of women is dictated by diet (Fidler and Koletzko, 2000), the loss of n-3 PUFA can be expected to have serious implications for the health of the neonate and adult. Probably the most important issue regarding metabolic programming is that any early deficiencies appear to be irreversible, even following repletion with the missing nutrient. For instance, n-3 PUFA deficiency in the perinatal period results in elevated blood pressure later in life, even when animals were subsequently repleted with these fatty acids (Weisinger et al., 2001).

Nutrition during the gestational and perinatal period seems to be a critical imprinting regulator of growth and development and, consequently, in the risk for diet-related adult chronic diseases (Godfrey and Barker, 2000). For example, during late gestation and throughout lactation, female rats fed an isocaloric diet containing 7% (by weight) fat as linseed oil (n-3 PUFA diet, ratio of n-6:n-3 PUFA = 0.4), soybean oil (ratio of n-6:n-3 PUFA = 9), or sunflower oil (n-6 diet PUFA, ratio of n-6:n-3 PUFA = 216) produced male and female pups having lower mean body weights than those of dams fed the n-6 PUFA diet containing soybean oil. As both male and female pups grew to 28 weeks of age, those given the sunflower diet (rich in n-6 PUFA) ended up being the heaviest, and the male pups from the sunflower-oil-fed dams had the highest systolic blood pressure (Korotkova et al., 2005). Femur length, cortical cross-sectional area, and BMC were significantly higher in the rat pups fed sources of n-3 PUFA (Korotkova et al., 2004).

As BMC may be programmed early in life, so too does skeletal muscle metabolism and fatigue resistance appear to be programmed during early life. Adults who were low-birth-weight infants and therefore had less muscle mass as children had significantly less resistance during adulthood to muscle fatigue than that of size-matched adults who were significantly larger at birth (Taylor et al., 1995).

Diets Rich in the n-3 PUFA DHA Attenuate Loss of Bone and Muscle Mass Associated with Skeletal Unloading

In our laboratory, 15-week-old male NIH Swiss mice (Harlan Labs, Indianapolis, IN) were fed either a diet supplemented with n-6 PUFA, one containing a combination of n-3 (DHA) and n-6 PUFA, or a control diet for 7 days (Watkins et al., 2007). Diets (AIN-93G basal diet) were isonitrogenous and isocaloric, varying only in the fat source. Skeletal-unloading-associated atrophy was then initiated in mice using hindlimb suspension (Warren et al., 1994), and mice continued on their respective diets during suspension. After 9 days of hindlimb suspension, mice were scanned by dual-energy X-ray absorptiometry (DXA), and regions of interest were defined as the whole body and a trapezoid area, which included the region of the hindlimb below the knee to the tarsus. In the n-6 PUFA diet group of mice, the bone mineral ash, as a percentage of dry weight in the femur, was 11.1% less in the suspended group as compared with the weight-bearing group. In contrast, in the n-3-PUFA-fed group of mice, the bone mineral ash/dry weight (femur) was reduced only 3.2% following suspension. These results demonstrate that, in comparison with an n-6 PUFA diet, consumption of an n-3-PUFA-supplemented diet significantly reduces the catabolic effect of hindlimb suspension on bone mineral loss. The bone-sparing effects of n-3 PUFA were also observed by DXA analysis. After 9 days of hindlimb suspension, a significant loss of whole-body and hindlimb BMD and BMC was observed. In contrast to the diet rich in n-6 PUFA, reduction in BMD and BMC was significantly attenuated in mice receiving the diet rich in DHA, the sole n-3 PUFA.

In addition to attenuating the loss of bone mass associated with skeletal unloading, consuming a diet rich in DHA also suppressed the loss of muscle associated with hindlimb suspension in mice (Watkins et al., 2007). Mice consuming the n-6 PUFA control diet lost approximately 26% of the gastrocnemius/soleus muscle wet weight following 9 days of suspension ($p < .05$ weight-bearing n-6 group versus the suspended n-6 group). Mice consuming the diet supplemented with n-3 PUFA lost only 11% of the gastrocnemius/soleus muscle wet weight following 9 days of suspension. Paralleling these wet weights, consumption of a diet rich in the n-3 PUFA DHA also attenuated the loss in fiber diameter observed with hindlimb suspension.

These results demonstrate that consumption of diets containing DHA attenuates loss of muscle associated with hindlimb suspension. The same experimental design was repeated with the n-3 PUFA EPA and in contrast to the results observed with DHA, EPA supplementation had no sparing effect with respect to bone loss associated with hindlimb suspension. Supplementing with DHA in the diet for only 7 days has been found in our hands to attenuate significantly the loss of bone mineral and muscle mass associated with disuse. Although these findings in mice are promising and potentially have significant and immediate importance to humans to help prevent adult bone loss associated with casting of limbs and in astronauts undergoing reduced gravity during spaceflight, much research is needed to establish a possible mechanism of action.

Endocannabinoids and the Musculoskeletal System

Recently, we found that DHA exerts actions on the endocannabinoid signaling pathway to attenuate the stimulation of the receptors and their actions on osteoclast numbers and osteoclastogenesis so as to favor bone formation during growth (Hutchins et al., 2009). The cannabinoid receptors, CB1 and CB2, were identified in the early and mid-1990s, and much attention has focused on the CB1 in brain because of its involvement in food intake and the use of antagonists to control weight and reverse obesity. The endogenous agonists for these receptors include *N*-arachidonoylethanolamide (anandamide or AEA) and 2-arachidonoylglycerol (2-AG). Both AEA and 2-AG are synthesized on demand from AA. The actions include food intake and influence obesity, insulin resistance, and osteoblast and osteoclast actions. We hypothesize that cross-talk between muscle and bone is communicated through the endocannabinoid signaling system, much like that between the recently described muscle and adipose interactions (Eckardt et al., 2008).

Although the EC system has been shown to regulate food intake, it has recently been found to be of great consequence to the skeletal system, especially to regulate bone mass (Idris et al., 2005, 2008; Tam et al., 2008). As described above, the EC is composed of two receptors, CB1 and CB2, and the main endogenous agonists for the receptors are AEA and 2-AG. Both agonists are derived from AA and can be synthesized in osteoblasts and muscle tissue. *In vitro* and *in vivo* modulation of the EC receptors has been shown to influence bone modeling. In fact, knockout mice that lack the CB2 endocannabinoid receptor have low BMC and lack capacity for bone formation (Ofek et al., 2006). The enzymes for the synthesis of agonists are expressed in osteoblasts, osteocytes, and bone lining cells (Bab and Zimmer, 2008).

The CB2 receptor has been identified in osteoblasts grown in an osteogenic medium for up to 28 days, whereas CB1 was not expressed in osteoblasts grown for this duration (Ofek et al., 2006; Tam et al., 2006). However, CB1 is expressed in sympathetic nerve fibers of trabecular bone (Tam et al., 2006). CB1 and CB2 are found in osteoclasts (Idris et al., 2005; Ofek et al., 2006; Scutt and Williamson, 2007). The expression of CB2 in osteoblasts mirrors that of osteoblast gene expression for tissue nonspecific ALP, runt-related transcription factor 2 (RUNX2), and parathyroid hormone receptor-1 (Ofek et al., 2006). The actions of the EC system in bone support our hypothesis that EC-related proteins are expressed during the development and growth of the musculoskeletal system and point to the need to investigate how DHA influences the actions of this system in bone and muscle.

The use of dietary manipulation of fatty acids that decreases AA levels and increases DHA in bone promotes bone formation (Watkins et al., 2000) and bone strength (Reinwald et al., 2004) in growing rats, and both dietary EPA + DHA (menhaden oil) and DHA alone conserve bone mineral in tibia and femur, respectively, in OVX rats (Watkins et al., 2005, 2006). Recently, we have reported that n-3 PUFA modifies the mRNA of receptors and biosynthetic and degradation enzymes of endogenous agonists of the EC system in osteoblast-like cells (Hutchins et al., 2009). In addition, DHA was found to reduce AA in specific cell and tissue compartments of murine muscle and bone (Watkins, unpublished findings) and to reduce cellular levels of AEA (Matias et al., 2008). Moreover, DHA may decrease osteoclast activity by decreasing AEA because this agonist is reported to stimulate osteoclast formation (Idris et al., 2008). The new findings demonstrating n-3 PUFA influence on the expression of EC receptors and enzymes are a promising area of investigation and will likely enhance our understanding of muscle and bone interactions to optimize health through lipid nutrition.

HUMAN STUDIES EVALUATING DIETARY N-3 PUFA ON BONE

Epidemiological studies on the relationship between dietary fatty acid intake and bone status in human subjects of various age groups confirm the concept that fatty acids are important modulators of skeletal health and that specific fatty acids, for example, n-3 and n-6 PUFA, affect bone metabolism differently. Rousseau and colleagues (2009) observed that in older adults aged 60 years and older (118 men and 129 women), higher self-reported n-3 PUFA intakes were positively related to femoral neck BMD. The mean reported intake of n-3 PUFA in this group of subjects was 1.27 g/day.

In a 6-year follow-up study of a cohort of 78 healthy young men (mean age 16.7 years at baseline), to evaluate factors that determine BMD, measurements of BMD (measured at baseline and at 22 years of age) of total body, hip, and spine and fatty acid concentrations (measured in the phospholipid fraction in serum at 22 years of age) showed that n-3 PUFA, especially DHA, were positively associated with BMD, and represented the peak BMD, in young men during this longitudinal study (Hogstrom et al., 2007).

In a follow-up study that measured BMD at baseline and 2 years later in 54 cystic fibrosis male and female patients (aged 6–33 years) and fatty acid composition of serum phospholipids, both EFA status and AA and DHA were associated with lumbar spine BMD Z-score (Gronowitz et al., 2006).

The BMD Z-score of lumbar spine was negatively correlated with the ratio of AA:DHA in serum phospholipids of children (n = 35, mean age in years after 2 years was 15.3 for boys and 13.9 for girls) but not in adults (n = 19). The lack of fatty acid associations with bone in adults is most likely because of significantly lower rates of bone growth, or a longer duration of study must be conducted (Gronowitz et al., 2006).

In a 2-year (mean 24.4 months) follow-up study of 22 recipients (22–65 years of age) of a first renal allograft, after 2 years, a strong positive correlation between the ratio of n-3 PUFA:AA in plasma phospholipids and BMD was observed (Baggio et al., 2005). The value calculated for n-3 PUFA in the ratio included EPA, DHA, and 22:5n-3. Based on multivariate regression analysis of the data, the femoral BMD change was negatively associated with AA in plasma phospholipids of the renal transplant patients (Baggio et al., 2005).

Several other human studies have examined the relationship of n-6 PUFA and bone mineral status. Eriksson et al. (2009) reported that serum fatty acid profiles are associated with bone mineralization in healthy 8-year-old children (50 boys and 35 girls). A general trend was that serum phospholipid LA (18:2n-6) was found to be negatively associated with BMD of total body and lumbar spine, and this same pattern was found for the total n-6 PUFA concentration and the ratio of n-6:n-3 PUFA.

Based on dietary intake from the Melbourne Collaborative Cohort Study, investigators examined dietary PUFA intakes with marrow and knee cartilage (Wang et al., 2008) in a cohort of 293 healthy adult subjects without knee pain or injury. The purpose of this study was to evaluate dietary fat intakes with predisease and early stages of osteoarthritis using magnetic resonance imaging as a diagnostic assessment of knee health. The researchers reported a significant association between n-6 PUFA intake and an increased risk of bone marrow lesions, suggesting the importance of maintaining an optimal balance between n-3 and n-6 PUFA in the diet (Wang et al., 2008).

In Spain, a case–control study (n = 167 with 1:1 matched controls) was conducted to examine the association of fatty acid intake and fracture risk in patients aged 65 years or older (80% women) suffering a low-energy fracture. Higher intakes of total PUFA and n-6 PUFA were reported to be associated with an elevated risk of fracture (p = .01 for the trend test), and a lower ratio of monounsaturated fatty acid:PUFA was associated with decreased fracture risk in these elderly subjects (Martinez-Ramirez et al., 2007).

Most studies examining the relationships of dietary intake or tissue levels of n-3 and n-6 PUFA in cell cultures or animals report some aspect of potential or confirmed regulatory function of these fatty acids on bone metabolism. In human subjects, especially in young individuals when bone formation rates are higher compared with adults, n-3 PUFA or a low ratio of n-6:n-3 PUFA in blood is positively associated with BMD and a negative association between n-6 PUFA or ratio of n-6:n-3 and BMD. In contrast, however, a study of aged Chinese patients undergoing elective orthopedic surgery (Griffith et al., 2009) did not find the same relationship between marrow fatty acids and BMD. In this study, the fatty acid composition of tissue samples of marrow fat and subcutaneous fat from 126 subjects (98 females, 34 males, mean age 69.7 ± 10.5 years) showed no difference in marrow fatty acid composition between subjects of varying BMD (normal, low bone mass, and osteoporosis). This study is confounded for any dietary association that could have taken place during bone growth that occurred in childhood and adolescence and remodeling of bone in adults. Also, a one-time measurement at the time of disease onset and orthopedic surgery is more likely to indicate changes after disease progression. An analysis of diet history or comparison with subjects who consumed diets that varied in types of fats would have improved the study, and it is less likely to observe a difference when BMD of lumbar spine is compared with the fatty acid composition of marrow samples taken from the femur.

Intervention studies in human subjects provide further support that n-3 PUFA intake is beneficial in reducing bone resorption and maintaining bone mass. Fish intake attenuated bone loss during long-term space flight, and higher n-3 PUFA intake led to lower N-telopeptide (NTx) urinary excretion during bed rest (Zwart et al., 2009). In a 6-week randomized 3-period crossover design study with 23 subjects, Griel et al. (2007) reported that supplementing diets with ALA from sources such as walnuts, walnut oil, and flaxseed oil significantly lowered the circulating NTx level (a reliable bone resorption marker), reflecting a protective effect of plant sources of dietary n-3 PUFA on bone metabolism via a decrease in bone resorption. Serum bone specific ALP activity, a bone formation marker, was not affected by the dietary treatments, which included an average American diet (control, ratio of n-6:n-3 PUFA = 9) and two high PUFA diets (one high in LA with a ratio of n-6:n-3 PUFA = 3.5 and the other high in ALA with a ratio of n-6:n-3 PUFA = 1.6).

STUDIES ON N-3 PUFA ACTIONS IN BONE CELL CULTURES

To elucidate the mechanism of n-3 PUFA action on bone metabolism, numerous research projects have been performed using the two major bone cell types (osteoblasts and osteoclasts) to reveal how these fatty acids affect bone metabolism on both the cellular and the genetic levels. Several studies have reported findings on the positive actions of n-3 PUFA as well as the negative influences asserted by the n-6 PUFA when in dietary abundance, specifically AA, on various cell culture models of osteoblasts. In a human osteoblast-like cell culture model, investigators (Musacchio et al., 2007) showed that both EPA and oleic acid increased gene expression of type I collagen and fibronectin, whereas AA diminished bone cell adhesion. In a study by Shen and coresearchers (2008), mouse bone marrow stromal cells (ST-2) were treated with AA, EPA, or ethanol as a control. AA treatment resulted in the highest value for PGE_2 production and elevated COX-2 mRNA expression in these ST-2 stromal cells. AA treatment also increased nitric oxide (NO) production in 7-day culture of these cells (early stage of osteoblastogenesis), whereas EPA showed a stronger stimulatory effect on NO production relative to AA treatment at near-mature osteoblast stages. The research implies that EPA could be supportive during early osteoblastogenesis through its suppressive actions on PGE_2 and the NO pathways. Osteoblast-derived NO has been suggested to mediate the localized bone destruction in certain inflammatory bone diseases (Hukkanen et al., 1995).

The process of osteoclastogenesis is known to be regulated, in part, by osteoblasts via the OPG/RANKL signaling system. OPG is a decoy receptor for RANKL, both produced by osteoblasts, but if RANK on preosteoclasts does not bind to RANKL, osteoclastogenesis is interrupted. In a study with MC3T3-E1 osteoblast-like cells (Coetzee et al., 2007), AA (5–20 μg/mL) treatment inhibited OPG secretion while stimulating the production of RANKL; however, this effect was attenuated by pretreatment with the COX inhibitor indomethacin, implying that PGE_2 is involved in the regulation of OPG/RANKL balance. In another study, EPA and DHA were shown to inhibit PGE_2-induced RANKL expression in MC3T3-E1 cells, implicating their antiosteoclastogenesis influence (Poulsen et al., 2008b). In cells not preinduced by PGE_2, neither EPA nor DHA showed any effect on RANKL expression. Some of these relationships and the role of n-3 PUFA in osteoclastogenesis are presented in Figure 16.3.

Many cell culture studies are showing a trend of distinct properties of n-3 and n-6 PUFA on osteoblast cell activity. However, because culture conditions are not consistent in the literature, some interpretation of data is difficult. As an example, one report that showed that ALP activity was inhibited when MC3T3-E1 osteoblast-like cells were exposed to either AA or DHA after short- and long-term exposure, although the mineralizing properties of these cells were not compromised under these conditions (Coetzee et al., 2009). Although cells were cultured for numerous days, and it is not clear if the high concentrations of fatty acids used in cell culture included albumin, the extended culture periods could have diminished osteoblast cell functions and protein synthesis because fatty acids (not bound to albumin) are toxic to cells in culture. More specific culturing conditions and physiological levels of fatty acids will help to resolve some of the inconsistent findings reported in the literature.

In addition to its influence on osteoclasts via its actions on osteoblasts, n-3 PUFA may also act upon osteoclasts directly by controlling their inflammatory responses in various testing models. Osteoclasts are recruited and activated upon the stimulation from osteoclastogenic cytokines that are increased in inflammatory joint disease, which leads to eventual bone destruction. In a cell culture study using the murine monocytic cell line RAW 264.7 (commonly used as an osteoclast precursor cell line), DHA was demonstrated to be much more effective than EPA in reducing RANKL-induced proinflammatory responses by decreasing TNFα production and the expressions of nuclear factor kappa B (NFκB) and p38 mitogen-activated protein kinases, factors that regulate the responses to inflammatory stimuli (Rahman et al., 2008). These findings suggest a great potential for DHA in decreasing osteoclast activation and bone resorption. In an experiment using the same preosteoclastic murine cell line RAW264.7, Zwart et al. (2009) reported that EPA inhibited NFκB activity and protein expression in a routine stationary culture as well as in a simulated microgravity system by culturing cells in a bioreactor that was rotated on a high aspect vessel that provides an environment in which the cells are in a continuous state of free fall, mimicking the state of weightlessness.

RECENT ANIMAL STUDIES SUPPORTING BENEFITS OF n-3 PUFA ON BONE

In animal feeding studies, n-3 PUFA have been shown to act alone or in concert with other dietary factors, such as isoflavones, estrogen, boron, and inulin, a prebiotic, to promote bone health. The animal models adopted in these experiments are mostly mouse and rat, and occasionally, pig and chicken. Although pure n-3 fatty acids (ALA, EPA, and DHA) are the best forms to be used in these feeding experiments (void of any confounding factors that originate from the diverse source of these fatty acids), for practical and economical reasons, oils (either of vegetables or marine fish) are the most common sources of n-3 PUFA used in the diets given to animals.

The effectiveness of various n-3 PUFA species, in particular, ALA, compared with the long chain, more biologically active EPA and DHA, is controversial because of its low conversion rate (0.2%) from ALA to EPA in healthy human subjects (Pawlosky et al., 2001). However, Sacco and coworkers demonstrated that ALA-rich flaxseed diet to OVX 3-month-old rats resulted in significantly higher levels of ALA and EPA and lower levels of LA, AA, and the ratio of n-6:n-3 PUFA compared with those of the control basal AIN-93M diet (Sacco et al., 2009). Furthermore, feeding these rats flaxseed (10% in the diet) plus a low-dose estrogen therapy (13 μg, 90-day release) led to the highest BMD and peak load at the lumbar vertebrae among the treatment groups; however, no such effect on BMD or bone strength was observed in the tibia and femur (Sacco et al., 2009). Another study (Poulsen et al., 2008a) found similar findings in an 18-week feeding experiment showing that dietary DHA (0.5 g/kg body weight/day) potentiated the mineral-sparing effect of 17β-estradiol (1 μg/day) in OVX rats. In either case, the combination treatment was more effective than either the n-3 PUFA or estrogen alone at maintaining bone mineral.

Fish oils are rich sources of long-chain n-3 PUFA EPA and DHA and have been widely used in both human and animal studies on their effectiveness in promoting and maintaining bone health. Most recent studies emphasize the synergistic or additive actions of n-3 PUFA from fish oil together with other nutritional factors. Feeding rats fish oil plus the prebiotic inulin-type fructans enhanced mineral absorption and resulted in increased BMC and bone strength in the tibia (Lobo et al., 2009). Others (Nielsen and Stoecker, 2009) showed that rats (either adequate or deficient in boron intake) fed fish oil had mechanically superior bones compared with the bones of those given safflower oil in the diet. Feeding OVX CD-1 mice fish oil (7% menhaden oil in the diet) led to higher BMD in lumbar vertebra, whereas combining fish oil with isoflavones (250 mg of genistein + 250 mg of daidzein/kg diet) resulted in a higher peak load of lumbar vertebra 4, showing that fish oil can act alone or potentiate the bone-protective effect of isoflavones (Ward and Fonseca, 2007).

Unlike any other animal model mentioned previously, the fat-1 mouse, a transgenic model that synthesizes n-3 PUFA from n-6 PUFA in its own tissue, provides a unique tool to illustrate how the same dietary source of fatty acids (safflower oil that contains about 70% LA and essentially void of any n-3 fatty acids) affects bone metabolism because of the different metabolic pathways the ingested fatty acids go through. In experiments with fat-1 mice and their wild-type counterparts (Lau et al., 2009a, 2009b), feeding an AIN-93 G diet containing 10% safflower oil from weaning until they were 12 weeks of age revealed that a lower ratio of n-6:n-3 PUFA was found in the vertebrae of fat-1 mice compared with the wild-type, and this ratio was negatively correlated with BMD and peak load in mechanical property testing, whereas total n-3 PUFA, including ALA, EPA, and

DHA, were positively correlated with BMD and the peak load in the vertebrae (Lau et al., 2009b). Similar findings were reported for the femur, suggesting that n-3 PUFA have a favorable effect on mineral accumulation and functional measures of bone in young mice (Lau et al., 2009a).

Differences have been established in how n-6 and n-3 PUFA affect bone metabolism in young modeling bone systems versus in older animals in which bone remodeling is the predominant process. In both animal and human studies, not only is n-3 PUFA (especially DHA) critical for bone mineral mass maintenance, but also AA is critical in bone mineral accretion during the rapid phase of growth that characterizes active bone modeling. Weiler et al. (2005) reported that whole-body BMC in human infants was positively predicted by cord RBC AA and that lumbar spine 1–4 and femur BMC was positively associated with cord RBC ratio of AA:EPA but negatively related to maternal DHA. This observation suggests the importance of a balanced maternal diet with respect to the n-6 and n-3 PUFA content of the diet. Furthermore, AA was found to be positively correlated with both total-body BMC and BMD in fast-growing Caucasian 8-year-old children (Eriksson et al., 2009). In animal studies, Kohut and coworkers reported that feeding low and very-low-birth-weight piglets a diet containing AA and DHA at a ratio of 6:1 (1.2 g AA + 0.2 g DHA/100 g dietary fat) for 15 days resulted in lowered bone resorption relative to the control group, whereas bone formation was not affected (Kohut et al., 2009).

STUDIES ON N-3 PUFA IN MODELS OF ARTHRITIS AND INFLAMMATION

The beneficial effects of n-3 PUFA EPA and DHA in alleviating symptoms of rheumatoid arthritis (RA) reside not only in their ability to change the eicosanoid precursors to those which are less inflammatory, compared with those derived from AA, that is, PGE_2, but also because both EPA and DHA give rise to resolvins that are anti-inflammatory and inflammation resolving (Calder, 2008). In addition, n-3 PUFA affect several other important aspects of immunity such as antigen presentation, T-cell reactivity, and inflammatory cytokine production that are important in RA development (Calder, 2008). Both intervention studies with n-3 long-chain PUFA and cross-sectional surveys support this notion. In a randomized double-blind placebo-controlled crossover study, 45 patients (43 females and 2 males) were divided into two groups and were given a placebo or n-3 long-chain PUFA-supplemented dairy products. At the end of the supplementation period (2 × 12 weeks), the n-3 long-chain PUFA supplements lowered triacylglycerol, decreased LPS-stimulated COX-2 expression, and suppressed the immune response as lymphocytes and monocytes were found to be significantly decreased in subjects who consumed the enriched dairy products (Dawczynski et al., 2009).

In rodent models of periodontitis, characterized by inflammation and infection of the ligaments and bones that support the teeth, n-3 PUFA have been shown to attenuate inflammation and minimize bone loss in the diseased area. In a feeding study using adult mice, diets containing 10% tuna oil resulted in significantly higher tissue n-3 PUFA concentrations in oral soft tissues compared with those in the control diet. Tuna oil also led to reductions in alveolar bone loss by more than 50% in mice with induced periodontitis compared with the control group that were fed a high n-6 PUFA Sunola oil (a sunflower oil with higher amount of monounsaturated fatty acids) diet, which exhibits an inverse relationship between alveolar bone loss and n-3 PUFA tissue levels (Bendyk et al., 2009). In a rat study using an LPS-induced periodontitis model, selective COX-2 inhibitor (Celecoxib), prophylactic n-3 PUFA, and a combination of these two agents inhibited gingival tissue MMP-8 expression, whereas the individual administration of therapeutic n-3 PUFA increased gingival TIMP-1 expression (Vardar-Sengul et al., 2008). Finally, one group (Hamazaki et al., 2006) reported a correlation between decreased tooth loss and EPA concentration in RBCs of humans.

CONCLUSIONS

Benefits of n-3 PUFA on bone modeling and remodeling have been shown in a number of human (Table 16.1) and animal (Table 16.2) investigations. A consistent observation in many, but not all, of these *in vivo* studies is that a negative relationship exists between n-6 PUFA and bone formation or BMD. It is not clear if the positive benefits from n-3 PUFA result from a reduction in the potency of the n-6 PUFA, that is, their negative effects on bone formation and resorption. Based on decades of research, the following questions must be addressed about the role of n-3 PUFA and bone.

What do we know after years of research on n-3 PUFA and bone biology? Early exposure of infants to DHA is vital for neural and retinal development, and in the case for children and young adults, DHA appears to support bone formation during modeling and the quality of mineral content. In mature adults, several positive relationships between bone quality and n-3 PUFA intakes are acknowledged, and in some cases, biomarkers of bone resorption are attenuated with the intake of n-3 PUFA.

Can we explain or better define the differences between n-3 PUFA (ALA, DHA, and EPA) and their individual actions on bone remodeling and modeling? Although an answer to this question is not yet possible, experimental data do support a role for DHA in promoting early bone growth, based on the positive observations in animals and what limited data are available for children. Certainly, the dietary studies in human subjects make a positive correlation between n-3 PUFA and bone quality measurements, and the data in animal studies suggest a biological basis for DHA in certain bone compartments and for bone formation. In contrast, some data in animals indicate that EPA is a potent n-3 PUFA that moderates the actions of AA and prostanoid production in bone that support osteoclastic activity (biochemical and gene expression). So, DHA and EPA appear to have different, but supporting, roles in bone metabolism throughout the life cycle. Also, an important balance between DHA and AA is vital to bone formation in the young so that replacing all n-6 PUFA with n-3 PUFA is not appropriate. The most optimal dietary ranges of n-6 and n-3 PUFA at the different stages of the life cycle remain to be determined.

What is the translational impact of the research on n-3 PUFA and bone? With convincing evidence that long-chain n-3 PUFA reduce cardiovascular disease, that DHA is essential for neural and retina development in the infant, and that positive associations of n-3 PUFA enhance bone health, a key role is emerging for the benefits of n-3 PUFA in bone metabolism. Future research with well-characterized test mixtures of PUFA and appropriate protocols for bone measurement endpoints should facilitate a better understanding of n-3 PUFA actions on bone in human subjects. Investigations of how EPA and DHA affect gene expression in both osteoblastogenesis and osteoclastogenesis are needed to advance the field. Discerning the relationships between the long-chain n-3 PUFA and eicosanoid production and the downstream signaling for these compounds may be critical for improving bone health. A final direction for this research is the study of n-3 PUFA actions in the endocannabinoid signaling pathways that impact muscle and bone physiology.

REFERENCES

Bab, I., Ofek, O., Tam, J., et al. 2008. Endocannabinoids and the regulation of bone metabolism. *J Neuroendocrinol* 20 Suppl 1:69–74.

Bab, I., and Zimmer, A. 2008. Cannabinoid receptors and the regulation of bone mass. *Br J Pharmacol* 153:182–8.

Baggio, B., Budakovic, A., Ferraro, A., et al. 2005. Relationship between plasma phospholipid polyunsaturated fatty acid composition and bone disease in renal transplantation. *Transplantation* 80:1349–52.

Barreiro, E., de la Puente, B., Busquets, S., et al. 2005. Both oxidative and nitrosative stress are associated with muscle wasting in tumour-bearing rats. *FEBS Lett* 579:1646–52.

Bartoccioni, E., Michaelis, D., and Hohlfeld, R. 1994. Constitutive and cytokine-induced production of interleukin-6 by human myoblasts. *Immunol Lett* 42:135–8.

Belec, L., Authier, F. J., Chazaud, B., et al. 1997. Interleukin (IL)-1 beta and IL-1 beta mRNA expression in normal and diseased skeletal muscle assessed by immunocytochemistry, immunoblotting and reverse transcriptase-nested polymerase chain reaction. *J Neuropathol Exp Neurol* 56:651–63.

Bendyk, A., Marino, V., Zilm, P. S., et al. 2009. Effect of dietary omega-3 polyunsaturated fatty acids on experimental periodontitis in the mouse. *J Periodontal Res* 44:211–6.

Blackwell, K. A., Hortschansky, P., Sanovic, S., et al. 2009. Bone morphogenetic protein 2 enhances PGE(2)-stimulated osteoclast formation in murine bone marrow cultures. *Prostaglandins Other Lipid Mediat* 90:76–80.

Calder, P. C. 2008. Session 3: Joint Nutrition Society and Irish Nutrition and Dietetic Institute Symposium on 'Nutrition and autoimmune disease' PUFA, inflammatory processes and rheumatoid arthritis. *Proc Nutr Soc* 67:409–18.

Carbo, N., Lopez-Soriano, J., Costelli, P. et al. 2000. Interleukin-15 antagonizes muscle protein waste in tumour-bearing rats. *Br J Cancer* 83:526–31.

Carmeli, E., Coleman, R., and Reznick, A. Z. 2002. The biochemistry of aging muscle. *Exp Geront* 37:477–89.

Coetzee, M., Haag, M., and Kruger, M. C. 2007. Effects of arachidonic acid, docosahexaenoic acid, prostaglandin E(2) and parathyroid hormone on osteoprotegerin and RANKL secretion by MC3T3-E1 osteoblast-like cells. *J Nutr Biochem* 18:54–63.

Coetzee, M., Haag, M., and Kruger, M. C. 2009. Effects of arachidonic acid and docosahexaenoic acid on differentiation and mineralization of MC3T3-E1 osteoblast-like cells. *Cell Biochem Funct* 27:3–11.

Dawczynski, C., Schubert, R., Hein, G., et al. 2009. Long-term moderate intervention with n-3 long-chain PUFA-supplemented dairy products: Effects on pathophysiological biomarkers in patients with rheumatoid arthritis. *Br J Nutr* 101:1517–26.

De Bleecker, J. L., Meire, V. I., Declercq, W., et al. 1999. Immunolocalization of tumor necrosis factor-alpha and its receptors in inflammatory myopathies. *Neuromuscul Disord* 9:239–46.

Eckardt, K., Sell, H., and Eckel, J. 2008. Novel aspects of adipocyte-induced skeletal muscle insulin resistance. *Archives Physiol Biochem* 114:287–98.

Ehrlich, P. J., and Lanyon, L. E. 2002. Mechanical strain and bone cell function: A review. *Osteoporos Int* 13:688–700.

Epker, B. N., and Frost, H. M. 1965. Correlation of bone resorption and formation with the physical behavior of loaded bone. *J Dental Res* 44:33–41.

Eriksson, S., Mellstrom, D., and Strandvik, B. 2009. Fatty acid pattern in serum is associated with bone mineralisation in healthy 8-year-old children. *Br J Nutr* 102:407–12.

Fernandes, G., Lawrence, R., and Sun, D. 2003. Protective role of n-3 lipids and soy protein in osteoporosis. *Prostaglandins Leukot Essent Fatty Acids* 68:361–72.

Fidler, N., and Koletzko, B. 2000. The fatty acid composition of human colostrum. *Eur J Nutr* 39:31–7.

Fricke, O., and Schoenau, E. 2007. The 'functional muscle–bone unit': Probing the relevance of mechanical signals for bone development in children and adolescents. *Growth Horm Igf Res* 17:1–9.

Frost, H. M. 1973. *Bone Modeling and Skeletal Modeling Errors*, vol. IV. Springfield, IL, Charles C. Thomas.

Frost, H. M. 2003a. Bone's mechanostat: A 2003 update. *Anat Rec A Discov Mol Cell Evol Biol* 275:1081–101.

Frost, H. M. 2003b. On the pathogenesis of osteogenesis imperfecta: Some insights of the Utah paradigm of skeletal physiology. *J Musculoskel Neuron Interact* 3:1–7.

Garg, A. K., and Aggarwal, B. B. 2002. Reactive oxygen intermediates in TNF signaling. *Mol Immunol* 39:509–17.

Giangregorio, L., and McCartney, N. 2006. Bone loss and muscle atrophy in spinal cord injury: Epidemiology, fracture prediction, and rehabilitation strategies. *J Spinal Cord Med* 29:489–500.

Godfrey, K. M., and Barker, D. J. 2000. Fetal nutrition and adult disease. *Am J Clin Nutr* 71:1344S–52S.

Godfrey, K. M., and Barker, D. J. 2001. Fetal programming and adult health. *Public Health Nutr* 4:611–24.

Gomes-Marcondes, M. C., and Tisdale, M. J. 2002. Induction of protein catabolism and the ubiquitin–proteasome pathway by mild oxidative stress. *Cancer Lett* 180:69–74.

Goossens, V., Grooten, J., De Vos, K., et al. 1995. Direct evidence for tumor necrosis factor-induced mitochondrial reactive oxygen intermediates and their involvement in cytotoxicity. *Proc Natl Acad Sci USA* 92:8115–9.

Gray, B., Hsu, J. D., and Furumasu, J. 1992. Fractures caused by falling from a wheelchair in patients with neuromuscular disease. *Dev Med Child Neurol* 34:589–92.

Griel, A. E., Kris-Etherton, P. M., Hilpert, K. F., et al. 2007. An increase in dietary n-3 fatty acids decreases a marker of bone resorption in humans. *Nutr J* 6:2.

Griffith, J. F., Yeung, D. K., Ahuja, A. T., et al. 2009. A study of bone marrow and subcutaneous fatty acid composition in subjects of varying bone mineral density. *Bone* 44:1092–6.

Grimble, R. F., and Tappia, P. S. 1998. Modulation of pro-inflammatory cytokine biology by unsaturated fatty acids. *Z Ernahrungswiss* 37:57–65.

Gronowitz, E., Lorentzon, M., Ohlsson, C., et al. 2008. Docosahexaenoic acid is associated with endosteal circumference in long bones in young males with cystic fibrosis. *Br J Nutr* 99:160–7.

Gronowitz, E., Mellstrom, D., and Strandvik, B. 2006. Serum phospholipid fatty acid pattern is associated with bone mineral density in children, but not adults, with cystic fibrosis. *Br J Nutr* 95:1159–65.

Haag, M., Magada, O. N., Claassen, N., et al. 2003. Omega-3 fatty acids modulate ATPases involved in duodenal Ca absorption. *Prostaglandins Leukot Essent Fatty Acids* 68:423–9.

Hamazaki, K., Itomura, M., Sawazaki, S., et al. 2006. Fish oil reduces tooth loss mainly through its antiinflammatory effects? *Med Hypotheses* 67:868–70.

Harrison, A. P., Rowlerson, A. M., and Dauncey, M. J. 1996. Selective regulation of myofiber differentiation by energy status during postnatal development. *Am J Physiol* 270:667–74.

Hogstrom, M., Nordstrom, P., and Nordstrom, A. 2007. n-3 Fatty acids are positively associated with peak bone mineral density and bone accrual in healthy men: The NO2 Study. *Am J Clin Nutr* 85:803–7.

Hukkanen, M., Hughes, F. J., Buttery, L. D., et al. 1995. Cytokine-stimulated expression of inducible nitric oxide synthase by mouse, rat, and human osteoblast-like cells and its functional role in osteoblast metabolic activity. *Endocrinology* 136:5445–53.

Hutchins, H. L., Zhao, D., Hannon, K. M., et al. 2009. Culture duration and PUFA treatment influence expression of endocannabinoid proteins in MC3T3-E1 osteoblast-like cells. *FASEB J* 23:543.

Idris, A. I., Sophocleous, A., Landao-Bassonga, E., et al. 2008. Regulation of bone mass, osteoclast function, and ovariectomy-induced bone loss by the type 2 cannabinoid receptor. *Endocrinology* 149:5619–26.

Idris, A. I., van't Hof, R. J., Greig, I. R., et al. 2005. Regulation of bone mass, bone loss and osteoclast activity by cannabinoid receptors. *Nat Med* 11:774–9.

Institute of Medicine. 2002. *Dietary References Intakes for Energy, Carbohydrate, Fiber, Fat, Fatty Acids, Cholesterol, Protein, and Amino Acids.* Washington, DC, The National Academies Press.

Judex, S., Boyd, S., Qin, Y., et al. 2003. Combining high-resolution micro-computed tomography with material composition to define the quality of bone tissue. *Curr Osteoporos Rep* 1:11–9.

Kang, J. X., and Weylandt, K. H. 2008. Modulation of inflammatory cytokines by omega-3 fatty acids. *Subcell Biochem* 49:133–43.

Khal, J., and Tisdale, M. J. 2008. Downregulation of muscle protein degradation in sepsis by eicosapentaenoic acid (EPA). *Biochem Biophys Res Commun* 375:238–40.

Kohut, J., Watkins, B., and Weiler, H. 2009. Enhanced lumbar spine bone mineral content in piglets fed arachidonic acid and docosahexaenoic acid is modulated by severity of growth restriction. *Br J Nutr* 102:1117–20.

Kondo, H., Nakagaki, I., Sasaki, S., et al. 1993. Mechanism of oxidative stress in skeletal muscle atrophied by immobilization. *Am J Physiol* 265:839–44.

Korotkova, M., Gabrielsson, B. G., Holmang, A., et al. 2005. Gender-related long-term effects in adult rats by perinatal dietary ratio of n-6/n-3 fatty acids. *Am J Physiol Regul Integr Comp Physiol* 288:575–9.

Korotkova, M., Ohlsson, C., Hanson, L. A., et al. 2004. Dietary n-6:n-3 fatty acid ratio in the perinatal period affects bone parameters in adult female rats. *Br J Nutr* 92:643–8.

Kris-Etherton, P. M., Taylor, D. S., Yu-Poth, S., et al. 2000. Polyunsaturated fatty acids in the food chain in the United States. *Am J Clin Nutr* 71:179S–88S.

Lau, B. Y., Ward, W. E., Kang, J. X., et al. 2009a. Femur EPA and DHA are correlated with femur biomechanical strength in young fat-1 mice. *J Nutr Biochem* 20:453–61.

Lau, B. Y., Ward, W. E., Kang, J. X., et al. 2009b. Vertebrae of developing fat-1 mice have greater strength and lower n-6/n-3 fatty acid ratio. *Exp Biol Med (Maywood)* 234:632–8.

Levine, B., Kalman, J., Mayer, L., et al. 1990. Elevated circulating levels of tumor necrosis factor in severe chronic heart failure. *N Engl J Med* 323:236–41.

Li, X., Moody, M. R., Engel, D., et al. 2000. Cardiac-specific overexpression of tumor necrosis factor-alpha causes oxidative stress and contractile dysfunction in mouse diaphragm. *Circulation* 102:1690–6.

Li, X., Pilbeam, C. C., Pan, L., et al. 2002. Effects of prostaglandin E2 on gene expression in primary osteoblastic cells from prostaglandin receptor knockout mice. *Bone* 30:567–73.

Li, Y., Greiner, R. S., Salem, N., Jr., et al. 2003a. Impact of dietary n-3 FA deficiency on rat bone tissue FA composition. *Lipids* 38:683–6.

Li, Y. P., Chen, Y., John, J., et al. 2005. TNF-alpha acts via p38 MAPK to stimulate expression of the ubiquitin ligase atrogin1/MAFbx in skeletal muscle. *Faseb J* 19:362–70.

Li, Y. P., Lecker, S. H., Chen, Y., et al. 2003b. TNF-alpha increases ubiquitin-conjugating activity in skeletal muscle by up-regulating UbcH2/E220k. *Faseb J* 17:1048–57.

Lingam, S., and Joester, J. 1994. Spontaneous fractures in children and adolescents with cerebral palsy. *BMJ* 309:265.

Lobo, A. R., Filho, J. M., Alvares, E. P., et al. 2009. Effects of dietary lipid composition and inulin-type fructans on mineral bioavailability in growing rats. *Nutrition* 25:216–25.

Martinez-Ramirez, M. J., Palma, S., Martinez-Gonzalez, M. A., et al. 2007. Dietary fat intake and the risk of osteoporotic fractures in the elderly. *Eur J Clin Nutr* 61:1114–20.

Matias, I., Carta, G., Murru, E., et al. 2008. Effect of polyunsaturated fatty acids on endocannabinoid and N-acyl-ethanolamine levels in mouse adipocytes. *Biochim Biophys Acta* 1781:52–60.

Mori, T. A., and Beilin, L. J. 2001. Long-chain omega 3 fatty acids, blood lipids and cardiovascular risk reduction. *Curr Opin Lipidol* 12:11–7.

Musacchio, E., Priante, G., Budakovic, A., et al. 2007. Effects of unsaturated free fatty acids on adhesion and on gene expression of extracellular matrix macromolecules in human osteoblast-like cell cultures. *Connect Tissue Res* 48:34–8.

Nielsen, F. H., and Stoecker, B. J. 2009. Boron and fish oil have different beneficial effects on strength and trabecular microarchitecture of bone. *J Trace Elem Med Biol* 23:195–203.

Ofek, O., Karsak, M., Leclerc, N., et al. 2006. Peripheral cannabinoid receptor, CB2, regulates bone mass. *Proc Natl Acad Sci USA* 103:696–701.

Ozdurak, R. H., Duz, S., Arsal, G., et al. 2003. Quantitative forearm muscle strength influences radial bone mineral density in osteoporotic and healthy males. *Technol Health Care* 11:253–61.

Pawlosky, R. J., Hibbeln, J. R., Novotny, J. A., et al. 2001. Physiological compartmental analysis of alpha-linolenic acid metabolism in adult humans. *J Lipid Res* 42:1257–65.

Poulsen, R. C., Firth, E. C., Rogers, C. W., et al. 2007. Specific effects of gamma-linolenic, eicosapentaenoic, and docosahexaenoic ethyl esters on bone post-ovariectomy in rats. *Calcif Tissue Int* 81:459–71.

Poulsen, R. C., Moughan, P. J., and Kruger, M. C. 2008a. Docosahexaenoic acid and 17 beta-estradiol co-treatment is more effective than 17 beta-estradiol alone in maintaining bone post-ovariectomy. *Exp Biol Med (Maywood)* 233:592–602.

Poulsen, R. C., Wolber, F. M., Moughan, P. J., et al. 2008b. Long chain polyunsaturated fatty acids alter membrane-bound RANK-L expression and osteoprotegerin secretion by MC3T3-E1 osteoblast-like cells. *Prostaglandins Other Lipid Mediat* 85:42–8.

Quinn, L. S., Haugk, K. L., and Grabstein, K. H. 1995. Interleukin-15: A novel anabolic cytokine for skeletal muscle. *Endocrinology* 136:3669–72.

Rahman, M. M., Bhattacharya, A., and Fernandes, G. 2008. Docosahexaenoic acid is more potent inhibitor of osteoclast differentiation in RAW 264.7 cells than eicosapentaenoic acid. *J Cell Physiol* 214:201–9.

Raisz, L. G., Alander, C. B., and Simmons, H. A. 1989. Effects of prostaglandin E3 and eicosapentaenoic acid on rat bone in organ culture. *Prostaglandins* 37:615–25.

Rauch, F., Bailey, D. A., Baxter-Jones, A., et al. 2004. The 'muscle–bone unit' during the pubertal growth spurt. *Bone* 34:771–5.

Reinwald, S., Li, Y., Moriguchi, T., et al. 2004. Repletion with (n-3) fatty acids reverses bone structural deficits in (n-3)-deficient rats. *J Nutr* 134:388–94.

Rousseau, J. H., Kleppinger, A., and Kenny, A. M. 2009. Self-reported dietary intake of omega-3 fatty acids and association with bone and lower extremity function. *J Am Geriatr Soc* 57:1781–8.

Sacco, S. M., Jiang, J. M., Reza-Lopez, S., et al. 2009. Flaxseed combined with low-dose estrogen therapy preserves bone tissue in ovariectomized rats. *Menopause* 16:545–54.

Saghizadeh, M., Ong, J. M., Garvey, W. T., et al. 1996. The expression of TNF alpha by human muscle. Relationship to insulin resistance. *J Clin Invest* 97:1111–6.

Sayer, A. A., and Cooper, C. 2005. Fetal programming of body composition and musculoskeletal development. *Early Hum Dev* 81:735–44.

Sayer, A. A., Syddall, H. E., Gilbody, H. J., et al. 2004. Does sarcopenia originate in early life? Findings from the Hertfordshire cohort study. *J Gerontol A Biol Sci Med Sci* 59:930–4.

Schoenau, E., and Frost, H. M. 2002. The "muscle–bone unit" in children and adolescents. *Calcif Tissue Int* 70:405–7.

Schulze, P. C., Gielen, S., Adams, V., et al. 2003. Muscular levels of proinflammatory cytokines correlate with a reduced expression of insulinlike growth factor-I in chronic heart failure. *Basic Res Cardiol* 98:267–74.

Scutt, A., and Williamson, E. M. 2007. Cannabinoids stimulate fibroblastic colony formation by bone marrow cells indirectly via CB2 receptors. *Calcif Tissue Int* 80:50–9.

Shen, C. L., Peterson, J., Tatum, O. L., et al. 2008. Effect of long-chain n-3 polyunsaturated fatty acid on inflammation mediators during osteoblastogenesis. *J Med Food* 11:105–10.

Shen, C. L., Yeh, J. K., Rasty, J., et al. 2006. Protective effect of dietary long-chain n-3 polyunsaturated fatty acids on bone loss in gonad-intact middle-aged male rats. *Br J Nutr* 95:462–8.

Shen, C. L., Yeh, J. K., Rasty, J., et al. 2007. Improvement of bone quality in gonad-intact middle-aged male rats by long-chain n-3 polyunsaturated fatty acid. *Calcif Tissue Int* 80:286–93.

Singhal, A., Cole, T. J., and Lucas, A. 2001. Early nutrition in preterm infants and later blood pressure: Two cohorts after randomised trials. *Lancet* 357:413–9.

Smith, H. J., Greenberg, N. A., and Tisdale, M. J. 2004. Effect of eicosapentaenoic acid, protein and amino acids on protein synthesis and degradation in skeletal muscle of cachectic mice. *Br J Cancer* 91:408–12.

Spate, U., and Schulze, P. C. 2004. Proinflammatory cytokines and skeletal muscle. *Curr Opin Clin Nutr Metab Care* 7:265–9.

Spiers, S., McArdle, F., and Jackson, M. J. 2000. Aging-related muscle dysfunction. Failure of adaptation to oxidative stress? *Ann N Y Acad Sci* 908:341–3.

Suda, K., Udagawa, N., Sato, N., et al. 2004. Suppression of osteoprotegerin expression by prostaglandin E2 is crucially involved in lipopolysaccharide-induced osteoclast formation. *J Immunol* 172:2504–10.

Tam, J., Ofek, O., Fride, E., et al. 2006. Involvement of neuronal cannabinoid receptor CB1 in regulation of bone mass and bone remodeling. *Mol Pharmacol* 70:786–92.

Tam, J., Trembovler, V., di Marzo, V., et al. 2008. The cannabinoid CB1 receptor regulates bone formation by modulating adrenergic signaling. *FASEB J* 22:285–94.

Taylor, D. J., Thompson, C. H., Kemp, G. J. et al. 1995. A relationship between impaired fetal growth and reduced muscle glycolysis revealed by 31P magnetic resonance spectroscopy. *Diabetologia* 38:1205–12.

Tisdale, M. J. 1996. Inhibition of lipolysis and muscle protein degradation by EPA in cancer cachexia. *Nutrition* 12:S31–33.

Tisdale, M. J. 2001. Loss of skeletal muscle in cancer: Biochemical mechanisms. *Front Biosci* 6:164–74.

Tisdale, M. J. 2002. Cachexia in cancer patients. *Nat Rev Cancer* 2:862–71.

Tisdale, M. J., and Dhesi, J. K. 1990. Inhibition of weight loss by omega-3 fatty acids in an experimental cachexia model. *Cancer Res* 50:5022–6.

Uauy, R., Hoffman, D. R., Peirano, P., et al. 2001. Essential fatty acids in visual and brain development. *Lipids* 36:885–95.

Valdez, H., and Lederman, M. M. 1997. Cytokines and cytokine therapies in HIV infection. *AIDS Clin Rev*187–228.

Vardar-Sengul, S., Buduneli, E., Turkoglu, O., et al. 2008. The effects of selective COX-2 inhibitor/celecoxib and omega-3 fatty acid on matrix metalloproteinases, TIMP-1, and laminin-5gamma2-chain immunolocalization in experimental periodontitis. *J Periodontol* 79:1934–41.

Wang, Y., Wluka, A. E., Hodge, A. M., et al. 2008. Effect of fatty acids on bone marrow lesions and knee cartilage in healthy, middle-aged subjects without clinical knee osteoarthritis. *Osteoarthritis Cartilage* 16:579–83.

Ward, W. E., and Fonseca, D. 2007. Soy isoflavones and fatty acids: Effects on bone tissue postovariectomy in mice. *Mol Nutr Food Res* 51:824–31.

Warren, G. L., Hayes, D. A., Lowe, D. A., et al. 1994. Eccentric contraction-induced injury in normal and hindlimb-suspended mouse soleus and EDL muscles. *J Appl Physiol* 77:1421–30.

Watkins, B. A., Jones, R., Li, Y., et al. 2007. Dietary long chain n-3 PUFA attenuates musculoskeletal atrophy associated with disuse in mice. *FASEB J* 21:A728.

Watkins, B. A., Li, Y., Allen, K. G. D., et al. 2000. Dietary ratio of (n-6)/(n-3) polyunsaturated fatty acids alters the fatty acid composition of bone compartments and biomarkers of bone formation in rats. *J Nutr* 130:2274–84.

Watkins, B. A., Li, Y., Lippman, H. E., et al. 2003. Modulatory effect of omega-3 polyunsaturated fatty acids on osteoblast function and bone metabolism. *Prostaglandins Leukot Essent Fatty Acids* 68:387–98.

Watkins, B. A., Li, Y., and Seifert, M. F. 2006. Dietary ratio of n-6/n-3 PUFAs and docosahexaenoic acid: Actions on bone mineral and serum biomarkers in ovariectomized rats. *J Nutr Biochem* 17:282–9.

Watkins, B. A., Lippman, H. E., Le Bouteiller, L., et al. 2001. Bioactive fatty acids: Role in bone biology and bone cell function. *Prog Lipid Res* 40:125–48.

Watkins, B. A., Reinwald, S., Li, Y., et al. 2005. Protective actions of soy isoflavones and n-3 PUFA on bone mass in ovariectomized rats. *J Nutr Biochem* 16:479–88.

Weiler, H., Fitzpatrick-Wong, S., Schellenberg, J., et al. 2005. Maternal and cord blood long-chain polyunsaturated fatty acids are predictive of bone mass at birth in healthy term-born infants. *Pediatr Res* 58:1254–8.

Weisinger, H. S., Armitage, J. A., Sinclair, A. J., et al. 2001. Perinatal omega-3 fatty acid deficiency affects blood pressure later in life. *Nat Med* 7:258–9.

Weiss, L. A., Barrett-Connor, E., and von Muhlen, D. 2005. Ratio of n-6 to n-3 fatty acids and bone mineral density in older adults: The Rancho Bernardo Study. *Am J Clin Nutr* 81:934–8.

Wohl, G. R., Loehrke, L., Watkins, B. A., et al. 1998. Effects of high-fat diet on mature bone mineral content, structure, and mechanical properties. *Calcif Tissue Int* 63:74–9.

Yamada, Y., Fushimi, H., Inoue, T., et al. 1995. Effect of eicosapentaenoic acid and docosahexaenoic acid on diabetic osteopenia. *Diabetes Res Clin Pract* 30:37–42.

Zwart, S. R., Pierson, D., Mehta, S., et al. 2009. Capacity of omega-3 fatty acids or eicosapentaenoic acid to counteract weightlessness-induced bone loss by inhibiting NF-kappaB activation: From cells to bed rest to astronauts. *J Bone Miner Res* 10.1359/JBMR091041.

17 Is There a Role for Dietary Potassium in Bone Health?

Susan Joyce Whiting

CONTENTS

INTRODUCTION

This chapter explores the question of the role of potassium in bone health, despite the specific reference to such an effect used in setting the current dietary reference intake recommendation for potassium by the Institute of Medicine (2005). Potassium has been associated with bone health (e.g., Lemann et al., 1989, 1991; Green and Whiting, 1994; Tucker et al., 1999; New et al., 2000; Jones et al., 2001; Sebastian et al., 2006) through its contribution to dietary alkalinity. Potassium is ingested mainly as a component of fruits and vegetables, but it is also found in lesser amounts in dairy foods, meats, and grains, especially whole grains. In Table 17.1, selected food sources of potassium in various food groups are shown. Unlike several nutrients that affect bone health directly through incorporation in bone mineral, such as calcium, phosphorus, magnesium, and fluoride, or through beneficial effects in bone cells, such as vitamins A, D, and K, potassium is classified as a nutrient which indirectly promotes bone health. Thus, uncertainty lies in whether a specific direct hypocalciuric effect of potassium exists or whether potassium serves primarily as a carrier for anions that promote bone health and also may possibly reduce sodium intake, assuming that potassium is consumed in its stead. In the former role, optimal potassium intake, but only as an alkaline salt, promotes the retention of calcium through countering the adverse effects of a mild metabolic acidosis that stimulates bone resorption. The latter role suggests that potassium itself plays no role and that several other cations (except sodium) are just as effective. This hypothesis is explored in this chapter in the context of bone health.

TABLE 17.1

Intakes of Nutrients Important for Bone Health according to Serving Sizes of Foods of the DASH Diet

Food Groups (Examples of a Serving)	DASH Diet (Minimum Servings/Day)	Approximate Calcium Intake (Not Fortified) (mg)	Approximate Sodium Intake (mg)	Approximate Potassium Intake (mg)	Approximate Protein Intake (g)
Milk products • Milk, 1% (250 mL—1 cup) • Cheese (50 g)	2	575	720	520	17
Grain products • Bread (1 slice) • Cereal (30 g—1 cup) • Rice (1 cup)	7	160	950	560	21
Vegetable group (raw leafy vegetable) • Lettuce (1 cup) • Spinach (1 cup)	4	200	100	970	6
Fruit group • Banana (medium size) • Orange (medium size) • Orange juice (1/2 cup)	4	95	10	1610	4
Meat • Lean meat (80 g) • Fish (80 g) • Poultry (80 g)	2 or less	50	135	550	19
Alternatives • Egg (1) • Cooked dry beans (125 g) • Tofu (100 g) • Peanut butter (2 tbsp—30 mL)	0.6 (4 servings / week from nuts, seeds, and dry beans)	30	35	180	8
Total	–	1110	1950[a]	4390	75

Source: Modified from Institute of Medicine. 2005. *Dietary Reference Intakes: Sodium, Chloride, Potassium and Sulphate.* National Academy Press, Washington, DC.

Notes: Calcium, potassium, and protein almost meet or exceed current recommendations, whereas sodium intake falls below its upper level. DASH diet = Dietary Approaches to Stop Hypertension diet.

[a] Consuming unsalted products reduces sodium intake further.

EFFECTS OF POTASSIUM ON CALCIUM METABOLISM

OBSERVATIONAL STUDIES OF POTASSIUM INTAKE AND BONE HEALTH

A role for dietary vegetables and fruit on bone health emerged in the literature. All age groups were implicated. For adults, several population-based studies reported that increased potassium intake through vegetables and fruits is associated with increased bone mineral density (BMD) (Tucker et al., 1999; New, 2003). Studies by New et al. (1997, 2000) of premenopausal British women found potassium as well as current and past intakes of fruit or milk to be positively associated with BMD. In the cross-sectional analyses performed by New and colleagues, generally, there were significant correlations between potassium intake (determined by food frequency questionnaire) and BMD at several skeletal sites, in contrast to calcium intake where a significant correlation was found at only one site. This and other findings indicated that fruit and vegetable intake was an important determinant for bone, possibly due to changes in acid–base status. Tucker et al. (1999) provided an epidemiologic examination of fruit and vegetable intake, as well as potassium content of the diet, on BMD. They used a cross-sectional as well as a prospective design, utilizing Framingham data from the 20th and 22nd visits. The age group was 69 to 97 years, and both men and women were included. Cross-sectional analyses showed that a greater potassium intake, a greater magnesium intake, as well as fruit and vegetable intake were significantly associated with greater BMD. The positive skeletal effects were observed at more bone sites for potassium, and magnesium intake was highly related to potassium intake (as their food sources are similar). Rates of change in bone loss were also examined. Potassium, magnesium, and fruit and vegetable intakes were related to a slower bone loss, but only in men. Thus, both cross-sectional and prospective research approaches provide strong evidence for a positive effect of potassium on BMD from fruit and vegetable intake.

A dietary plan promoting fruit and vegetable intake, the DASH (Dietary Approaches to Stop Hypertension) diet, emphasizes intake of vegetables, fruits, and low-fat diary products, and it avoids the consumption of processed foods (Table 17.1). A 3-month trial among 186 middle-aged men and women (Lin et al., 2003) reported that the DASH diet significantly reduced bone turnover, indicating that the DASH diet has beneficial effects on bone health (Doyle and Cashman, 2004). One disadvantage of using the DASH diet as evidence for a potassium effect is that the DASH diet incorporates many important healthful changes, that is, meeting calcium and protein recommendations (1000 mg and > 75 g, respectively) and keeping sodium intakes below the upper level of 2300 mg. High dietary sodium intakes cause hypercalciuria, which, in the absence of compensatory increases in enteric calcium absorption, would lead to negative calcium balance and loss of skeletal calcium. Overall, a diet rich in fruits and vegetables also supplies magnesium, vitamin C, polyphenols, and other plant compounds, which play roles in bone metabolism. As such, potassium may represent a marker for the beneficial components of such a healthful diet. Alternatively, potassium may be a marker for an alkaline-DASH diet, which has also been associated with both skeletal and cardiovascular health.

A recent study corroborates this dietary effect of increasing fruits and vegetables, thus improving potassium intakes. McTiernan and coworkers (2009) examined whether dietary advice to improve fruit and vegetable intake could improve indices of bone, that is, BMD, and falls. In the Women's Health Initiative Dietary Modification study, a low-fat and increased fruit, vegetable, and grain educational intervention in close to 50,000 postmenopausal women was evaluated with respect to incident hip, other site-specific, and total fractures and self-reported falls, and, in a subset, BMD. After an 8-year follow-up, the intervention group had a lower rate of reporting two or more falls than that of the comparison group. Thus, a dietary intervention which promoted increased fruit and vegetable consumption modestly reduced the risk of multiple falls and slightly lowered hip BMD of women.

In children, Jones et al. (2001) first reported cross-sectional data that showed a positive link between potassium from fruit and vegetable consumption and BMD in 10-year-old girls. Tylavsky et al. (2004), studying girls aged 8 to 13 years, also found a positive relationship of fruit and vegetable consumption to bone area and BMD. McGartland et al. (2004) examined whether usual intake of fruit and vegetable influenced BMD in boys and girls aged 12 and 15 years; they found a significantly higher heel BMD only in 12-year-old girls who consumed high amounts of fruit. In contrast, however, vegetable and fruit intake had a significant independent effect on total body bone mineral content (BMC), development in boys but not girls (Vatanparast et al., 2005). In the latter study, it was predicted that total body (BMC) could be increased by about 50 g in a boy who had 10 servings/day intake of vegetable and fruit compared with a boy who had only one serving/day of these plant sources. Together, these studies suggest that both boys and girls likely benefit from the added fruit and vegetable intake, and potentially a lifetime beneficial effect may result.

THE PALEOLITHIC DIET IMPLICATES A HIGH POTASSIUM DIET

The diet of Paleolithic humans has been proposed as a model for the amounts and types of foods and nutrients that humans have evolved to consume (Eaton, 2006). Many differences exist between that diet, which is high in plant-based foods and meat but low in grains and dairy, compared with modern diets. Relevant to the potassium hypothesis, the Paleolithic diet was high in potassium, high in bicarbonate-producing anions, extremely low in sodium (<5 mEq/day), yet high in protein (Sebastian et al., 2006). The Paleolithic diet is calculated to have a net base urinary production that induces a low-grade metabolic alkalosis, in contrast to the modern diet which is net acid producing and may generate a low-grade metabolic acidosis (Frassetto et al., 2008). For most of the past 200,000 years, hominids and modern humans have consumed the diet of hunter-gatherers; uncultivated plant food sources, intermittent animal sources of protein, and rarely cereal grains or legumes. With the advent of the agricultural age approximately 10,000 years ago, cereal-based diets became established, along with the ingestion of protein from domesticated animals. It is generally believed that the humans from earlier times such as the Paleolithic era had low incidence of chronic diseases including osteoporosis (Eaton, 2006; Sebastian et al., 2006). The Paleolithic diet has been estimated to contain 400 mEq (400 mmol) per day of potassium (Sebastian et al., 2006).

In contrast, the contemporary North American diet induces a mild metabolic acidosis through foods typically containing low amounts of bicarbonate precursors, high amounts of acid-forming protein, and a high sodium intake that can alter acid–base balance through "dilutional-type" acidosis caused by the expansion of extracellular fluid volume. Even cultivated cereal grains yield net acid on metabolism, and these foods displace potassium- and bicarbonate-precursor-rich plant foods (Frasseto et al., 2008). The ratio of inorganic salts of potassium to sodium chloride has also been reversed with this dietary shift. As potassium- and bicarbonate-precursor-rich plant food consumption has declined, sodium chloride has been increasingly consumed largely because of its use in food processing for specific functions, such as preservation and enhancement of taste (Frassetto et al., 2008). Thus, not only has a deficit of dietary potassium become commonplace in the modern diet, but also an excess intake of sodium chloride has become the rule, and an altered sodium-to-potassium ratio exists (see below).

ROLE OF THE ANION IN POTASSIUM STUDIES

STUDIES USING DIFFERENT POTASSIUM SALTS

In the early 1980s, several reports indicated that potassium salts were effective in the treatment of renal stone disease. For example, five male patients, with documented uric acid lithiasis, were given 60 mmol/day of potassium citrate for 3 weeks (Sakhaee et al., 1983), and during this period, their 24-hour urinary calcium significantly declined from the control level of 154 ± 47 mg/day by one third. Further investigation revealed, however, that providing any source of potassium would not produce hypocalciuria. Then, they compared the effects of different anions, that is, 80 mmol of potassium bicarbonate, potassium citrate, and potassium chloride, on the urine chemistries of eight patients with kidney stones (Sakhaee et al., 1991). After 2 weeks, 24-hour urinary calcium fell significantly during both potassium bicarbonate and potassium citrate administration: from 4.5 ± 1.0 to 3.0 ± 0.8 and 3.6 ± 1.0 mg/day, respectively. This study revealed that potassium chloride had no significant effect on reducing urinary calcium excretion, whereas bicarbonate and citrate salts had similar hypocalciuric actions. The finding that potassium chloride had no effect on urinary calcium loss suggests that either it is the anion associated with potassium that is the major dietary factor or that the anion accompanying the potassium can modify the response to potassium in some way.

One might predict that providing a source of citrate or bicarbonate would cause hypocalciuria, but that did not happen either. Lemann and coworkers compared potassium and sodium bicarbonate salts and then evaluated potassium versus sodium with either a fixed anion (chloride) or a metabolizable anion (bicarbonate). In their first study (Lemann et al., 1989), they gave 60 mmol/day of potassium bicarbonate to nine healthy males for 12 days. Twenty-four-hour urinary calcium declined significantly during treatment with potassium bicarbonate, that is, from 4.4 ± 2.0 (control) to 3.5 ± 1.9 mmol/day. Daily calcium balance also significantly improved from −2.3 ± 1.9 to 1.4 ± 1.8 mg with potassium but not sodium bicarbonate treatment. Lemann et al. (1991) then compared potassium and sodium bicarbonate salts, evaluating each cation (potassium vs. sodium) with either a fixed anion (chloride) or a metabolizable anion (bicarbonate). They gave 13 healthy adults 90 mmol/day in a crossover design, measuring 24-hour urinary excretion at day 5. A schematic depiction of the results is shown in Table 17.2. Differences in 24-hour urinary calcium excretion were significant in rank order of lowest calcium excretion: potassium bicarbonate < potassium chloride = sodium bicarbonate < sodium chloride. Fasting calcium excretion, a measure of bone resorption, was also significantly reduced during potassium bicarbonate administration. These data support the contention that alkaline potassium, but not potassium paired with chloride, may slow bone breakdown and conserve bone mass.

Depleting the body of potassium, independent of anion, promotes urinary calcium excretion. Lemann et al. (1991) examined the effect of removing either potassium bicarbonate or potassium chloride from the diet. Eight subjects were fed a formula diet low in potassium (2 mmol) for 5 days, which met their nutritional needs and contained added potassium as either potassium chloride or potassium bicarbonate at 1.0 mmol/kg/day. After a 5-day control period, the potassium salts were removed from the diet for 5 days and then reintroduced for a final 5-day recovery period. The removal of either potassium chloride or potassium bicarbonate from the diet resulted in a significant increase in urinary calcium excretion, which averaged 1.31 ± 0.25 mmol/day (p < .005) for both groups when potassium-depleted. Further evidence for the effect of potassium on urinary calcium was generated in a study of the effect of potassium depletion on essential hypertension (Krishna and Kapoor, 1991). In this randomized, crossover study, 12 patients were given either a placebo or potassium chloride (80 mmol/day) for 10 days, with a background dietary intake of only 16 mmol potassium. Urinary calcium was significantly lower during the potassium depletion phase (placebo)

TABLE 17.2
The Effect of Various Combinations of Salts from Two Cations, Potassium or Sodium and Two Anions, a Nonmetabolizable One (Chloride) or a Metabolizable One (Bicarbonate)

Cation	Anion	Effect on Urinary Calcium Excretion
Sodium	Chloride	↑
Sodium	Bicarbonate	↔
Potassium	Chloride	↔
Potassium	Bicarbonate	↓

Note: Data represent results from a study of these salts on calcium balance and calcium excretion in human volunteers.

Source: Lemann, J.J., Pleuss, J.A., Gray, R.W., and Hoffman, R.G., *Kidney Int*, 39, 973–83, 1991.

than during potassium chloride administration. These studies suggest that potassium deficiency may be an important determinant of bone loss and that this role is independent of its anion.

THE ALKALINE POTASSIUM HYPOTHESIS

The Paleolithic diet is suggested to be the model for preserving bone integrity through its high potassium and bicarbonate precursors. This idea has led to the alkaline potassium hypothesis in which dietary potassium at levels of 400 mmol/day (close to five times the current adequate intake [AI] for potassium) are advocated to maintain bone integrity due to counter the high acid-forming potential of the modern Western diet (Sebastian et al. 2002, 2006). Frassetto and coworkers (2008) have suggested that the modern diet is low in alkaline potassium which in turn is coupled with an excess of acid-forming compounds as well as of sodium chloride, which promotes an increase in urinary potassium excretion. These factors are considered to make major contributions to the pathogenesis of age-related disorders, including hypertension, renal stones, and osteoporosis.

To return to a more favorable ratio of potassium (K) to sodium (Na) in the diet, that is, to a ratio that is comparable with what humans ate in preagricultural diets, both an increase in potassium and an avoidance or severe restriction of sodium chloride are necessary (Frassetto et al., 2008). They proposed that the diet can return to its evolutionary norms of net base production inducing low-grade metabolic alkalosis and a high potassium-to-sodium ratio by (1) greatly reducing content of energy-dense nutrient-poor foods and potassium-poor acid-producing cereal grains, which would entail increasing consumption of potassium-rich net-base-producing fruits and vegetables for maintenance of energy balance, and (2) greatly reducing sodium chloride consumption. Recent food guide revisions have reduced the amount of cereal grains servings and increased the amounts of fruit and vegetable servings, for example, Eating Well with Canada's Food Guide (released in 2007) and MyPyramid (released in 2005). Both of these food guides resemble the DASH diet. As illustrated in Table 17.1, the DASH diet (and food guides that resemble it) is probably the "best" dietary pattern that can be achieved today using largely unprocessed foods available in the marketplace. By following the DASH diet, one can attain a dietary Na:K ratio of approximately 1:1. This ratio is a marked improvement over dietary intakes that typically occur, i.e., ~2:1, in the United States and Canada. Recent dietary surveys indicate that sodium intakes are higher than the upper level for sodium of 2.3 g and much lower than the AI for potassium of 4.7 g in Canada (Dolega-Cieszowski et al., 2006) and the United States (U.S. Department of Agriculture, 2008).

CAN POTASSIUM BE REPLACED BY OTHER CATIONS?

The adverse effect of chloride on calcium retention has been related to the provision of a nonmetabolizable anion, in contrast to citrate which is a metabolic bicarbonate precursor. Barzel (1995), in making a recommendation for taking calcium carbonate, indicated that both the calcium and the carbonate would be beneficial to bone. This recommendation leads to the question: can the cation in a alkaline potassium salt be replaced by other cations (except sodium, as noted above)? Recently, the question of potassium versus calcium has been investigated.

Karp and coworkers (2009) compared the effects of calcium carbonate, calcium citrate, and potassium citrate on markers of calcium and bone metabolism in young women. At the beginning of each of four 24-hour measurements, subjects received a single dose of calcium carbonate (calcium = 1000 mg), calcium citrate (calcium = 1000 mg), potassium citrate (potassium = 2250 mg; citrate equal to that of calcium citrate), or a placebo in random order. Potassium citrate and calcium carbonate significantly decreased the bone resorption marker N-terminal collagen peptide (Figure 17.1). The results suggest that potassium citrate has a positive effect on bone despite the low calcium intake during the session. These results suggest that a diet high in fruits and vegetables is protective to bone in the short-term. However, a low calcium diet cannot be replaced by alkaline

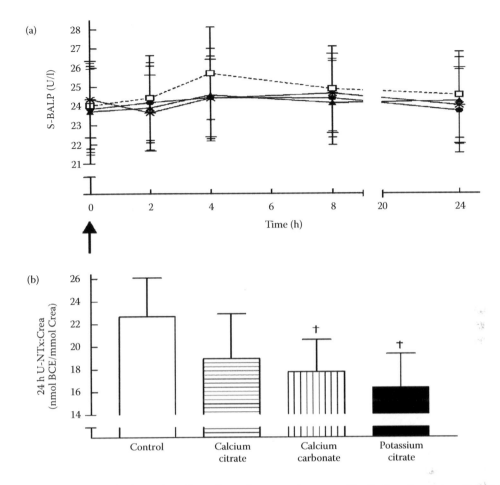

FIGURE 17.1 Changes in the marker of bone formation, serum bone-specific alkaline phosphatase (S-BALP) activity (a), and the marker of bone resorption 24-hour urinary excretion of N-terminal telopeptide of type I collagen (U-NTx/Crea) (b) during the four study sessions in young women. A: control (□), calcium citrate (▲), calcium carbonate (*), potassium citrate (●). The supplement administration time is indicated with an arrow. The supplements did not affect S-BALP (marker of bone formation) but did affect 24-hour U-NTx/Crea (marker of bone resorption as indicated by symbol [+]); (a) indicates significantly different from control session. Crea = creatinine. (From Karp, H.J., et al., *Br J Nutr* 102, 1341–1347, 2009. With permission.)

potassium in the long-term, as indicated by studies in which vegetarians having a low calcium intake were found to have low bone mass (Barr et al., 1998).

POTASSIUM'S ROLE IN BONE EXAMINED

THE AI VALUE FOR POTASSIUM

The current recommended intake for potassium for those aged 14 years and over is 4.7 g (120 mmol) (Institute of Medicine 2005). This value is an AI, meaning that not enough evidence was available to set an estimated average requirement. The criterion for setting this high AI value was to help blunt the salt sensitivity prevalent in African American men and to decrease the risk of kidney stones in the entire population. Also, an indication that "higher levels of potassium intake from foods are associated with decreased bone loss" had an impact in arriving at the potassium AI (Institute of Medicine, 2005). A further statement emphasized that "the beneficial effects of potassium ... [are] from the forms of potassium that are associated with bicarbonate precursors." Although these caveats are important, they do not get readily incorporated into tables where dietary recommendations are provided. As shown in Table 17.1, it is possible to achieve the AI for potassium, but it requires a diet emphasizing fruits and vegetables and lacking in packaged and most processed foods, such as the DASH diet, to achieve an intake even close to the AI value.

Potassium Salts versus Fruits and Vegetables

Few studies have directly compared the effects of an alkaline potassium salt associated with the ingestion of fruits and vegetables. Macdonald and coworkers (2008) completed a trial of potassium from either citrate or fruit and vegetable consumption in postmenopausal women. This randomized controlled trial, blinded for two levels of potassium citrate against a placebo, involved 276 women and lasted 2 years. Results from the trial were disappointing in that neither the potassium salt nor the additional fruits and vegetables improved bone turnover markers. One possible reason for the lack of an effect of the potassium salt was that habitual dietary calcium was likely to be adequate, that is, atypically low. Similarly, the women may have already been consuming fairly adequate numbers of servings of fruits and vegetable, which meant that the effect of ingesting more could not be detected. Compliance of study participants is also an issue for investigating dietary change. Thus, it may be difficult to conclude that an increase in fruit and vegetable intake, or an increase in alkaline potassium salts, has beneficial long-term effects on bone. Hopefully, better study designs in the future will be able to overcome some of the common limitations of these investigations.

Does Potassium Intake Alone Predict Bone Health?

Several lines of evidence suggest that the relationship between potassium and preservation of bone mass is not straightforward. In establishing the definition of the AI value, the Institute of Medicine stressed that potassium intake should be obtained from foods, that is, fruits and vegetables, that provide potassium with bicarbonate precursors. Nevertheless, one would still expect that if potassium intake is protective to bone mass, then a good relationship between potassium intake and maintenance of bone should exist during aging. Rafferty et al. (2005) tested this relationship under steady-state conditions, using data from a total of 644 inpatient balance studies. Dietary potassium was highly significantly associated with urinary calcium excretion in a negative direction; yet, dietary potassium was negatively correlated with calcium absorption, and the effect of potassium on urinary calcium was lost when adjusted for enteric calcium absorption. The authors concluded that dietary potassium does not seem to exert a net positive influence on calcium retention. The source of potassium in these subjects was primarily from milk and meat, indicating that when the alkaline precursors were not with potassium, then potassium has no net effect on bone.

A second line of evidence suggests that potassium itself is not the "active" part of alkaline potassium salts, according to a study from Dawson-Hughes and coinvestigators (2009). Unlike other studies in which bone loss or gain was attributed to changes in urinary calcium excretion alone, the Dawson-Hughes et al. study used changes in bone resorption markers to determine the effects of potassium on bone. In this study, 171 older adults (>50 years) were randomized to receive 67.5 mmol potassium bicarbonate (equivalent to 2600 mg potassium), sodium bicarbonate, potassium chloride, or a placebo. Subjects were measured at entry and after 3 months. The investigators were thus able to examine the effects of the anion (bicarbonate vs. chloride) and of the cation (sodium vs. potassium). Results are shown in Figure 17.2. Potassium chloride clearly did not prevent bone resorption, in contrast to potassium bicarbonate. The authors concluded that bicarbonate alone is the active component protecting against the loss of bone mineral, that is, calcium. However, the results with respect to sodium bicarbonate were equivocal because the skeletal effect of the bicarbonate was less than that of potassium bicarbonate, as previously reported (Lemann et al., 1989, 1991; Green and Whiting, 1994). Theoretically, the sodium cation may have caused an increase in urinary calcium excretion, which would nullify the beneficial effect of the

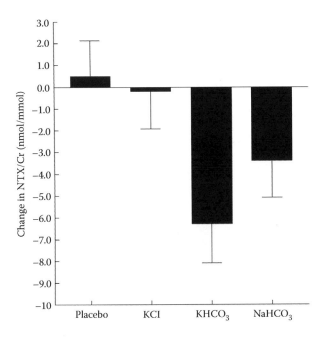

FIGURE 17.2 Mean 3-month change in the marker of bone resorption urinary N-terminal telopeptide of type I collagen NTX per creatinine (Cr) excretion by treatment group, adjusted for sex and baseline NTX/Cr. Subjects were men and women over 50 years old. (From Dawson-Hughes, B., et al., *J Clin Endocrinol Metab* 94, 96–102, 2009. With permission.)

bicarbonate anion on bone remodeling. Obviously, the use of sodium bicarbonate as an alkalizing food ingredient or supplement would not be desirable.

CONCLUSIONS

The question addressed in this chapter was whether dietary potassium intake plays a role in bone health. From depletion studies, it is apparent that low levels of potassium, which could arise from low intakes, contribute to an increase in calcium excretion and, thus, promote bone loss via resorption should a negative calcium balance persist. This effect is independent of anion. Therefore, adequate dietary potassium is required for optimal bone health. However, the question is often phrased as being whether a higher than typical potassium intake is required for bone health, that is, one that is similar to or higher than the current recommendation of 4700 mg. Here, attention has been given to the concept that alkaline potassium salts promote calcium retention. This concept arose from two lines of research: (1) epidemiological studies in which fruit and vegetable intake was demonstrated to be positive for BMD or other markers of bone health and (2) experimental studies either in laboratory animals or human volunteers showing that alkaline potassium salts promoted a more positive calcium balance or reduced markers of bone resorption, in comparison with alkaline sodium salts or with acid-forming potassium salts. The data, however, are not so clear-cut as higher potassium intake does not always protect against bone loss. Also, the question has arisen as to whether the alkaline salt must have potassium as the cation, although sodium clearly would not benefit bone health because of other mechanisms. Thus, current recommended intake (AI) for potassium of 4700 mg (120 mmol) for 14 years and older, which is based, in part, on the alkaline potassium hypothesis, is providing an optimal cation level, but this cation does not have to be potassium. Meeting this high level of potassium necessitates choosing a healthy diet emphasizing fruits and vegetables, such as the DASH diet, Canada's Food Guide, and MyPyramid. This dietary choice, and not intake of an alkaline potassium salt, ensures that bone health is optimized.

REFERENCES

Barr, S.I., Prior, J.C., Janelle, K.C., et al. 1998. Spinal bone mineral density in premenopausal vegetarian and nonvegetarian women: Cross-sectional and prospective comparisons. *J Am Diet Assoc* 98:760–765.

Barzel, U. 1995.The skeleton as an ion exchange system: Implications for the role of acid–base imbalance in the genesis of osteoporosis. *J Bone Miner Res* 10:1431–1436.

Dawson-Hughes, B., Harris, S.S., Palermo, N.J., et al. 2009. Treatment with potassium bicarbonate lowers calcium excretion and bone resorption in older men and women. *J Clin Endocrinol Metab* 94:96–102.

Dolega-Cieszowski, J., Bobyn, P.J., and Whiting, S.J. 2006. Dietary Intakes of Canadians in the 1990s using population weighted data derived from the Provincial Nutrition Surveys. *Appl Physiol Nutr Metab* 31:753–758.

Doyle, L., and Cashman, K.D. 2004. The DASH diet may have beneficial effects on bone health. *Nutr Rev* 62:215–220.

Eaton, S.B. 2006. The ancestral human diet: What was it and should it be a paradigm for contemporary nutrition? *Proc Nutr Soc* 65:1–6.

Frassetto, L.A., Morris, C.R., Sellmeyer, D.E., et al. 2008. Adverse effects of sodium chloride on bone in the aging human population resulting from habitual consumption of typical American diets. *J Nutr* 138:419S–422S.

Green, T.J., and Whiting, S.J. 1994. Potassium bicarbonate reduces high protein-induced hypercalciuria in adult men. *Nutr Res* 14:991–1002.

Institute of Medicine. 2005. *Dietary Reference Intakes: Sodium, Chloride, Potassium and Sulphate*. National Academy Press, Washington, DC.

Jones, G., Riley, M.D., and Whiting, S.J. 2001. Association between urinary potassium, urinary sodium, current diet, and bone density in prepubertal children. *Am J Clin Nutr* 73:839–844.

Karp, H.J., Ketola, M.E., and Lamberg-Allardt, C.J. 2009. Acute effects of calcium carbonate, calcium citrate, and potassium citrate on calcium and bone metabolism in young women. *Br J Nutr* 102:1341–1347.

Krishna, G.G., and Kapoor, S.C. 1991. Potassium depletion exacerbates essential hypertension. *Ann Int Med* 115:77–83.

Lemann, J.J., Gray, R.W., and Pleuss, J.A. 1989. Potassium bicarbonate, but not sodium bicarbonate, reduces urinary calcium excretion and improves calcium balance in healthy men. *Kidney Int* 35:688–695.

Lemann, J.J., Pleuss, J.A., Gray, R.W., and Hoffman, R.G. Potassium administration decreases and potassium deprivation increases urinary calcium excretion in healthy adults. *Kidney Int* 39:973–983.

Lin, P.H., Ginty, F., Appel, L.J., et al. 2003. The DASH diet and sodium reduction improve markers of bone turnover and calcium metabolism in adults. *J Nutr* 133:3130–3136.

Macdonald, H.M., Black, A.J., Aucott, L., et al. 2008. Effect of potassium citrate supplementation or increased fruit and vegetable intake on bone metabolism in healthy post menopausal women: A randomized controlled trial. *Am J Clin Nutr* 88:465–474.

McGartland, C.P., Robson, P.J., Murray, L.J., et al. 2004. Fruit and vegetable consumption and bone mineral density: The Northern Ireland Young Hearts Project. *Am J Clin Nutr* 80:1019–1023.

McTiernan, A., Wactawski-Wende, J., Wu, L.L., et al. 2009. Low-fat, increased fruit, vegetable, and grain dietary pattern, fractures, and bone mineral density: The Women's Health Initiative Dietary Modification Trial. *Am J Clin Nut* 89:1864–1876.

New, S.A. 2003. Intake of fruit and vegetables: Implications for bone health. *Proc Nutr Soc* 62:889–899.

New, S.A., Boulton-Smith, C., Grubb, D.A., et al. 1997 Nutritional influences on bone mineral density: A cross-sectional study in premenopausal women. *Am J Clin Nutr* 65:1831–1839.

New, S.A., Robins, S.P., Campbell, M.K., et al. 2000. Dietary influences on bone mass and bone metabolism: Further evidence of a positive link between fruit and vegetable consumption and bone health. *Am J Clin Nutr* 71:142–151.

Rafferty, K., Davies, M., and Heaney, R.P. 2005. Potassium intake and the calcium economy. *J Am Coll Nutr* 24:99–106

Sakhaee, K., Alpern, R., Jacobson, H.R., et al. 1991. Contrasting effects of various potassium salts on renal citrate excretion. *J Clin Endocrinol Metab* 72:396–400.

Sakhaee, K., Nicar, M., Hill, K., et al. 1983. Contrasting effects of potassium citrate and sodium citrate on urinary chemistries and crystallization of stone-forming salts. *Kidney Int* 24:348–352.

Sebastian, A., Frassetto, L.A., Sellmeyer, D.E., et al. 2002. Estimation of the net acid load of the diet of ancestral preagricultural *Homo sapiens* and their hominid ancestors. *Am J Clin Nutr* 76:1308–1316.

Sebastian, A., Frassetto, L.A., Sellmeyer, D.E., et al. 2006. The evolution-informed optimal dietary potassium intake of human beings greatly exceeds current and recommended intakes. *Sem Nephrol* 26:447–453.

Tucker, K.L., Chen, H., Hannan, M.T., et al. 1999. Potassium, magnesium, and fruit and vegetable intakes are associated with greater bone mineral density in elderly men and women. *Am J Clin Nutr* 69:727–736.

Tylavsky, F.A., Holliday, K., Danish, R.K., et al. 2004. Fruit and vegetable intake is an independent predictor of bone mass in early-pubertal children. *Am J Clin Nutr* 79:311–317.

U.S. Department of Agriculture, Agricultural Research Service. 2008. *Nutrient Intakes from Food: Mean Amounts Consumed per Individual, One Day, 2005–2006*. Available at www.ars.usda.gov/ba/bhnrc/fsrg

Vatanparast, H., Whiting, S.J., Baxter-Jones, A., et al. 2005. The positive effect of vegetable and fruit consumption on bone mineral accrual of boys during growth from childhood to adolescence in the University of Saskatchewan Pediatric Bone Mineral Accrual Study. *Am J Clin Nutr* 82:700–706.

18 Acid–Base Balance

Susan A. Lanham-New

CONTENTS

INTRODUCTION

Nutritional strategies for optimizing bone health throughout the life cycle are vital because prevention of osteoporosis rather than its treatment is the preferred approach. As an exogenous factor, nutrition is amenable to change and has relevant public health implications and hence deserves special attention. With the growing increase in the age of life expectancy, that is, 1:4 in the adult population will be aged 65 years and over by 2030, hip fractures are predicted to rise exponentially in the next decade and hence an urgent need for the implementation of public health strategies to target prevention of poor skeletal health on a population-wide basis. The role that the skeleton plays in acid–base homeostasis has been gaining increasing prominence in the literature over the last few decades. Theoretical considerations of the role alkaline bone mineral may play in the defense against acidosis date as far back as the late 19th century. Natural, pathological, and experimental states of acid loading/acidosis have long been associated with hypercalciuria and negative calcium balance. More recently, the detrimental effects of acid from the diet on bone mineral have been demonstrated.

At the cellular level, a reduction in extracellular pH has been shown to have a direct effect on osteoclastic activity, resulting in increased resorption pit formation in bone. Although scientists thought that vegetarianism may be protective against bone loss, studies over the last two decades have demonstrated that such an eating practice is not protective. The amount of dietary alkali in vegetarian diets, however, may be a key component obtained from the consumption of high-potassium, high-bicarbonate foods, such as fruits and vegetables. A low intake of dietary acidity has been shown to be protective to the skeleton, and numerous observational, experimental, clinical, and intervention studies, over the last decade have supported a positive link between fruit-and-vegetable consumption and preservation of the skeleton. Further research on fracture prevention, particularly with respect to the influence of dietary manipulation using alkali-forming foods, is required.

FUNDAMENTALS OF ACID–BASE MAINTENANCE: CRITICALITY TO HEALTH

> Life is a struggle, not against sin, not against the money power, not against malicious animal magnetism, but against hydrogen ions.
>
> **H.L. Mencken, 1880–1956**

As noted by Kraut and Coburn (1994), these famous words by Mencken in the early 20th century about the meaning of life and death may also apply to the struggle of the healthy skeleton against the deleterious effects of retained acid. As shown in Figure 18.1, acid–base homeostasis is critical to health. The pH of extracellular fluid ranges between 7.38 and 7.42, and it is a major challenge to the body's balance to defend against changes in hydrogen ion (H+ ion) concentrations between 0.035 and 0.045 mEq/L (Green and Kleeman, 1991). Maintaining the H+ concentration within such narrow limits is essential to survival, and the body's adaptive response involves three specific mechanisms: (1) buffer systems, (2) exhalation of CO_2, and (3) kidney excretion. On a daily basis, humans eat substances that both generate and consume H+ ions (protons), and as a net result, adult humans on a normal Western diet generate ~1 mEq of acid (as H+ ions) per kilogram lean body mass (LBM) per day. The more acid precursors a diet contains, the greater the degree of systemic acid load (Kurtz et al., 1983). Furthermore, as people age, the overall renal function declines, including the ability to excrete hydrogen ion (acid) in the form of ammonium ion (Frassetto et al., 1996a). Thus, with increasing age, humans become significantly (albeit slightly) more acidic (Frassetto et al., 1996b), that is, less than pH 7.38, which is the lower end of the normal range. The question arises: Should not the elderly with reduced ammoniagenesis and decreased H+ secretion defend normal pH by increasing pulmonary ventilation and thus decrease their pCO_2? Probably not. So, the elderly with decreased H+ ion excretory capacity likely depend on bone to buffer the retained H+ ions and

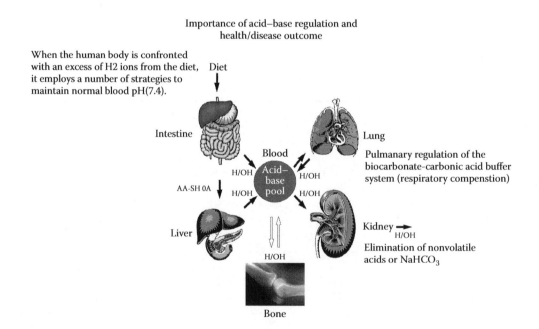

FIGURE 18.1 Acid–base homeostasis: The components of the control of blood and tissue pH are critical to life. (*Source*: Green, J. and Kleeman, R., *Kidney Int*, 39, 9–26, 1991. With permission.)

present with hypercalciuria even in the face of a normal arterial pH of 7.40. This point, however, has not been adequately addressed by current research.

A Role for the Skeleton in Acid–Base Homeostasis: Early Reports

The theoretical considerations of the role alkaline bone mineral may play in the defense against acidosis go as far back as the late 1880s (Goto, 1918; Irving and Chute, 1933; Albright and Reifenstein, 1948). In those early years, a number of studies were published that provided evidence that in natural (e.g., starvation), pathological (e.g., diabetic acidosis), and experimental (e.g., ammonium chloride ingestion) metabolic acidosis caused by fixed acid loading, an association exists between H+ ion loading on one hand and hypercalciuria and negative calcium balance on the other (Gastineau et al., 1960; Reidenberg et al., 1966). The pioneering work of Jacob Lemann and Uriel Barzel over 30 years ago showed extensively the effects of acid from the diet on bone mineral in both man and in the animal model (Lemann et al., 1966; Barzel, 1969).

In the 1960s, Wachman and Bernstein (1968) put forward a hypothesis linking the daily diet to the development of osteoporosis based on the role of bone in acid–base balance. They hypothesized "the increased incidence of osteoporosis with age may represent, in part, the results of a life-long utilisation of the buffering capacity of the basic salts of bone for the constant assault against pH homeostasis" (Wachman and Bernstein, 1968). The intake of acid is a way of everyday life, and it is known that animal proteins but also cereals and grains are rich sources of phosphoric and sulfuric acid and are recognized as acid ash foods (Barzel and Massey, 1998). Sources of the net production of acid are H+ ions produced by endogenous cell metabolism and from dietary proteins and other components. A gross quantitative relationship exists between the amount of acid generated from dietary protein sources (as reflected by urine pH) and the amount of acid ash consumed in the diet.

Quantitative Loss of Bone: Ratio of Calcium to Fixed Acid Load

Chronic metabolic acidosis exists, such as resulting from distal tubular renal acidosis (d-RTA), and is associated with hypercalciuria and loss of considerable amounts of skeletal calcium. Under such high degrees of hydrogen ion retention and resultant systemic metabolic acidosis, 2 mEq of Ca/kg/day is required to buffer each mEq of fixed acid/kg/day; over a period of 10 years (and assuming a total body Ca of approximately 1 kg), this would account for 15% loss of inorganic bone mass in an average individual (Widdowson et al., 1951). To lessen the skeletal calcium loss from high dietary acid exposure in d-RTA, the consumption of a diet consisting of large quantities of fruit and vegetables, that is, alkaline ash diet, may be important for bone health maintenance. Although unproven, this diet may also benefit skeletal health in older persons in the general population with age-related defects in renal H+ ion secretion (Barzel, 1995).

SYSTEMIC ACIDOSIS AND THE SKELETON: POTENTIAL MECHANISMS OF ACTION?

The novel work by Arnett and Dempster in 1986 demonstrated a direct enhancement of osteoclastic activity following a reduction in extracellular pH, an effect that was independent of parathyroid hormone (Arnett and Dempster, 1986, 1990; Arnett et al., 1994). Osteoclasts and osteoblasts appear to respond independently to small changes in pH in the culture media in which they are growing (Kreiger et al., 1992), and evidence exists that a small drop in pH, close to the lower limit of the physiological range, causes a tremendous burst in bone resorption (Arnett and Spowage, 1996; Bushinsky, 1996). The recent work by Arnett's group has shown that metabolic acidosis stimulates resorption by activating mature osteoclasts already present in calvarial bone rather than by inducing formation of new osteoclasts (Meghji et al., 2001). Almost all the bone mineral, that is, calcium and phosphate ions, released in response to acidosis results from osteoclast activation and increased formation of resorption pits on bone surfaces. Also, the organic matrix is destroyed at the same time (Dr. T.R. Arnett, University College London, personal communication). Some evidence has been reported that excess hydrogen ions directly induce physicochemical calcium release from bone (Bushinsky et al., 1994), but most agree that osteoclasts must be involved.

VEGETARIANISM AND SKELETAL HEALTH

Following the recognition of the role that bone plays in acid–base balance and the hypothesis linking diet to osteoporosis, it was proposed that long-term ingestion of vegetable-based diets may have a beneficial effect on bone mineral mass. In general, the earlier studies (published before 1990) appeared to support the hypothesis that plant foods had positive effects on bone, that is, bone mineral mass was found to be higher in the vegetarian group compared with their omnivorous counterparts (Table 18.1) (Ellis et al., 1972; Marsh et al., 1980, 1983, 1988; Tylavsky and Anderson, 1988; Hunt et al., 1989). However, two important points concerning these data require consideration. First, a fundamental error existed in the interpretation of the photographic density measurements in the first article published by Ellis et al. (1972); their conclusions should have been the opposite of what they claimed (Meema, 1973; Ellis et al., 1974; Meema, 1996; Barzel, 1996). Second, many subjects in several of the published studies were Seventh-Day Adventists who had a different lifestyle compared with that of the omnivorous group. The lifestyle variable was likely to have had an important confounding influence because almost all SDAs refrained from smoking and taking alcohol and caffeine and their physical activity levels were higher than those of comparator omnivores.

Studies published in the last two decades suggest no differences in BMD between vegetarians and omnivores (Lloyd et al., 1991; Tesar et al., 1992; Reed et al., 1994) (Table 18.2). In a 5-year prospective study of changes in radial bone density of elderly white American women, no differences were seen in bone loss rates between the lacto-ovo vegetarians and the omnivorous group (Reed et al., 1994). Furthermore, in the most recently published studies, bone mass was found to be significantly lower in the Asian vegetable-based dietary groups (Chiu et al., 1997; Lau et al., 1998), although it is likely that protein undernutrition may account for some of these differences (Rizzoli et al., 1998). In a recent meta-analysis of vegetarianism and bone, Ho-Pham and colleagues (2009) found no clinically significant effects of vegetarianism on bone health, and in

TABLE 18.1
Vegetarianism and Bone Health—Review of Earlier Work (Pre-1989)

Author	Year	Journal Source	Key Findings	Overall Summary
Ellis et al.	1972	*Am J Clin Nutr* 25: 555–558	BMD ↑ in vegetarian group	✓
Ellis et al.	1974	*Am J Clin Nutr* 27: 769–770	BMD ↓ in vegetarian group	✗
Mazess and Mather	1974	*Am J Clin Nutr* 27: 916–919	BMC ↓ in North Alaskan Eskimos	✓
Mazess and Mather	1975	*Human Biol* 47: 45	BMC ↓ in Canadian Eskimos	✓
Marsh et al.	1980	*JAMA* 76: 148–151	Bone loss ↑ in omnivores	✓
Marsh et al.	1983	*Am J Clin Nutr* 37: 453–456	BMD ↑ in vegetarians	
Marsh et al.	1988	*Am J Clin Nutr* 48: 837–841	BMD ↑ in elderly vegetarians	✓
Tylavsky et al.	1988	*Am J Clin Nutr* 48: 842–849	No difference in BMD between groups	–
Hunt et al.	1989	*Am J Clin Nutr* 50: 517–523	No difference in BMD between groups	–

TABLE 18.2
Vegetarianism and Bone Health: Summary of Studies—Later Work (1990 and Beyond)

Author	Year	Source	Findings	Summary
Lloyd et al.	1991	*Am J Clin Nutr* 54: 1005–1010	No difference in BMD between groups	–
Tesar et al.	1992	*Am J Clin Nutr* 56: 699–704	No difference in BMD between groups	–
Reed et al.	1994	*Am J Clin Nutr* 59: 1997–1202	Bone loss rates similar	–
Chui et al.	1997	*Calcified Tissue Int* 60: 245–249	BMD ↓ in vegan group	×
Lau et al.	1998	*Eur J Clin Nutr* 52: 60–64	Hip BMD lower in vegetarian group	×
Ho-Pham et al.	2009	*Am J Clin Nutr* 90: 943–950	Meta-analysis—no clinically significant difference	–

an accompanying editorial, it was concluded that vegetarianism is not a significant risk factor for osteoporosis (Lanham-New, 2009).

OMNIVORES AND BONE HEALTH

Very few studies have focused attention with respect to bone health on populations consuming a diet highly dependent on animal foods, particularly that of meat (Hammond and Storey, 1970). Mazess and Mather (1974) examined the bone mineral content of forearm bones in a sample of 217 children, 89 adults, and 107 elderly Eskimo natives of the north coast of Alaska (Mazess and Mather, 1974). After the age of 40 years, the Eskimos of both sexes were found to have a deficit of bone mineral of 10% to 15% relative to white standards. An even greater aging bone loss was found in Canadian Eskimos (Mazess and Mather, 1975). The issue of dietary change among the Eskimo population, particularly the increased utilization of refined carbohydrates, was raised (Mann, 1975), but the high-acid ash diet based on animal meat was considered a major factor contributing to bone loss of Eskimo adults. Clearly, these findings are of considerable interest to the interaction between diet and bone in the regulations of systemic acid–base balance, and further work in this area is clearly warranted (New, 2001a).

QUANTIFYING THE ACIDITY OF FOODS: POTENTIAL RENAL ACID LOAD

Of considerable interest is the finding that vegetable-based proteins generate a large amount of acid in the urine. The work by Remer and Manz (1995) examining the potential renal acid loads (PRALs) of a variety of foods has found that many grain products and some cheeses have a high PRAL level (Remer and Manz, 1995) (Table 18.3). These foods, which are likely to be consumed in large quantities by lacto-ovo vegetarians, may provide an explanation for the lack of a positive effect on bone health indices in studies comparing lacto-ovo vegetarians versus omnivores.

NET ENDOGENOUS ACID PRODUCTION AND ITS EFFECTS ON BONE

Determination of the acid–base content of diets consumed by individuals and populations groups is a useful way forward concerning the role of the skeleton in acid–base homoeostasis. Because 24-hour urine collections, considered as the gold standard for acid–base research, are difficult to perform in large population-based studies, an alternative approach is to examine the net acid content of the diet. Research from Sebastian et al. (1990) has found that the protein-to-potassium ratio predicts net acid excretion, and in turn, net renal acid excretion predicts calcium excretion.

TABLE 18.3
Potential Renal Acid Load (PRAL) Values of a Variety of Foods and Food Groups

Food/Food Group	PRAL mEq/100 g Edible Portion
Cheese with high protein content	26.4
Meat and meat products	9.5
Cheese with low protein content	8.0
Bread	3.5
Milk and non-cheese products	1.0
Fruits and fruit juices (without dried fruit)	−3.1
Vegetables	−2.8

Source: Adapted from Remer, T. and Manz, F., *J Am Diet Assoc*, 95, 791–7, 1995.

They proposed a simple algorithm to determine the net rate of endogenous noncarbonic acid production (NEAP) from considerations of the acidifying effect of protein and the alkalizing effect of potassium (Frassetto et al., 1998). High intakes of NEAP have been shown to be associated with poorer indices of bone health throughout the life cycle (New et al., 2004). In the most recent meta-analysis of protein and bone, Darling and coworkers (2009) have shown that the overriding finding is that animal protein is positively associated with bone health (Kerstetter, 2009), yet other reports have shown that too much animal protein in the diet may also result in increased acid generation and bone loss.

INTERPRETATIONS

The diet of the modern-age human is widely believed to be considerably different from that consumed by our Paleolithic ancestors (Eaton and Konner, 1985). Reflections on the dietary content of preagricultural man estimate intakes of sodium to be 2 to 5 mEq/day and potassium to be at levels reaching 200 mEq/day. This ratio is in stark contrast to current dietary data that estimate population intakes of sodium and potassium at levels of approximately 170 and 65 mEq/day, respectively, in the United Kingdom, United States, and Australia. Eaton and coinvestigators (1996) stated that the kidneys of our hunter-gatherer ancestors were designed to excrete potassium and conserve sodium. This evolutionary mechanism still exists despite the almost total dietary reversal of consuming more sodium than potassium; hence the term "today's diet, yesterday's genes" is most fitting. Although our Paleolithic forbears occasionally ate animal protein, their choice of foods was predominantly fruits, vegetables, and other plant sources. This alkali ash diet meant that they had lower renal H+ excretory demands than that of humans living over the last 10,000 years when agriculture and animal husbandry has flourished.

CONCLUSIONS

The evidence currently available from experimental, clinical, and observational studies suggests a role for the skeleton in acid–base balance. An acidic dietary load appears to have an adverse effect on the retention of bone mass, whereas an alkaline dietary load appears to help conserve bone mass. Future research should focus attention on intervention trials centered specifically on fruits and vegetables as the supplementation vehicle and assessing a wide range of bone health indices, including fracture risk. Reanalyses of existing dietary and bone mass/metabolism datasets to examine, in particular, the impact of dietary acidity on the skeleton, also are valuable data sources for future research.

REFERENCES

Albright, F., and Reifenstein, E.C., Jr. 1948. *The Parathyroid Glands and Metabolic Bone Disease.* Williams and Wilkins, Baltimore, 241–247.

Arnett, T.R., Boyde, A., Jones, S.L., et al. 1994. Effects of medium acidification by alteration of carbon dioxide or bicarbonate concentrations on the resorptive activity of rat osteoclasts. *J Bone Miner Res* 9: 375–379.

Arnett, T.R., and Dempster, D.W. 1986. Effect of pH on bone resorption by rat osteoclasts in vitro. *Endocrinology* 119: 119–124.

Arnett, T.R., and Dempster, D.W. 1990. Perspectives: Protons and osteoclasts. *J Bone Miner Res* 5: 1099–1103.

Arnett, T.R., and Spowage, M. 1996. Modulation of the resorptive activity of rat osteoclasts by small changes in extracellular pH near the physiological range. *Bone* 18: 277–279.

Barzel, U.S. 1969. The effect of excessive acid feeding on bone. *Calcif Tissue Res* 4: 94–100.

Barzel, U.S. 1995. The skeleton as an ion exchange system: Implications for the role of acid–base imbalance in the genesis of osteoporosis. *J Bone Miner Res* 10: 1431–1436.

Barzel, U.S. 1996. Nevertheless, an acidogenic diet may impair bone. *J Bone Miner Res* 11: 704. [Letter]

Barzel, U.S., and Massey, L.K. 1998. Excess dietary protein can adversely affect bone. *J Nutr* 128: 1051–1053.

Bernstein, D.S., Wachman, A., and Hattner, R.S. 1970. Acid–base balance in metabolic bone disease. In *Osteoporosis*, Barzel, U.S., ed. Grune and Stratton, New York, 207–216.

Bushinsky, D.A. 1996. Metabolic alkalosis decreases bone calcium efflux by suppressing osteoclasts and stimulating osteoblasts. *Am J Physiol (Renal Fluid Electrolyte Physiol)* 271: F216–F222.

Bushinsky, D.A., Lam, B.C., Nespeca, R., et al. 1993. Decreased bone carbonate content in response to metabolic, but not respiratory, acidosis. *Am J Physiol (Renal Fluid Electrolyte Physiol)* 265: F530–F536.

Chiu, J.F., Lan, S.J., Yang, C.Y., et al. 1997. Long term vegetarian diet and bone mineral density in postmenopausal Taiwanese women. *Calcif Tissue Int* 60: 245–249.

Darling, A.L., Millward, D.M., Torgerson, D.T., et al. 2009. Dietary protein and bone health: A systematic review and meta-analysis. *Am J Clin Nutr* 90: 1674–1692.

Eaton, B.S., Eaton, B.S., III, Konner, M.J., et al. 1996. An evolutionary perspective enhances understanding of human nutritional requirements. *J Nutr* 126: 1732–1740.

Eaton, B.S., and Konner, M. 1985. Paleolithic nutrition. A consideration of its nature and current implications. *New Engl J Med* 312: 283–290.

Ellis, F.R., Holesh, S., and Ellis, J.W. 1972. Incidence of osteoporosis in vegetarians and omnivores. *Am J Clin Nutr* 25: 555–558.

Ellis, F.R., Holesh, S., and Sanders, T.A 1974. Osteoporosis in British vegetarians and omnivores. *Am J Clin Nutr* 27: 769–770.

Frassetto, L.A., Morris, R.C., Jr., and Sebastian, A. 1996a. Effect of age on blood acid–base composition in adult humans: Role of age-related renal functional decline. *Am J Physiol (Renal Fluid Electrolyte Physiol)* 271: F1114–F1122.

Frassetto, L.A., and Sebastian, A. 1996b. Age and systemic acid–base equilibrium: Analysis of published data. *J Gerontol* 51A: B91–B99.

Frassetto, L., Todd, K., Morris, R.C., Jr., et al. 1998. Estimation of net endogenous noncarbonic acid production in humans from dietary protein and potassium contents. *Am J Clin Nutr* 68: 576–583.

Gastineau, C.F., Power, M.H., and Rosevear, J.W. 1960. Metabolic studies of a patient with osteoporosis and diabetes mellitus: Effects of testosterone enanthate and strontium lactate. *Proc Mayo Clin* 35: 105–111.

Goto, K. 1918. Mineral metabolism in experimental acidosis. *Journal Biol Chem* 36: 355–376.

Green, J., and Kleeman, R. 1991. Role of bone in regulation of systematic acid–base balance. *Kidney Int* 39: 9–26. [Editorial Review]

Hammond, R.H., and Storey, E. 1970. Measurement of growth and resorption of bone in rats fed meat diet. *Calcif Tissue Res* 4: 291.

Ho-Pham, L.T., Nguyen, D.N., and Nguyen, T.V. 2009. Effect of vegetarian diets on bone mineral density: A Bayesian meta-analysis. *Am J Clin Nutr* 90: 943–950.

Hunt, I.F., Murphy, N.J., Henderson, C, et al. 1989. Bone mineral content in postmenopausal women: Comparison of omnivores and vegetarians. *Am J Clin Nutr* 50: 517–523.

Irving, L., and Chute, A.L. 1933. The participation of the carbonates of bone in the neutralisation of ingested acid. *J Cell Comp Physiol* 2: 157.

Kerstetter, J.E. 2009. Dietary protein and bone: A new approach to an old problem. *Am J Clin Nutr* 90: 1451–1452. [Editorial]

Kraut, J.A., and Coburn, J.W. 1994. Bone, acid and osteoporosis. *New Engl J Med* 330: 1821–1822.

Kreiger, N.A., Sessler, N.E., and Bushinsky, D.A. 1992. Acidosis inhibits osteoblastic and stimulates osteoclastic activity in vitro. *Am J Physiol* 262: F442–F448.

Kurtz, I., Maher, T., Hulter, H.N., et al. 1983. Effect of diet on plasma acid–base composition in normal humans. *Kidney Int* 24: 670–680.

Lanham-New, S.A. 2009. Is "vegetarianism" a serious risk factor for osteoporotic fracture? *Am J Clin Nutr* 90: 910–911. [Editorial]

Lau, E.M., Kwok, T., Woo, J., et al. 1998. Bone mineral density in Chinese elderly female vegetarians, vegans, lactoovovegetarians and omnivores. *Eur J Clin Nutr* 52: 60–64.

Lemann, J., Jr., Adams, N.D., and Gray, R.W. 1979. Urinary calcium excretion in humans. *New Engl J Med* 301: 535–541.

Lemann, J., Jr., Litzow, J.R., and Lennon, E.J. 1967. Studies of the mechanisms by which chronic metabolic acidosis augments urinary calcium excretion in man. *J Clin Invest* 46: 1318–1328.

Lloyd, T., Schaeffer, J.M., Walker, M.A., et al. 1991. Urinary hormonal concentrations and spinal bone densities of premenopausal vegetarian and nonvegetarian women. *Am J Clin Nutr* 54: 1005–1010.

Mann, G. 1975. Bone mineral content of North Alaskan Eskimos. *Am J Clin Nutr* 28: 566–567. [Letter]

Marsh, A.G., Sanchez, T.V., Chaffee, F.L., et al. 1983. Bone mineral mass in adult lactoovovegetarian and omnivorous males. *Am J Clin Nutr* 83: 155–162.

Marsh, A.G., Sanchez, T.V., Micklesen, O., et al. 1980. Cortical bone density of adult lactoovovegetarians and omnivorous women. *J Am Diet Assoc* 76: 148–151.

Marsh, A.G., Sanchez, T.V., Michelsen, O., et al. 1988. Vegetarian lifestyle and bone mineral density. *Am J Clin Nutr* 48: 837–841.

Mazess, R.B., and Mather, W.E. 1974. Bone mineral content of North Alaskan Eskimos. *Am J Clin Nutr* 27: 916–925.

Mazess, R.B., and Mather, W.E. 1975. Bone mineral content in Canadian Eskimos. *Human Biol* 47: 45.

Meema, H.E. 1973. Photographic density versus bone density. *Am J Clin Nutr* 26: 687. [Letter]

Meema, H.E. 1996. What's good for the heart is not good for the bones? *J Bone Miner Res* 11: 704. [Letter]

Meghji, S., Morrison, M.S., Henderson, B., et al. 2001. PH dependence of bone resorption: Mouse calvarial osteoclasts are activated by acidosis. *Am J Physiol (Endocrinol and Metab)* 280: E112–E119.

Mencken, H. L. 1880–1956. www.quotationspage.com

New, S.A. 2001a. Nutrition, exercise and bone health. *Proc Nutr Soc* 60(2): 265–274.

New, S.A. 2001b. Impact of food clusters on bone. In *Nutritional Aspects of Osteoporosis 2000*, Dawson-Hughes, B., Burckhardt, P., and Heaney, R.P., eds. *Challenges of Modern Medicine*. Proceedings of the 4th International Symposium on Nutritional Aspects of Osteoporosis. Ares-Serono Symposia Publications, Academic Press, London, 379–397.

New, S.A., MacDonald, H.M., Campbell, M.K., Martin, J.C., Garton, M.J., Robins, S.P., and Reid, D.M. 2004. Lower estimates of net endogenous non-carbonic acid production are positively associated with indexes of bone health in premenopausal and perimenopausal women. *AM J Clin Nutr* 79: 131–138.

Reed, J.A., Anderson, J.J.B., Tylavsky, F.A., et al. 1994. Comparative changes in radial bone density of elderly female lactoovovegetarians and omnivores. *Am J Clin Nutr* 59: 1197S–1202S.

Reidenberg, M.M., Haag, B.L., Channick, B.J., et al. 1966. The response of bone to metabolic acidosis in man. *Metabolism* 15: 236–241.

Remer, T., and Manz, F. 1995. Potential renal acid load of foods and its influence on urine pH. *J Am Diet Assoc* 95: 791–797.

Rizzoli, R., Schurch, M.A., Chevalley, T., et al. 1998. Protein intake and osteoporosis. In *Nutritional Aspects of Osteoporosis 1997*, Burckhardt, P., Dawson-Hughes, B., Heaney R.P., eds. Proceedings of the 3rd International Symposium on Nutritional Aspects of Osteoporosis. Ares-Serono Symposia Publications, Springer-Verlag, New York, 141–154.

Sebastian, A., Hernandez, R.E., Portale, A.A., et al. 1990. Dietary potassium influences kidney maintenance of serum phosphorus concentrations. *Kidney Int* 37: 1341–1349.

Tesar, R., Notelovitz, M., Shim, E., et al. 1992. Axial and peripheral bone density and nutrient intakes of postmenopausal vegetarian and omnivorous women. *Am J Clin Nutr* 56: 699–704.

Tylavsky, F., and Anderson, J.J.B. 1988. Bone health of elderly lactoovovegetarian and omnivorous women. *Am J Clin Nutr* 48: 842–849.

Wachman, A., and Bernstein, D.S. 1968. Diet and osteoporosis. *Lancet* I: 958–959.

Widdowson, E.M., McCance, R.A., and Spray, C.M. 1951. The chemical composition of the human body. *Clin Sci* 10: 113–125.

Wood, R.J. 1994. Potassium bicarbonate supplementation and calcium metabolism in postmenopausal women: Are we barking up the wrong tree? *Nutr Rev* 52: 278–280.

19 Antioxidants and Bone Health

Martin Kohlmeier

CONTENTS

INTRODUCTION

Antioxidants have long been touted as an insurance against cancer, cardiovascular disease, and other chronic ailments. Much less attention has been given to the ability of antioxidants to protect against accelerated bone mineral loss and bone fracture. Now that robust evidence has burst the bubble of exuberant expectations for the health benefits of antioxidants, more sober considerations still point to an important role of antioxidants in foods for the protection of bone health. Consistent experimental and clinical evidence leaves little doubt that several food-derived antioxidants protect critical events in bone cell differentiation and function. The most important question for every individual is then whether additional intakes can improve bone health and reduce fracture risk. A slowly growing number of high-quality human studies can now provide some answers and guide the selection of healthy foods for strong bones.

This chapter reviews the known effects of the antioxidants in human bone, and some questions about what is not known are raised.

PHYSICOCHEMICAL AND METABOLIC FEATURES OF ANTIOXIDANTS

Antioxidants are defined by their ability to neutralize or otherwise counteract oxidants, such as reactive oxygen molecules (superoxide anion, hydrogen peroxide, and the hydroxyl radical), transition metals (particularly, iron and copper), hypochlorite, and reactive nitrogen compounds (e.g., peroxynitrite). Some of these oxidants are free radicals, meaning that they contain unpaired electrons. All of them are highly reactive, with the potential for damaging DNA, proteins, and lipids. Several vital processes naturally generate significant amounts of free radicals. The super-oxide anion, for instance, is a regular side product of oxidative phosphorylation due to unavoid-able mechanistic inefficiencies (Sun and Trumpower, 2003). Intense and prolonged physical exertion (Hattori et al., 2009) slightly increases the release of reactive oxygen species (ROS). Significant amounts of ROS also come from the breakdown of purines (superoxide anion gen-erated by xanthine oxidase), the production of prostanoid mediators (peroxides leaked from lipoxygenases), and the cellular immune response (myeloperoxidase-generated hypochlorous acid and hypobromous acid). Macrophages and eosinophils release highly corrosive bursts of hypochlorous acid and hypobromous acid, which can neutralize bacteria and parasites. These natural immune defense reactions highlight the fact that several oxidants have important physi-ological functions.

Harmful amounts of free radicals also come from exposure to external influences. Both active (Bloomer, 2007) and passive (Valkonen and Kuusi, 2000) cigarette smoke inhalation constitutes a particularly consequential source. Exposure to industrial pollutants, such as polycyclic aro-matic hydrocarbons and toluene, is another potential inducer of ROS, usually in a work-related context.

Oxidant free radicals also function as modulators of intracellular signaling events. In particu-lar, receptor activator of NF-κB ligand (RANKL) uses ROS to induce long-lasting oscillations of intracellular concentration of ionized calcium, which promotes the differentiation of monocytes from bone marrow into osteoclasts (Ha et al., 2004; Kim et al., 2010) and increases the rate of bone resorption (Darden et al., 1996). It is no surprise, therefore, that antioxidants slow osteoclast activity and motility by their ability to remove ROS (Bax et al., 1992). For example, the potent endogenous antioxidant lipoic acid was found to inhibit osteoclast differentiation (Kim et al., 2006). Exposure of osteoblasts, on the other hand, to ROS appears to slow proliferation by inducing cell cycle arrest (Li et al., 2009) and limit differentiation by heightened NF-κB p65 phosphorylation (Zhong et al., 2009).

Additional complexity comes from extracellular ROS signaling. Superoxide anion generated during muscle contraction, for instance, appears to enhance maximal force generation (Gomez-Cabrera et al., 2010), which might impact bone health indirectly. Furthermore, ROS can increase expression of free-radical scavenging enzymes, such as superoxide dismutase, through activation of specific redox-sensitive transcription factors (Hollander et al., 2001).

Antioxidants have diverse physicochemical properties. Vitamin E and the carotenoids are highly lipophilic due to their aliphatic nature. They are transported in blood with lipoproteins, fit well into cell membranes, and accumulate in adipose tissue. Vitamin C, on the other hand, is a hydrophilic sugar alcohol, which is transported in blood plasma and distributes in cells mainly to the cytosol. Uric acid is another potent hydrophilic antioxidant, particularly in blood (Beretta et al., 2006). The major antioxidant metabolite in cells is glutathione, which mediates the enzyme-catalyzed reactiva-tion of antioxidants.

The metabolic interactions of antioxidants are often complex. For example, the reaction of alpha-tocopherol with superoxide anion neutralizes the free radical but converts alpha-tocopherol itself to tocopherylquinone epoxides, potent free radicals themselves (Podmore et al., 1998). Similarly, the reaction of ascorbic acid with a hydroxyl radical gives rise to semidehydroascorbic acid, which is a free radical itself. This may explain why excessive intakes of both vitamin C and vitamin E appear to increase free-radical load under some circumstances and promote diseases usually associated with free-radical exposure (Terentis et al., 2002; Levy et al., 2004).

Selenium is an essential cofactor of several enzymes with antioxidant properties and of others that reactivate antioxidant compounds. Both tocopheryl quinone and the ascorbyl radical have to be detoxified by a system that relies on the reductant glutathione and the selenoenzyme thioredoxin reductase. The importance of the glutathione redox system for bone health is exemplified by the observation that consumption of N-acetylcysteine, which increases tissue glutathione levels, inhibits bone loss after ovariectomy (Lean et al., 2003).

Many natural food constituents also are potent antioxidants. The overwhelming majority comes from plant foods and herbal teas and includes hundreds of different molecular species of carotenoids and flavonoids. The vibrant colors of fruits and vegetables usually indicate the presence of carotenoids, anthocyanines, and other antioxidants.

FUNCTIONS OF ANTIOXIDANTS IN BONE METABOLISM

The four major nutrient antioxidants, that is, vitamin C, carotenoids, vitamin E, and selenium, have important functions in bone cells that impact on both bone formation and resorption.

VITAMIN C

Ascorbic acid is needed for collagen maturation. The reduced form acts in concert with iron as an essential cofactor of procollagen-proline dioxygenase and procollagen-lysine 5-dioxygenase. Inadequate vitamin C availability slows collagen synthesis and thereby bone growth and remodeling. Vitamin C is also the precursor of ascorbate 2-sulfate, which is needed for the synthesis of bone glucosaminoglycans, such as chondroitin and dermatansulfate.

CAROTENOIDS

An enzyme in the intestinal wall, 16,16'-oxygenase, cleaves a small percentage of ingested beta-carotene, alpha-carotene, and a few other provitamin A carotenoids into retinol (vitamin A). An adequate supply of the vitamin A is important for bone health, not the least because its metabolite retinoic acid acts on multiple gene targets, either alone through retinoic acid receptors or through retinoic acid X receptors in combination with vitamin D and other cofactors. Even a slight excess of preformed vitamin A, on the other hand, is likely to promote osteoclastic activity and ultimately jeopardize bone health (Crandall, 2004).

The majority of carotenoids in foods are not vitamin A precursors because their cleavage product does not yield retinol. An important example of such non-provitamin A carotenoids is lycopene, which lacks the conjugated rings of beta-carotene. Lycopene appears to promote proliferation and differentiation of osteoblast-like cells *in vitro* (Park et al., 1997; Kim et al., 2003). Osteoclastic activity of cultured cells, on the other hand, was found to be inhibited by lycopene (Rao et al., 2003).

VITAMIN E

At least 10 natural compounds possess characteristic vitamin E features, including their lipophilic character and their strong antioxidant activity. The major forms in plant-based foods are alpha-tocopherol and gamma-tocopherol, whereas beta- and delta-tocopherol are present in minor amounts. There are also four tocotrienols, which are tocopherol analogs with three instead of two double bonds in their side chain. Rice oil and palm oil are particularly rich in tocotrienols. People who maintain a low-fat diet and avoid fatty foods cannot meet recommended intake levels because these vitamin E-like compounds come mainly from high-fat foods, such as oils, seeds, and nuts. Much of the vitamin E added to foods (to protect them against oxidation) and dietary supplements is synthetic alpha-tocopherol. The chemical synthesis produces a racemic mixture of stereoisomers with reduced bioavailability and activity.

Just like other antioxidants, vitamin E appears to limit ROS-induced RANKL signaling and thereby slow excessive osteoclast activation. The hydrophilic vitamin E analog Trolox was found to counteract the induction of RANKL, possibly due to inhibition of cyclooxygenase-2 activity (Lee et al., 2009). Judging by cell culture studies, vitamin E also may protect against the inhibitory effect of oxidized lipoproteins on osteoblast differentiation and osteopontin expression (Maziere et al.,

2010). These findings are somewhat at odds with other *in vitro* observations suggesting an inhibitory effect of vitamin E on early osteoblast differentiation (Soeta et al., 2010).

Selenium

Selenium, in the form of the amino acid selenocysteine, is present in several enzymes that maintain normal redox status, reduce oxidized lipids, and reactivate antioxidants. Several versions of glutathione peroxidase defang hydrogen peroxide and other ROS, repair lipids, and reactivate oxidized vitamin C. A closely related mitochondrial enzyme, phospholipid hydroperoxide glutathione peroxidase (GPX4), uses glutathione to detoxify lipid hydroperoxides. This enzyme protects cell membranes against damage from the highly corrosive effects of oxidative phosphorylation.

Thioredoxin reductases are unusually ubiquitous enzymes that all known organisms use. The mammalian versions are selenoproteins and contribute to the reactivation of vitamin C, maintain the functional thiol groups of proteins in their optimal redox state, and activate NF-κB and other transcription factors.

Which of these enzyme functions specifically contributes to bone health remains unclear. Protection against oxidative damage and ensuing cell death is likely to play a factor. The recycling of oxidized vitamin C may be of even greater importance.

A strict ceiling effect of selenium intake on enzyme function can be expected a priori because the selenium content of the enzymes is governed by constant stochiometric ratios.

HUMAN DATA

Human investigations of the four types of nutrient antioxidants are reviewed.

Vitamin C

Mechanistic considerations certainly argue for an important role of vitamin C status in maintaining bone health. However, it is not even clear whether people with scurvy have an increased risk of osteoporosis or bone fracture. Data from healthy populations are sparse.

The prospective observation of more than 11,000 postmenopausal women indicated a statistically significant effect of vitamin C consumption levels on bone mineral density, which disappeared after adjustments for bone-related factors (Wolf et al., 2005). Nonetheless, women with the highest quartile of vitamin C intake had a persistently greater bone-density-promoting effect of hormone replacement therapy than women with lower intakes. Low vitamin C concentration in blood, but not vitamin C intake level, appeared to be related to increased risk of osteoporotic fractures (Martinez-Ramirez et al., 2007). In a cross-sectional study of postmenopausal women in Japan, radial bone mineral density was found to be highest in participants with high vitamin C consumption (Sugiura et al., 2010). A 4-year prospective cohort study found that higher vitamin C intake slowed bone mineral loss in elderly men, but not in women (Sahni et al., 2008).

To put these effects into perspective, it has been suggested that 1% decrease in BMD translates into a 12% increase of hip fracture risk (Nguyen et al., 2005). One might then assume that when men with relatively low vitamin C intake get an extra 60 mg, their hip fracture risk might decrease by as much as 18%. Adding about 200 mg per day might lower hip fracture risk by 34% (see Table 19.1).

Carotenoids

Data from most prospective cohort studies are compatible with a beneficial effect of high carotenoid intake with fruits and vegetables on bone health. The strongest effect appears to be attributable to lycopene, and more modest effects, if any, may be associated with beta-carotene. In an investigation of healthy postmenopausal women, for instance, women with osteoporosis had lower serum

TABLE 19.1
Daily Food Amount That on Its Own Might Reduce Hip Fracture Risk by 20% When Added to a Diet with Modest Vitamin C Content

Food Amount	Vitamin C (mg)	Energy (kcal)
Guava, 1/3 cup (83 g)	126	37
Red papaya, 1 cup cubes (140 g)	87	55
Strawberries, 1 cup (144 g)	85	46
Orange juice, medium glass (180 ml)	93	85
Grapefruit, whole small fruit (200 g)	69	64
Broccoli, 3 spears (96 g)	87	32

TABLE 19.2
Daily Food Amount That on Its Own Might Reduce Hip Fracture Risk by 20% When Added to a Low-Carotenoid Diet

Food Amount	Lycopene (μg)	Carotenoids (μg)	Energy (kcal)
Water melon, 1/4 of a wedge (75 g)	3241	3520	22
Red papaya, 1 cup cubes (140 g)	3122	4678	55
Guava, 1/3 cup (83 g)	2862	3068	37
Tomato juice, 2 tablespoons (30 ml)	2745	2845	5
Spaghetti sauce, 1 tablespoon (15 ml)	2628	2681	6
Pepperoni pizza, 2 slices	2536	2696	394

lycopene and cryptoxanthin concentrations than those in women with higher bone mineral density, whereas the concentration of beta-carotene tended to be higher in women with osteoporosis (Yang et al., 2008). In the Women's Health Initiative study (Wolf et al., 2005), on the other hand, only beta-carotene intake was associated with bone mineral density at the femoral neck and at all sites combined, whereas no association was observed for alpha-carotene, lycopene, lutein, or cryptoxanthin.

The benefits from other carotenoids may well be obscured by a lack of reliable dietary data. Smokers may have the greatest bone health benefit from carotenoids (Melhus et al., 1999; Zhang et al., 2006), but high carotenoid intake from foods also was related to bone mineral density in non-smoking elderly women (Barker et al., 2005; Pasco et al., 2006).

The strongest and practically most applicable data come from the Framingham cohort study (Sahni et al., 2009b). These findings suggest that adding about one table spoon of tomato sauce daily (providing about 2600 μg lycopene/day) to the diet of someone with low intake may decrease the long-term hip fracture risk by about 20% (see Table 19.2). Adding daily half a cup (10,000 μg) might cut this risk nearly in half. The same 50% risk reduction might be achieved by adding to the daily menu two medium carrots or half a cup of cooked spinach (each providing 15,000 μg total carotenoids). In real life, of course, the benefit should accrue from any combination of foods rich in total carotenoids and/or lycopene. A correspondingly slower rate of bone mineral loss in the same cohort fully explains the reduced fracture risk (Sahni et al., 2009a). A recent clinical trial investigated the potential clinical benefit of several dietary supplements providing 15,000–70,000 μg of lycopene to postmenopausal women for 4 months. The reportedly lower excretion of N-telopeptide is consistent with slower bone resorption as a potential mechanism (Mackinnon et al., 2010).

Although at least some carotenoids may lower osteoporosis risk, it is important to remember that several studies have observed accelerated bone mineral loss in people with high retinol intake (Melhus et al., 1998; Feskanich et al., 2002; Promislow et al., 2002), although the absence of such an effect was also found (Ballew et al., 2001). This issue becomes important when choosing a multivitamin supplement because both retinyl esters and beta-carotene are available as vitamin A sources in commercial products.

Vitamin E

Age-adjusted data from the Women's Health Initiative (Wolf et al., 2005) demonstrated higher bone mineral density in women with higher than average vitamin E intake (mostly from dietary supplements). However, further adjustment for multiple relevant factors abolished the statistical significance of this association. A greatly underpowered randomized controlled study of vitamin C (1000 mg/day) and vitamin E (400 mg) of only 6 months duration failed to show clinically relevant benefit (Chuin et al., 2009).

Selenium

Among the participants of a large population-based case–control study, risk of osteoporotic hip fracture was inversely associated with selenium intake in smokers, but not at all in those who never smoked (Zhang et al., 2006).

A WELL BALANCED ANTIOXIDANT DIET

Making a habit of including fruits and vegetables with most meals is a solid basis for protecting bone health. Diverse population studies consistently find that high fruit and vegetable intakes protect bone mineral density (Tucker et al., 1999; Macdonald et al., 2004; Prynne et al., 2006). The high content of several antioxidant nutrients, particularly of vitamin C and lycopene, explains the beneficial effect of fruits and vegetables on bone health to a significant degree, in addition and in synergy with other favorable nutrients. This is the main reason foods should be the preferred source of these antioxidants.

The availability of vitamin E from foods alone is much more limited (Chun et al., 2010). Americans get on average less than 8 mg of alpha-tocopherol from foods, about half of what is recommended. Vegetables and whole-grain foods are an important source of vitamin E, but it would be difficult to meet requirements with these foods alone. Additional vitamin E sources are oils, nuts, and seeds. People who avoid fatty foods have a particularly hard time to get enough vitamin E from foods alone. Although moderate amounts of supplemental vitamin E are likely to be beneficial, high-dosed products (>200 IU/day) should be avoided in light of slightly increased mortality and health risks (Bjelakovic et al., 2007).

A mixed diet is also a solid foundation to get enough selenium, but the amounts in foods vary greatly by region of origin. Americans get on average 109 μg selenium from foods, which is well above the 55 μg that most adults should get. Good foods for boosting selenium intakes are ocean fish and other sea food.

For foods and beverages rich in phenolic antioxidants, the picture is more mixed and often inconclusive due to confounding by other food constituents.

The polyphenols in soy (mainly the isoflavones genistein, daidzein, and glycetin) and other legumes have received probably the most attention and are discussed elsewhere.

Drinkers of tea (*Camellia sinensis*), who consume several hundred milligrams of polyphenols per cup (including ellagic acid, catechins, theaflavins, and thearubigins), may protect the structural integrity of their bones, most importantly at the hip, nonetheless (Hegarty et al., 2000; Devine et al., 2007).

No such beneficial effect can be expected from coffee despite its very high content of phenolic antioxidants (a hundred milligrams or more of chlorogenic acid per cup). If anything, consumption of several cups of caffeinated coffee may accelerate bone mineral loss and increase bone fracture risk, particularly in women with low calcium intake (Rapuri et al., 2001; Hallstrom et al., 2006). However, the results of the numerous reported studies are divergent and do not allow for a final conclusion, yet (Higdon and Frei, 2006).

Particularly disappointing for many may be the apparently unfavorable effect of chocolate consumption, which was associated in a linear fashion with lower bone density in one prospective cohort study despite its very high content of catechins, epicatechins, procyandins, and other flavonoids with antioxidant properties (Hodgson et al., 2008).

CONCLUSIONS

What we know are the following: ROS participate in cell signaling and other physiological events, but exposure to excessive ROS concentrations endangers bone health by inappropriately promoting osteoclastic activity and interfering with normal osteoblast differentiation and function. Various antioxidant nutrients help to inactivate ROS and protect normal function and regulation of bone cells. Generous intakes of vitamin C and lycopene with a diet rich in fruits and vegetables reduce the risk of accelerated bone mineral loss and osteoporosis more than generally appreciated. Even modest targeted intake adjustments that are easy to implement will reduce bone fracture risk by more than 20%. Such benefits are less ensured if most of these nutrients come from dietary supplements.

What we do not know are the following: Adequate amounts of vitamin E and selenium may also promote bone health, but the available human data are weak and inconsistent across populations and bone sites. Troubling questions about the use of high-dosed supplements as the main source of these nutrients, particularly for vitamin E, remain. Some flavonoids and other polyphenols with antioxidant properties in fruits, vegetables, and green tea may well have beneficial effects, but more high-quality studies will be required to substantiate claims.

REFERENCES

Ballew, C., Galuska, D., and Gillespie, C., 2001. High serum retinyl esters are not associated with reduced bone mineral density in the Third National Health And Nutrition Examination Survey, 1988–1994. *J Bone Miner Res* 16, 2306–2312.

Barker, M.E., McCloskey, E., Saha, S., et al., 2005. Serum retinoids and beta-carotene as predictors of hip and other fractures in elderly women. *J Bone Miner Res* 20, 913–920.

Bax, B.E., Alam, A.S., Banerji, B., et al., 1992. Stimulation of osteoclastic bone resorption by hydrogen peroxide. *Biochem Biophys Res Commun* 183, 1153–1158.

Beretta, G., Aldini, G., Facino, R.M., et al., 2006. Total antioxidant performance: A validated fluorescence assay for the measurement of plasma oxidizability. *Anal Biochem* 354, 290–298.

Bjelakovic, G., Nikolova, D., Gluud, L.L., et al., 2007. Mortality in randomized trials of antioxidant supplements for primary and secondary prevention: Systematic review and meta-analysis. *JAMA* 297, 842–857.

Bloomer, R.J., 2007. Decreased blood antioxidant capacity and increased lipid peroxidation in young cigarette smokers compared to nonsmokers: Impact of dietary intake. *Nutr J* 6, 39.

Chuin, A., Labonte, M., Tessier, D., et al., 2009. Effect of antioxidants combined to resistance training on BMD in elderly women: A pilot study. *Osteoporos Int* 20, 1253–1258.

Chun, O.K., Floegel, A., Chung, S.J., et al., 2010. Estimation of antioxidant intakes from diet and supplements in U.S. adults. *J Nutr* 140, 317–324.

Crandall, C., 2004. Vitamin A intake and osteoporosis: A clinical review. *J Womens Health (Larchmt)* 13, 939–953.

Darden, A.G., Ries, W.L., Wolf, W.C., et al., 1996. Osteoclastic superoxide production and bone resorption: Stimulation and inhibition by modulators of NADPH oxidase. *J Bone Miner Res* 11, 671–675.

Devine, A., Hodgson, J.M., Dick, I.M., et al., 2007. Tea drinking is associated with benefits on bone density in older women. *Am J Clin Nutr* 86, 1243–1247.

Feskanich, D., Singh, V., Willett, W.C., et al., 2002. Vitamin A intake and hip fractures among postmenopausal women. *JAMA* 287, 47–54.

Gomez-Cabrera, M.C., Close, G.L., Kayani, A., et al., 2010. Effect of xanthine oxidase-generated extracellular superoxide on skeletal muscle force generation. *Am J Physiol Regul Integr Comp Physiol* 298, R2–R8.

Ha, H., Kwak, H.B., Lee, S.W., et al., 2004. Reactive oxygen species mediate RANK signaling in osteoclasts. *Exp Cell Res* 301, 119–127.

Hallstrom, H., Wolk, A., Glynn, A., et al., 2006. Coffee, tea and caffeine consumption in relation to osteoporotic fracture risk in a cohort of Swedish women. *Osteoporos Int* 17, 1055–1064.

Hattori, N., Hayashi, T., Nakachi, K., et al., 2009. Changes of ROS during a two-day ultra-marathon race. *Int J Sports Med* 30, 426–429.

Hegarty, V.M., May, H.M., Khaw, K.T., 2000. Tea drinking and bone mineral density in older women. *Am J Clin Nutr* 71, 1003–1007.

Higdon, J.V., and Frei, B., 2006. Coffee and health: A review of recent human research. *Crit Rev Food Sci Nutr* 46, 101–123.

Hodgson, J.M., Devine, A., Burke, V., et al., 2008. Chocolate consumption and bone density in older women. *Am J Clin Nutr* 87, 175–180.

Hollander, J., Fiebig, R., Gore, M., et al., 2001. Superoxide dismutase gene expression is activated by a single bout of exercise in rat skeletal muscle. *Pflügers Arch* 442, 426–434.

Kim, H.J., Chang, E.J., Kim, H.M., et al., 2006. Antioxidant alpha-lipoic acid inhibits osteoclast differentiation by reducing nuclear factor-kappaB DNA binding and prevents in vivo bone resorption induced by receptor activator of nuclear factor-kappaB ligand and tumor necrosis factor-alpha. *Free Radic Biol Med* 40, 1483–1493.

Kim, L., Rao, A.V., and Rao, L.G., 2003. Lycopene II—Effect on osteoblasts: The carotenoid lycopene stimulates cell proliferation and alkaline phosphatase activity of SaOS-2 cells. *J Med Food* 6, 79–86.

Kim, M.S., Yang, Y.M., Son, A., et al., 2010. RANKL-mediated reactive oxygen species pathway that induces long lasting Ca2+ oscillations essential for osteoclastogenesis. *J Biol Chem* 285, 6913–6921.

Lean, J.M., Davies, J.T., Fuller, K., et al., 2003. A crucial role for thiol antioxidants in estrogen-deficiency bone loss. *J Clin Invest* 112, 915–923.

Lee, J.H., Kim, H.N., Yang, D., et al., 2009. Trolox prevents osteoclastogenesis by suppressing RANKL expression and signaling. *J Biol Chem* 284, 13725–13734.

Levy, A.P., Friedenberg, P., Lotan, R., et al., 2004. The effect of vitamin therapy on the progression of coronary artery atherosclerosis varies by haptoglobin type in postmenopausal women. *Diabetes Care* 27, 925–930.

Li, M., Zhao, L., Liu, J., et al., 2009. Hydrogen peroxide induces G2 cell cycle arrest and inhibits cell proliferation in osteoblasts. *Anat Rec (Hoboken)* 292, 1107–1113.

Macdonald, H.M., New, S.A., Golden, M.H., et al., 2004. Nutritional associations with bone loss during the menopausal transition: Evidence of a beneficial effect of calcium, alcohol, and fruit and vegetable nutrients and of a detrimental effect of fatty acids. *Am J Clin Nutr* 79, 155–165.

Mackinnon, E.S., Rao, A.V., Josse, R.G., et al., 2010. Supplementation with the antioxidant lycopene significantly decreases oxidative stress parameters and the bone resorption marker N-telopeptide of type I collagen in postmenopausal women. *Osteoporos Int* Jun 15. [Epub ahead of print]

Martinez-Ramirez, M.J., Palma Perez, S., Delgado-Martinez, A.D., et al., 2007. Vitamin C, vitamin B12, folate and the risk of osteoporotic fractures. A case–control study. *Int J Vitam Nutr Res* 77, 359–368.

Maziere, C., Savitsky, V., Galmiche, A., et al., 2010. Oxidized low density lipoprotein inhibits phosphate signaling and phosphate-induced mineralization in osteoblasts. Involvement of oxidative stress. *Biochim Biophys Acta* Jul 25. [Epub ahead of print]

Melhus, H., Michaelsson, K., Holmberg, L., et al., 1999. Smoking, antioxidant vitamins, and the risk of hip fracture. *J Bone Miner Res* 14, 129–135.

Melhus, H., Michaelsson, K., Kindmark, A., et al., 1998. Excessive dietary intake of vitamin A is associated with reduced bone mineral density and increased risk for hip fracture. *Ann Intern Med* 129, 770–778.

Nguyen, T.V., Center, J.R., and Eisman, J.A., 2005. Femoral neck bone loss predicts fracture risk independent of baseline BMD. *J Bone Miner Res* 20, 1195–1201.

Park, C.K., Ishimi, Y., Ohmura, M., et al., 1997. Vitamin A and carotenoids stimulate differentiation of mouse osteoblastic cells. *J Nutr Sci Vitaminol (Tokyo)* 43, 281–296.

Pasco, J.A., Henry, M.J., Wilkinson, L.K., et al., 2006. Antioxidant vitamin supplements and markers of bone turnover in a community sample of nonsmoking women. *J Womens Health (Larchmt)* 15, 295–300.

Podmore, I.D., Griffiths, H.R., Herbert, K.E., et al., 1998. Vitamin C exhibits pro-oxidant properties. *Nature* 392, 559.

Promislow, J.H., Goodman-Gruen, D., Slymen, D.J., et al., 2002. Retinol intake and bone mineral density in the elderly: The Rancho Bernardo Study. *J Bone Miner Res* 17, 1349–1358.

Prynne, C.J., Mishra, G.D., O'Connell, M.A., et al., 2006. Fruit and vegetable intakes and bone mineral status: A cross sectional study in 5 age and sex cohorts. *Am J Clin Nutr* 83, 1420–1428.

Rao, L.G., Krishnadev, N., Banasikowska, K., et al., 2003. Lycopene I—Effect on osteoclasts: Lycopene inhibits basal and parathyroid hormone-stimulated osteoclast formation and mineral resorption mediated by reactive oxygen species in rat bone marrow cultures. *J Med Food* 6, 69–78.

Rapuri, P.B., Gallagher, J.C., Kinyamu, H.K., et al., 2001. Caffeine intake increases the rate of bone loss in elderly women and interacts with vitamin D receptor genotypes. *Am J Clin Nutr* 74, 694–700.

Sahni, S., Hannan, M.T., Blumberg, J., et al., 2009a. Inverse association of carotenoid intakes with 4-y change in bone mineral density in elderly men and women: The Framingham Osteoporosis Study. *Am J Clin Nutr* 89, 416–424.

Sahni, S., Hannan, M.T., Blumberg, J., et al., 2009b. Protective effect of total carotenoid and lycopene intake on the risk of hip fracture: A 17-year follow-up from the Framingham Osteoporosis Study. *J Bone Miner Res* 24, 1086–1094.

Sahni, S., Hannan, M.T., Gagnon, D., et al., 2008. High vitamin C intake is associated with lower 4-year bone loss in elderly men. *J Nutr* 138, 1931–1938.

Soeta, S., Higuchi, M., Yoshimura, I., et al., 2010. Effects of vitamin E on the osteoblast differentiation. *J Vet Med Sci* 72, 951–957.

Sugiura, M., Nakamura, M., Ogawa, K., et al., 2010. Dietary patterns of antioxidant vitamin and carotenoid intake associated with bone mineral density: Findings from post-menopausal Japanese female subjects. *Osteoporos Int* May 18. [Epub ahead of print]

Sun, J., and Trumpower, B.L., 2003. Superoxide anion generation by the cytochrome bc1 complex. *Arch Biochem Biophys* 419, 198–206.

Terentis, A.C., Thomas, S.R., Burr, J.A., et al., 2002. Vitamin E oxidation in human atherosclerotic lesions. *Circ Res* 90, 333–339.

Tucker, K.L., Hannan, M.T., Chen, H., et al., 1999. Potassium, magnesium, and fruit and vegetable intakes are associated with greater bone mineral density in elderly men and women. *Am J Clin Nutr* 69, 727–736.

Valkonen, M.M., and Kuusi, T., 2000. Vitamin C prevents the acute atherogenic effects of passive smoking. *Free Radic Biol Med* 28, 428–436.

Wolf, R.L., Cauley, J.A., Pettinger, M., et al., 2005. Lack of a relation between vitamin and mineral antioxidants and bone mineral density: Results from the Women's Health Initiative. *Am J Clin Nutr* 82, 581–588.

Yang, Z., Zhang, Z., Penniston, K.L., et al., 2008. Serum carotenoid concentrations in postmenopausal women from the United States with and without osteoporosis. *Int J Vitam Nutr Res* 78, 105–111.

Zhang, J., Munger, R.G., West, N.A., et al., 2006. Antioxidant intake and risk of osteoporotic hip fracture in Utah: An effect modified by smoking status. *Am J Epidemiol* 163, 9–17.

Zhong, Z.M., Bai, L., and Chen, J.T., 2009. Advanced oxidation protein products inhibit proliferation and differentiation of rat osteoblast-like cells via NF-kappaB pathway. *Cell Physiol Biochem* 24, 105–114.

Part III

Effects of Life Cycle Changes on Bone

20 Diet and Bone Changes in Pregnancy and Lactation

Frances A. Tylavsky

CONTENTS

INTRODUCTION

Over the past 80 years, strong interest has centered on the question as to whether the net effect of pregnancy and lactation on the human skeleton is positive, negative, or zero. Pregnancy and lactation are times of high nutrient demand. During the course of a normal, full-term, singleton pregnancy, approximately 25 g (range 13–33 g) of calcium is deposited in the skeleton of the fetus (Kovacs and Kronenberg, 1997), and between 280 and 400 mg of calcium per day is expressed in breast milk (Kovacs and Kronenberg, 1997). Along with calcium, 16 mg of phosphorus, 750 mg of magnesium, and 50 mg zinc are concomitantly deposited in the fetus, primarily during the last trimester (Prentice and Bates, 1994). During the first 6 months of lactation, approximately 140 mg of calcium, 70 mg of phosphorus, 3 mg of magnesium, and 0.4 mg of zinc are deposited in the growing infant skeleton. Table 20.1 summarizes the recommended intakes set by the dietary reference intakes for these nutrients for women of child-bearing age (Institute of Medicine, Food and Nutrition Board, 1997).

In the 1997 report, the Institute of Medicine has made no recommendations for increases in allowances for calcium, phosphorus, or vitamin D during pregnancy or lactation. The recommendations for these three nutrients were based on evidence that adaptive increases in intestinal absorption and renal conservation can provide adequate minerals to meet the needs for transfer to the fetus or for milk production. Yet, no scientific evidence supports compensatory changes in the maternal metabolism to meet the increased requirements for magnesium and zinc. Increases in requirements for magnesium (Institute of Medicine, Food and Nutrition Board, 1997) and zinc were based on meeting the needs of the growing fetus and infant during the first 6 months of life without regard to skeletal needs. These assumptions of maternal adaptation are based on the consumption of a relatively adequate nutrient intake from foods, but they may not be applicable to all ethnic groups, socioeconomic levels, and those with different eating patterns (Northstone et al., 2008b; Rifas-Shiman et al., 2009). Research underscoring the importance of single nutrients, nutrient–nutrient interactions, and summary estimates of diet quality on bone metabolism makes evaluating how diet affects bone changes during pregnancy and lactation very complex.

TABLE 20.1
Dietary Reference Intake Levels for Females of Child-Bearing Age

Nutrient	Normal Age Group			Percentage Change—Pregnancy Age Group			Percentage Change—Lactation Age Group		
	<18	19–31	31–50	<18	19–30	31–50	<18	19–30	31–50
Vitamins									
A, μg	700	700	700	7	10	10	71	86	86
C, mg	65	75	75	23	13	13	77	60	60
D, μg	5	5	5	0	0	0	0	0	0
K, μg	75	90	90	0	0	0	0	0	0
Minerals									
Calcium, mg	1300	1000	1000	0	0	0	0	0	0
Fluoride, mg	3	3	3	0	0	0	0	0	0
Magnesium, mg	360	310	320	11	13	13	0	0	0
Phosphorus, mg	1250	700	700	0	0	0	0	0	0
Potassium, mg	4700	4700	4700	0	0	0	9	9	9
Zinc, mg	9	8	8	33	38	38	44	50	50

Sources: Institute of Medicine, Food and Nutrition Board. 1997. *Dietary Reference Intakes for Calcium, Phosphorus, Magnesium, Vitamin D and Fluoride*; 2000. *Dietary Reference Intakes for Vitamin C, Vitamin E, Selenium, and Carotenoids: A Report of the Panel on Micronutrient, Subcommittees on Upper Reference Levels of Nutrients and of Interpretation and Uses of Dietary Reference Intakes, and the Standing Committee on the Scientific Evaluation of Dietary Reference Intakes*; 2001. *Dietary Reference Intakes for Vitamin A, Vitamin K, Arsenic, Boron, Chromium, Copper, Iodine, Iron, Manganese, Molybdenum, Nickel, Silicon, Vanadium, and Zinc: A Report of the Panel on Micronutrient, Subcommittees on Upper Reference Levels of Nutrients and of Interpretation and Uses of Dietary Reference Intakes, and the Standing Committee on the Scientific Evaluation of Dietary Reference Intakes*; 2002. *Dietary Reference Intakes for: Energy, Carbohydrate, Fiber, Fat, Fatty Acids, Cholesterol, Protein, and Amino Acids: A Panel on Micronutrient, Subcommittees on Upper Reference Levels of Nutrients and of Interpretation and Uses of Dietary Reference Intakes, and the Standing Committee on the Scientific Evaluation of Dietary Reference Intakes*; 2005. *Dietary Reference Intakes for Water, Potassium, Sodium, Chloride, and Sulfate: A Panel on Micronutrient, Subcommittees on Upper Reference Levels of Nutrients and of Interpretation and Uses of Dietary Reference Intakes, and the Standing Committee on the Scientific Evaluation of Dietary Reference Intakes*. National Academy Press, Washington, DC.

TIMING OF ASSESSING FUNCTIONAL MARKERS

The skeleton has a normal remodeling cycle, during which old bone is resorbed and new bone is formed. The remodeling process is intended to replace old bone or to liberate minerals to meet metabolic needs. A 3- to 12-month lag exists between the time that bone is resorbed and is fully replaced, depending on age across the life cycle. Approximately 25% of the skeleton is undergoing remodeling; thus, a measurement of bone mineral density (BMD) at any given time will reflect this status. In the case of pregnancy and lactation, an uncoupling of this cycle permits mobilization of calcium to meet increased needs. A measurement at the beginning of this cycle and one midway would suggest a relative loss of bone. A measurement made, however, when resorption and formation are recoupled (Heaney, 1994) would show skeletal gain to approximately the original level if no adverse effects contributed to bone loss. In the two phases of reproduction, the decline in bone evidenced at the end of pregnancy and during early lactation results most likely in an apparent loss due to a high initiation of resorption. Once the coupling of the remodeling cycle is restored after sufficient time, bone gains occur and the BMD appears to have recovered. This phenomenon has been well described for calcium supplementation studies using BMD as an endpoint. Similarly, research which examines bone indices before and after pregnancy without sufficient follow-up time shows a loss of bone (Kolthoff et al., 1998; Ritchie et al., 1998). When the same women are then followed a minimum of 3 to12 months after the completion of pregnancy, the results show practically no change compared with prepregnancy measurements (Kolthoff et al., 1998; Ritchie et al., 1998). Examining how diet can affect bone changes during pregnancy and lactation by integrating the remodeling flux, however, is a formidable task.

CONSIDERATION IN STUDY DESIGN OF ESTIMATING DIET EFFECTS ON BONE CHANGES

Optimal research designs with functional outcomes, such as BMD or estimates of microarchitecture, are needed to evaluate how dietary factors interact to affect changes in bone mass during pregnancy and lactation. The randomized prospective clinical trial is the penultimate design used to establish cause and effect. Because of the nature of pregnancy and lactation, ethical constraints would not permit randomization of pregnant women to an optimal dietary regimen versus one that would not be considered to be optimal. Thus, researchers are forced to examine this topic using observational studies. A major limitation of observational studies is the ability to recruit women planning a pregnancy, obtain functional measures, and follow them through pregnancy, lactation, and after pregnancy/lactation. This approach entails considerable effort following participants for long periods, it may require a substantial respondent burden, usually it is quite expensive, and the investigator cannot control the course or outcome of pregnancy or the length of time of lactation. These constraints often result in small sample sizes for final publication. Well-designed cohort, case–control, or time-series studies have provided a consensus on bone changes: a deflection downward of BMD during pregnancy that may further decrease with lactation and then a return to baseline within 3 to 6 months after pregnancy/lactation ends or with the resumption of menses (Ensom et al., 2002).

CHANGES IN BONE WITH PREGNANCY/LACTATION

Histomorphometry studies comparing nonpregnant controls to pregnant women suggest an increase in thinning and separation of trabeculae at the iliac crest in the first trimester and an increase in trabecular thickness and connectivity in the third trimester (Shahtaheri et al., 1999b). Using calcium and vitamin D-replete animal models, this same flux in trabecular volume, number and length has been well described (Shahtaheri et al., 1999a). A net increase in volumetric lumbar spine BMD from before to after pregnancy in humans has been captured by quantitative computed tomography (Ritchie et al., 1998). Studies using dual-energy x-ray absorptiometry (DXA) have reported a return to prepregnant levels of BMD at the lumbar spine (Laskey and Prentice, 1997; Kolthoff et al., 1998). In contrast, measurement of the os calcis (90% trabecular) by ultrasound evidenced a loss of bone from early to late pregnancy or within 6 weeks of delivery (Sowers et al., 2000; To et al., 2003). Without sufficient follow-up, the true change in bone at the os calcis cannot be determined by these studies. Not factored in most studies are lifestyle, body composition, and weight gain during pregnancy (To et al., 2003) and the timing of the measurements and use of different bone assessment techniques that yield variable results that make studies incomparable.

ESTIMATING DIET EFFECTS ON SKELETAL CHANGES

Much of what we know about how diet affects the mineralization of the fetus and the composition of breast milk has focused on calcium and/or vitamin D. Kinetic and metabolic studies have shown that adolescent women absorb more calcium from the diet, excrete less calcium into urine and feces, and have higher bone turnover rates and higher daily net calcium retention than do adults with similarly high-calcium intakes (≥1000 mg/day) (Wastney et al., 1996; Weaver et al., 1996). In a cross-sectional study of low-calcium consumers (<500 mg/day), pregnant adolescents had lower serum calcium, lower overnight-fasting urine calcium, higher parathyroid hormone, higher dexoy-pryridoline, yet similar bone-specific alkaline phosphatase, compared with those of pregnant adults (Bezerra et al., 2002). Chan et al. (1987) reported that U.S. adolescents consuming a high-calcium diet prevented the loss of bone mineral content (BMC) at 4 months of lactation compared with those on a low-calcium diet. These studies suggest that the pregnant adolescent appears to have an increased ability to retain calcium, but in the absence of adequate intake, detrimental effects may occur in bone mass in this vulnerable population.

The few trials which examined the effect of calcium supplementation on BMD during pregnancy and prolonged lactation have reported variable results across skeletal sites (Cross et al., 1995; Kalkwarf et al., 1999). The findings were consistent with a 2% to 3% reduction in the remodeling transient associated with calcium supplementation. A lack of effect due to calcium supplementation in the ultradistal radius in a randomized clinical trial in low-calcium-consuming Gambian women during lactation could be due to the lack of sensitivity associated with single-photon absorptiometry or to a greatly increased efficiency of intestinal absorption needed to meet the increased calcium needs (Prentice et al., 1995). Functional outcomes of bone indices throughout pregnancy and lactation in two studies were not different between habitually high-calcium consumers (>1200 mg/day) (Ritchie et al., 1998) and low-calcium consumers (<500 mg/day) (Vargas Zapata et al., 2004). Collectively, these studies clearly demonstrated that the adjusted differences in intestinal absorption of calcium responding to divergent calcium intakes meet the mineral requirements for placental transfer to the fetus. In lactation, however, the conservation of urinary calcium typically accounts for the estimated amount of calcium transferred to the growing infant through breast milk (Chan et al., 1987; Cross et al., 1995; Prentice et al., 1995; Bezerra et al., 2002).

In the United States, 42% of African American and 4% of Caucasian females of child-bearing age were considered to be vitamin D insufficient or deficient (Nesby-O'Dell et al., 2002). In pregnant females, estimates are even higher; approximately 54% of African American and 46% of Caucasian residing in Northern United States were considered to have insufficient vitamin D levels (Bodnar et al., 2007). The effect of vitamin D on bone metabolism during human pregnancy and lactation has not been specifically addressed by any studies. Only observational and supplementation studies provide the basis for examining the effect of vitamin D status during reproduction. Vitamin D supplementation clearly increases serum concentrations of 25(OH)D in the mother (Wagner et al., 2006), but no systematic reports on outcomes exist on the maternal or fetal skeleton when serum 25(OH)D levels are insufficient.

In animal studies, it appears that adaptations to conserve calcium in the mother and the transfer of calcium to the fetus are independent of vitamin D status. Pregnant rats with severe vitamin D deficiency have increased intestinal calcium absorption, and skeletal BMDs of the mother and fetus are not affected. During lactation in animals, low serum vitamin D levels do not stimulate maternal demineralization, reduce calcium content of breast milk, or limit recovery from modest skeletal losses (Prentice, 2003; Kovacs, 2008). No data are available to support or refute these findings in humans. Furthermore, insufficient evidence exists to show that exclusively-breast-fed infants are at risk for vitamin D deficiency and rickets. The American Academy of Pediatrics is recommending vitamin D supplementation via drops for infants exclusively breast fed (Kovacs, 2008).

Other nutrients which have been shown to be associated with BMD in adults have not been consistently reported in the studies of bone metabolism during pregnancy and lactation. Most studies report energy, vitamin D, calcium, phosphorus, caffeine, and sodium. The role of caffeine and sodium is well acknowledged but has small effects on calcium balance. Unless the intake of foods containing these nutrients increases dramatically, they will have little or no effect on the metabolism of bone during pregnancy and lactation. Vitamin A is shown to increase fracture risk in some but not all studies (Crandall, 2004) and may depend on the adequacy of vitamin D (Ribaya-Mercado and Blumberg, 2007). The source of vitamin A may be important, whereas the excess may be terato-genic to the fetus and may affect mineralization.

Increased magnesium during pregnancy and lactation was set without regard to skeletal metabolism. The increase in requirements for pregnancy and lactation reflects increase in maternal lean body mass during pregnancy and fetal requirements for growth. In older populations, magnesium has been shown to affect BMD (Ryder et al., 2005). Although no scientific articles have examined how magnesium affects BMD in pregnancy and lactation, a few reports show that the magnesium density of the diet during pregnancy is associated with bone mass at aged 9 and 16 years (Jones et al., 2000; Yin et al., 2009). This finding suggests that perhaps alteration in calcium homeostasis that results from suboptimal magnesium intake may influence bone metabolism of the fetus and exert lifelong effects on the bone metabolism of the offspring. Data evaluating the effect of magnesium on bone metabolism during pregnancy and lactation are needed.

The preponderance of evidence on the effects of vitamin K on BMD or fracture risk of older adults is conflicting (Gundberg, 2009). Insufficient scientific evidence on vitamin K effects exists for studies focusing on pregnancy and lactation. In young girls, a high value of undercarboxy-lated osteocalcin was shown to be negatively related to whole-body BMC (O'Connor et al., 2007). Improvement in BMC in girls with a higher value of carboxylated osteocalcin has been reported (van Summeren et al., 2008). Further research capturing vitamin K status by examining undercarboxylated to carboxylated fractions of osteocalcin is warranted.

Zinc is involved in the promotion of skeletal growth and bone formation and has been shown to be positively related to BMD in men (Hyun et al., 2004). With 30% of zinc contained in the skeleton, how suboptimal intake affects bone metabolism in the mother during pregnancy and lactation is lacking.

High or low energy balance as indicated by excess or limited weight gain during pregnancy has been tied to adverse outcomes. To et al. (2003) have reported less loss of bone at the os calcis for those with high body fat accumulation from early to late pregnancy. Whether this reduction in bone loss is due to excess weight gain or the shift in increasing cortical tissues associated with increased weight is not discernable from this study (Tylavsky et al., 2002). Ultrasound measurements have recently come under scrutiny because of insensitivity in detecting changes in bone compared with DXA measurements. Intervention trials clearly show that bone metabolism is integrally linked to insufficient energy intake and can increase bone resorption but decrease bone formation in the presence of adequate calcium intake (Ihle and Loucks, 2004). Exactly how energy metabolism during pregnancy and lactation affects bone mineralization remains to be elucidated.

Nutrient antioxidants (vitamins A, E, and C) have been positively linked to bone metabolism and BMD in older adults (Sahni et al., 2009a, 2009b, 2009c) and, through fruit and vegetable intake, in adults (New et al., 2000) and growing children (Tylavsky et al., 2004; Alexy et al., 2005). Potassium has been shown to be positively related to BMD in adult studies. The promotion of potassium's role has been through fruit and vegetable intake and a significant component of modulating net endogenous acid production. Collectively, these nutrients are concentrated and coexist in selected foods, primarily fruits and vegetables, underscoring the importance of investigating dietary patterns on bone changes during pregnancy. In adult women, there are qualitative changes in foods during the first trimester and in the third trimester that suggest efforts to increase nutrient-dense and caloric-dense food items, respectively (Crozier et al., 2009). Principal component analyses have provided evidence that qualitative components of the diet can be tracked during pregnancy and lactation (Rifas-Shiman et al., 2006; Crozier et al., 2009). Dietary patterns that described intakes as health conscious, traditional, processed, confectionery, and vegetarian explained 32% of the variability in overall food intake during pregnancy (Northstone et al., 2008a). More importantly, the health-conscious and traditional diets were positively associated with intakes of protein, vitamins C and K, calcium, potassium, magnesium, zinc, iron, and folate, all modifiers of bone metabolism at one or more levels. The processed and confectionary patterns were negatively associated with these same nutrients as well as with higher fat (total and saturated), sugar, and sodium intakes. This approach to exploring how a dietary pattern affects bone changes in pregnancy and lactation provides an opportunity to investigate the advantages of patterns that contain suboptimal intakes of critical nutrients for bone health specifically and for health generally.

Only in the last few years has research examined how diet during pregnancy has a potential long-term impact on bone mass of offspring in mid-childhood and adolescents (Jones et al., 2000; Ganpule et al., 2006; Yin et al., 2009). These data suggest that dietary intake may have epigenetic influences, such as altering the child's ability to accrue bone mass during childhood. Whether these effects result from metabolic adaptations or stable long-term dietary patterns of the mothers is not yet discernable. This added dimension on how diet during pregnancy may affect the programming of a child's BMD brings a new meaning to the importance of diet during pregnancy on bone mass.

SUMMARY

Although many design limitations are evident in currently published research, results suggest that compensatory metabolic mechanisms conserve calcium during pregnancy and lactation, and, hence, little or no change in BMD occurs in adult women. In adolescents, the same mechanisms are operative, but low-calcium intake during pregnancy and lactation may be detrimental to the skeleton. A paucity of human data is available to support a role for vitamins A, C, D, and K as well as for magnesium and zinc in affecting changes in bone mass during pregnancy and lactation. Principal component analysis holds promise for evaluating how various dietary patterns affect changes in bone density. A major limitation of investigations of skeletal changes during pregnancy and lactation is the examination of BMD rather than assessment of bone architecture, especially of trabecular bone tissue. Increased resolution in magnetic resolution imaging may provide needed estimates on what structural changes occur during the increased remodeling activity of these dynamic reproductive processes that may be beneficial or deleterious to the skeleton. Thus, numerous avenues remain open for research efforts to advance our understandings of how diet affects bone tissue during pregnancy and lactation.

REFERENCES

Alexy, U., Remer, T., Manz, F., et al. 2005. Long-term protein intake and dietary potential renal acid load are associated with bone modeling and remodeling at the proximal radius in healthy children. *Am J Clin Nutr* 82: 1107–1114.

Bezerra, F.F., Laboissiere, F.P., King, J.C., et al. 2002. Pregnancy and lactation affect markers of calcium and bone metabolism differently in adolescent and adult women with low calcium intakes. *J Nutr* 132: 2183–2187.

Bodnar, L.M., Simhan, H.N., Powers, R.W., et al. 2007. High prevalence of vitamin D insufficiency in black and white pregnant women residing in the northern United States and their neonates. *J Nutr* 137: 447–452.

Chan, G.M., McMurry, M., Westover, K., et al. 1987. Effects of increased dietary calcium intake upon the calcium and bone mineral status of lactating adolescent and adult women. *Am J Clin Nutr* 46: 319–323.

Crandall, C. 2004. Vitamin A intake and osteoporosis: A clinical review. *J Womens Health (Larchmt)* 13: 939–953.

Cross, N.A., Hillman, L.S., Allen, S.H., et al. 1995. Changes in bone mineral density and markers of bone remodeling during lactation and postweaning in women consuming high amounts of calcium. *J Bone Miner Res* 10: 1312–1320.

Crozier, S.R., Robinson, S.M., Godfrey, K.M., et al. 2009. Women's dietary patterns change little from before to during pregnancy. *J Nutr* 139: 1956–1963.

Ensom, M.H., Liu, P.Y., and Stephenson, M.D. 2002. Effect of pregnancy on bone mineral density in healthy women. *Obstet Gynecol Surv* 57: 99–111.

Ganpule, A., Yajnik, C.S., Fall, C.H., et al. 2006. Bone mass in Indian children—Relationships to maternal nutritional status and diet during pregnancy: The Pune Maternal Nutrition Study. *J Clin Endocrinol Metab* 91: 2994–3001.

Gundberg, C.M. 2009. Vitamin K and bone: Past, present, and future. *J Bone Miner Res* 24: 980–982.

Heaney, R.P. 1994. The bone-remodeling transient: Implications for the interpretation of clinical studies of bone mass change. *J Bone Miner Res* 9: 1515–1523.

Hyun, T.H., Barrett-Connor, E., and Milne, D.B. 2004. Zinc intakes and plasma concentrations in men with osteoporosis: The Rancho Bernardo Study. *Am J Clin Nutr* 80: 715–721.

Ihle, R., and Loucks, A.B. 2004. Dose–response relationships between energy availability and bone turnover in young exercising women. *J Bone Miner Res* 19: 1231–1240.

Institute of Medicine, Food and Nutrition Board. 1997. *Dietary reference intakes for calcium, phosphorus, magnesium vitamin D and fluoride.* National Academy Press, Washington, DC.

Institute of Medicine, Food and Nutrition Board. 2000. *Dietary reference intakes for Vitamin C, Vitamin E, Selenium, and Carotenoids: A Report of the Panel on Micronutrient, Subcommittees on Upper Reference Levels of Nutrients and of Interpretation and Uses of Dietary Reference Intakes, and the Standing Committee on the Scientific Evaluation of Dietary Reference Intakes.* National Academy Press, Washington, DC, 139.

Institute of Medicine, Food and Nutrition Board. 2001. *Dietary Reference Intakes for Vitamin A, Vitamin K, Arsenic, Boron, Chromium, Copper, Iodine, Iron, Manganese, Molybdenum, Nickel, Silicon, Vanadium and Zinc: A Report of the Panel on Micronutrient, Subcommittees on Upper Reference Levels of Nutrients and of Interpretation and Uses of Dietary Reference Intakes, and the Standing Committee on the Scientific Evaluation of Dietary Reference Intakes.* National Academy Press, Washington, DC, 113.

Institute of Medicine, Food and Nutrition Board. 2002. *Dietary Reference Intakes for Energy, Carbohydrate, Fiber, Fat, Fatty Acids, Cholesterol, Protein, and Amino Acids: A Panel on Micronutrient, Subcommittees on Upper Reference Levels of Nutrients and of Interpretation and Uses of Dietary Reference Intakes, and the Standing Committee on the Scientific Evaluation of Dietary Reference Intakes.* National Academy Press, Washington, DC, 936.

Institute of Medicine, Food and Nutrition Board. 2005. *Dietary Reference Intakes for Water, Potassium, Sodium, Chloride and Sulfate: A Panel on Micronutrient, Subcommittees on Upper Reference Levels of Nutrients and of Interpretation and Uses of Dietary Reference Intakes, and the Standing Committee on the Scientific Evaluation of Dietary Reference Intakes.* National Academy Press, Washington, DC, 71–145.

Jones, G., Riley, M.D., and Dwyer, T. 2000. Maternal diet during pregnancy is associated with bone mineral density in children: A longitudinal study. *Eur J Clin Nutr* 54: 749–756.

Kalkwarf, H.J., Specker, B.L., and Ho, M. 1999. Effects of calcium supplementation on calcium homeostasis and bone turnover in lactating women. *J Clin Endocrinol Metab* 84: 464–470.

Kolthoff, N., Eiken, P., Kristensen, B., et al. 1998. Bone mineral changes during pregnancy and lactation: A longitudinal cohort study. *Clin Sci (Lond)* 94: 405–412.

Kovacs, C.S. 2008. Vitamin D in pregnancy and lactation: Maternal, fetal, and neonatal outcomes from human and animal studies. *Am J Clin Nutr* 88: 520S–528S.

Kovacs, C.S., and Kronenberg, H.M. 1997. Maternal–fetal calcium and bone metabolism during pregnancy, puerperium, and lactation. *Endocr Rev* 18: 832–872.

Laskey, M.A., and Prentice, A. 1997. Effect of pregnancy on recovery of lactational bone loss. *Lancet* 349: 1518–1519.

Nesby-O'Dell, S., Scanlon, K.S., Cogswell, M.E., et al. 2002. Hypovitaminosis D prevalence and determinants among African American and white women of reproductive age: Third National Health and Nutrition Examination Survey, 1988–1994. *Am J Clin Nutr* 76: 187–192.

New, S.A., Robins, S.P., Campbell, M.K., et al. 2000. Dietary influences on bone mass and bone metabolism: Further evidence of a positive link between fruit and vegetable consumption and bone health? *Am J Clin Nutr* 71: 142–151.

Northstone, K., Emmett, P.M, and Rogers, I. 2008a. Dietary patterns in pregnancy and associations with socio-demographic and lifestyle factors. *Eur J Clin Nutr* 62: 471–479.

Northstone, K., Emmett, P.M., and Rogers, I. 2008b. Dietary patterns in pregnancy and associations with nutrient intakes. *Br J Nutr* 99: 406–415.

O'Connor, E., Molgaard, C., Michaelsen, K.F., et al. 2007. Serum percentage undercarboxylated osteocalcin, a sensitive measure of vitamin K status, and its relationship to bone health indices in Danish girls. *Br J Nutr* 97: 661–666.

Prentice, A. 2003. Micronutrients and the bone mineral content of the mother, fetus and newborn. *J Nutr* 133: 1693S–1699S.

Prentice, A., and Bates, C.J. 1994. Adequacy of dietary mineral supply for human bone growth and mineralisation. *Eur J Clin Nutr* 48 (Suppl 1): S161–S176; discussion, S177.

Prentice, A., Jarjou, L.M., Cole, T.J., et al. 1995. Calcium requirements of lactating Gambian mothers: Effects of a calcium supplement on breast-milk calcium concentration, maternal bone mineral content, and urinary calcium excretion. *Am J Clin Nutr* 62: 58–67.

Ribaya-Mercado, J.D., and Blumberg, J.B. 2007. Vitamin A: Is it a risk factor for osteoporosis and bone fracture? *Nutr Rev* 65: 425–438.

Rifas-Shiman, S.L., Rich-Edwards, J.W., Kleinman, K.P., et al. 2009. Dietary quality during pregnancy varies by maternal characteristics in Project Viva: A US cohort. *J Am Diet Assoc* 109: 1004–1011.

Rifas-Shiman, S.L., Rich-Edwards, J.W., Willett, W.C., et al. 2006. Changes in dietary intake from the first to the second trimester of pregnancy. *Paediatr Perinat Epidemiol* 20: 35–42.

Ritchie, L.D., Fung, E.B., Halloran, B.P., et al. 1998. A longitudinal study of calcium homeostasis during human pregnancy and lactation and after resumption of menses. *Am J Clin Nutr* 67: 693–701.

Ryder, K.M., Shorr, R.I., Bush, A.J., et al. 2005. Magnesium intake from food and supplements is associated with bone mineral density in healthy older white subjects. *J Am Geriatr Soc* 53: 1875–1880.

Sahni, S., Hannan, M.T., Blumberg, J., et al. 2009a. Inverse association of carotenoid intakes with 4-y change in bone mineral density in elderly men and women: The Framingham Osteoporosis Study. *Am J Clin Nutr* 89: 416–424.

Sahni, S., Hannan, M.T., Blumberg, J., et al. 2009b. Protective effect of total carotenoid and lycopene intake on the risk of hip fracture: A 17-year follow-up from the Framingham Osteoporosis Study. *J Bone Miner Res* 24: 1086–1094.

Sahni, S., Hannan, M.T., Gagnon, D., et al. 2009c. Protective effect of total and supplemental vitamin C intake on the risk of hip fracture—A 17-year follow-up from the Framingham Osteoporosis Study. *Osteoporos Int* 20: 1853–1861.

Shahtaheri, S.M., Aaron, J.E., Johnson, D.R., et al. 1999a. The impact of mammalian reproduction on cancellous bone architecture. *J Anat* 194 (Pt 3): 407–421.

Shahtaheri, S.M., Aaron, J.E., Johnson, D.R., et al. 1999b. Changes in trabecular bone architecture in women during pregnancy. *Br J Obstet Gynaecol* 106: 432–438.

Sowers, M.F., Scholl, T., Harris, L., et al. 2000. Bone loss in adolescent and adult pregnant women. *Obstet Gynecol* 96: 189–193.

To, W.W., Wong, M.W., and Leung, T.W. 2003. Relationship between bone mineral density changes in pregnancy and maternal and pregnancy characteristics: A longitudinal study. *Acta Obstet Gynecol Scand* 82: 820–827.

Tylavsky, F.A., Carbone, L.D., and Bush, A.J. 2002. Effects of ethnicity and gender on reliable measurements using the Sahara ultrasonometer. *J Clin Densitom* 5: 411–419.

Tylavsky, F.A., Holliday, K., Danish, R., et al. 2004. Fruit and vegetable intakes are an independent predictor of bone size in early pubertal children. *Am J Clin Nutr* 79: 311–317.

van Summeren, M.J., van Coeverden, S.C., Schurgers, L.J., et al. 2008. Vitamin K status is associated with childhood bone mineral content. *Br J Nutr* 100: 852–858.

Vargas Zapata, C.L., Donangelo, C.M., Woodhouse, L.R., et al. 2004. Calcium homeostasis during pregnancy and lactation in Brazilian women with low calcium intakes: A longitudinal study. *Am J Clin Nutr* 80: 417–422.

Wagner, C.L., Hulsey, T.C., Fanning, D., et al. 2006. High-dose vitamin D3 supplementation in a cohort of breastfeeding mothers and their infants: A 6-month follow-up pilot study. *Breastfeed Med* 1: 59–70.

Wastney, M.E., Ng, J., Smith, D., et al. 1996. Differences in calcium kinetics between adolescent girls and young women. *Am J Physiol* 271: R208–R216.

Weaver, C.M., Peacock, M., Martin, B.R., et al. 1996. Calcium retention estimated from indicators of skeletal status in adolescent girls and young women. *Am J Clin Nutr* 64: 67–70.

Yin, J., Dwyer, T., Riley, M., et al. 2009. The association between maternal diet during pregnancy and bone mass of the children at age 16. *Eur J Clin Nutr* 64: 131–137.

21 Calcium Intake Influences the Bone Response to Exercise in Growing Children

Bonny L. Specker, Ramu Sudhagoni, and Natalie W. Thiex

CONTENTS

INTRODUCTION

Bone gained during childhood and the rate of bone loss later in life are considered important predictors for osteoporosis and fracture risk. Both exercise and nutrition are recognized as important, independent, modifiable lifestyle factors essential for optimal bone health during growth. Although the majority of pediatric exercise trials do not simultaneously evaluate the effect of calcium intake on bone response to exercise, there are several trials that were designed in this manner. The results of these trials indicate that the beneficial skeletal effects of exercise may only occur with adequate calcium intake. This exercise-by-calcium intake interaction is important to consider when recommending lifestyle changes in either of these factors.

The purpose of this chapter is to review the meaning of *interaction*, methods used for assessing bone during growth, and the published literature on the effect of exercise on bone during growth, with discussion of how calcium intake may modify the relationship between bone and exercise.

MEANING OF A CALCIUM-BY-EXERCISE INTERACTION

Interactions result from complex biological relationships, with individual factors interacting with each other to "modify" the effect that another factor has on the response. Interactions explain why it is not possible to separate the variation within a population into individual factors whose variances sum to 100%; some of the variation attributed to one factor may be a function of how that factor interacts with other factors. The complexity of these interactions is likely one of the reasons for inconsistent bone findings among pediatric exercise trials.

The presence of an interaction implies that the effects of two factors are multiplicative rather than additive. Figure 21.1a shows a hypothetical example in which increasing calcium intake is correlated with areal bone mineral density (aBMD), but no effect of exercise is present. Figure 21.1b shows a benefit of exercise on aBMD, but no relationship between aBMD and calcium intake exists. These two examples illustrate what is termed significant individual *main effects*. Figure 21.1c shows an example in which both main effects are significant, but no interaction is found. In other words, both exercise and calcium intake have positive effects on aBMD, but these effects are not "modified" by each other. In this case, the effect of exercise on aBMD is the same at all levels of calcium intake, or the effect of calcium intake on aBMD is the same regardless of exercise group. An example of an interaction or effect modification is shown in Figure 21.1d, which shows that the response to exercise varies depending on the calcium intake or vice versa (the response to calcium varies depending on whether there is exercise).

It is apparent from these examples that, if biological interactions among individual factors are not considered in study designs or in the statistical analyses of data pertaining to bone outcomes, conflicting results may arise among different studies. In addition, estimates of the amount of variance attributed to these individual factors are not valid when interactions among the variables are present but not taken into account (Rockhill et al., 1998). Interactions should be considered during the study design phase rather than post hoc because the sample sizes needed to detect interactions are often significantly greater than those needed to detect main effects (Lachenbruch, 1988).

From a biological perspective, an interaction between exercise and calcium intake on bone makes sense. Bone responds and adapts to mechanical stimulus, or loading, by increasing mass or

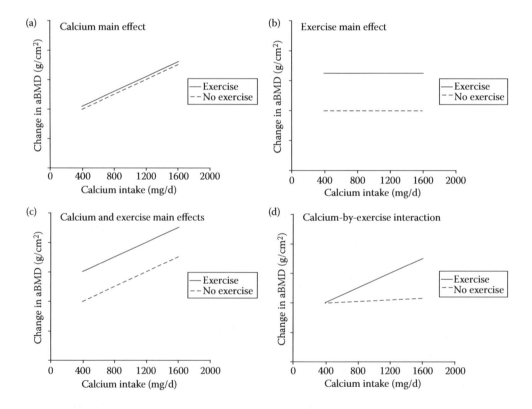

FIGURE 21.1 Graphical illustration of main effects of calcium (a), exercise (b), both calcium and exercise (c), and a calcium-by-exercise interaction on change in aBMD (d).

size (Frost, 1987), and calcium is one of the major substrates needed for bone mineralization. If no stimulus to increase bone mass or size exists, increased mineralization will not occur, no matter how much calcium is consumed. However, in the presence of mechanical loading, bone will respond by increasing its mass or size to strengthen bone. If a substrate, such as calcium, needed for this increase in mineralization is not available, then bone will not adequately adapt. This example is overly simplified because it does not take into account the effect of bone growth that occurs in pediatric populations. One can envision an even more complex relationship, in which the interaction between exercise and calcium intake on aBMD may also be a function of the age of the population, that is, a three-way interaction.

BONE GROWTH

Childhood is a period of rapid longitudinal bone growth and increase in bone width. Longitudinal bone growth occurs when prechondrocytes in the growth plates at the proximal and distal ends of bones differentiate into columns of proliferative and then hypertrophic chondrocytes. The cartilage that is formed is eventually replaced with bone in the adjacent metaphyses. The growth in bone width occurs through bone modeling.

Modeling allows individual bones to grow in width by the formation of new bone on the outer or periosteal surface, whereas resorption occurs on the inside, or endosteal surface, of the bone. Bones ultimately achieve a shape and size that best fits their function (Forwood and Turner, 1995). Although the degree of modeling is determined in part by genetics, it also is influenced by the strains on bone from physical activity and gains in body weight during growth.

Bone remodeling, which differs from modeling, occurs throughout life and does not change the shape of bone. Remodeling occurs on the same bone surface, with bone being removed from either the surface of trabeculae or on the inner cortex by osteoclasts and replaced along the same surface by osteoblasts. Remodeling is important for bone maintenance and reparation of bone damage.

Bone growth is measurable with certain imaging devices, but not with others. Increases in the periosteal circumference, or cross-sectional area of bone, and cortical thickness are both functions of increased modeling, whereas cortical volumetric BMD (vBMD) is a function of remodeling. Changes in these parameters can be measured by quantitative computed tomography (QCT), but not dual-energy x-ray absorptiometry (DXA). The rapid increase in bone size and the high rates of bone modeling and remodeling that occur during rapid growth lead to larger bones and lower cortical vBMD. This rapid increase in bone size and lower cortical vBMD that is observed during the pubertal growth spurt is thought to be associated with the increased fracture risk that is observed during adolescence (Bailey et al., 1989; Rauch et al., 2004).

Whether exercise during periods of rapid bone growth in children has the same effect on bone as exercise during periods of slower growth is not known. Tanck and coworkers showed a time lag between increases in trabecular density and adaptation of trabecular architecture in rapidly growing pigs (Tanck et al., 2001). During periods of rapid growth, body weight increases faster than does bone cross-sectional area, and it increases the mechanical loads on bones. Trabecular bone responds to these loads with increased trabecular deposition, leading to increased trabecular density. Once growth slows, trabeculae alignment occurs to increase the efficiency of distributing mechanical loads and trabecular density decreases. Some of the pediatric studies on the effects of exercise on bone have used peripheral QCT (pQCT) methods for assessing trabecular vBMD, but these methods only measure the trabecular region of the distal ends of the long bones, not the density or alignment of trabeculae.

PEDIATRIC BONE MEASUREMENT ISSUES

Density is defined as mass per unit volume. The ratio of the amount of matter in an object compared with its volume seems straightforward, but *bone density* is anything but straightforward. Bone is made up of an organic collagen protein and inorganic mineral hydroxyapatite. The arrangement of these components determines two types of bone tissue: trabecular bone tissue found mainly in the vertebrae and ends of the long bones and cortical bone tissue found mainly in the shafts of the long bones. When defining *bone density*, it is important to consider the type of bone tissue that is being measured and the mass and volume that are being used. Rauch and Schoenau (2001) suggested considering three levels when interpreting bone density depending on the biological organization of bone: material bone density, compartment bone density, and total bone density. Material bone density considers the mass of the extracellular organic bone matrix, whether it is mineralized or not, and the volume of the bone matrix exclusive of the marrow spaces, osteonal canals, lacunae, and canaliculi. During bone growth, or bone modeling, the new bone on the periosteal surface has a higher material density than that of existing bone, even though it is younger. During remodeling, the recently deposited matrix has a lower material density than that of the existing matrix, and lower material density is an indication of increased bone remodeling of existing bone. Mineralization enhances the overall bone density.

Trabecular and cortical bone compartments are defined by the endocortical surface of the bone. The space within the endocortical surface is considered the trabecular compartment, and the space between the endocortical and periosteal surface is considered the cortical compartment. Both compartments contain bone matrix and non-bone tissues; however, the trabecular compartment has more non-bone tissue than does the cortical compartment. The analysis of compartmental BMD uses the same mass as material BMD, but the volume used is greater because the compartment volume includes all the spaces that are excluded in material density. Compartmental BMD of trabecular bone increases as the number and thickness of the trabeculae increase. During remodeling, osteonal canals increase in size and the compartmental density of cortical bone decreases. This compartmental BMD is always lower than the material density. For example, the trabecular material BMD at age 10 years is approximately 1050 mg/cm^3, whereas the trabecular compartment BMD is approximately 150 mg/cm^3. The total BMD is determined using both trabecular and cortical compartments and their relative volumes. Changes in total BMD are noted during growth because the relative volumes of each compartment change as bone grows. Interpretation of bone density measures in children must be based on these definitions, with an understanding of how they differ in relation to bone physiology, modeling, remodeling, and growth. Complicating these interpretations are the different methods for measuring BMD that are in the literature.

The most common measurement method that has been used in pediatrics is DXA. DXA measures bone in two rather than three dimensions. Because only two dimensions are measured, a true volumetric density cannot be obtained, but rather an aBMD results. A larger bone size may artificially inflate aBMD measurements. This difference between two- and three-dimensional bone assessments is illustrated in studies that show that aBMD increases with age, but vBMD measured in girls by QCT is relatively constant during childhood until the time of puberty when a large increase occurs between Tanner stages 2 and 3 (Gilsanz et al., 1991).

A variety of mathematical methods have been proposed to adjust this two-dimensional aBMD to more closely reflect vBMD (Prentice et al., 1994; Cowell et al., 1995). These methods include the calculation of bone mineral apparent density for the spine or femoral neck, which divides bone mineral content (BMC) by the projected bone area to the power of 1.5 for spine (Carter et al., 1992) and 2.0 for the femoral neck (Katzman et al., 1991). Including bone and body size parameters in a regression model approach (size-adjusted BMC) or expressing BMC for bone area or BMC for height also have been suggested for correcting for the influence of size on aBMD measures (Prentice et al., 1994).

QCT assesses bone in three dimensions and allows for separation of cortical and trabecular bone. This method also provides assessment of bone size and geometry, both of which are known to significantly influence bone strength (Burr and Turner, 2003). vBMD of the trabecular and cortical bone compartments at both peripheral and axial bone sites can be measured with QCT scanners; vBMD at peripheral sites can be measured with pQCT scanners.

The importance of bone size and geometry, in addition to mass, is apparent from an evolutionary viewpoint. If optimizing bone mass were of primary importance, then evolutionary processes would have led to the formation of bones with solid, not hollow, diaphyses. The anatomical structure of bone suggests that bone development is set to attain peak bone strength by using as little material as possible while still supporting red marrow. For a bone with a given structure, bone mass usually correlates with strength. However, structural strength will differ depending on the size of the structure and where the material or mass is located. The polar moment of inertia is a measure of the distribution of material around the center of the structure. The polar moment of inertia and the section modulus are used in bone biomechanical studies and have been found to be good indicators of bone strength (Turner and Burr, 1993; Van Der Meulen et al., 2001) and can be easily and precisely determined at peripheral bone sites using pQCT (Augat et al., 1996). The importance of these structural measures illustrates that the structural strength of bone is dependent upon size and not the sole function of mass. Because bone loading activities should theoretically increase bone size, it is important to have measurements of cross-sectional area or bone size when evaluating the bone response to exercise during growth.

PEDIATRIC EXERCISE TRIALS

A summary of pediatric exercise studies is shown in Table 21.1. Sample sizes ranged from 32 to 481, and the interventions were of varying length, ranging from 3 to 36 months. Some of the studies randomized individual children, but the majority of studies were trials or observational studies where one school or more were assigned to a specific exercise program, whereas other schools were assigned to a control intervention. Although studies that assign schools or classrooms to the intervention are the easiest to conduct, they present both epidemiological and statistical problems. First, confounding factors may vary among the schools; this would occur if the populations that attend the different schools vary in some factor that might be associated with bone mass accrual. Such factors include race or ethnicity and baseline activity levels or dietary intakes of nutrients that influence bone, which may or may not differ by socioeconomic status. Second, a statistical issue with these types of studies is that the number of independent observations is not the number of subjects participating in the study because subjects attending the same school are not independent, and the school as a unit needs to be taken into account in the statistical analysis. In addition to the issues of whether the child or school were assigned to treatment, pediatric exercise studies often measure different bone sites with different technologies, making the comparison of studies difficult.

As shown in Table 21.1, a wide assortment of bone sites was measured using different imaging equipment and various statistical methods to adjust for bone size. DXA technology was used in the majority of studies, although hip structural analysis (HSA) and pQCT technology were used in some of the studies to assess the effect of activity on bone size (Bradney et al., 1998; Heinonen et al., 2000; Petit et al., 2002; Specker and Binkley, 2003).

In general, no consistent effect of bone loading exercises on bone accrual measured by DXA was found (Table 21.2). No studies, however, have reported an overall adverse effect of exercise on bone changes. The most consistent finding is an increase in BMC, not aBMD or bone area, as measured by DXA. The standardized differences between means in intervention and control groups are illustrated in Figure 21.2 for spine BMC. Although one study did not report a bone size effect with exercise using DXA technology (MacKelvie et al., 2001), a further analysis of the same cohort using HSA found an greater increase in femoral neck cross-sectional area among pubertal girls randomized to jumping than that in sedentary girls (Petit et al., 2002). One study using pQCT reported a greater periosteal circumference at the 20% distal tibia among young prepubertal children and suggested that this result supported the findings of animal studies showing an effect of exercise at more distal bone sites (Specker and Binkley, 2003).

Numerous factors may be influencing the bone response to activity or bone loading. The amount, frequency, and type of load that is applied to the skeleton may influence its response to the load, as

TABLE 21.1
Summary of Pediatric Intervention Studies

References	Additional Publications	Numbers Random, Unit Sex, Age	Intervention Description Study Length	Bone Method Sites	Covariates	Ca Intake (mg/day)	Completion and Compliance Rate	Main Findings and Comments
Blimkie et al., 1993		N = 32 I = 16 C = 16 Yes, I F, 14–18 y	I = 3×/week resistance training C = no training 6 mo	DPA aBMD and BMC: TB and LS BMAD: LS	None	919	89% completed 50% had >80% compliance 50% had 50%–80% compliance	Largest increases in first half of study Significant strength gains, no changes in bone
Morris et al., 1997		N = 71 I = 38 C = 33 No, S F, 9–10 y	I = 30 min PA, 3×/ week + weight training C = no change in activity 10 mo	DXA aBMD and BMC: TB, PF, FN, LS BMAD: FN and LS	Height, weight change	1001	I: 95% C: 100% Completed 92% compliance	TB, LS, PF, and FN BMC; LS BMAD and FN BA greater in I vs. C
Bradney et al., 1998		N = 38 I = 19 C = 19 Yes, S M, 8–12 y	I = 30 min PA, 3×/ week C = regular PE (2 h/week) 8 mo	DXA aBMD and BMC: TB, LS	None	ND	95% completed 96% compliance	TB, LS, and leg aBMD greater in I vs. C Baseline FSH higher in I vs. C
Heinonen et al., 2000	Heinonen et al., 2001: MRI results; Kontulainen et al., 2002: measures 12 mo after the program ended	N = 126 I = 64 (25 pre, 39 post) C = 62 (33 pre, 29 post) no, S F, 10–15 y	I = 50 min, 2×/ week step-aerobics with additional jumps C = no training 9 mo	DXA, pQCT BMC: FN, trochanter, LS Cortical vBMD: tibia	Baseline bone values, age	1042	91% completed 65% compliance	Premenarcheal: LS and FN BMC greater in I vs. C; no group differences in postmenarcheal girls

Study	Sample	Intervention	Measurement	Adjustments/Matching	Ca intake	Completion/Compliance	Results
Witzke and Snow, 2000	N = 53 I = 25 C = 28 no, I F, 13–15 y	I = plyometric jump training 30–45 min, 3×/week C = no training 9 mo	DXA BMC: TB, LS, PF, FN, femoral shaft	I and C matched for age and mo postmenarche	1338	95% completed 86% compliance	Greater increase in trochanter BMC in I vs. C—no other measures significant. C group participated in exercise outside of intervention more before and during study than did the I group
McKay et al., 2000	N = 144 I = 63 C = 81 yes, S both, 7–10 y	I = PE class 2×/week incorporating load-bearing exercise C = regular PE class 8 mo	DXA aBMD: TB, LS, PF, FN, trochanter	Baseline aBMD; change in height and lean mass; avg activity and Ca intake, sex, ethnicity	953	87% completed compliance not measured	Greater increase in trochanter aBMD in I vs. C—no other measures significant
Fuchs et al., 2001 Building Growing Skeletons in Youth Study Fuchs and Snow, 2002: change 7 mo after intervention stopped Gunter et al., 2008b: results of 43 mo of follow-up with more children. Gunter et al., 2008a: results of 8 y of follow-up	N = 89 I = 45 (25 boys) C = 44 (26 boys) Later papers report: I = 101 (47 boys) C = 104 (51 boys) yes, I both 6–10 y	I = jumping activities 10 min/day, 3×/week C = nonimpact, stretching 7 mo	DXA BMC, BA, and aBMD: FN and LS	Baseline age, baseline bone, changes in height and weight Later papers adjusted for baseline bone; race; sex; maturity; change in height, lean mass, fat mass, weight-bearing activity	1251	90% completed 96% compliance	Greater increase in FN and LS BMC, LS aBMD, and FN BA in I vs. C. Gain in FN BMC and BA persisted 7 mo after intervention stopped. In later papers, greater increases in TB, PF, FN, and LS BMC in I vs. C at study completion and 3 y after study completion reported. Difference in PF BMC persisted after 8 y. % change estimated from pre and post means. Results not consistent between papers (i.e., paper in bone states 8.5% greater % change in PF BMC over controls, yet JBMR paper in same year states 3.5%.

continued

TABLE 21.1 (Continued)
Summary of Pediatric Intervention Studies

References	Additional Publications	Numbers Random, Unit Sex, Age	Intervention Description Study Length	Bone Method Sites	Covariates	Ca Intake (mg/day)	Completion and Compliance Rate	Main Findings and Comments
Nichols et al., 2001		N = 67 I = 46 (5 completed) C = 21 (11 completed) yes, I F, 14–17 y	I = 30–45 m/day, 3 day/week of resistance training C = no exercise 15 mo	DXA aBMD: TB, PF, FN, TR, LS	Weight	I = 563 C = 714	I = 5% C = 52% completed 73% compliance for those completing the study	No group differences
MacKelvie et al., 2001	Healthy Bones II Petit et al., 2002: HSA results. MacKelvie et al., 2003 extended to 2 y	N = 177 I = 87 C = 90 End of 2 years: I = 32 C = 43 yes, S F, 9–12 y	I = jumping activities 10 min/day, 3x/week C = stretching, no jumping 7 mo	DXA BMC: TB, PF, LS, FN, TR aBMD: PF, LS, FN, TR BMAD: FN	Baseline age and bone measure, change in height (and BA for BMC) and pubertal stage. 2-y analysis: baseline BMC and height, change in height, physical activity, and final pubertal stage	I = 826 C = 742	93% completed 80% compliance	Among early pubertal girls, greater change in FN and LS BMC and aBMD and BMAD FN in I vs. C. No differences in prepubertal girls. After 20-mo LS and FN BMC greater in I vs. C. 2-y results: greater increase in FN and LS BMC in I vs. C. Stratified analysis into prepubertal and early pubertal. Later HSA analysis found increased CSA and reduced endosteal expansion at the FN in I vs. C early pubertal girls

Study	Sample	Intervention	Measurement	Covariates	Calcium intake	Compliance	Results
MacKelvie et al., 2002 Healthy Bones II MacKelvie et al., 2004 extended to 2 y	N = 121 I = 61 C = 60 yes, S M, 9–12 y	I = jumping activities 10 min/day, 3×/week C = stretching, no jumping 7 mo	DXA BMC: TB, PF, LS, FN, and TR aBMD: PF, LS, FN, TR BMAD: FN HSA: FN	Age, baseline weight, change in height, and activity levels	I = 883 mg/day C = 842 mg/day	91% completed 80% compliance	Greater change in TB and LS BMC, PF and TR aBMD in I vs. C. 2-y results: greater increases in FN BMC and HSA results in I vs. C Secondary analysis by baseline BMI and ethnicity. No bone differences in I vs. C among boys with high BMI at baseline
Van Langendonck et al., 2003	N = 42 I = 21 I = 21 yes, I F, avg 9 y	I = 10 min high impact 3×/week C = no exercise 9 mo	DXA aBMD and BMC: TB, PF, FN, LS, and right arm (regional from TB)	None monozygotic twins	ND		No differences between I and C unless analysis limited to twins (n = 12) who did not participate in high-impact sports (greater changes in aBMD and BMC of PF in I vs. C). Monozygotic twins randomized
McKay et al., 2005 Bounce at the Bell & Healthy Bones II above (controls)	N = 124 I = 51 (23 boys) C = 73 (36 boys) no, S both, 9–11 y	I = 10 jumps 3×/day, 5 day/week C = no jumps 8 mo	DXA BMC and BA: TB, PF, FN, TR, and LS HSA: FN	Baseline bone value and weight; change in height, final pubertal stage	827 mg/day	100% completed 60% compliance	Greater increase in TB BMC in C vs. I. Greater increase in PF BMC in I vs. C. No differences in HSA
Valdimarsson et al., 2006 POP Study Linden et al. 2006: 2-y data; Alwis et al., 2008b: HSA 2-y data.	N = 103 I = 53 C = 50 2-y analysis: I = 49 C = 50 HSA: I = 42 C = 43 no, S F, 7–9 y	I = 200 m/week C = 60 m/week 12 mo	DXA BMC and aBMD: TB, FN, LS, and leg BMAD: FN HSA: FN	Baseline age, change in height and weight	ND	I = 96% C = 78% completed 90% compliance	Greater change in LS and L3 BMC and aBMD and L3 BA in I vs. C. 2-y results: greater change in LS and L3 BMC; TB, LS, L3, and leg aBMD; L3 and FN bone width. No between-group differences in FN HSA analyses. All girls at Tanner 1 throughout study; p values provided for adjusted and unadjusted covariates

continued

TABLE 21.1 (Continued)
Summary of Pediatric Intervention Studies

References	Additional Publications	Numbers Random, Unit Sex, Age	Intervention Description Study Length	Bone Method Sites	Covariates	Ca Intake (mg/day)	Completion and Compliance Rate	Main Findings and Comments
Linden et al., 2007	POP Study Alwis et al., 2008a presented 2-y data.	N = 138 I = 81 C = 57 no, S M, 7–9 y	I = 200 min/week of PE C = 60 min/week of PE 12 mo	DXA aBMD, BMC: TB, L3, and FN Bone width: L3 and FN BMAD: FN and L3 HSA at 2 y	ND	ND	91%	Greater increases in aBMD, BMC, and bone width of L3 in I vs. C. 2-y: increases persisted in BMC and bone width of L3. No group differences in HSA measures. All boys in Tanner stage 1. Excluded 32 scans as outliers or obvious errors
Macdonald et al., 2007	AS!BC Macdonald et al., 2008 HSA results	N = 401 I = 281 (145 boys) C = 120 (64 boys) yes, S both, avg 10 y	I = additional 60 min/week PA + 5–36 jumps/week C = regular PE 14 mo	pQCT: 8 and 50% tibia BSI, total area, and total vBMD at 8% site; SSI, total and cortical area, and cortical vBMD at 50% site DXA BMC: TB, PF, and LS	Boys: baseline bone value, change in tibia length, and MCSA Girls: same as boys + final Tanner stage	867 mg/day	I = 78% C = 83% completed Teacher log compliance: 97% Bounce at Bell: 74%	Greater change in BSI (8% tibia) in I vs. C among prepubertal boys only; greater change in LS BMC in I vs. C boys; greater FN-Z in I vs. C girls if compliance >80%. Controls not studied concurrently (controls for Healthy Bones II)
Hasselstrom et al., 2008	Copenhagen School Child Interventions Study	N = 481 I = 243 (135 boys) C = 138 (62 boys) no, S both, 6–8 y	I = 180 min/week of PE C = 90 min/week of PE 36 mo	DXA aBMD, BMC, and BA: radius and calcaneus	Baseline height, weight, bone mass (BMC or BMD), and change in height	ND	87% completed compliance not stated	Greater increases in radius BMC and BA in I vs. C girls. Analysis stratified by sex. Participants and nonparticipants similar

Study	Sample	Intervention	Measurements	Covariates	Calcium intake	Completion/compliance	Results
Weeks et al., 2008 — Power PE Study	N = 81; I = 43 (22 boys); C = 38 (15 boys); yes, I both, avg 14 y	I = 10 min of jumping (300 jumps) in place of regular PE warm-up 2×/week; C = regular PE warm-up controls regular warm-up (walking, light jogging, stretching); 8 mo	DXA aBMD, BMC, and BA: TB, FN, TR, and LS; BMAD: FN and LS; QUS calcaneus	Height, weight, and age at peak height velocity	ND	82% completion; compliance not stated	Greater increases in FN and LS BMAD in I vs. C girls; greater increase in TB BMC in I vs. C boys. Analysis stratified by sex.

Studies investigating calcium-by-exercise interaction:

Study	Sample	Intervention	Measurements	Covariates	Calcium intake	Completion/compliance	Results
Specker and Binkley, 2003 — Binkley and Specker, 2004: residual bone change	N = 178; I = 88; C = 90; yes, I both, 3–5 y	I = 30 min loading/day, 5 day/week; C = 30 min fine motor activities/day, 5 day/week; 12 mo	DXA BMC and BA: TB and leg; pQCT—20% tibia; Periosteal and endosteal circumferences; Cortical area and thickness	Age, history of preterm birth; childcare center, changes in weight, height, and % body fat	Ca = 1354; Plac = 940	74% completed; I = 92% C = 94% compliance	Interaction between activity and Ca for leg BMC changes and cortical thickness and area at study completion (exercise effect more pronounced with Ca). 2 × 2 factorial design including Ca vs. placebo
Iuliano-Burns et al., 2003 — Melbourne Study	N = 70; I = 34 (16 with Ca); C = 36 (14 with Ca); yes, I both, F, 7–11 y	I = 20 min 3×/week moderate–high impact exercises; C = 20 min 3×/week low impact; 8.5 mo	DXA BMC: TB, LS, and regional from TB [leg (femur, tibia/fibula) and arm (humerus, ulna/radius)]	Baseline regional BMC, change in limb length	Ca = 980; Plac = 675	88% completed; 93% compliance	Exercise-by-calcium interaction at the femur; greater increases in BMC at tibia/fibula, humerus and radius/ulna in I vs. C. 2 × 2 with Ca vs. placebo in addition to exercise.

continued

TABLE 21.1 (Continued)
Summary of Pediatric Intervention Studies

References	Additional Publications	Numbers Random, Unit Sex, Age	Intervention Description Study Length	Bone Method Sites	Covariates	Ca Intake (mg/day)	Completion and Compliance Rate	Main Findings and Comments
Bass et al., 2007	Melbourne Study	N = 88 I = 41 (20 with Ca) C = 47 (21 with Ca) yes, I both, 7–11 y	I = 20 min 3×/ week moderate–high impact exercises C = 20 min 3×/ week low impact 8.5 mo	DXA BMC: TB, LS, and regional from TB [leg (femur, tibia/ fibula) and arm (humerus, ulna/ radius)]	None	Ca = 1302 Plac = 913	88% completed 89% compliance	Greater increase in PF BMC in I + Ca vs. other 3 groups. No group effect at LS BMC. 2 × 2 with Ca vs. placebo in addition to exercise
Stear et al., 2003		N = 131 I = 65 C = 66 yes, I F, 16–18 y	I = 45 min 3×/ week C = no exercise 16 mo	DXA BMC and BA: TB, PF, FN, TR, LS, and radius	Baseline BMC, change and avg BA, change and avg weight, change and avg height	Ca = 1685 Plac = 907	91% completed 36% compliance with exercise 70% with calcium supplement	Greater increases in size-adjusted BMC at PF and TR in I vs. C among girls with good compliance (>50%) only. 2 × 2 with Ca vs. placebo in addition to exercise
Courteix et al., 2005		N = 113 Exercise was not randomized, Ca supplementation trial Ex/Ca N = 12 Ex/Plac N = 42 Control/Ca N = 10 Control/Plac N = 21 no F, 8–13 y		DXA BMC and aBMD: TB, LS, FN, TR, and radius	Lean mass; exercise was based on activity questionnaire at baseline (exercise group ≥ 6 h/ week exercise)	Ca = 1783 Plac = 972	75% completed compliance not stated	Greater changes in TB, LS, and FN aBMD in exercise + Ca group vs. other 3 groups

Study	Subjects	Exercise	Measurements	Baseline measures	Ca intake	Compliance	Results
Johannsen et al., 2003	N = 54 I = 28 C = 26 yes, I both, 3–18 y	I = 25 jumps/day, 5 days/week C = no jumps 3 mo	DXA BMC and BA: TB, LS, FN, and leg pQCT—4% and 20% tibia Periosteal and endosteal circumference Cortical area Total BMD, BMC, and BA at 4%	Baseline weight, Ca intake and gender	I = 965 C = 1295	98% completed 76% compliance	Change in TB and leg BMC greater in I vs. C; BMC and vBMD at 4% tibia and spine BMC appeared to be lower in I vs. C during peripubertal period. Had prepubertal, peripubertal, and postpubertal groups. Bone change correlated to Ca intake in exercise but not control group
Specker et al., 1999	N = 69 I = 34 C = 35 yes, I both, 6 mo at enrollment	I = 15–20 min/day, 5 day/week, 52 weeks of tension, bending, torsion, and compression exercises C = fine motor exercises for 15–20 min/day, 5 day/week, 52 week	DXA BMC: TB	Weight, length, bone area, and Ca intake	Approximately 530 at 6 mo and 840 at 18 mo in both groups	96% completed 65% in I	No effect of exercise at high Ca intake, but exercise at low Ca intake resulted in less BMC gain

continued

TABLE 21.1 (Continued)
Summary of Pediatric Intervention Studies

References	Additional Publications	Numbers Random, Unit Sex, Age	Intervention Description Study Length	Bone Method Sites	Covariates	Ca Intake (mg/day)	Completion and Compliance Rate	Main Findings and Comments
Ianc et al., 2006		N = 53 I = 77 (38 Ca, 39 Plac) C = 76 (36 Ca, 40 Plac) yes, I both, 8–11 y	I = 50 min/day, 2 day/week C = no exercise 6 mo	Ultrasound phalanges, SOS, and Hmean (fractal analysis reflects trabecular microarchitecture)	Baseline Ca intake	Ca = 1579 Plac = 733	96% completed Compliance not stated	SOS greater in Ca vs. Plac; Hmean greater in I vs. C. Hmean gain greater in I + Ca vs. C + Plac

Notes: Randomization unit: I = individual; S = school or class; Sex: M = males; F = females.
I = intervention; C = control; PA = physical activity; FSH = follicle-stimulating hormone; ND = not determined; Plac = placebo.
DPA = dual-photon absorptiometry; DXA = dual-energy x-ray absorptiometry; pQCT = peripheral quantitative computed tomography; SOS = speed of sound.
aBMD = areal bone mineral density; BMC = bone mineral content; BA = bone area; BMAD = bone mineral apparent density; HSA = hip structural analysis; BSI = bone strength index; vBMD = volumetric bone mineral density; SSI = stress strain index.
TB = total body; LS = lumbar spine; PF = proximal femur; FN = femoral neck; TR = trochanter.
avg = average; Ca = calcium supplement; min = minute; mo = months; MRI = magnetic resonance imaging; POP = Pediatric Osteoporosis Prevention; y = year.
AS!BC = Action Schools! British Columbia; CSA = cross-sectional area; FN-Z = femoral neck section modulus (Z, cm³); MCSA = muscle cross-sectional area; PE = physical education; QUS = quantitative ultrasound

TABLE 21.2
Summary of Findings among Pediatric Exercise Studies

	Positive Effect	Negative Effect	No Effect	Number of Studies Reporting	Not Reported
aBMD					
Hip	3 (43%)	0	4 (57%)	7	15
Femoral neck	1 (10%)	0	9 (90%)	10	11
Trochanter	2 (33%)	0	4 (67%)	6	15
Spine	5 (38%)	0	8 (62%)	13	9
Total body	1 (10%)	0	9 (90%)	10	12
Leg	1 (33%)	0	2 (67%)	3	18
BMC					
Hip	5 (56%)	0	4 (44%)	9	11
Femoral neck	4 (31%)	0	9 (69%)	13	7
Trochanter	2 (29%)	0	5 (71%)	7	13
Spine	8 (44%)	0	10 (56%)	18	3
Total body	5 (28%)	0	13 (72%)	18	4
Leg	3 (75%)	0	1 (25%)	4	16
Bone area					
Hip	0 (0%)	0	4 (100%)	4	16
Femoral neck	2 (33%)	0	4 (67%)	6	14
Trochanter	0 (0%)	0	5 (100%)	5	15
Spine	1 (14%)	0	6 (86%)	7	14
Total body	0 (0%)	0	5 (100%)	5	15
BMAD					
Femoral neck	2 (33%)	0	4 (67%)	6	12
Spine	2 (50%)	0	2 (50%)	4	15

Notes: Some of the positive results were only seen in certain subpopulations (e.g., prepubertal but not postpubertal children; only if population limited to children who did not participate in sports; only in boys, not girls; etc.) These are discussed in greater detail in the text. aBMD = areal bone mineral density; BMC = bone mineral content; BMAD = bone mineral apparent density.

well as other factors that modify the relationship between bone and loading. Calcium intake has been proposed to influence the bone response to loading in adults (Specker, 1996), and a few pediatric studies have tried to examine how calcium intake may modify the bone response to loading activities.

PEDIATRIC EXERCISE AND CALCIUM TRIALS

Calcium is a primary bone mineral constituent and is a critical nutrient for optimal bone mineral accrual during growth. Calcium requirements increase during growth, but there is some disagreement on the amount needed to optimize bone health. Calcium is well established to be a "threshold nutrient," and there is some evidence that maximal calcium retention plateaus at intakes around 1300 mg/day in adolescent girls (Jackman et al., 1997). However, defining the optimal amount of calcium at different stages of the lifespan is difficult due, in part, to the complexity of how calcium may interact with other factors in determining bone mass, including other nutrients, for example, vitamin D, protein, sodium, and phosphorus, as well as with physical activity levels.

As described previously, a physiological basis exists for an interactive effect of calcium and exercise on bone in children; exercise is necessary to stimulate bone modeling and remodeling,

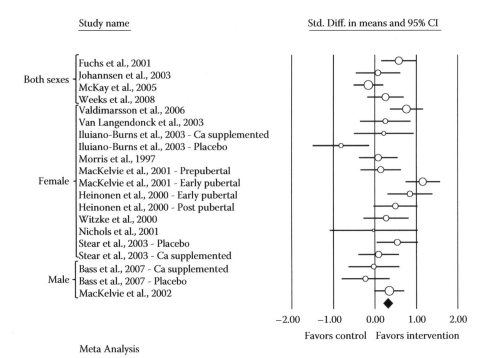

FIGURE 21.2   Meta-analysis of exercise intervention on annual percentage change in spine BMC. The studies are sorted by sex and age at enrollment.

and calcium is a required substrate for bone mineralization. A review of adult exercise studies showed a possible interaction between exercise and calcium intake on changes in spine aBMD in adults (Specker, 1996). In this analysis, which included a combination of randomized and nonrandomized trials mostly involving perimenopausal and postmenopausal women, the mean annualized rates of change in spine aBMD at different calcium intakes were examined for groups of individuals assigned to either an exercise intervention or a control group. This analysis showed what appeared to be a benefit of exercise in preventing bone loss, but only at calcium intakes greater than 1000 mg/day.

Despite the theoretical basis for an interaction between exercise and dietary calcium, relatively few well-designed, randomized, controlled pediatric studies have tested this hypothesis. As indicated in a recent review, many studies examining whether calcium enhances the effect of exercise on bone have included both factors in multivariate analyses, but these studies failed to report an interaction between these two factors (Welch and Weaver, 2005).

Five pediatric exercise trials were specifically designed to test for a calcium-by-exercise interaction (Iuliano-Burns et al., 2003; Specker and Binkley, 2003; Stear et al., 2003; Ianc et al., 2006; Bass et al., 2007); one of these studies used ultrasound speed of sound and broadband attenuation measures as the bone outcomes (Ianc et al., 2006). Two other studies were randomized exercise intervention trials (Specker et al., 1999; Johannsen et al., 2003), and a third one was a calcium supplementation trial (Courteix et al., 2005). These last five studies conducted post hoc analyses to investigate calcium-by-exercise interactions.

RANDOMIZED CALCIUM-BY-EXERCISE PEDIATRIC TRIALS

In a study of 239 preschool children designed specifically to test for a calcium-by-exercise interaction (Specker and Binkley, 2003), half the children were randomized to a gross motor activity program involving bone loading activities for 30 minutes per day, 5 days per week for 1 year, and the other half to a fine motor activity program that was designed to keep them sitting quietly. Within each of these groups, the children were further randomized to receive either a calcium supplement or placebo. The main findings from this study were that calcium intake modified the DXA leg BMC and bone geometry in response to physical activity in young children. These analyses revealed that gross motor activity increases periosteal circumference, or bone diameter, whereas calcium supplementation appeared to decrease the endosteal expansion that normally occurs with aging, but only among the gross motor exercise group (Specker and Binkley, 2003). Overall, the greatest bone benefit from exercise or calcium supplementation was observed when both factors were present, that is, there was a significant calcium-by-exercise interaction. Consistent with previous findings from supplementation trials, the bone benefit of calcium supplementation did not persist beyond the intervention period, whereas the increase in bone size with exercise was still significant 12 months after the intervention had ceased (Binkley and Specker, 2004). It was unclear, however, whether this increase in bone size was a result of a persistent effect of exercise on bone or an increase in baseline activity levels observed 6 months after the intervention ceased.

Stear et al. (2003) conducted a 15-month, 2 × 2 randomized trial among 144 females aged 16 to 18 years. Participants were randomly assigned, double blind, to receive either a calcium supplement or placebo. They were further randomized within each supplement group to one of two exercise groups. The exercise group attended three 45-minute exercise sessions a week, whereas the other group did not participate in any exercise program. The average attendance at the exercise classes was only 36%. Overall, no benefit of exercise was observed, but a greater increase in total hip BMC among the exercise compared with that in the control group was observed when the analysis was limited to only those girls with greater than 50% attendance (N=76). Calcium supplementation also was associated with greater bone mineral accrual at multiple skeletal sites. The authors noted a trend toward a significant exercise-by-calcium interaction but acknowledged that their sample size was insufficient to detect an interaction.

Iuliano-Burns et al. (2003) conducted an 8.5 month, 2 × 2 randomized trial among 72 prepubertal girls aged 7 to 11 years whose calcium intakes were <700 mg/day. Girls were assigned to either a moderate-impact exercise group or a low-impact exercise group. Approximately half of each of these groups received supplemental calcium (mean 434 mg/day) supplied through food products, whereas the placebo group received the same foods but without added calcium. The moderate-impact exercise group participated in a progressive 20-minute exercise program consisting of skipping and jumping activities performed three times per week; the low-impact exercise group followed the same format but only participated in stretching and low-impact dance activities. Sixty-six girls completed the study, and the mean attendance at the exercise sessions was 93%, and the average compliance with the food products was 70%. A significant calcium-by-exercise interaction was detected at the femur.

The authors also reported an exercise effect, but not a calcium effect, in the tibia–fibula, and a calcium effect, but not an exercise effect, in the arms. In a similar study conducted by the same researchers that involved 88 prepubertal boys aged 7 to 11 years using the same design, exercise and calcium combined (four-group analysis) found a greater increase in hip BMC in the exercise plus calcium group compared with the other three groups (Bass et al., 2007). The authors proposed that the lower skeletal responses in boys compared with those in girls may have been partly attributed to the higher baseline calcium intakes and background loading history in the boys.

An additional 6-month randomized trial of calcium and exercise was completed by Ianc et al. (2006), who used ultrasound bone measures as outcome variables. In this study, 160 children aged 8 to 11 years were randomized to an additional 50 minutes of physical exercises twice a week for 6 months, whereas the control group received the usual physical education classes. The fractal "Hmean" parameter, which is obtained using ultrasound and is a measure of trabecular bone texture quality, was significantly greater in the calcium with exercise group compared with the no calcium, no exercise group (Figure 21.3).

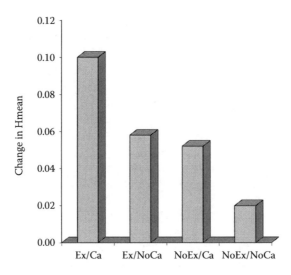

FIGURE 21.3   The fractal Hmean parameter, a measure of trabecular bone texture obtained by ultrasound, was significantly greater in the exercise plus calcium (Ex/Ca) group after 6 months of exercise compared with the no exercise, no calcium (NoEx/NoCa) group. (Data from Ianc, D., et al., *Int J Sport Nutr Exer Metab*, 16, 580–96.)

Exercise or Calcium Supplementation Pediatric Trials

Several additional pediatric exercise trials have found results consistent with the hypothesis that greater exercise-induced changes occur in individuals with high compared with low dietary calcium intakes (Specker et al., 1999; Johannsen et al., 2003; Courteix et al. 2005).

One of the first pediatric exercise trials was conducted in 72 infants who were aged 6 months at the time of randomization into either a gross motor (bone loading) or fine motor group and followed for 12 months (Specker et al., 1999). Total body BMC and bone area were measured at 6, 9, 12, 15, and 18 months. BMC was associated with weight, length, and bone area and correlated with earlier calcium intakes. Calcium intake, measured every 3 months by 3-day diet records, appeared to modify the effect of gross motor activity on bone mass accretion: infants in both groups had similar bone accretion at moderately high calcium intakes, but at low calcium intakes, the infants in the gross motor group had less bone accretion than that of infants in the fine motor group. This age (6 months) is a time of rapid linear growth velocity, and the authors speculated that participation in gross motor activities during rapid bone growth may lead to reduced bone accretion in the presence of a moderate to low–moderate calcium intake.

Johannsen and coworkers, in a study of 54 children aged 3 to 18 years, found a relationship between change in leg BMC by calcium intake (Johannsen et al., 2003). In this study, children were randomized to either a jumping program 5 days per week for 12 weeks or to a control group. Total body, spine and hip DXA, and pQCT measurements at the 4% (trabecular) and 20% (cortical) distal tibia site were measured. Overall, jumpers had a greater increase in DXA leg BMC than nonjumpers did. Although calcium intake was not controlled in this study, post hoc analysis showed a significant correlation between the change in leg BMC and calcium intake among the jumping group, but not the control group. Although the overall sample size was small, which makes detection of a statistical interaction difficult, these findings support the hypothesis that the bone response to exercise may be modified by calcium intake.

Courteix et al. (2005) enrolled 113 premenarcheal girls who were randomly assigned to receive either 800 mg/day of calcium phosphate or placebo that was added to milk. Each of the girls was classified into an exercise or a sedentary group based on an activity questionnaire that recorded the

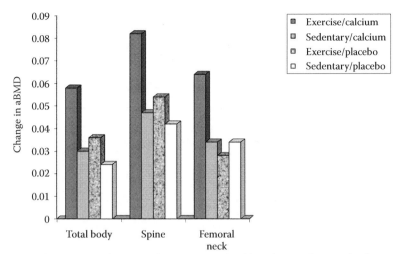

Gain in aBMD after a 1–year calcium supplementation trial and based on usual activity levels. Exercise + clacium group had greater gains than the other 3 groups (all, $p<0.05$)

FIGURE 21.4   Gain in aBMD after a 1-year calcium supplementation trial, with usual activity levels categorized as "exercise" or "sedentary." The group randomized to receive calcium and who were active had statistically significant greater changes in aBMD than the other three groups did. (Data from Courteix, D., et al., *Int J Sports Med*, 20, 328–33, 1999.)

frequency and duration of previous sports participation. Although this study was not a randomized trial of exercise and the investigators did not test for exercise-by-calcium interactions, the calcium exercise group had significantly greater gains in aBMD at the total body, spine, and hip sites than the other three groups did after 1 year of intervention (Figure 21.4). As a result, the authors concluded that a beneficial combined effect of exercise and calcium supplementation on bone accretion exists in premenarcheal girls.

COMBINING TRIAL RESULTS

To compare study findings, the results for each treatment and control group were expressed as percentage change from baseline and then annualized. The difference between the percentage change in the exercise and control groups was then determined and plotted against the mean calcium intake for the calcium and placebo groups, as shown in Figure 21.5. This graphical representation illustrates the effect of exercise on bone changes and how calcium may modify the response.

Figure 21.6 shows that the increase in the annual percentage change in BMC of the total body and spine as a result of exercise was not consistently above zero, nor does it appear to be influenced by the mean calcium intake. Two studies found a greater benefit of exercise in the calcium-supplemented group than that in the placebo group (Courteix et al., 1999; Iuliano-Burns et al., 2003), but the other two studies found no beneficial effect of calcium on the percentage change resulting from exercise (Specker and Binkley, 2003; Bass et al., 2007). The total body and spine results differ from those seen in the femoral neck, legs, or arms, where almost all the studies found a greater effect of exercise on bone accretion with higher calcium intakes (see Figure 21.5). The only study that did not show a greater benefit was by Stear and coresearchers, which had a low mean compliance with the exercise program of 36% and a small difference in mean calcium intakes between the exercise and control groups (Stear et al., 2003). These results suggest that, at least at some bone sites, higher calcium intake increases the bone response to bone loading exercises in children.

Some investigators have suggested that calcium requirements may actually be increased with increased physical activity. Significant dermal loss of calcium through sweat has been observed

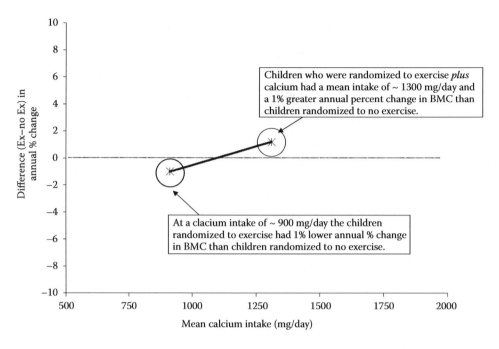

FIGURE 21.5   Graphical illustration of the difference between the percentage change in the exercise and controls groups of the same study that also had different calcium intake groups.

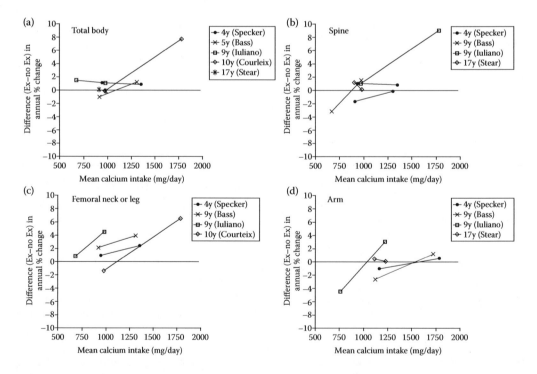

FIGURE 21.6   Differences in annual percentage change between exercise and control groups for (a) total body, (b) spine, (c) femoral neck or leg, and (d) arm BMC. The lines connect placebo and calcium-supplemented groups from the same study. Points above 0 show a positive effect of exercise, whereas the direction of the lines shows the effect that increasing calcium intake has on the bone response to exercise.

in collegiate athletes (Klesges et al., 1996), as well as increased urinary calcium excretion during intensive training in adult men (Ashizawa et al., 1997). The increased urinary calcium excretion was speculated to be related to metabolic acidosis that may occur during intense exercise. Whether these changes would be expected in the types of exercise programs implemented in pediatric populations is not known.

FACTORS OTHER THAN CALCIUM THAT MAY MODIFY BONE RESPONSE TO EXERCISE

A variety of other factors have been suggested to modify the bone response to activity. These factors are noted for the individual studies listed in Table 21.1 and include pubertal status, body mass index (BMI), and baseline activity levels.

Different responses to bone loading activities among prepubertal and pubertal children, especially with regard to the effect on bone size, have been identified. None of the studies conducted in pubertal children has found a benefit of bone loading activities on bone size. However, many of the studies conducted in pubertal children did not measure distal sites, that is, lower legs, which are thought to be more likely to increase in periosteal circumference in response to bone loading activities (Mosley et al., 1997; Heinonen et al., 2001). Some of the difficulty with assessing the influence of puberty on bone response to loading is that the definition of puberty varies from one study to the other. Some studies define puberty based on menarcheal status, whereas other studies use Tanner staging.

A few investigators have proposed that estrogen augments the bone response to loading (Bassey et al., 1998). If estrogen modifies the bone response to loading, it may explain why MacKelvie et al. found beneficial bone effects in early pubertal but not prepubertal girls (MacKelvie et al., 2001). Other trials report beneficial bone effects of activity in prepubertal children but not in pubertal children (Morris et al., 1997; Bradney et al., 1998; Fuchs et al., 2001). Increased activity has been speculated to enhance bone formation during the prepubertal years by acting synergistically with growth hormone (Bass, 2000). The study by Johannsen and coworkers (2003) compared the bone response to exercise among prepubertal, peripubertal, and postpubertal children, but the numbers in each pubertal group were so small that minimal power to detect a pubertal stage-by-exercise interaction was not reached.

MacKelvie and coworkers found that the bone benefit in prepubertal boys varied depending upon the child's BMI (MacKelvie et al., 2002). Boys with a low or average BMI who were in the exercise intervention had greater increases in hip and trochanter aBMD and total body and spine BMC compared with controls, whereas no exercise effect was found among boys with a high BMI. The authors speculated that the skeleton of the heavy boys with high BMIs may not respond to an exercise program because the skeleton is under substantial adaptive stress because of greater body weight.

The idea that the loads the skeleton is accustomed to determine the bone response to exercise also would explain the findings of Van Langendonck and coworkers who found that the bone benefit from exercise was only significant when the analysis was limited to girls who had minimal weight-bearing activity during their leisure time (Van Langendonck et al. 2003). The bones of these girls would not have been under adaptive stress prior to intervention, which may lead to a greater response to bone loading activities during the intervention.

SUMMARY

Exercise and nutrition are recognized as important modifiable lifestyle factors essential for optimal bone health during growth. However, results of pediatric exercise interventions are conflicting, and there is increasing evidence that other factors may modify the bone response to exercise. The effects of exercise and calcium may vary both by sex and bone site. These interactions are important to understand and to consider when recommending lifestyle changes. Overall, current evidence suggests that both regular adequate calcium intake and weight-bearing exercise are required to optimize bone health.

REFERENCES

Alwis, G., Linden, C., Ahlborg, H.G., et al. 2008a. A 2-year school-based exercise programme in pre-pubertal boys induces skeletal benefits in lumbar spine. *Acta Paediatr* 97:1564–1571.

Alwis, G., Linden, C., Stenevi-Lundgren, S., et al. 2008b. A school-curriculum-based exercise intervention program for two years in pre-pubertal girls does not influence hip structure. *Dynamic Med* 7:8.

Ashizawa, N., Fujimura, R., Tokuyama, K., et al. 1997. A bout of resistance exercise increases urinary calcium independently of osteoclastic activation in men. *J Appl Physiol* 83:1159–1163.

Augat, P., Reeb, H., and Cales, L.E. 1996. Prediction of fracture load at different skeletal sites by geometric properties of the cortical shell. *J Bone Miner Res* 11:1356–1363.

Bailey, D.A., Wedge, J.H., McCulloch, R.G., et al. 1989. Epidemiology of fractures of the distal end of the radius in children is associated with growth. *J Bone Joint Surg Am* 71:1225–1230.

Bass, S.L. 2000. The prepubertal years: A uniquely opportune stage of growth when the skeleton is most responsive to exercise. *Sports Med* 30:73–78.

Bass, S.L., Naughton, G., Saxon, L., et al. 2007. Exercise and calcium combined results in a grater osteogenic effect than either factor along: A blinded randomized placebo-controlled trial in boys. *J Bone Miner Res* 22:458–464.

Bassey, E.J., Rothwell, M.C., Littlewood, J.J., et al. 1998. Pre- and postmenopausal women have different bone mineral density responses to the same high-impact exercise. *J Bone Miner Res* 13:1805–1813.

Binkley, T., and Specker, B. 2004. Increased periosteal circumference remains present 12 months after an exercise intervention in preschool children. *Bone* 35:1383–1388.

Blimkie, C.J.R., Lefevre, J., Beunen, G.P., et al. 1993. Fractures, physical activity, and growth velocity in adolescent Belgian boys. *Med Sci Sports Exer* 25:801–808.

Bradney, M., Pearce, G., Naughton, G., et al. 1998. Moderate exercise during growth in prepubertal boys: Changes in bone mass, size, volumetric density, and bone strength: A controlled prospective study. *J Bone Miner Res* 13:1814–1821.

Burr, D.B., and Turner, C.H.. 2003. Section I: Anatomy and biology of bone matrix and cellular elements. Chapter 8: Biomechanics of bone. In *Primer on the Metabolic Bone Diseases and Disorders of Mineral Metabolism*, edited by J.B. Lian and S.R. Goldring. Washington, DC: American Society for Bone and Mineral Research.

Carter, D.R., Bouxsein, M.L., and Marcus, R. 1992. New approaches for interpreting projected bone densitometry data. *J Bone Miner Res* 7:137–145.

Courteix, D., Jaffre, C., Lespessailles, E., et al. 2005. Cumulative effects of calcium supplementation and physical activity on bone accretion in premenarcheal children: A double-blind randomised placebo-controlled trial. *Int J Sports Med* 26:332–338.

Courteix, D., Lespessailles, E., Obert, P., et al. 1999. Skull bone mass deficit in prepubertal highly-trained gymnast girls. *Int J Sports Med* 20:328–333.

Cowell, C.T., Lu, P.W., Lloyd-Jones, S.A., et al. 1995. Volumetric bone mineral density—A potential role in paediatrics. *Acta Paediatr Suppl* 411:12–16.

Forwood, M.R., and Turner, C.H. 1995. Skeletal adaptations to mechanical usage. *Bone* 17:197S–205S.

Frost, H.M. 1987. Bone "mass" and the "mechanostat": A proposal. *Anat Rec* 219:1–9.

Fuchs, R.K., Bauer, J.J., and Snow, C.M. 2001. Jumping improves hip and lumbar spine bone mass in prepubescent children: A randomized controlled trial. *J Bone Miner Res* 16:148–156.

Fuchs, R.K., and Snow, C.M. 2002. Gains in hip bone mass from high-impact training are maintained: A randomized controlled trial in children. *J Pediatr* 141:357–362.

Gilsanz, V., Roe, T.F., Mora, S., et al. 1991. Changes in vertebral bone density in black girls and white girls during childhood and puberty. *N Engl J Med* 325:1597–1600.

Gunter, K., Baxter-Jones, A.D.G., Mirwald, R.L., et al. 2008a. Impact exercise increases BMC during growth: An 8-year longitudinal study. *J Bone Miner Res* 23:986–993.

Gunter, K., Baxter-Jones, A.D.G., Mirwald, R.L., et al. 2008b. Jump starting skeletal health: A 4-year longitudinal study assessing the effects of jumping on skeletal development in pre and circum pubertal children. *Bone* 42:710–718.

Hasselstrom, H.A., Karlsson, M.K., Hansen, S.E., et al. 2008. A 3-year physical activity intervention program increases the gain in bone mineral and bone width in prepubertal girls but not boys: The Prospective Copenhagen School Child Interventions Study (CoSCIS). *Calcif Tissue Int* 83:243–250.

Heinonen, A., McKay, H.A., MacKelvie, K.J., et al. 2001. High-impact exercise and tibial polar moment of inertia in pre-and early pubertal girls: A quantitative MRI study. *J Bone Miner Res* 16 (S1):S482.

Heinonen, A., Sievaenen, H., Kannus, P., et al. 2000. High-impact exercise and bones of growing girls: A 9-month controlled trial. *Osteoporos Int* 11:1010–1017.

Ianc, D., Serbescu, C., Bembea, M., et al. 2006. Effects of an exercise program and a calcium supplementation on bone in children: A randomized control trial. *Int J Sport Nutr Exer Metab* 16:580–596.

Iuliano-Burns, S., Saxon, L., Naughton, G., et al. 2003. Regional specificity of exercise and calcium during skeletal growth in girls: A randomized controlled trial. *J Bone Miner Res* 18:156–162.

Jackman, L.A., Millane, S.S., Martin, B.R., et al. 1997. Calcium retention in relation to calcium intake and postmenarcheal age in adolescent females. *Am J Clin Nutr* 66:327–333.

Johannsen, N., Binkley, T., Englert, V., et al. 2003. Bone response to jumping is site-specific in children: A randomized trial. *Bone* 33:533–539.

Katzman, D.K., Bachrach, L.K., Carter, D.R., et al. 1991. Clinical and anthropometric correlates with bone mineral acquisition in healthy adolescent girls. *J Clin Endocrinol Metab* 73:1332–1339.

Klesges, R.C., Ward, K.D., Shelton, M.L., et al. 1996. Changes in bone mineral content in male athletes: Mechanisms of action and intervention effects. *JAMA* 276:226–230.

Kontulainen, S.A., Kannus, P., Pasanen, M.E., et al. 2002. Does previous participation in high-impact training results in residual bone gain in growing girls? *Int J Sports Med* 23:575–581.

Lachenbruch, P.A. 1988. A note on sample size computation for testing interactions. *Stat Med* 7:467–469.

Linden, C., Ahlborg, H.G., Besjakov, J., et al. 2006. A school curriculum-based exercise program increases bone mineral accrual and bone size in prepubertal girls: Two-year data from the Pediatric Osteoporosis Prevention (POP) Study. *J Bone Miner Res* 21:829–835.

Linden, C., Alwis, G., Ahlborg, H.G., et al. 2007. Exercise, bone mass and bone size in prepubertal boys: One-year data from the pediatric osteoporosis prevention study. *Scand J Med Sci Sports* 17:340–347.

Macdonald, H.M., Kontulainen, S., Khan, K.M., et al. 2007. Is a school-based physical activity intervention effective for increasing tibial bone strength in boys and girls? *J Bone Miner Res* 22:434–446.

Macdonald, H.M., Kontulainen, S., Petit, M.A., et al. 2008. Does a novel school-based physical activity model benefit femoral neck bone strength in pre- and early pubertal children? *Osteoporos Int* 19:1445–1456.

MacKelvie, K.J., Khan, K.M., Petit, M.A., et al., 2003. A school-based exercise intervention elicits substantial bone health benefits: A 2-year randomized controlled trial in girls. *Pediatrics* 112:e447–e452.

MacKelvie, K.J., McKay, H.A., Khan, K.M., et al. 2001. A school-based exercise intervention augments bone mineral accrual in early pubertal girls. *J Pediatr* 139:501–508.

MacKelvie, K.J., McKay, H.A., Petit, M.A., et al. 2002. Bone mineral response to a 7-month randomized controlled, school-based jumping intervention in 121 prepubertal boys: Associations with ethnicity and body mass index. *J Bone Miner Res* 17:834–844.

MacKelvie, K.J., Petit, M.A., Khan, K.M., et al. 2004. Bone mass and structure are enhanced following a 2-year randomized controlled trial of exercise in prepubertal boys. *Bone* 34:755–764.

McKay, H.A., MacLean, L., MacKelvie-O-Brien, K. et al. 2005. "Bounce at the Bell": A novel program of short bouts of exercise improves proximal femur bone mass in early pubertal children. *Br J Sports Med* 39:521–526.

McKay, H.A., Petit, M.A., Schutz, R.W., et al. 2000. Augmented trochanteric bone mineral density after modified physical education classes: A randomized school-based exercise intervention study in prepubescent and early pubescent children. *J Pediatr* 136:156–162.

Morris, F.L., Naughton, G.A., Gibbs, J.L., et al. 1997. Prospective ten-month exercise intervention in premenarcheal girls: Positive effects on bone and lean mass. *J Bone Miner Res* 12:1453–1462.

Mosley, J.R., March, B.M., Lynch, J., et al. 1997. Strain magnitude related changes in whole bone architecture in growing rats. *Bone* 20:191–198.

Nichols, D.L., Sanborn, C.F., and Love, A.M. 2001. Resistance training and bone mineral density in adolescent females. *J Pediatr* 139:494–500.

Petit, M.A., McKay, H.A., MacKelvie, K.J., et al. 2002. A randomized school-based jumping intervention confers site and maturity-specific benefits on bone structural properties in girls: A hip structural analysis study. *J Bone Miner Res* 17:363–372.

Prentice, A., Parsons, T.J., and Cole, T.J.. 1994. Uncritical use of bone mineral density in absorptiometry may lead to size related artifacts in the identification of bone mineral determinants. *Am J Clin Nutr* 60:837–842.

Rauch, F., Bailey, D.A., Baxter-Jones, A.R., et al. 2004. The 'muscle–bone unit' during the pubertal growth spurt. *Bone* 34:771–775.

Rauch, F., and Schoenau, E.. 2001. Changes in bone density during childhood and adolescence: An approach based on bone's biological organization. *J Bone Miner Res* 16:597–604.

Rockhill, B., Newman, B., and Weinberg, C. 1998. Use and misuse of population attributable fractions. *Am J Public Health* 88:15–19.

Specker, B.L. 1996. Evidence for an interaction between calcium intake and physical activity on changes in bone mineral density. *J Bone Miner Res* 11:1539–1544.

Specker, B.L., and Binkley, T. 2003. Randomized trial of physical activity and calcium supplementation on bone mineral content in 3–5 year old children. *J Bone Miner Res* 18:885–892.

Specker, B.L., Mulligan, L., and Ho, M.L.. 1999. Longitudinal study of calcium intake, physical activity, and bone mineral content in infants 6–18 months of age. *J Bone Miner Res* 14:569–576.

Stear, S.J., Prentice, A., Jones, S.C., et al. 2003. Effect of a calcium and exercise intervention on the bone mineral status of 16–18 y old adolescent girls. *Am J Clin Nutr* 77:985–992.

Tanck, E., Hommingaa, J., van Lenthea, G.H., et al. 2001. Increase in bone volume fraction precedes architectural adaptation in growing bone. *Bone* 28:650–654.

Turner, C.H., and Burr, D.B. 1993. Basic biomechanical measurements of bone: A tutorial. *Bone* 14:595–608.

Valdimarsson, O., Linden, C., Johnell, O., et al. 2006. Daily physical education in the school curriculum in prepubertal girls during 1 year is followed by an increase in bone mineral accrual and bone width—Data from the prospective controlled Malmo Pediatric Osteoporosis Prevention Study. *Calcif Tissue Int* 78:65–71.

Van Der Meulen, M.C.H., Jepsen, K.J., and Mikic, B. 2001. Understanding bone strength: Size isn't everything. *Bone* 29:101–104.

Van Langendonck, L., Claessens, A.L., Vlietinck, R., et al. 2003. Influence of weight-bearing exercises on bone acquisition in prepubertal monozygotic female twins: A randomized controlled prospective study. *Calcif Tissue Int* 72:666–674.

Weeks, B.K., Young, C.M., and Beck, B.R. 2008. Eight months of regular in-school jumping improves indices of bone strength in adolescent boys and girls: The POWER PE Study. *J Bone Miner Res* 23:1002–1011.

Welch, J.M., and Weaver, C.M. 2005. Calcium and exercise affect the growing skeleton. *Nutr Rev* 63:361–373.

Witzke, K.A., and Snow, C.M. 2000. Effects of plyometric jump training on bone mass in adolescent girls. *Med Sci Sports Exerc* 32:1051–1057.

22 Obesity, Adipose Tissue, and Bone

Sue A. Shapses, Norman K. Pollock, and Richard D. Lewis

CONTENTS

INTRODUCTION

It is well established that a higher body weight or obesity has a positive correlation with bone, and a low body weight or loss of weight is associated with bone loss and fracture risk. The greater bone mass in obesity may result from the greater mechanical load on bone due to excess weight, an altered dietary intake, or hormones/adipokines produced by the excess adipose tissue. Furthermore, the regional distribution of fat may also influence bone mass independently of obesity (Tarquini et al., 1997; Warming et al., 2003; Kuwahata et al., 2008). Whereas obesity may affect specific bones differently, specific bone sites may also be affected differently due to weight bearing or the cortical:trabecular content of a particular bone. This weight–bone relationship is not gender specific, and it is also found in children, although severe obesity at greater levels of adiposity observed typically only in Western countries may attenuate the positive effect on bone and/or bone quality in children. Obesity is associated with higher areal bone mineral density (aBMD), yet the impact of excess adiposity on bone quality, especially modification of the trabecular and cortical compartments, presents a more complicated picture that may actually lead to an increase in fracture risk.

Our findings in overweight adolescents suggest lower cortical bone mass and bone strength (Pollock et al., 2007), which is consistent with our data in adults (Shapses et al., 2007).

This chapter briefly reviews the relationships between fat and bone at a cellular and hormonal level and then discusses in each section the independent influences of total weight and body composition on bone and fracture during bone modeling (children) and remodeling (adults).

OSTEOBLASTS AND ADIPOCYTES: THE CELLULAR BASIS FOR A RELATIONSHIP

Factors that signal pluripotent stromal cells to differentiate into their mature cell types will eventually constitute the balance between bone, adipose tissue, and muscle mass (see Chapter 7). Undifferentiated mesenchymal stem cells can differentiate into osteoblasts, chondrocytes, and adipocytes. For example, cultured myoblasts will differentiate into osteocytes or adipocytes following treatment with bone morphogenetic proteins or adipogenic inducers, respectively (Asakura et al., 2001). In addition, the number of transgenic or gene-deficient mice has increased, with phenotypes reflecting altered bone marrow adipogenesis and/or osteogenesis (Gimble et al., 2006). Runx2/Cbfa1 and osterix are examples of several bone-specific transcription factors required for osteoblast differentiation (Rosen and Bouxsein, 2006). The peroxisome proliferator activated receptor δ (PPARδ) plays a central role in initiating adipogenesis and inhibits osteoblastogenesis (Takada et al., 2009). Thiazolidinedione PPARδ ligands are used in the treatment of type 2 diabetes to increase insulin sensitivity (Tontonoz et al., 2008), yet they also increase adiposity, reduce bone mass, and increase fracture risk.

In addition, skeletal unloading increases adipocyte differentiation and inhibits osteoblast differentiation that can be reversed by transforming growth factor-ß2 (Ahdjoudj et al., 2002). Also, low-density lipoprotein oxidation products promote osteoporotic loss of bone by directing progenitor marrow stromal cells to undergo adipogenic instead of osteogenic differentiation (Parhami et al., 1999). Adipocytes are known to secrete biologically active hormonal factors known as adipokines (e.g., leptin, adiponectin, resistin, adipsin, tumor necrosis factor, and interleukins), which some studies suggest could be important mediators in bone–fat relationship (Klein et al., 1998; Roemmich et al., 2003; Lorentzon et al., 2006; Shapses and Reidt 2006; Zhao et al., 2008; do Prado et al., 2009; Pollock et al., 2009b). Adipose tissue might also influence both adult and pediatric bone through the production of estrogen or through an effect on the secretion of bone-active hormones from the pancreas (e.g., insulin, amylin, and preptin) (Reid, 2008). In vivo, extra weight in the form of fat mass has been shown to stimulate bone growth through increased production of the hormones insulin, estrogen, and leptin (Grodin et al., 1973; Ducy et al., 2000; Cornish et al., 2002; Hamrick et al., 2008). Alternatively, excess adipose tissue has also been shown to hinder bone growth, in vitro, by enhancing the role of oxidized lipids in accelerating atherogenesis, thus activating calcifying vascular cells and inhibiting osteoblastic differentiation (Parhami et al., 1997).

Finally, both osteoporosis and aging-related bone loss increase marrow adiposity and suggest a switch in differentiation of stromal cells from the osteoblastic to the adipocytic lineage (Verma et al., 2002). Overall, the plasticity between adipose and osteoblast cells is an interesting area showing the relationship between different components of body composition. Continued study in this area could potentially result in drugs that inhibit marrow adipogenesis and further our understanding of obesity and osteoporosis related to aging and to abnormal conditions.

FAT, LEAN, AND BONE IN CHILDREN

Pediatric obesity has reached epidemic proportions globally (Wang and Lobstein, 2006). The dire consequence of childhood obesity is the increased risk for metabolic conditions such as hypertension, type 2 diabetes, and cardiovascular diseases (Weiss, 2004). Now, increasing concern has been expressed that being overweight may be associated with suboptimal bone growth and development as mounting evidence is accruing that links childhood obesity to skeletal fractures (Table 22.1).

TABLE 22.1
Pediatric Investigations of Adiposity and Skeletal Fractures

		Childhood Fracture Reports Related to Obesity			
References	**Population**	**Obesity Definition/ Adiposity Measure**	**Bone Measure/Site and Fracture Assessment**	**Methodological/ Statistical Approach**	**Results**
Goulding et al. (1998)	200 white females with (*n* = 100) and without (*n* = 100) distal forearm fractures (average time of 47 days postfracture); age: 3–15 years	• BMI • Total fat mass assessed by DXA	• Total body aBMD • Spine aBMD • Hip aBMD • Radial aBMD • Medical record of skeletal fracture	Forearm fracture cases vs. controls, matched for age and height	Young females with forearm fractures had greater BMI, higher levels of fat mass, and lower aBMD at all skeletal sites than controls.
Goulding et al. (2000a)	170 white females with (*n* = 82) and without (*n* = 88) prior distal forearm fracture; age: 3–15 years at baseline	BMI	• Total body aBMD • Spine aBMD • Medical record of skeletal fracture	To determine risk factors for occurrence of new skeletal fractures over a 4-year period	In young females, previous forearm fracture, low total body aBMD, low spine aBMD, and high BMI each increase the risk of new skeletal fracture within 4 years.
Goulding et al. (2001)	200 Caucasian males with (*n* = 100) and without (*n* = 100) distal forearm fractures (average time of 4 weeks post-fracture); age: 3–19 years	• BMI • Total fat mass assessed by DXA	• Total body aBMD • Spine aBMD • Medical record of skeletal fracture	To determine factors associated with forearm fractures in young males	Low total body aBMD, low spine aBMD, high BMD, and high adiposity each increased the risk of forearm fracture in young males.
Skaggs et al. (2001)	100 white females with (*n* = 50) and without (*n* = 50) distal forearm fracture (average time of 4 weeks postfracture); age: 4–15 years	BMI	At the radius, the following CT-derived bone parameters were assessed at the distal site: • Trab vBMD • Total CSA	Forearm fracture cases vs. controls, matched for age, height, weight, and pubertal stage	Young females with forearm fractures had a significantly smaller bone size (total CSA) than controls. More importantly, compared with established normative data for BMI-for-age percentiles, the girls with fractures were overweight.

continued

TABLE 22.1 (Continued)
Pediatric Investigations of Adiposity and Skeletal Fractures

Childhood Fracture Reports Related to Obesity

References	Population	Obesity Definition/ Adiposity Measure	Bone Measure/Site and Fracture Assessment	Methodological/ Statistical Approach	Results
Davidson et al. (2003)	50 white males; age: 4–17 years	BMI	• Medical record of skeletal fracture	To compare the relative likelihood of forearm fractures between obese (≥95th BMI percentile) and nonobese (<85th BMI percentile) male children and adolescents; matched for age, pubertal stage, and height	Obese male children and adolescents were shown to have 1.7 times greater risk of forearm fracture compared with their nonobese counterparts.
Goulding et al. (2005)	90 children and adolescents having experienced ≥2 forearm fractures (47 F, 43 M); age: 5–19 years	BMI	• Radial aBMD and BMC • Medical record of skeletal fracture	To determine factors associated with multiple forearm fractures during childhood	A greater number of forearm fractures were associated with a higher BMI and lower radial aBMD and BMC.
Taylor et al. (2006)	355 children and adolescents (198 F, 157 M), (210 W, 145 B); age: 12.2 ± 2.8 yeares	BMI	• Medical record of skeletal fracture	Non-overweight (5th–95th BMI percentile) vs. overweight (>95th BMI percentile)	Overweight/obese children and adolescents were found to have greater prevalence of skeletal fractures than non-overweight peers.
Pollack et al. (2008)	3232 children and adolescents (1754 F, 1478 M); age: 9–15 years	BMI	• Medical record of skeletal fracture of the lower and upper extremities caused by motor vehicle crashes	To compare the relative likelihood of skeletal fractures between overweight/obese and normal-weight children and adolescents	The risk of skeletal fractures of the lower and upper extremities (due to motor vehicle crashes) was 2.5 times as great in overweight/obese vs. normal-weight children.

| Dimitri et al. (2009) | 103 children and adolescents; age: 11.7 ± 2.8 years | • BMI
• Total fat mass assessed by DXA | • Total body BMC, bone area, and aBMD
• Lumbar spine BMC, bone area, and aBMD
• Radial BMC, bone area, and aBMD
• Medical record of skeletal fracture | To determine relations between total fat mass and bone parameters in four groups of children and adolescents: obese (≥99th BMI percentile) with and without prior fracture and normal-weight (<85th BMI percentile) with and without prior fracture; statistical control for gender, age, and weight or gender, height and weight, or lean mass | There was a consistent pattern of differences in BMC, bone area, and aBMD at the skeletal sites according to both obesity and prior skeletal fracture. Specifically, children and adolescents who fracture have smaller bones; the difference is substantially increased in those children and adolescents who have a history of skeletal fracture and are obese. |

Notes: F, female; M, male; W, white/Caucasian; B, black/African American; DXA, dual-energy X-ray absorptiometry; CT/QCT, axial quantitative computed tomography; BMI, body mass index; aBMD, areal bone mineral density; BMC, bone mineral content; vBMD, volumetric BMD; CSA, cross-sectional area; trab, trabecular.

Inevitably, the potential for increasing adiposity to negatively affect pediatric skeletal integrity is a subject of growing interest.

In adults, a high body mass index (BMI) or being excessively fat has long been thought to be protective against osteoporosis and related fractures (Reid, 2002, 2008). Contrary to the notion that excess fat may also protect youth from fractures, Taylor and colleagues (2006) reported that overweight children (BMI ≥95% for age) had significantly more documented skeletal fractures than non-overweight children did (Figure 22.1). In a fracture study of females 4 to 15 years of age conducted by Skaggs and coworkers (2001), those who sustained a fracture were more overweight and had a smaller cross-sectional area at the nonfractured forearm compared with the nonfracture group. A higher fracture risk in obese children may be the result of greater forces generated during a fall, a lifestyle contraindicative to strong bones, and/or excess fat tissue that impairs bone growth and development (Frost, 1997). Given the current state of increasing pediatric obesity along with reports of high fracture rates in obese children, it is vital to understand the effects of adiposity on the skeleton because achieving optimal bone mass and size during growth will presumably reduce the risk of osteoporotic fractures later in life (Hui et al., 2003).

With the emergence of dual-energy X-ray absorptiometry (DXA) in the 1990s as a clinical instrument to assess aBMD and soft tissue mass, great strides were made in furthering our understanding of the impact of fat mass on aBMD in adults and bone mineral accrual in the growing skeleton. DXA has proven to be a valuable two-dimensional bone imaging technique, although because DXA generates areal and not volumetric measures, interpretation of the data is complex in the developing skeleton, particularly when statistically adjusting bone variables for body size, sex, and/or maturity (Gordon et al., 2004; Petit et al., 2005a). Moreover, DXA does not measure geometrical properties of bone, nor does it differentiate between cortical and trabecular compartments. Because whole bone strength, defined as the amount of loading force required to cause the material to fail under a certain loading condition (Turner and Burr, 1993; van der Meulen et al., 2001), reflects not merely the amount of mineralized material but also its spatial distribution or geometrical properties (Wainwright et al., 1976; Rauch and Schoenau, 2002), other three-dimensional (3-D) methodologies are preferred in childhood studies compared with DXA.

The utilization of 3-D bone-measuring tools such as axial quantitative computed tomography (QCT or CT) and peripheral QCT (pQCT), in particular, has increased in pediatric bone research over the past few years. Unlike DXA, QCT and pQCT have the technical capability to assess vBMD and bone structural parameters, distinguish between cortical and trabecular bone, and perhaps more importantly, provide bone-site-specific information about the muscle (e.g., muscle cross-sectional area [MCSA]). Because of the strong relationship between bone and muscle, it has been proposed

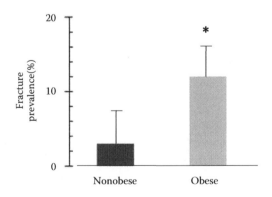

FIGURE 22.1 Prevalence of documented fractures in overweight children and adolescents based on medical chart review. Solid (black) and open (white) bars indicate nonoverweight and overweight subjects, respectively. [a]$p < .01$. (Adapted from Taylor, E.D., et al., *Pediatrics* 117, 2167–74, 2006.)

that bone measurements, irrespective of how they are measured, should be considered in relation to muscle size or strength (Rauch and Schoenau, 2001; Klein et al., 2005). Although no clinically defined recommendations are available to consider muscle-related parameters in pediatric bone assessments, future studies using 3-D bone techniques will provide greater insight. In addition, with the increasing use of pQCT and QCT, investigators have the tools to ascertain more accurately the independent influence of adiposity on the developing skeleton. The following sections summarize the cross-sectional and prospective DXA, pQCT, and QCT studies addressing the relationships between childhood and adolescent obesity and bone mass on fractures. Then, the differential effects of sex are discarded. Finally, the limitations of previous studies along with considerations for future pediatric fat–bone investigations are addressed.

DXA Cross-Sectional Studies

The close relationship between the skeleton and muscle mass/size has been known for nearly four decades (Doyle et al., 1970). Over the years, a plethora of pediatric studies have confirmed this positive influence of muscle mass/size on skeletal development. For instance, cross-sectional (Faulkner et al., 1993; Ogle et al., 1995; Young et al., 1995; Manzoni et al., 1996; Schoenau et al., 1996, 2000; Courteix et al., 1998; Valdimarsson et al., 1999; Witzke and Snow, 1999; McKay et al., 2000; Rittweger et al., 2000; Hogler et al., 2003; Arabi et al., 2004; Petit et al., 2005b; Janicka et al., 2006) and prospective (Morris et al., 1997; Heinonen et al., 2000; Schoenau et al., 2002, 2004; Specker et al., 2004; MacKelvie et al., 2004; Macdonald et al., 2005, 2006; Rauch et al., 2004; Baxter-Jones et al., 2008; Rauch and Schoenau, 2008) childhood investigations have shown that measures of muscle mass, that is, fat-free soft tissue (FFST) or lean tissue, and/or muscle size, i.e., MCSA, are either strongly related or independent predictors of bone parameters assessed by DXA, pQCT, and QCT. Although studies agree on the robust relationship between muscle and bone, the effect of body fatness on the developing skeleton is still debated.

Much of what is known about childhood fat and bone relationships emerged from the early cross-sectional body composition studies examining total FFST, fat mass, and total body aBMD. These studies and their findings are summarized in Table 22.2. Obese children have been reported to have either lower bone mass when corrected for their body weight or lean mass (Goulding et al., 2000b; Weiler et al., 2000) or higher bone mass relative to height, maturation, and/or FFST mass (Ellis et al., 2003; Leonard et al., 2004; Petit et al., 2005b). Goulding et al. (2000b, 2002) observed that obese children have lower lumbar spine and total body BMC relative to weight compared with normal-weight children. Furthermore, these investigators found that a high body weight, independent of total lean mass, contributed to fracture risk in children and adolescents who had fractured their forearms repeatedly (Goulding et al., 2005). More recently, Dimitri et al. (2009) reported that obese children, with or without a fracture, had lower total body, lumbar spine, and radius aBMD than nonobese children did when corrected for weight and/or height.

Other studies, however, challenge these observations and suggest that childhood overweight has no effect on bone mass or is linked to higher bone mass (Faulkner et al. 1993; Young et al 1995; Ellis et al., 2003; Leonard et al., 2004; Petit et al., 2005b; Ackerman et al., 2006; do Prado et al., 2009; El Hage et al., 2009a, 2009b; Timpson et al., 2009). Faulkner et al. (1993) found in males and females aged 8 to 16 years that age, height, and FFST were the strongest predictors of total body BMD and that fat mass did not account for any additional variance. Furthermore, Leonard et al. (2004) observed in boys and girls 4 to 20 years of age that obesity, based on BMI-for-age percentiles, was predictive of higher lumbar spine aBMD when corrected for height. Ellis et al. (2003) grouped children by percentage body fat (<25%, 25%–30%, and >30% body fat) and found that the >30% body fat group had significantly higher total body BMC relative to height. Additional support for a positive effect of fat on bone mass was presented in a recent study of almost 5000 European children. In this study, Timpson et al. (2009) reported that total fat mass was a positive predictor of total body, spine, and upper and lower limb BMC when adjusting for age, height, and sitting height.

TABLE 22.2
Adiposity and Bone Relationships in Children and Adolescents by Bone Imaging Technique and Cross-Sectional/Prospective Design

References	Population	Obesity Definition/ Adiposity Measure	Site and Bone Measure	Methodological/ Statistical Approach	Results
			DXA Cross-Sectional Investigations		
McCormick et al. (1991)	335 white, black, and Hispanic children and adolescents; age: 5–18 years	BMI	• Lumbar spine aBMD	Obese vs. non-obese group; statistical control for body weight	Young obese females, but not males, were shown to have lower lumbar spine aBMD than their do non-obese peers, after controlling for body weight.
Faulkner et al. (1993)	234 children and adolescents; age: 8–16 years	Total fat mass assessed by DXA	• Total body aBMD	To determine the relation between fat mass and total body aBMD	Age, height, and fat-free soft tissue mass were the strongest predictors of total body aBMD. Body weight and total body fat mass did not account for any additional variance.
Young et al. (1995)	215 female twin pairs; age: 10–26 years	Total fat mass assessed by DXA	• Total body BMC • Total hip BMC	To determine the independent contribution of fat mass and lean mass to total body BMC and total hip BMC; covariates included height, weight, menarche, dietary calcium, and activity levels	Fat mass and lean mass were independent predictors of total body BMC. Lean mass, but not fat mass, was an independent predictor of total hip BMC.
De Schepper et al. (1995)	59 children and adolescents; Age: 11.8 ± 2.7 years	BMI	• Lumbar spine aBMD	Obese vs. non-obese group; matched for sex, age, and height	Lumbar spine aBMD was not different between the obese and non-obese groups.
Klein et al. (1998)	48 children (23 F, 25 M); Age: 9.45 ± 1.9 years	BMI	• Total body aBMD	Obese vs. non-obese group; statistical control for age or bone age	Total body aBMD was not different between the obese and non-obese groups, even when controlling for age or bone age.

Reference	Sample	Measure	Outcome	Comparison	Findings
Goulding et al. (2000b)	336 children and adolescents (200 F, 136 M); age: 3–19 years	BMI	• Total body BMC and bone area	Normal weight vs. overweight vs. obese; statistical control for age and weight	Overweight and obese children have lower total body BMC and bone area compared with normal-weight children, after controlling for age and weight.
Weiler et al. (2000)	60 female children and adolescents; age: 10–19 years	Percentage body fat assessed by DXA	• Total body aBMD and BMC	To determine the relation between percentage body fat and total body aBMD and BMC; statistical control for age, weight, and height	Percentage body fat was negatively related with total body aBMD and BMC, after controlling for age, weight, and height.
Goulding et al. (2002)	362 children and adolescents (160 F, 202 M); age: 3–19 years	BMI	• Lumbar spine BMC	Normal weight vs. overweight vs. obese; statistical control for total body bone area, height, weight, and Tanner stage	Overweight girls had 8% less, obese girls 12% less, and obese boys 13% less bone mineral at the spine than did normal-weight controls, after controlling for total body bone area, height, weight, and Tanner stage.
Ellis et al. (2003)	865 children and adolescents (444 F, 421 M), (359 W, 249 B, and 257 H); age: 11.3 ± 3.4 years	Percentage body fat assessed by DXA	• Total body BMC	<25% vs. 25%–30% vs. >30% body fat; statistical control for gender, ethnicity, age, and height or lean tissue	The >30% body fat group had significantly higher total body BMC than did the other two groups, after controlling for gender, ethnicity, age, and height, or lean mass.
Leonard et al. (2004)	235 children and adolescents (140 F, 95 M), (145 W, 91 B); age: 4–20 years	BMI	• Total body BMC and aBMD • Lumbar spine BMC and aBMD	Non-obese (5th–85th BMI percentile) vs. obese (>95th BMI percentile); statistical control race, height, Tanner stage, total body bone area, or lean mass	In the male and female obese groups, BMC and aBMD of the total body and lumbar spine were significantly greater than those in the non-obese groups, after controlling for race, height, Tanner stage, total body bone area, or lean mass.

continued

TABLE 22.2 (Continued)
Adiposity and Bone Relationships in Children and Adolescents by Bone Imaging Technique and Cross-Sectional/Prospective Design

References	Population	Obesity Definition/ Adiposity Measure	Site and Bone Measure	Methodological/ Statistical Approach	Results
Nagasaki et al. (2004)	1070 obese Japanese children and adolescents; age: 7–15 years	Percentage body fat by bioelectric impedance	• aBMD of the second metacarpal bone in left hand assessed by digital image processing	To determine the relation between metacarpal BMD and percentage body fat; statistical control for bone age	In boys 12 years and older, percentage body fat was negatively related to metacarpal BMD of the hand, after controlling for bone age. No relationships were found between percentage body and metacarpal BMD of the hand in either the boys younger than 12 years or the females.
Petit et al. (2005b)	134 children and adolescents (80 F, 54 M), (74 W, 60 B); age: 4–20 years	• BMI • Total fat mass assessed by DXA	• DXA-derived bone geometry and strength parameters at the femoral shaft and narrow neck (i.e., total CSA and section modulus)	Healthy weight (5th–85th BMI percentile) vs. overweight (>85th BMI percentile); statistical control sex, pubertal stage, and fat mass or lean mass	Hip structural and strength indices (bone CSA and section modulus, an index of bone bending strength) were greater in the overweight vs. healthy weight group, after controlling for sex and maturational stage. When fat mass was added as a covariate, the bone differences between groups remained. However, when lean mass was included as a covariate, group differences in bone parameters no longer remained. Thus, the higher bone values observed in the overweight vs. healthy weight group were attributed to the greater level of lean mass rather than fat mass observed in the overweight vs. healthy weight group.

Study	Sample	Exposure measure	Outcome	Objective	Findings
Ackerman et al. (2006)	926 children and adolescents (446 F, 482 M), (306 W, 274 B, and 346 A); age: 6–18 years	Total fat mass assessed by DXA	• Total body BMC	To determine the relationship between fat mass and total body BMC at different stages of puberty, separately for females and males; statistical control for height, age, or ethnicity	In both prepubertal females and males, fat mass was positively related to total body BMC, after controlling for height, age, or ethnicity. In pubertal (stages 2–5) females only, fat mass was positively related to total body BMC, after controlling for the same covariates.
Afghani and Goran (2006)	184 children and adolescents (116 F, 65 M), (99 W, 82 B); age: 5–10 years	VAT and SAAT assessed by CT	• Total body BMC	To determine the relationship between central adiposity (i.e., VAT + SAAT, VAT, SAAT) and total body BMC, separately for whites and blacks; statistical control for gender, age, height, total fat mass, and lean mass	In white and black children, central adiposity (VAT + SAAT) was negatively related to total body BMC, after controlling for gender, age, height, fat mass, and lean mass. However, there appears to be racial differences with regard to the separate contributions of VAT and SAAT to total body BMC.
Goulding et al. (2008)	194 children and adolescents (81 F, 113 M), age: 4–5 years	Total fat mass assessed by DXA	• Total body less head (TBLH) BMC and bone area	To determine the relationship between total fat mass and TBLH bone area; statistical control for height and lean mass	In females and males, total fat mass was positively associated with TBLH BMC and bone area, after controlling for height and lean mass.
Rocher et al. (2008)	46 children (20 F, 23 M); age: 9–12 years	BMI	• Total body BMC • Total body bone area • Lumbar spine BMC and bone area	Obese vs. normal-weight group; statistical control for weight or lean mass	Obese children had lower BMC and bone area of the total body and lumbar spine compared with their normal-weight peers, after controlling for weight or lean mass.

continued

TABLE 22.2 (Continued)
Adiposity and Bone Relationships in Children and Adolescents by Bone Imaging Technique and Cross-Sectional/Prospective Design

References	Population	Obesity Definition/ Adiposity Measure	Site and Bone Measure	Methodological/ Statistical Approach	Results
Afghani and Goran (2009)	256 overweight Hispanic American children and adolescents (111 F, 145 M); age: 8–14 years	VAT and SAAT assessed by CT	• Total body BMC	To determine the relationship between central adiposity (i.e., VAT + SAAT, VAT, SAAT) and total body BMC, separately for females and males; statistical control for age, pubertal stage, fat mass, and VAT or SAAT	In Hispanic American females and males, central adiposity (VAT + SAAT) was negatively related to total body BMC, after controlling for age, pubertal stage, and weight. SAAT was inversely related to total body BMC in both females and males, after controlling for age, pubertal stage, fat mass, and SAAT. VAT was inversely related to total body BMC in females only, after controlling for age, pubertal stage, fat mass, and SAAT.
do Prado et al. (2009)	109 Brazilian obese adolescents (41 F, 68 M); age: 13–18 years	Total fat mass assessed by DXA	• Total body aBMD and BMC	To determine the relationship between total fat mass and total body aBMD and BMC, separately for females and males	In Brazilian females and males, no significant relations were found between total fat mass and total body aBMD and BMC.
El Hage et al. (2009a)	42 Lebanese female adolescents; Age: 12–20 years	BMI	• Total body aBMD • Lumbar spine aBMD • Total hip aBMD • Femoral neck aBMD	Overweight vs. normal weight; statistical control for body weight, lean mass, or fat mass	Total body aBMD, lumbar spine aBMD, total hip aBMD, and femoral neck aBMD were not different between groups, after controlling for body weight, lean mass, or fat mass.

Study	Population	Fat mass measure	Bone outcomes	Objective	Findings
El Hage et al. (2009b)	100 adolescents (35 F, 65 M; age: 14–16 years	Total fat mass assessed by DXA	• Total body aBMD • Lumbar spine aBMD	To determine the relationship between total fat mass and total body aBMD and lumbar spine aBMD, separately for females and males	In males, total fat mass was not related to either total body aBMD or lumbar spine aBMD. In contrast, there were significant positive relations of total fat mass with total body aBMD and spine aBMD in the females. In multiple regression analyses, fat mass vs. lean mass was found to be a stronger positive predictor of total body aBMD in females; whereas in males, fat mass was a negative determinant and lean mass a positive determinant of total body BMD and lumbar spine aBMD.
Timpson et al. (2009)	7470 white children and adolescents; age: mean 9.8 years	Total fat mass assessed by DXA	• Total body BMC and bone area	To determine the independent predictive role of total fat mass on total body BMC; covariates included in the model were sitting height, height, sex, pubertal stage, or total body bone area	Total fat mass was a positive predictor of total body BMC, after adjusting for sex, sitting height, height, or total body bone area.
			DXA Prospective Investigations		
Nelson et al. (1997)	721 children and adolescents (355 F, 366 M), (288 W, 433 B); age: 8–11 years	Total fat mass assessed by DXA	• Total body aBMC and BMC • Lumbar spine aBMC and BMC	• To assess the independent contribution of change in fat mass and lean mass to change in bone parameters; other covariates included height, weight, gender, age, and ethnicity • Follow-up was at 12 months	Over 12 months, change in fat mass and change in lean mass were both positively associated with change in all bone parameters, but change in lean mass vs. fat mass was the stronger predictor. These findings were independent of height, weight, gender, age, and ethnicity.

continued

TABLE 22.2 (Continued)
Adiposity and Bone Relationships in Children and Adolescents by Bone Imaging Technique and Cross-Sectional/Prospective Design

References	Population	Obesity Definition/ Adiposity Measure	Site and Bone Measure	Methodological/ Statistical Approach	Results
Young et al. (2001)	286 white female twins pairs; age: 8–26 years	Total fat mass assessed by DXA	• Total body aBMC and BMC • Lumbar spine aBMC and BMC • Total hip aBMC and BMC	• To assess the independent contribution of change in fat mass and lean mass to change in bone parameters; other covariates included height and menarche • Follow-up was at 1.8 years (range 0.7–6.7 years)	During linear growth, change in fat mass and change in lean mass were independent positive predictors of bone change in all parameters, with the lean mass as the stronger predictor. During postlinear growth, change in fat mass and change in lean mass were still positive predictors of bone change in all parameters, but fat mass, rather than lean mass, was the stronger predictor.
Clark et al. (2006)	3082 children (1684 F, 1398 M), (173 W, 41 B); age: 9–11 years	Total fat mass assessed by DXA	• TBLH BMC and bone area	• To determine the relation between change in fat mass and bone mineral accrual, separately for females and males; covariates in model were age, ethnicity, socioeconomic status, height, or lean mass • At baseline and follow-up, mean ages were 9.9 and 11.8 years, respectively	In pubertal males (stages 1–3) and prepubertal females (stage 1), males (stages 1–3) and prepubertal (females stage 1), change in fat mass was a positive independent predictor of TBLH BMC and bone area over 2 years, after adjusting for sex, height, and lean mass. However, change in fat mass was negatively associated with change in TBLH BMC and bone area among females in pubertal stages 2 and 3 at the 2-year follow-up

Wosje et al. (2009)	214 children (105 F, 109 M), (173 W, 41 B); age: 3–7 years	Total fat mass assessed by DXA	• Total body BMC • Total body bone area	• To determine the relation between change in fat mass and bone mineral accrual; covariates included in the model were age, sex, race, height, lean mass, calcium intake, physical activity, or TV viewing • At baseline and follow-up, mean ages were 3.5 and 7.0 years, respectively	Greater fat mass in children mass at age 3.5 years at baseline was associated with smaller increases in total body bone area and BMC over 3.5 years, after controlling for sex, race, height, physical activity, and calcium intake.

pQCT Cross-Sectional Investigations

Lorentzon et al. (2006)	1068 late adolescent males, age: 18.9 ± 0.02 years	Total fat mass assessed by DXA	At the radius and tibia, the following trabecular bone parameter was assessed at the 4% site of the bone length in the proximal direction of the distal end: • Trab vBMD At the radius and tibia, the following cortical bone parameters were assessed at the 25% site of the bone length in the proximal direction of the distal end: • Cort vBMD • Total CSA • Cort thk • Peri circ • Endo circ	To determine the independent predictive role of total fat mass on cortical and trabecular bone parameters at the radius and tibia; covariates included in the model were age, height, leptin, calcium intake, physical activity, and smoking	Total fat mass was a positive predictor of trabecular vBMD and cortical bone size (total CSA, cort thk, peri circ, and endo circ) of the tibia, after adjusting for age, height, leptin, calcium intake, and smoking. However, total fat mass was a negative predictor of cort vBMD of the tibia. At the radius, no significant relations were observed between total fat mass and bone parameters.

continued

TABLE 22.2 (Continued)
Adiposity and Bone Relationships in Children and Adolescents by Bone Imaging Technique and Cross-Sectional/Prospective Design

References	Population	Obesity Definition/ Adiposity Measure	Site and Bone Measure	Methodological/ Statistical Approach	Results
Pollock et al. (2007)	115 late adolescent females (78 W, 2 B, 3 H, and 10 A); age: 18–19 years	Total fat mass and percentage body fat assessed by DXA	At the radius and tibia, the following trabecular bone parameters were assessed at the 4% site of the bone length in the proximal direction of the distal end: • Total vBMD • Trab vBMD • Total CSA At the radius and tibia, the following cortical bone parameters were assessed at the 20% site of the bone length in the proximal direction of the distal end: • Cort vBMD • Total CSA • Cort BMC • Cort CSA • Cort thk • Peri circ • Endo circ • SSI	Normal fat (<32% body fat) vs. High fat groups (≥32% body fat), and to determine relations between total fat mass on cortical and trabecular bone parameters at the radius and tibia in the total sample; statistical control for site-specific limb length and/or MCSA (66% bone site)	The high fat group vs. normal fat group had significantly lower cortical (cort CSA, total CSA, cort BMC, and SSI), but not trabecular, bone parameters at the radius and tibia, after controlling for MCSA. In the total sample, total fat mass was inversely correlated with total CSA and cort BMC at the radius and tibia, after controlling for limb length and MCSA.

Reference	Subjects	Adiposity measure	Bone parameters	Objective	Results
Fricke et al. (2008)	295 children and adolescents (156 F, 139 M); age: 5–19 years	• Percentage body fat assessed by skinfold calipers • pQCT-derived fat CSA at 65% site	At the radius, the following trabecular bone parameters were assessed at the 4% site of the bone length in the proximal direction of the distal end: • Total vBMD • Trab vBMD • Total CSA. At the radius, the following cortical bone parameters were assessed at the 65% site of the bone length in the proximal direction of the distal end of the bone: • Cort vBMD • Cort BMC • Cort CSA • Peri circ • Endo circ • SSI	To determine relations of percentage body fat and fat CSA with trabecular and cortical bone parameters at the radius, separately for females and males and for prepubertal (Tanner 1) and pubertal (Tanner 2–5) stages; statistical control for height and MCSA	In prepubertal and pubertal females, percentage body fat was positively associated with trab vBMD, after controlling for height and MCSA. Although percentage body fat was positively related to trab vBMD in prepubertal males, an inverse association was found between percentage body fat and vBMD in pubertal males. No significant relations were found of either percentage body fat or fat CSA with other bone parameters, after controlling for height and MCSA.
Ducher et al. (2009)	427 children (221 F, 206 M); age: 7–10 years	BMI	At the radius and tibia, the following trabecular bone parameters were assessed at the 4% site of the bone length in the proximal direction of the distal end: • Total vBMD • Trab vBMD • Total CSA • Cort thk • BSI	Overweight vs. normal-weight group; statistical control for MCSA	Overweight vs. normal-weight children had significantly higher bone values at all sites, except cort vBMD and cort thk at the tibia and radius. After control for MCSA, trab vBMD, cort CSA, and cort thk (66% site) at the tibia remained significantly greater in the overweight children, whereas at the trabecular site of the radius, total CSA and cortical thickness were significantly smaller in the overweight children.

continued

TABLE 22.2 (Continued)
Adiposity and Bone Relationships in Children and Adolescents by Bone Imaging Technique and Cross-Sectional/Prospective Design

References	Population	Obesity Definition/ Adiposity Measure	Site and Bone Measure	Methodological/ Statistical Approach	Results
			At the radius and tibia, the following cortical bone parameters were assessed at the 66% site of the bone length in the proximal direction of the distal end: • Cort vBMD • Total CSA • Cort CSA • Cort thk • SSI		
Sayers and Tobias (2009)	4005 adolescents (2154 F, 1851 M); age: 15.5 ± 0.29 years	Total fat mass assessed by DXA	At the tibia, the following cortical bone parameters were assessed at the 50% site of the bone length in the proximal direction of the distal end: • Cort vBMD • Cort BMC • Total CSA • Cort CSA • Peri circ • Endo circ • Cort thk	To determine the independent predictive role of total fat mass on cortical bone parameters at the tibia, separately in females and males; covariate included height	Although total fat mass was a positive predictor of the cortical bone parameters in males and females, the beneficial effect of adiposity on cortical bone was greater in females.

pQCT Prospective Investigations

Study	Sample	Measure	Bone parameters	Design	Results
Wetzsteon et al. (2008)	445 children (219 F, 226 M); age: 9–11 years	BMI	At the tibia, the following trabecular bone parameters were assessed at the 8% site of the bone length in the proximal direction of the distal end: • Total vBMD • Total CSA • BSI At the tibia, the following cortical bone parameters were assessed at the 50% and 66% sites of the bone length in the proximal direction of the distal end of the bone: • Cort vBMD • Total CSA • Cort CSA • SSI	16-month follow-up to compare change in bone parameters in healthy weight (<75th BMI percentile) vs. overweight (≥85th BMI percentile); statistical control sex, ethnicity, baseline pubertal stage, and change in tibia length	Over 16 months, the overweight group had a greater increase in bone size (total CSA) but similar increases in estimated bone compressive strength (BSI) at the trabecular site of the tibia, after controlling for sex, ethnicity, baseline pubertal stage, and change in tibia length. At both cortical bone sites (50% and 66% sites), the overweight group had a significantly greater change in SSI because of greater increases in total CSA and cort CSA compared with the healthy weight group. Importantly, change in estimated torsional bone strength (SSI) was significantly related with change in lean mass and muscle CSA, but not fat mass.
Pollock et al. (2009a)	71 late adolescent to young adult white females; age: 18–21 years	Total fat mass and percentage body fat assessed by DXA	At the radius and tibia, the following trabecular bone parameters were assessed at the 4% site of the bone length in the proximal direction of the distal end: • Total vBMD • Trab vBMD • Total CSA	3-year follow-up to compare change in bone parameters in normal fat (<32% body fat) vs. high fat group (≥32% body fat); statistical control for baseline lean mass and height	At baseline and 3-year follow-up, the high vs. normal fat group had lower bone structure and strength parameters at the radius and tibia, after controlling for baseline lean mass and height. Cort CSA and cort thk at the radius and tibia increased more in the high vs. normal fat group, whereas there were no differences in change for other bone parameters.

continued

TABLE 22.2 (Continued)
Adiposity and Bone Relationships in Children and Adolescents by Bone Imaging Technique and Cross-Sectional/Prospective Design

References	Population	Obesity Definition/ Adiposity Measure	Site and Bone Measure	Methodological/ Statistical Approach	Results
			At the radius and tibia, the following cortical bone parameters were assessed at the 20% site of the bone length in the proximal direction of the distal end: • Cort vBMD • Total CSA • Cort BMC • Cort CSA • Cort thk • Peri circ • Endo circ • SSI		
			QCT Cross-Sectional Investigations		
Janicka et al. (2007)	300 early adolescent to young adult whites (150 F, 150 M); age: 13–21 years	Total fat mass assessed by DXA	Lumbar spine • Trab vBMD • Total CSA Femoral midshaft • Total CSA • Cort CSA	To determine the independent determinant role of total fat mass on vBMD and CSA of the lumbar spine and femoral midshaft, separately in females and males; covariates in model were lean mass, leg length, or trunk height	In males, fat mass was a negative predictor of lumbar spine trab vBMD and femoral midshaft cort CSA, after adjusting for lean mass and trunk height or leg length. In females, there were no associations between fat mass and bone measurements.

| Gilsanz et al. (2009) | 100 late adolescent to young adult white females; age: 17.9 ± 1.9 years (range: 15–25 years) | VAT and SAAT assessed by CT | Femoral midshaft
• Total CSA
• Cort CSA
• Principal max and min moment
• Polar moment | To determine the relations of VAT and SAAT with bone structure and strength parameters of the femoral midshaft; covariates were leg length and MCSA of the midthigh. | VAT and SAAT have strong but opposing relations with bone structure and strength. Whereas VAT had negative relations with all bone parameters, SAAT had positive relations with them, after controlling for leg length and midthigh MCSA. |

Notes: F, female; M, male; W, white/Caucasian; B, black/African American; H, Hispanic American; A, Asian American. DXA, dual-energy X-ray absorptiometry; pQCT, peripheral quantitative computed tomography; CT/QCT, axial quantitative computed tomography; BMI, body mass index; aBMD, areal bone mineral density; BMC, bone mineral content; VAT, visceral adipose tissue; SAAT, subcutaneous abdominal adipose tissue; TBLH, total body less head; vBMD, volumetric BMD; CSA, cross-sectional area; cort, cortical; trab, trabecular; thk, thickness; peri, periosteal; circ, circumference; endo, endosteal; MCSA, muscle cross-sectional area; SSI, strength-strain index; BSI, bone strength index.

The discrepancies observed in the above studies are primarily related to the use of body weight, height, or both as confounders in the statistical analyses. When weight is used in the statistical adjustments, bone mass appears to be lower in overweight or obese children. When height is used in the model, bone mass is either similar or higher in overweight/obese children. Another important consideration is that when assessing total body bone in children and adolescents, it is preferable to report BMC rather than aBMD because of its reproducibility and lack of areal-density-related errors (Gordon et al., 2008). Likewise, when evaluating the relationships between fat and bone, it is ideal to examine BMC rather than aBMD.

DXA PROSPECTIVE STUDIES

Overall, the prospective DXA studies support the notion that changes in total body fat are positively associated with changes in total body BMC with growth using unadjusted data (Nelson et al., 1997) or when correcting for height, maturation, or FFST (Young et al., 2001; Clark et al., 2006) (Table 22.2). Strong positive correlations were reported by Nelson et al. (1997) for annual changes in total body BMC and fat mass in third-grade students. Young et al. (2001) reported that changes in both FFST and fat mass were strong predictors of changes in lumbar spine and hip aBMD and total body BMC in female twins, 8 to 26 years of age. However, puberty had an influence in how much FFST and fat mass affected the skeleton such that in prepubertal girls, FFST was the strongest predictor, but following the pubertal growth spurt, fat mass was the strongest predictor (Young et al., 2001). In another study that included 9-year-old children and followed for 2 years, fat mass was positively related to changes in total body less head (TBLH) bone area in both boys and girls and to TBLH BMC in boys and Tanner stage 1 girls after adjusting for either height or FFST (Clark et al., 2006).

In contrast to these findings, Wosje et al. (2009) found that a higher fat mass at 3.5 years of age resulted in less BMC accrual over the next 3.5 years, when adjusting for BMC, race, sex, age, height, or lean mass at baseline and/or follow-up. The primary difference in these prospective studies that may explain discrepancies could be related to the maturation and age of the subjects, with some being prepubertal, early pubertal, or postpubertal. These studies raise questions regarding the differential responses that may occur based on sex and maturational status.

pQCT/QCT CROSS-SECTIONAL INVESTIGATIONS

Because of their 3-D assessment capability, peripheral and axial QCT have contributed significantly to our understanding of the pediatric bone–fat relationship. In late adolescent males, Lorentzon et al. (2006) found that total fat mass was positively related with cortical bone structural parameters of the tibia, after adjusting for age, height, serum leptin concentrations, dietary calcium intake, and cigarette smoking. Similar results were observed in a study of over 4000 adolescents in which fat mass was found to be a positive predictor of cortical bone structure and density at the tibia, after controlling for height (Sayers and Tobias, 2009). These two pQCT studies suggest that increasing adiposity may be beneficial to the skeleton. Because fat mass is a component of body weight, it is indeed possible that adiposity may have a protective effect on bone due to the extra weight it mechanically "loads" on the skeleton. However, these positive findings between fat and adolescent bone must be interpreted with caution because muscle-related parameters (e.g., FFST, MCSA, etc.) were not considered in the analyses. In general, obese or overweight individuals not only have higher levels of fat than do normal-weight individuals, but they also have greater amounts of muscle.

Because of the strong relationship between muscle and bone, the higher amount of muscle in the obese participants may have confounded the relation between fat and bone. Indeed, when studies consider muscle-related parameters in the fat and bone relationship, a different picture emerges. For instance, Janicka et al. (2007) reported that total fat mass was a negative predictor of QCT-derived trabecular density at the lumbar spine and cortical bone size at the femoral midshaft, after adjusting for lean mass. In late adolescent females, Pollock et al. (2007) found that a body fat percentage greater than 32% was associated with lower pQCT-derived cortical bone structural parameters at both the tibia and radius, after controlling for MCSA (Figure 22.2). When Ducher et al. (2009) took into account MCSA in the comparison of pQCT-derived bone parameters between overweight and normal-weight children (aged 7 to 10 years), lower cortical bone structural parameters at the radius, but not at the tibia, in the overweight children were observed. This particular finding has profound clinical significance as the distal radius is the most frequent site of fracture in children approaching adolescence (Khosla et al., 2003). A recent report in children and adolescents that total fat mass was positively associated with trabecular vBMD at the radius when controlling for MCSA (Fricke et al., 2008) further supports the idea that bone size and geometry, rather than bone density, at non-weight-bearing sites may be negatively influenced by obesity when muscle-related parameters are taken into account.

pQCT PROSPECTIVE INVESTIGATIONS

Currently, only two prospective pQCT investigations have studied pediatric bone and fat relationships. In a 16-month follow-up study in 9- to 11-year-old children, Wetzsteon et al (2008) observed that increases in cortical bone geometry and strength indices at the tibia were associated with increases in FFST and MCSA, not fat mass. In late adolescent white females, Pollock et al. (2009a) observed that 3-year changes in fat mass were positively associated with changes in cortical bone size and thickness, but this relationship no longer remained statistically significant once accounting for changes in FFST and MCSA. These findings support Frost's mechanostat theory that bone adapts primarily to dynamic forces produced by muscle and not static forces imposed by extra fat mass (Frost, 1987). The significant implication of this bone adaptive response is that traumatic impact forces generated from atypical falls or other traumas depend directly on body weight (Davidson et al., 2003). Thus, if a heavier child or adolescent fell on an outstretched hand, he or she may be more likely to fracture. This example may help explain the recent evidence linking childhood obesity to skeletal fractures.

LIMITATIONS AND FUTURE DIRECTIONS FOR PEDIATRICS

A limitation of the aforementioned pediatric bone and fat investigations is that biochemical parameters indicative of metabolic abnormalities in the overweight/obese children have not been reported. Comorbidities associated with adult obesity, such as dyslipidemia, insulin resistance, and type 2 diabetes mellitus, also occur in children and adolescents (Gower et al., 1999; Weiss et al., 2004), and more importantly, the prevalence of these metabolic abnormalities is increasing alongside childhood obesity (Sinha et al., 2002; Davis et al., 2005; Sakarcan and Jerrell, 2007; Li et al., 2009). Recently, it was reported that 16% of the U.S. pediatric population have diagnosed pre-diabetes (Li et al., 2009).

Because impaired glucose metabolism, along with other metabolic abnormalities, has shown unfavorable effects on bone metabolism (Katayama et al., 1996; Miyata et al., 1997; Ahmad et al., 2003), discrepancies in prior pediatric bone–fat studies may have been attributed to metabolic abnormalities in some but not all obese subjects. Obesity-related metabolic abnormalities are more strongly related to centralized rather than total adiposity, and they lead to another potential explanation for the large body of conflicting data (Wisse, 2004). To date, only three childhood studies have considered this topic, and it seems that the influence of adiposity on bone may be dependent on the site in which fat accumulates (Afghani and Goran, 2006, 2009; Gilsanz et al., 2009).

A final explanation for the inconsistent data linking childhood adiposity and bone can be attributed to study design. The uneven spread in maturity status in children and adolescents of the same age creates one of the most difficult challenges facing researchers studying bone growth and development. At any given age, a wide variation exists among children in stature, body composition, rate of

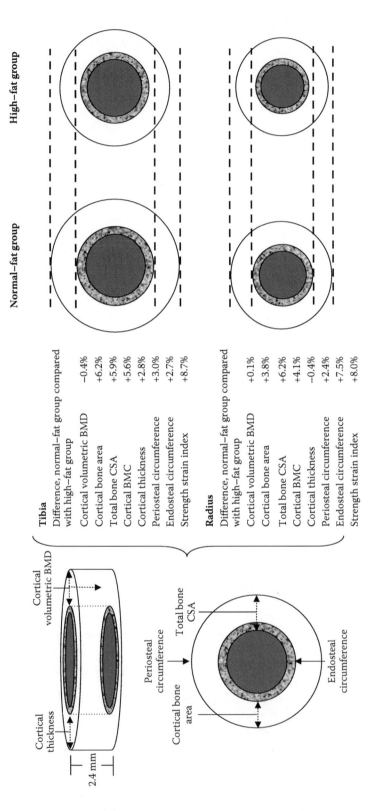

FIGURE 22.2 Schematic representation of the average magnitude of difference [A − B / (A + B) / 2 × 100] at the 20% site of the tibia and radius, after controlling for muscle cross-sectional area (CSA), in adolescent females in the normal fat group (n = 93) compared with the high fat group (n = 22). (From Pollock, N.K., et al., *Am J Clin Nutr*, 86, 1530–8, 2007. With permission.)

growth, and timing and tempo of biological maturation. Because overweight compared with normal-weight children of the same age are generally further advanced in maturation, their skeletal development is likewise more advanced, because of increased hormonal activity, than that of their normal-weight peers.

Although childhood obesity is a major public health concern and risk factor for many adult diseases, it has been difficult to determine whether adiposity is either beneficial or detrimental to the growing skeleton. Future pediatric bone–fat investigations should be innovative in study design when approaching the intricate nature of maturation. Perhaps more importantly, future studies should take into consideration the complex nature of development of the adipocyte and the osteoblast as both originate from mesenchymal stem cells in bone marrow, as described earlier in the chapter.

RELATIONSHIPS BETWEEN BONE AND BODY COMPOSITION IN ADULTS

The influence of lean or fat tissue mass on bone mass in adults, not uniformly reported in the literature, is summarized in Table 22.3. An important determinant of bone mass may be the amount of lean tissue mass (lean body mass), as a reflection of weight-bearing activity, or fat mass because it is known to influence bone density as a peripheral site of estrogen synthesis and other hormones in women and men (Baumgartner et al., 1996; Shapses and Reidt, 2006; Zhao et al., 2008). Low muscle mass is a risk factor for low BMD in young adult women, whereas higher fat accrual is protective only when it is associated with substantial muscle mass (Sowers and Reidt 1992). Consistent with this muscle–fat linkage, premenopausal and perimenopausal women show a beneficial effect of increased body weight on bone mass, but only when the weight gain is composed primarily of lean mass (Salamone et al., 1995). In studies with a wide range of ages, lean mass and strength are important predictors of bone (Aloia et al., 1995; Travison et al., 2008 a). In two populations ($n = 6477$, mean ages of 27 and 48 years for Chinese and Caucasian, respectively), a higher percentage of body fat within a BMI category diminished the beneficial effect of excess weight on total body bone (Zhao et al., 2007). A fat threshold may exist whereby the higher amounts of fat are detrimental because they release higher amounts of adipokines and inflammatory markers, or lower amounts of lean mass may permit the threshold to be attained more readily.

The strong association between lean body mass and BMD in younger women may be attributed to exercise, lifestyle factors, estrogen sufficiency, or a combination of these factors. Some studies suggest a positive influence of fat mass on bone with aging (Lindsay et al., 1992; Chen et al., 1997; Douchi et al., 2000 a), and these findings are consistent with most other studies showing that fat mass influences bone more in postmenopausal women. The influence of adiposity to increase bone in late postmenopausal years may be attributed to higher adipose-derived estrogen levels (Baumgartner et al., 1996), but other hormones may also play a role (Shapses and Reidt, 2006; Zhao et al., 2008). It is interesting that postmenopausal women on hormone replacement therapy show a greater influence of lean mass on BMD (Arabi et al., 2003). In addition, whereas osteoporosis may influence the relationship of body composition with bone mass (Gillette-Guyonnet et al., 2000; Gnudi et al., 2007), the effect of race/ethnicity shows inconsistent results (Aloia et al., 1995; Taaffe et al., 2000, 2001; Zhao et al., 2007; Travison et al., 2008a). A few studies include men (Adami et al., 2004; Makovey et al., 2005; Zhao et al., 2007; Gjesdal et al., 2008), and two show a greater relationship between BMD and greater lean tissue (Travison et al., 2008a, 2008b). Establishing the relative importance of fat versus lean mass in different populations is important because it may lead to measures that help prevent bone loss in certain physiological states.

TRABECULAR AND CORTICAL BONE AND BODY COMPOSITION

The influence of lean versus fat tissue on bone mass is complicated by the fact that this effect varies depending on the bone site being evaluated (Hla et al., 1996; Takata et al., 1999; Blain

TABLE 22.3
Body Composition and Bone in Adults

References	Population: Gender, Age, Location	Site of BMC/BMD measure	Number	Result/Conclusion	Fat or Lean, Importance to BMD
Compston et al. (1992)	Female, post age: 58 years (49–65 years) Britain	Regional bone density in the lumbar spine and femur	97	FM is the greatest predictor of bone in postmenopausal women. Both FM and LM are related to total and regional bone mass in postmenopausal women, the relationship being strongest for fat mass.	Fat
Di Monaco et al. (2007)	Female, post age: 80 years after hip fracture Italy	Neck, total femur, trochanter, intertrochanteric	293	FM, but not LM, was the pivotal determinant of BMD in our sample of hip fracture women. This may suggest that reduced LM does not have a wide enough range in this older and likely sedentary population to influence BMD.	Fat
Reid et al. (1994)	Female, post age: 60 years New Zealand	Lumbar spine	119	FM was a better predictor than lean for LS vBMD.	Fat
Reid (1992)	Female, post age: 58 years (45–71 years) New Zealand	Total body (and subregions, spine, femur)	140	FM is the most significant predictor of BMD	Fat
Reid et al. (1995)	Female, pre nonexercising and exercising Age: 33 years New Zealand	Total body	99: non-exercising subjects (36), exercising subjects (63)	In non-exercisers, the percent fat tended to be positively related to areal BMD, whereas the percent lean was inversely related to this index. For exercisers, bone density is only associated with FM in sedentary women. In exercisers, femoral neck density is related to LM, possibly through the effects of weight-bearing exercise on both of these variables.	Fat for sedentary, lean for exercisers
Aloia et al. (1995)	Female (pre and post) Age: 24–79 years Black, Caucasian USA	Total body	165	In black and white healthy women, although bone mass may be partially influenced by fatness or race, the major determinant of bone mass is fat-free mass. FM may play a more important role in postmenopausal women.	Lean

continued

Reference	Subjects	Measurement	Sample	Findings	
Zhao et al. (2007)	Male and female Chinese Pre, men Age: 27 years (19–45 years) China Caucasians: Pre, post, men Age: 47 years (19–90 years) USA	Lumbar spine and femoral neck; total Body BMC	1988 Chinese 878 pre, 1110 men 4489 Caucasians 2667 pre and post; 1822 male	Higher FM does not increase bone mass when the mechanical loading effects of overall body weight are statistically controlled. Further multivariate analyses in subjects stratified by body weight confirmed the inverse relationship between bone mass and FM, after mechanical loading effects due to total body weight were controlled. Increasing FM may not have a beneficial effect on bone mass.	Lean
Travison et al. (2008a, 2008b)	Male, age: 30–79 years Black, Caucasian, Hispanic USA	Hip, spine, forearm Femur strength (2008a)	1209 subjects: 363 non-Hispanic Black, 397 Hispanic, 449 non-Hispanic white n = 1171 in 2008a article	Weight, BMI, waist circumference, and FM were associated with BMC only up to certain thresholds, whereas lean mass exhibited more consistent associations. Results did not vary by race/ethnicity. The protective effect of increased body size on bone mass is likely due to the influence of LM, which increases femoral strength measures.	Lean
Arabi et al. (2003)	Female, post age: 48–60 years on hormone replacement therapy France	Total and Regional BMD	109	Both FM and LM are related to BMD in postmenopausal women, but the relationship is strongest with LM.	Lean
Gjesdal et al. (2008)	Male and female, post age: 47–50 years and 71–75 years Norway	Hip, femoral neck	5205	Compared with FM, LM was generally more strongly related to BMD of the femoral neck in middle-aged and elderly men and women.	Lean
Bedogni et al. (2002)	Female (pre and post) Age: 63 years (37–88 years) Caucasian Italy	Total Body BMD	2009	In Caucasian women, (1) LM is a stronger predictor of BMC than FM, but (2) Wt is a better predictor of BMC than body composition for practical purposes; however, weight and body composition are not able to explain more than 46% of BMC variance.	Lean
Liu et al. (2004)	Female, pre age: 35 years China	BMD at lumbar spine (L2–L4), total hip, and total body	282	LM is an important factor determining BMD in young and premenopausal women.	Lean

TABLE 22.3 (Continued)
Body Composition and Bone in Adults

References	Population: Gender, Age, Location	Site of BMC/BMD measure	Number	Result/Conclusion	Fat or Lean, Importance to BMD
Sowers et al. (1992)	Female, pre age: 20–40 years USA	Proximal femur, including femoral neck and trochanter	246	Low muscle mass is a risk factor for low bone mineral density in young adult women, whereas higher fat is protective only when it is associated with substantial muscle mass (Sowers et al., 1992).	Lean
Salamone et al. (1995)	Female (pre peri) Age: 44–50 years USA	Femoral neck, lumbar spine, and whole-body	334	Premenopausal and perimenopausal women show a beneficial effect of increased body weight on bone mass, but only when it is comprised primarily of LM. In premenopausal and early perimenopausal women, body weight alone may not be associated with increased bone mass unless a significant proportion of that weight is composed of LM.	Lean
Douchi et al. (2000a)	Female, pre age: 39 years, post: 62 years Japan	Lumbar spine	296 pre and 233 post	Significant determinants of lumbar spine BMD Pre: LM and age at menarche Post: Years since menopause, FM, LM, height Effect of adiposity on BMD is more prominent in post compared with pre.	Both in post, lean in pre
Gnudi et al. (2007)	Female, post age: 62 years Italy	Total Body BMD	770 total osteoporotic (307) and nonosteoporotic (463)	In nonosteoporotic postmenopausal women, lean mass was significantly associated with BMD, BMC, and BMD/height ($p < .001$), whereas fat mass was not. In osteoporotic women, both LM and FM were associated with BMD to the same extent.	Lean for nonosteoporotic; both for osteoporotic
Blum et al. (2003)	Female, pre age: 42 years USA	Total hip, lumbar spine, and total body	153	Results suggest that for a given body weight, a higher proportion of fat and a higher serum leptin concentration have negative associations with bone mass in premenopausal women.	Lean, negative association with fat

Reference	Subjects	Measurement	N	Findings	Fat or lean more important
Khosla et al. (1996)	Female (pre and post) Age: pre 35 years Age: post 68 years USA	BMC at the total body, lumbar spine, proximal femur, and forearm	351 total 138 pre 213 post	LM had a dominant effect on spine and hip BMC in both groups and hip BMC in premenopausal women, whereas both LM and FM predicted hip BMC in postmenopausal women. Both LM and FM predicted total body BMC in premenopausal and postmenopausal women. However, when BMC was adjusted for bone or body size using BMD, BMAD, or BMD/height, FM tended to become more important than LM.	Fat, but varied depending on where measured (i.e., lean in premenopausal in non-weight-bearing sites)
Gillette-Guyonnet et al. (2000)	Female, post age: 78–89 years Osteoporotic France	Total body BMD	129	FM alone, in a multivariate model, was correlated with whole body BMD, whereas femoral BMD was associated with both fat mass and lean tissue mass. There were significant positive correlations between BMD in all areas and body measurements (weight, fat mass, lean tissue mass), but FM accounted for more of the variance in total body and femoral BMD than lean tissue mass.	Fat, but also varied depending on where measured
Glauber et al. (1995)	Female, post age: 65 years and older USA	Total body, fat mass by BIA	6705	For older women, the effect of weight on BMD is important at weight-bearing sites (femur, calcaneous) via total weight rather than adiposity, but at non-weight-bearing sites, such as the radius, adiposity exerts more important effects.	Fat but only on non-weight-bearing sites
Taaffe et al. (2000)	Female, post age: 60–86 years Mexican American and non-Hispanic Caucasians USA	Lumbar spine, hip (femoral neck, trochanter, Ward's triangle), and total body	116	LM influenced BMD at the spine and hip in non-Hispanic Caucasian women, with FM also contributing at the femoral neck. In Mexican American women, LM influenced spine and trochanter BMD, and both LM and FM contributed to whole body BMD. However, the effects of LM and FM were removed in both groups when BMD was adjusted for body or bone size.	LM and FM were associated with BMD depending on the bone site index and primarily explained by sex and not race/ethnicity.
Taaffe et al. (2001)	Female and male Age: 70–79 years White and Black USA	Femoral neck and total body	2619	LM was a significant determinant of BMD in all. In women, FM was a significant determinant of BMD at the femoral neck; FM and muscle strength contributed to limb BMD. LM and FM were associated with BMD depending on the bone site index and primarily explained by sex, not race.	

continued

TABLE 22.3 (Continued)
Body Composition and Bone in Adults

References	Population: Gender, Age, Location	Site of BMC/BMD measure	Number	Result/Conclusion	Fat or Lean, Importance to BMD
Makovey et al. (2005)	Male and female (pre and post) 45 pairs aged <50 years and 48 pairs aged >50 years) Australia	Total body and hip BMD	186 total 93 pairs of twins	LM had stronger positive relationships with the most bone variables than did fat mass in both genders at all ages. FM had positive relationships with total body and hip BMD in women aged <50, but not >50, years. There was no significant relationship between FM and total or regional BMD in men <50 years, but men >50 years showed positive relationships between FM measures and total and some regional BMD measures.	Varied depending on where measured, age, gender

Notes: Table is sorted by importance of relationship to BMD (fat or lean) then both. Studies with >96 total subjects (does not include those with small subgroups unless unique questions were addressed). DXA for all studies unless otherwise indicated. BIA, bioimpedence; BMC, bone mineral content; BMD, bone mineral density; BMAD, bone mineral apparent density; pre, premenopausal; post, postmenopausal; peri, perimenopausal. LM, lean mass; FM, fat mass; DXA, dual-energy vBMD = volumetric bone mineral density; Wt = weight; X-ray absorptiometry.

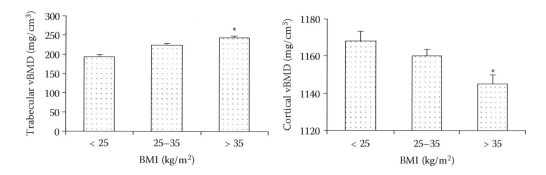

FIGURE 22.3 Influence of BMI on trabecular and cortical vBMD in women. *Differs from BMI <25 kg/ m^2, $p < .05$; volumetric bone mineral density (vBMD); body mass index (BMI). (From Nutritional Aspects of Osteoporosis: Shapses, S.A., Riedt, C.S., Schlussel, Y., et al., Body weight and menopausal status influence trabecular and cortical BMD, pp. 231–40, Copyright 2007, with permission from Elsevier.)

et al., 2001). Differences in trabecular or cortical content of bone, as well as weight bearing of the specific site, may confound the observations. For example, a study in older women showed that total weight influenced BMD at weight-bearing sites, yet adiposity (and not total weight) influenced non-weight-bearing sites, such as the radius (Glauber et al., 1995). In addition, the excess fat tissue surrounding the bone in obesity may result in potential errors in the DXA measurement (Hangartner and Johnston, 1990; Bolotin, 1998; Tothill, 2005). In clinical trials, pQCT, which measures true volumetric (v) bone density (mg/cm^3) and uses the density of fat tissue as zero, has been found to reduce artifacts associated with a two-dimensional measurement of areal bone density (g/cm^2) by DXA. In addition, potential BMD artifacts in obesity may be attenuated or removed by measuring a peripheral site (rather than axial) because less soft tissue surrounds the bone of the forearm or leg.

Some reports suggest that fat mass has a negative influence on BMD (Blum et al., 2003; Hsu et al., 2006; Zhao et al., 2007; Sukumar et al., 2011) or no significant influence on the strength of cortical bone as measured in obese rodent models (Stevenson et al., 2009). In our laboratory, we have found that a greater adiposity in women was associated with higher trabecular BMD but lower cortical BMD (Figure 22.3). Even when corrected for a greater muscle area, a negative relationship exists between fat mass and cortical bone, and a positive association of fat mass with trabecular bone and strength indices is no longer observed (Shapses et al., 2007; Sukumar et al., 2011). These data in adults are consistent with findings in overweight children (Pollock et al., 2007; Ducher et al., 2009). Although a lower cortical vBMD is typically associated with greater fracture risk, it is possible that compensation by increased cortical area, BMC, and periosteal circumference in obese individuals positively affects the biomechanical properties because bone size has been shown to contribute to bone strength (Ducher et al., 2009; Uusi-Rasi et al., 2009a). Nevertheless, the lower cortical BMD in obesity may help to explain why others have found that even when BMD T score is in the normal range in obese individuals, it is associated with an increased fracture risk (Premaor et al., 2009). Higher serum parathyroid hormone (PTH) and lower 25-hydroxyvitamin D (25OHD) in the obese population may contribute to reduced bone quality and fracture risk independent of other factors.

VISCERAL COMPARED WITH SUBCUTANEOUS FAT AND BMD

The distribution of adipose tissue in the body is more clinically relevant for metabolic syndrome than the increased total body adipose tissue per se. Yet, less is known about its specific influence of metabolic syndrome on bone. In postmenopausal overweight and obese women, visceral fat, estimated by waist:hip ratio, was a better predictor of bone at the radius (Tarquini et al., 1997). In addition, trunk fat or abdominal fat, but not peripheral fat mass, was found to be the most important predictor of BMD in women (Douchi et al., 2000b; Warming et al., 2003; Makovey et al., 2005; Kuwahata et al., 2008). Others have suggested that the low blood concentration of adiponectin in obesity plays a role in the protective effects of visceral fat on BMD (Lenchik et al., 2003). One study examining the ultradistal radius in men found that greater visceral adiposity was associated with reduced BMD (Jankowska et al., 2001). In healthy young women (mean age of 18 years; BMI 17–34 kg/m^2), subcutaneous fat is beneficial to bone structure and strength, whereas visceral fat serves as a unique pathogenic fat depot and negatively correlates with bone structure and strength (Gilsanz et al., 2009).

Although studies in postmenopausal women consistently suggest a positive relationship between visceral fat and bone, the influence of fat on bone may differ in children or men or depend on the specific bone site. Therefore, the site in which fat accumulates may help explain the large body of conflicting data on the link between body adiposity and bone mass.

Total Weight, Composition, and Fracture Risk

Obesity is associated with numerous comorbidities, but osteoporosis, as defined by low bone mineral density, is not one characteristic of excess body weight. In fact, it is well established that lean individuals are at greater risk of fracture than the obese. De Laet et al. (2005) showed almost a two-fold greater risk of fracture in men and women with BMI of 20 kg/m^2 compared with 25 kg/m^2. The association between BMI and fracture is so closely linked that, when BMD T score are not available, BMI is used to predict fracture risk (Kanis et al., 2008). However, empirical evidence suggests that the obese individuals are not protected from fracture at all sites (Table 22.4). For example, a population-based longitudinal study which included 10,902 women showed that high BMI significantly increased the risk of proximal humerus and ankle fractures, whereas, by contrast, a high BMI lowered the risk of forearm, vertebral, and hip fractures (Holmberg et al., 2006) (Figure 22.4). In addition, other researchers have also found a higher humerus fracture risk in obese women (Gnudi et al., 2009). High BMI was associated with a lower risk of fracture at most sites (including the proximal humerus) in 22,444 men (Holmberg et al., 2006). In addition, De Laet et al. (2005) found that, when BMI is adjusted for BMD, the risk of fracture increases when BMI is greater than 35 kg/m^2. This high BMI–fracture link suggests that obesity may differentially diminish bone quality at specific bone sites, in addition to the mechanical disadvantage of falling.

The influence of body composition on incident fractures is less well understood, although an increase in fat and a decrease in lean tissue are associated with functional decline and metabolic dysfunction in the elderly. In men (30–79 years), the protective effect of high BMI in preventing fractures (as estimated by femoral strength measures) was mediated by the influence of increased muscle mass, and not by additional adipose tissue (Travison et al., 2008b). Combination of a higher percentage fat and lower lean mass was associated with non-spine fractures (Hsu et al., 2006). In another study, 59% of obese and 73% of morbidly obese women had normal BMD, and only 12% and 5%, respectively, had osteoporosis (Premaor et al., 2009). However, although BMI was associated with higher hip T score, it was also associated with a greater rate of a previous fracture. The explanation of these results is not clear from this trial, yet the possibility that excess adiposity overestimates BMD in obese subjects because of measurement artifacts cannot be excluded. However, the normal BMD and higher risk of fracture in obesity is either a result of compromised bone quality or greater mechanical forces on the bone during a fall, despite the extra padding of body fat.

In 2941 elderly white and black women and men where hip fracture was validated over a 7-year period, it was found that individuals with fractures were older and had lower percentage fat, lower muscle strength and physical performance score, and lower total hip BMD (Lang et al., 2009), which is similar to other studies. This study also found that a decrease of one standard deviation in thigh muscle Hounsfield Unit (an indicator of intramuscular fat) conferred a nearly 40% increase in

TABLE 22.4
Effect of Body Weight or Composition on Fracture Risk

References	Population and Location	Duration	Methods	Result/Conclusion
Hsu et al. (2006)	Men (n = 7137) Pre (n = 2248) Post (n = 4585) China	Cross-sectional	Non-spine fx (reported in questionnaire) and body composition. Analyzed in fat quartiles	Greater percent fat mass is associated with greater risk of non-spine fx: Fat mass for third and fourth quartiles (Q3 and Q4): Men—Q3 1.7 (0.9, 3.2); Q4 2.3 (1.1, 4.9) Premenopausal women—Q3 2.1 (0.8, 5.1); Q4 3.0 (1.1, 7.8) Postmenopausal women—Q3 1.7 (0.7, 4.3); Q4 1.3 (0.4, 3.4) Lean mass Q3 and Q4 for postmenopausal women only: Q3 0.6 (0.3, 1.1); Q4 0.5 (0.2, 1.0)
De Laet et al. (2005)	12 prospective trials (~60,000 men and women) USA and Europe	250,000 person years (3- to 20-year follow-up)	Any fx and BMI	Compared with BMI (kg/m^2) of 25, hip fx RR for: BMI of 20 is 1.95 (CI 1.71–2.22), whereas BMI of 30 RR is 0.83 (CI 0.69–0.99) No difference between gender for risk of fx based on BMI
Premaor et al. (2009)	Post (n = 805) 62 years Fracture clinic UK	Cross-sectional	Spine and hip BMD history of low trauma fracture, BMI quartile, T score	High prevalence of low trauma fx in obese and morbidly obese postmenopausal women with normal BMD. As expected, fx rate was highest in leaner women.
Holmberg et al. (2006)	Post (n = 10,902) 50 years at baseline Sweden 22,444 men (age 44 years at baseline	~15-year follow-up 19 years follow-up	Fracture (forearm, vertebral, proximal humerus, ankle, hip)	Women: Higher BMI increased the risk of proximal humerus and ankle fx (RR 1.21–1.33) and lowered the risk of forearm fx (RR 0.88, CI 0.81–0.96) and hip fx (RR 0.63, CI 0,51–0.78) Men: Higher BMI reduced fx risk at all sites except ankle (trend for increased RR at ankle)
Gnudi et al. (2009)	Post (n = 2235) 63 years Italy	Cross-sectional	Hip, proximal humerus, ankle, wrist, separated by BMI categories (lean, overweight, obese)	Leanness predicted hip fx OR 3.8 (CI, 2.035–7.168), but not overweight and obesity. Only the obese group predicted proximal humerus fx OR 3.5 (CI, 1.8–6.7)
Lang et al. (2009)	Men (n = 1286) Post (n = 1345) 70–79 years Black and white	6.6 years follow-up	Hip fx and tertiles of thigh muscle Hounsfield Unit (a measure of intramuscular fat)	↓ thigh muscle Hounsfield Unit = ↑ risk of hip fx RR of 1.58 (CI 1.1, 1.99) at 3rd tertile

Notes: Measurement with DXA except Lang et al. (2009). Fx, fracture; CI, 95% confidence interval; OR, odds ratio pre, premenopausal; post, postmenopausal; RR, relative risk; BMD, bone mineral density; BMI, body mass index.

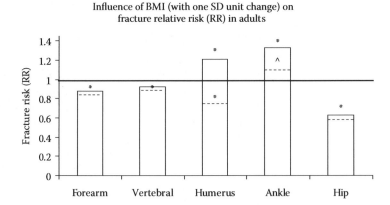

Influence of BMI (with one SD unit change) on
fracture relative risk (RR) in adults

FIGURE 22.4   Data represent women (bar graph) and men (dashed line); SD, standard deviation. *Differs from RR of 1.0, $p \leq .01$, ^$p = .07$. (Adapted from Holmberg, A.H., et al., *Osteoporos Int* 17, 1065–1077, 2006.)

the risk of hip fracture. Hence, measurement of total fat or lean mass by DXA may not be able to adequately capture changes in muscle composition in older individuals, suggesting that thigh muscle fat may provide a better estimate of muscle strength and hip fracture risk (Lang et al., 2009).

Overall, obesity is associated with lower hip fracture but higher risk of proximal humerus fracture and possibly ankle fracture in women, and these findings are consistent with higher forearm fracture risk in children (Goulding et al., 2005). In older men, obesity has not specifically been shown to increase fracture risk (Holmberg et al., 2006), although some evidence suggests that further analysis may be needed to establish a fat–fracture relationship in older men (Lang et al., 2009; Premaor et al., 2009). Unfortunately, evidence has been published that once an obese child or adult fractures, recovery involves more complications or is longer in duration (Leet et al., 2005; Di et al., 2006).

EXERCISE INFLUENCES BONE AND FRACTURE RISK

The effects of physical activity or mechanical forces on bone have a positive effect (Nordström et al., 1997), and the greater mechanical load on bone due to excess weight has been suggested to increase bone mass in obesity. In premenopausal women divided into exercisers and non-exercise groups, bone density is conclusively associated only with fat mass in sedentary women (Reid et al., 1995). In exercisers, femoral neck density is related to lean mass, possibly through the effects of weight-bearing exercise on both of these variables (Reid et al., 1995). In men, lean mass is influenced by physical activity and is the single most important correlate with BMD (Hill et al., 2008). In elderly women with low bone mass, impact exercise was randomly assigned over a 30-month period (home-based and supervised) compared with no intervention (Korpelainen et al., 2006). Exercise reduced loss of BMD at the trochanter and femoral neck compared with the control group, and importantly, only six falls were reported in the exercise group that resulted in fractures compared with 16 falls/fractures in the control group (Korpelainen et al., 2006). Other investigators have shown that resistance exercise in a randomized double-blind study (98 women aged 75–85 years) increases cortical BMD compared with agility training or stretching exercise (Liu-Ambrose et al., 2004).

BODY WEIGHT PREDICTS SUBSEQUENT BONE LOSS

In a prospective observational study (Nguyen et al., 1998) in postmenopausal women over a period of almost 3 years, researchers observed more rapid bone loss in those weighing less than 60 kg

(−1.5 ± 0.2%) and in women weighing between 61 and 70 kg (−0.6 ± 0.2%), compared with women weighing more than 70 kg who showed no significant bone loss. The effect of weight on bone loss was independent of age in this study. Another longitudinal study in postmenopausal women over 3 years confirms these findings (Tremollieres et al., 1993), showing a reduced annual rate of bone loss in overweight compared with lean women. From a regression analysis in this study, annual spinal BMD loss was estimated to be >1.0% in normal-weight women (BMI <25), 0.5%–1.0% in overweight women (BMI 25–30), and less than 0.5% in obese women (BMI >30) (Tremollieres et al., 1993). These findings suggest an almost linear relationship between bone loss and initial body weight. In addition, a prospective study in postmenopausal women showed that women with a lower baseline body weight showed significantly greater 5-year bone loss at the radius (Sowers et al., 1993). Holmberg et al. (2006) found that weight gain of >10 kg because the age 30 years reduces fracture risk at the hip (37%) but increases fractures at the ankle (54%).

Studies examining how body fat, rather than total weight, influence future bone loss are limited, but at least two studies (Reid et al., 1994; Chen et al., 1997) found that BMD loss correlates significantly with loss of fat mass. In addition, in older adults, an association between sarcopenia (estimated by relative skeletal muscle mass) and lower BMD, thinner cortices (Szulc et al., 2005), and greater bone loss has become well established.

WEIGHT REDUCTION AND BONE

Epidemiological studies have consistently shown that loss of body weight in older men or women, whether voluntary or involuntary, is associated with reduced BMD. Furthermore, studies showing that this decline in BMD resulting from weight reduction will increase susceptibility to fracture have been reported for animal studies (Talbott et al., 2001; Hamrick et al., 2008) and for hip fracture risk in clinical trials of women (Langlois et al., 2001; Ensrud et al., 2003) and men (Mussolino et al., 1998; Meyer et al., 2008). In addition, Omsland et al. (2009) found that a 5% weight loss increases fracture risk at the distal forearm by 33% (1.33, 95% confidence interval: 1.09, 1.62) in a study of 7817 postmenopausal women.

In intervention trials with voluntary weight reduction, a 1%–2% loss of bone at the hip and lumbar spine with about 10% weight reduction in older women (Shapses and Reidt 2006) has been reported. Nevertheless, we have found that moderate amount of weight loss in older women primarily results in loss of fat tissue (17% loss) and surprisingly, little lean mass (3% loss) (Riedt et al., 2005). Loss of bone due to moderate weight reduction is not consistently reported in younger women (< 45 years) or in men (Shapses et al., 2001; Riedt et al., 2007; Redman et al., 2008). This is consistent with findings in a short-term weight reduction study (3 months) using pQCT in obese premenopausal women (Uusi-Rasi et al., 2009a), where there was no bone loss, and may be attributed to the well-maintained muscle performance in men and young women (Uusi-Rasi et al., 2009b). Similar to severe weight loss in humans at any age (Fleischer, et al., 2008) (~30% weight loss), caloric restriction in rodents over 10 weeks results in significant bone loss (Hamrick et al., 2008; Hawkins et al., 2010) that may be primarily from cortical regions (Hamrick et al., 2008). More moderate compared with extreme weight reduction may possibly differentially influence bone quality. Both obesity (Shapses et al., 2007; Pollck et al., 2007) and weight reduction (Hamrick et al., 2008) are associated with reduced cortical bone density so that the combination of dieting in obese individuals may pose a risk to cortical bone.

Maintaining weight reduction over a long duration versus weight cycling may be important considerations for bone loss. For example, preliminary data show that obese older women who maintain their lower body weight after 2 years exhibit a faster rate of bone loss compared with women who regain their lost weight (Shapses, unpublished data). Fogelholm et al. (1997) found that women with a history of weight cycling are associated with lower spine and distal radius BMD compared with noncyclers. Importantly, Meyer et al. (1998) showed that greater weight variability was associated with increased hip fracture incidence in women and men over a 12-year period (aged 49–61 years). Change in BMD may be regulated by changes in fat mass (Reid, 2002). Nevertheless, in a cohort that included an older population of 2163 men and women over a 4-year period, greater loss of lean mass was found with weight reduction and only a small gain in lean mass with weight gain compared with no weight stable individuals (Newman et al., 2005). Other researchers have not found an effect of weight cycling on bone, such as a cross-sectional study in younger women (aged 37 years) (Gallagher et al., 2002) and in weight cycling athletes (Prouteau et al., 2006). Again, the preservation of muscle mass likely plays an important role in maintaining bone in younger individuals.

EXERCISE DURING WEIGHT REDUCTION

Exercise training can slow or prevent the loss and/or increase of BMD (Prince et al., 1991). A decrease in mechanical loading on the skeleton could contribute to bone loss associated with weight loss, whereas the addition of exercise to weight loss regimens may help to maintain lean body mass and attenuate bone loss (Ryan et al., 1998; Villareal et al., 2006; Silverman et al., 2009). In weight loss studies that address the level of physical activity, resistance training has not shown a significant improvement on bone compared with diet alone in premenopausal women (Andersen et al., 1997), nor has it been observed in other studies with aerobic and anaerobic exercise (Svendsen et al., 1993; Redman et al., 2008; Villareal et al., 2008). Perhaps a limited number of subjects, or variable age, calcium intake, or duration of the weight loss programs contributes to the inconsistent findings of the effect of exercise on bone during weight loss.

Overall, strong evidence supports the loss of bone related to weight reduction in older women, but not in younger women or in men, and with weight regain, partial recovery of bone may occur, yet fracture risk may be increased by partial loss of bone mass (Meyer et al., 1998). Studies addressing cortical and trabecular bone changes resulting from weight reduction in long-term trials are needed to determine whether the bone quality, in addition to mass, is altered with changes in body weight and composition.

SUMMARY

The assumption that obesity is beneficial to bones by protecting against fragility fractures can no longer be assumed. Measures of bone quality can be assessed with computed tomography and magnetic resonance imaging to better understand the relationship with body fat during growth and with aging, as has been addressed in our laboratories. It is possible that hormones and adipokines synthesized by adipose tissue are influencing bone, whereas the mechanical advantage of excess adipose tissue on bone may be reducing the risk of fracture at some sites. In adults, excess weight can prevent bone loss with aging, and although overweight individuals may be protected against fracture risk, excessive adiposity may not, such as when BMI is greater than 35 kg/m^2. Moderate weight reduction decreases bone in older obese women, whereas severe weight and fat loss result in a proportional loss of bone in individuals at any age. Many questions, however, about fat–bone relationships still remain. Answers to some questions will likely require longitudinal studies with large sample size, a suitably powered design, and careful data analysis, but also further advances in our ability to measure and interpret bone quality and integrity. The need to improve understandings of the fat–bone relationship will generate substantial research interest in the coming years.

ACKNOWLEDGMENTS

Thanks to D. Sukumar for her review of the literature and assistance in creating the figures and to and L. Blade, M. Slane, and K. Tomaino for their editorial assistance.

REFERENCES

Ackerman A., J. C. Thornton, J. Wang, et al. 2006. Sex difference in the effect of puberty on the relationship between fat mass and bone mass in 926 healthy subjects, 6 to 18 years old. *Obesity* 14:819–825.

Adami S., V. Braga, M. Zamboni, et al. 2004. Relationship between lipids and bone mass in 2 cohorts of healthy women and men. *Calcif Tissue Int* 74:136–142.

Afghani A., M.I. Goran. 2006. Racial differences in the association of subcutaneous and visceral fat on bone mineral content in prepubertal children. *Calcif Tissue Int* 79:383–388.

Afghani A., and M.I. Goran. 2009. The interrelationships between abdominal adiposity, leptin and bone mineral content in overweight Latino children. *Horm Res* 72:82–87.

Ahdjoudj S., F. Lasmoles, X. Holy, et al. 2002. Transforming growth factor beta2 inhibits adipocyte differentiation induced by skeletal unloading in rat bone marrow stroma. *J Bone Miner Res* 17:668–677.

Ahmad T., C. Ohlsson, M. Saaf, et al. 2003. Skeletal changes in type-2 diabetic Goto-Kakizaki rats. *J Endocrinol* 178:111–116.

Aloia J. F., A. Vaswani, R. Ma, et al. 1995. To what extent is bone mass determined by fat-free or fat mass? *Am J Clin Nutr* 61:1110–1114.

Andersen R. E., T. A. Wadden, R. J. Herzog. 1997. Changes in bone mineral content in obese dieting women. *Metabolism* 46: 857–861.

Arabi A., P. Garnero, R. Porcher, et al. 2003. Changes in body composition during post-menopausal hormone therapy: A 2 year prospective study. *Hum Reprod* 18:1747–1752.

Arabi A., H. Tamim, M. Nabulsi, et al. 2004. Sex differences in the effect of body-composition variables on bone mass in healthy children and adolescents. *Am J Clin Nutr* 80:1428–1435.

Asakura A., M. Komaki, M. Rudnicki. 2001. Muscle satellite cells are multipotential stem cells that exhibit myogenic, osteogenic, and adipogenic differentiation. *Differentiation* 68:245–253.

Baumgartner R. N., P. M. Stauber, K. M. Koehler, et al. 1996. Associations of fat and muscle masses with bone mineral in elderly men and women. *Am J Clin Nutr* 63:365–372.

Baxter-Jones A.D., S.A. Kontulainen, R.A. Faulkner, D.A. Bailey. 2008. A longitudinal study of the relationship of physical activity to bone mineral accrual from adolescence to young adulthood. *Bone* 43: 1101–1107.

Bedogni G., C. Mussi, M. Malavolti, et al. 2002. Relationship between body composition and bone mineral content in young and elderly women. *Ann Hum Biol* 29:559–565.

Blain H., A. Vuillemin, A. Teissier, et al. 2001. Influence of muscle strength and body weight and composition on regional bone mineral density in healthy women aged 60 years and over. *Gerontology* 47:207–212.

Blum M., S. S. Harris, A. Must, et al. 2003. Leptin, body composition and bone mineral density in premenopausal women. *Calcif Tissue Int* 73:27–32.

Bolotin H. H. 1998 A new perspective on the casual influence of soft tissue composition on DXA-measured in vivo bone mineral density. *J Bone Miner Res* 13:1739–1746.

Chen Z., T. G. Lohman, W. A. Stini, et al. 1997. Fat or lean tissue mass: Which one is the major determinant of bone mineral mass in healthy postmenopausal women? *J Bone Miner Res* 12:144–151.

Clark E. M., A. R. Ness, J. H. Tobias. 2006. Adipose tissue stimulates bone growth in prepubertal children. *J Clin Endocrinol Metab* 91:2534–2541.

Compston J. E., M. Bhambhani, M. A. Laskey, et al. 1992. Body composition and bone mass in post-menopausal women. *Clin Endocrinol* (Oxf). 37(5):426–431.

Cornish J., K. E. Callon, U. Bava, et al. 2002. Leptin directly regulates bone cell function in vitro and reduces bone fragility in vivo. *J Endocrinol* 175:405–415.

Courteix D., E. Lespessailles, S. Loiseau-Peres, et al. 1998. Lean tissue mass is a better predictor of bone mineral content and density than body weight in prepubertal girls. *Rev Rhum Engl Ed* 65:328–336.

Davidson P. L., A. Goulding, D. J. Chalmers. 2003. Biomechanical analysis of arm fracture in obese boys. *J Paediatr Child Health* 39:657–664.

Davis C. L., B. Flickinger, D. Moore, et al. 2005. Prevalence of cardiovascular risk factors in schoolchildren in a rural Georgia community. *Am J Med Sci* 330:53–59.

De Laet C., J. A. Kanis, A. Odén, et al. 2005. Body mass index as a predictor of fracture risk: A meta-analysis. *Osteoporos Int* 16:1330–1338.

De Schepper J., M. Van den Broeck, M. H. Jonckheer. 1995. Study of lumbar spine bone mineral density in obese children. *Acta Paediatr* 84:313–315.

Di M. M., F. Vallero, M. R. Di, et al. 2006. Body mass index and functional recovery after hip fracture: A survey study of 510 women. *Aging Clin Exp Res* 18:57–62.

Dimitri P., J. Wales, N. Bishop. 2009. Fat and bone in children—differential effects of obesity on bone size and mass according to fracture history. *J Bone Miner Res* DOI:10.1359/jbmr.090823.

Di Monaco M., F. Vallero, R. Di Monaco, et al. 2007. Skeletal muscle mass, fat mass, and hip bone mineral density in elderly women with hip fracture. *J Bone Miner Metab* 25:237–242.

Do Prado W. L., A. de Piano, M. Lazaretti-Castro, et al. 2009. Relationship between bone mineral density, leptin and insulin concentration in Brazilian obese adolescents. *J Bone Miner Metab* 27:613–619.

Douchi T., S. Yamamoto, T. Oki, et al. 2000a. Relationship between body fat distribution and bone mineral density in premenopausal Japanese women. *Obstet Gynecol* 95:722–725.

Douchi T., S. Yamamoto, T. Oki, et al. 2000b Difference in the effect of adiposity on bone density between pre- and postmenopausal women. *Maturitas* 34:261–266.

Doyle F., J. Brown, C. Lachance. 1970. Relation between bone mass and muscle weight. *Lancet* 17(643):391–393.

Ducher G., S. L. Bass, G. A. Naughton, et al. 2009. Overweight children have a greater proportion of fat mass relative to muscle mass in the upper limbs than in the lower limbs: Implications for bone strength at the distal forearm. *Am J Clin Nutr* 90:1104–1111.

Ducy P., M. Amling, S. Takeda, et al. 2000. Leptin inhibits bone formation through a hypothalamic relay: A central control of bone mass. *Cell* 100:197–207.

El Hage R., C. Jacob, E. Moussa, et al. 2009a. Total body, lumbar spine and hip bone mineral density in overweight adolescent girls: Decreased or increased? *J Bone Miner Metab* 27:629–633.

El Hage R. P., D. Courteix, C. L. Benhamou, et al. 2009b. Relative importance of lean and fat mass on bone mineral density in a group of adolescent girls and boys. *Eur J Appl Physiol* 105:759–764.

Ellis K. J., R. J. Shypailo, W. W. Wong, et al. 2003. Bone mineral mass in overweight and obese children: Diminished or enhanced? *Acta Diabetol* 40 (Suppl 1):S274–S277.

Ensrud K. E., S. K. Ewing, K. L. Stone, et al. 2003. Study of Osteoporotic Fractures Research Group. Intentional and unintentional weight loss increase bone loss and hip fracture risk in older women. *J Am Geriatr Soc* 51:1740–1747.

Faulkner R. A., D. A. Bailey, D. T. Drinkwater, et al. 1993. Regional and total body bone mineral content, bone mineral density, and total body tissue composition in children 8–16 years of age. *Calcif Tissue Int* 53:7–12.

Fogelholm M., H. Sievänen, A. Heinonen, et al. 1997. Association between weight cycling history and bone mineral density in premenopausal women. *Osteoporos Int* 7:354–358.

Fricke O., C. Land, O. Semler, et al. 2008. Subcutaneous fat and body fat mass have different effects on bone development at the forearm in children and adolescents. *Calcif Tissue Int* 82:436–444.

Frost H. M. 1987. Bone mass and the mechanostat: A proposal. *Anat Rec* 219:1–9.

Frost H. M. 1997. Obesity, and bone strength and mass: A tutorial based on insights from a new paradigm. *Bone* 21:211–214.

Gallagher K. I., J. M. Jakicic, D. P. Kiel, et al. 2002. Impact of weight-cycling history on bone density in obese women. *Obes Res* 10:896–902.

Gillette-Guyonnet S., F. Nourhashemi, S. Lauque, et al. 2000.Body composition and osteoporosis in elderly women. *Gerontology* 46:189–193.

Gilsanz V., J. Chalfant, A. O. Mo, et al. 2009 Reciprocal relations of subcutaneous and visceral fat to bone structure and strength. *J Clin Endocrinol Metab* 94:3387–3393.

Gimble J. M., S. Zvonic, Z. E. Floyd, et al. 2006. Playing with bone and fat. *J Cell Biochem* 15(98):251–266.

Gjesdal C. G., J. I. Halse, G. E. Eide, et al. 2008. Impact of lean mass and fat mass on bone mineral density: The Hordaland Health Study. *Maturitas* 20(59):191–200.

Glauber H. S., W. M. Vollmer, M. C. Nevitt, et al. 1995. Body weight versus body fat distribution, adiposity, and frame size as predictors of bone density. *J Clin Endocrinol Metab* 80:1118–1123.

Gnudi S., E. Sitta, N. Fiumi. 2007. Relationship between body composition and bone mineral density in women with and without osteoporosis: Relative contribution of lean and fat mass. *J Bone Miner Metab* 25(5):326–332.

Gnudi S., E. Sitta, L. Lisi. 2009. Relationship of body mass index with main limb fragility fractures in postmenopausal women. *J Bone Miner Metab* 27:479–484.

Gordon C. M., L. K. Bachrach, T. O. Carpenter, et al. 2004. Bone health in children and adolescents: A symposium at the annual meeting of the Pediatric Academic Societies/Lawson Wilkins Pediatric Endocrine Society, May 2003. *Curr Probl Pediatr Adolesc Health Care* 34:226–242.

Gordon C. M., L. K. Bachrach, T. O. Carpenter, et al. 2008. Dual energy X-ray absorptiometry interpretation and reporting in children and adolescents: The 2007 ISCD Pediatric Official Positions. *J Clin Densitom* 11:43–58.

Goulding A., R. Cannan, S. M. Williams, et al. 1998. Bone mineral density in girls with forearm fractures. *J Bone Miner Res* 13:143–148.

Goulding A., A. M. Grant, S. M. Williams. 2005. Bone and body composition of children and adolescents with repeated forearm fractures. *J Bone Miner Res* 20:2090–2096.

Goulding A., I. E. Jones, R. W. Taylor, et al. 2000a. More broken bones: A 4-year double cohort study of young girls with and without distal forearm fractures. *J Bone Miner Res* 15:2011–2018.

Goulding A., I. E. Jones, R. W. Taylor, et al. 2001. Bone mineral density and body composition in boys with distal forearm fractures: A dual-energy X-ray absorptiometry study. *J Pediatr* 139:509–515.

Goulding A., R. W. Taylor, A. M. Grant, et al. 2008. Relationship of total body fat mass to bone area in New Zealand five-year-olds. *Calcif Tissue Int* 82:293–299.

Goulding A., R. W. Taylor, I. E. Jones, et al. 2002. Spinal overload: A concern for obese children and adolescents? *Osteoporos Int* 13:835–840.

Goulding A., R. W. Taylor, I. E. Jones, et al. 2000b. Overweight and obese children have low bone mass and area for their weight. *Int J Obes Relat Metab Disord* 24:627–632.

Gower B. A., T. R. Nagy, M. I. Goran. 1999. Visceral fat, insulin sensitivity, and lipids in prepubertal children. Diabetes 48:1515–1521.

Grodin J. M., P. K. Siiteri, P. C. MacDonald. 1973. Source of estrogen production in postmenopausal women. *J Clin Endocrinol Metab* 36:207–214.

Hamrick M. W., K. H. Ding, S. Ponnala, et al. 2008. Caloric restriction decreases cortical bone mass but spares trabecular bone in the mouse skeleton: Implications for the regulation of bone mass by body weight. *J Bone Miner Res* 23:870–878.

Hangartner T. N., C. C. Johnston. 1990. Influence of fat on bone measurements with dual-energy absorptiometry. *Bone Miner* 9:71–81.

Heinonen A., H. Sievanen, P. Kannus, et al. 2000. High-impact exercise and bones of growing girls: A 9-month controlled trial. *Osteoporos Int* 11:1010–1017.

Hill D. D., J. A. Cauley, Y. Sheu, et al. 2008. Correlates of bone mineral density in men of African ancestry: The Tobago bone health study. *Osteoporos Int.* 19:227–234.

Hla M. M., J. W. Davis, P. D. Ross, et al. 1996. A multicenter study of the influence of fat and lean mass on bone mineral content: Evidence for differences in their relative influence at major fracture sites. Early Postmenopausal Intervention Cohort (EPIC). *Am J Clin Nutr* 64:354–360.

Hogler W., J. Briody, H. J. Woodhead, et al. 2003. Importance of lean mass in the interpretation of total body densitometry in children and adolescents. *J Pediatr* 143:81–88.

Holmberg A. H., O. Johnell, P. M. Nilsson, et al. 2006. Risk factors for fragility fracture in middle age. A prospective population-based study of 33,000 men and women. *Osteoporos Int* 17:1065–1077.

Hsu Y. H., S. A. Venners, H. A. Terwedow, et al. 2006. Relation of body composition, fat mass, and serum lipids to osteoporotic fractures and bone mineral density in Chinese men and women. *Am J Clin Nutr.* 83:146–154.

Hui S. L., L. A. Dimeglio, C. Longcope, et al. 2003. Difference in bone mass between black and white American children: Attributable to body build, sex hormone levels, or bone turnover? *J Clin Endocrinol Metab* 88:642–649.

Janicka A., T. A. Wren, M. M. Sanchez, et al. 2007. Fat mass is not beneficial to bone in adolescents and young adults. *J Clin Endocrinol Metab* 92:143–147.

Jankowska E. A., E. Rogucka, M. Medraś. 2001 Are general obesity and visceral adiposity in men linked to reduced bone mineral content resulting from normal ageing? A population-based study. *Andrologia* 33:384–389.

Kanis J. A., O. Johnell, A. Oden, et al. 2008. FRAX and the assessment of fracture probability in men and women from the UK. *Osteoporos Int* 19:385–397.

Katayama Y., T. Akatsu, M. Yamamoto, et al. 1996. Role of nonenzymatic glycosylation of type I collagen in diabetic osteopenia. *J Bone Miner Res* 11:931–937.

Kuwahata A., Y. Kawamura, Y. Yonehara, et al. 2008. Non-weight-bearing effect of trunk and peripheral fat mass on bone mineral density in pre- and post-menopausal women. *Maturitas* 60:244–247.

Khosla S., E. J. Atkinson, B. L. Riggs, et al. 1996. Relationship between body composition and bone mass in women. *J Bone Miner Res.* 11:857–863.

Khosla S., L. J. Melton, 3rd, M. B. Dekutoski, et al. 2003. Incidence of childhood distal forearm fractures over 30 years: A population-based study. *JAMA* 290:1479–1485.

Klein G. L., L. A. Fitzpatrick, C. B. Langman, et al 2005. The state of pediatric bone: Summary of the ASBMR pediatric bone initiative. *J Bone Miner Res* 20:2075–2081.

Klein K. O., K. A. Larmore, E. de Lancey, et al. 1998. Effect of obesity on estradiol level, and its relationship to leptin, bone maturation, and bone mineral density in children. *J Clin Endocrinol Metab* 83:3469–3475.

Korpelainen R., S. Keinänen-Kiukaanniemi, J. Heikkinen, et al. 2006. Effect of impact exercise on bone min-
    eral density in elderly women with low BMD: A population-based randomized controlled 30-month
    intervention. *Osteoporos Int* 17:109–118.
Lang T. F., J. Cauley, F. Tylavsky, et al. 2009, for the Health ABC Study. Computed tomography measurements
    of thigh muscle cross-sectional area and attenuation coefficient predict hip fracture: The Health, Aging
    and Body Composition Study. *J Bone Miner Res* 25: 513–519.
Langlois J. A., M. E. Mussolino, M. Visser, et al. 2001. Weight loss from maximum body weight among mid-
    dle-aged and older white women and the risk of hip fracture: The NHANES I epidemiologic follow-up
    study. *Osteoporos Int* 12:763–768.
Leet A. I., C. P. Pichard, M. C. Ain. 2005. Surgical treatment of femoral fractures in obese children: Does
    excessive body weight increase the rate of complications? *J Bone Joint Surg Am* 87:2609–2613.
Lenchik L., T. C. Register, F. C. Hsu, et al. 2003 . Adiponectin as a novel determinant of bone mineral density
    and visceral fat. *Bone*.33:646-51.
Leonard M. B., J. Shults, B. A. Wilson, et al. 2004. Obesity during childhood and adolescence augments bone
    mass and bone dimensions. *Am J Clin Nutr* 80:514–523.
Li C., E. S. Ford, G. Zhao, et al. 2009. Prevalence of pre-diabetes and its association with clustering of car-
    diometabolic risk factors and hyperinsulinemia among U.S. adolescents: National Health and Nutrition
    Examination Survey 2005–2006. Diabetes Care 32:342–347.
Lindsay R., F. Cosman, B. S. Herrington, et al. 1992. Bone mass and body composition in normal women. *J
    Bone Miner Res*. 7:55–63.
Liu J. M., H. Y. Zhao, G. Ning, et al. 2004. Relationship between body composition and bone mineral density
    in healthy young and premenopausal Chinese women. *Osteoporos Int* 15:238–242.
Liu-Ambrose T. Y., K. M. Khan, J. J. Eng, et al. 2004. Both resistance and agility training increase cortical bone
    density in 75- to 85-year-old women with low bone mass: A 6-month randomized controlled trial. *J Clin
    Densitom* 7:390–398.
Lorentzon M., K. Landin, D. Mellstrom, et al. 2006. Leptin is a negative independent predictor of areal BMD
    and cortical bone size in young adult Swedish men. *J Bone Miner Res* 21:1871–1878.
Macdonald H. M., S. A. Kontulainen, K. J. Mackelvie-O'Brien, et al. 2005. Maturity- and sex-related changes
    in tibial bone geometry, strength and bone-muscle strength indices during growth: A 20-month pQCT
    study. *Bone* 36:1003–1011.
Macdonald H., S. Kontulainen, M. Petit, et al. 2006. Bone strength and its determinants in pre- and early puber-
    tal boys and girls. *Bone* 39:598–608.
MacKelvie K. J., M. A. Petit, K. M. Khan, et al. 2004. Bone mass and structure are enhanced following a 2-year
    randomized controlled trial of exercise in prepubertal boys. *Bone* 34:755–764.
Makovey J., V. Naganathan, P. Sambrook. 2005. Gender differences in relationships between body composi-
    tion components, their distribution and bone mineral density: A cross-sectional opposite sex twin study.
    Osteoporos Int 16:1495–505.
Manzoni P., P. Brambilla, A. Pietrobelli, et al. 1996. Influence of body composition on bone mineral content in
    children and adolescents. *Am J Clin Nutr* 64:603–607.
McCormick D. P., S. W. Ponder, H. D. Fawcett, et al. 1991. Spinal bone mineral density in 335 normal
    and obese children and adolescents: Evidence for ethnic and sex differences. *J Bone Miner Res*
    6:507–513.
McKay H. A., M. A. Petit, K. M. Khan, et al. 2000. Lifestyle determinants of bone mineral: A comparison
    between prepubertal Asian- and Caucasian-Canadian boys and girls. *Calcif Tissue Int* 66:320–324.
Meyer H.E., Søgaard, A.J., Falch, J.A., Jørgensen, L., Emaus, N. 2008. Weight change over three decades and
    the risk of osteoporosis in men: The Norwegian Epidemiological Osteoporosis Studies (NOREPOS). *Am
    J Epidemiol* 168: 454–460.
Miyata T., K. Notoya, K. Yoshida, et al. 1997. Advanced glycation end products enhance osteoclast-induced
    bone resorption in cultured mouse unfractionated bone cells and in rats implanted subcutaneously with
    devitalized bone particles. *J Am Soc Nephrol* 8:260–270.
Morris F. L., G. A. Naughton, J. L. Gibbs, et al. 1997. Prospective ten-month exercise intervention in premenar-
    cheal girls: Positive effects on bone and lean mass. *J Bone Miner Res* 12:1453–1462.
Mussolino M. E., A. C. Looker, J. H. Madans, et al. 1998. Risk factors for hip fracture in white men: The
    NHANES I epidemiologic follow-up study. *J Bone Miner Res* 13:918–924.
Nagasaki K., T. Kikuchi, M. Hiura, et al. 2004. Obese Japanese children have low bone mineral density after
    puberty. *J Bone Miner Metab* 22:376–381.
Nelson D. A., P. M. Simpson, C. C. Johnson, et al. 1997. The accumulation of whole body skeletal mass in third-
    and fourth-grade children: Effects of age, gender, ethnicity, and body composition. *Bone* 20:73–78.

Newman A. B., J. S. Lee, M. Visser, et al. 2005. Weight change and the conservation of lean mass in old age: The Health, Aging and Body Composition Study. *Am J Clin Nutr* 82:872–878

Nguyen T. V., P. N. Sambrook, J. A. Eisman. 1998. Bone loss, physical activity, and weight change in elderly women: The Dubbo Osteoporosis Epidemiology Study. *J Bone Miner Res* 13:1458–1467.

Nordström P., G. Nordström, R. Lorentzon. 1997. Correlation of bone density to strength and physical activity in young men with a low or moderate level of physical activity. *Calcif Tissue Int* 60:332–327.

Ogle G. D., J. R. Allen, I. R. Humphries, et al. 1995. Body-composition assessment by dual-energy X-ray absorptiometry in subjects aged 4–26 y. *Am J Clin Nutr* 61:746–753.

Omsland T. K., B. Schei, A. B. Grønskag, et al. 2009. Weight loss and distal forearm fractures in postmenopausal women: The Nord-Trøndelag health study, Norway. *Osteoporos Int* 20: 2009–2016.

Parhami F., S. M. Jackson, Y. Tintut, et al. 1999. Atherogenic diet and minimally oxidized low density lipoprotein inhibit osteogenic and promote adipogenic differentiation of marrow stromal cells. *J Bone Miner Res* 14:2067–2078.

Parhami F., A. D. Morrow, J. Balucan, et al. 1997. Lipid oxidation products have opposite effects on calcifying vascular cell and bone cell differentiation. A possible explanation for the paradox of arterial calcification in osteoporotic patients. *Arterioscler Thromb Vasc Biol* 17:680–687.

Petit M. A., T. J. Beck, S. A. Kontulainen. 2005a. Examining the developing bone: What do we measure and how do we do it? *J Musculoskelet Neuronal Interact* 5:213–224.

Petit M. A., T. J. Beck, J. Shults, et al. 2005b. Proximal femur bone geometry is appropriately adapted to lean mass in overweight children and adolescents. *Bone* 36:568–576.

Pollack K. M., D. Xie, K. B. Arbogast, et al. 2008. Body mass index and injury risk among US children 9–15 years old in motor vehicle crashes. *Inj Prev* 14:366–371.

Pollock, N. K., A. Ferira, E. M. Laing, et al. 2009a. Adiposity and bone structural development in young adult females: A 3-year follow-up study. *J Bone Miner Res* 24 (Suppl 1):S95.

Pollock N. K., Y. Dong, B. Gutin, et al. 2009b. Lower bone mass and adiponectin in overweight adolescents with cardiovascular risk factors. *J Bone Miner Res* 24 (Suppl 1):S151.

Pollock N. K., E. M. Laing, C. A. Baile, et al. 2007. Is adiposity advantageous for bone strength? A peripheral quantitative computed tomography study in late adolescent females. *Am J Clin Nutr* 86:1530–1538.

Premaor M. O., L. Pilbrow, C. Tonkin, et al. 2009. Obesity and fractures in postmenopausal women. *J Bone Miner Res* 25: 292–297.

Prince R. L., M. Smith, I. M. Dick, et al. 1991. Prevention of postmenopausal osteoporosis. A comparative study of exercise, calcium supplementation, and hormone-replacement therapy. *N Engl J Med* 325:1189–1195.

Prouteau S., A. Pelle, K. Collomp, et al. 2006.Bone density in elite judoists and effects of weight cycling on bone metabolic balance. *Med Sci Sports Exerc* 38:694–700.

Rauch F., D. A. Bailey, A. Baxter-Jones, et al. 2004. The 'muscle–bone unit' during the pubertal growth spurt. *Bone* 34:771–775.

Rauch F., E. Schoenau. 2001. The developing bone: Slave or master of its cells and molecules? *Pediatr Res* 50:309–314.

Rauch F., E. Schonau. 2002. Skeletal development in premature infants: A review of bone physiology beyond nutritional aspects. *Arch Dis Child* 86:F82–F85.

Rauch F., E. Schoenau. 2008. Peripheral quantitative computed tomography of the proximal radius in young subjects—new reference data and interpretation of results. *J Musculoskelet Neuronal Interact* 8:217–226.

Redman L. M., J. Rood, S. D. Anton, et al. 2008. Comprehensive Assessment of Long-Term Effects of Reducing Intake of Energy (CALERIE) Research Team. Calorie restriction and bone health in young, overweight individuals. *Arch Intern Med.* 22(168):1859–1866.

Reid I. R. 2002 Relationships among body mass, its components, and bone. *Bone.* 31:547–555.

Reid I. R. 2008. Relationships between fat and bone. *Osteoporos Int* 19:595–606.

Reid I. R., R. W. Ames, M. C. Evans, et al. 1994. Determinants of the rate of bone loss in normal postmenopausal women. *J Clin Endocrinol Metab* 79:950–954.

Reid I. R., M. Legge, J. P. Stapleton, et al. 1995. Regular exercise dissociates fat mass and bone density in premenopausal women. *J Clin Endocrinol Metab* 80:1764–1768.

Riedt C. S., M. Cifuentes, T. Stahl, et al. 2005. Overweight postmenopausal women lose bone with moderate weight reduction and 1 g/d calcium intake. *J Bone Min Res* 20:455–463.

Riedt C. S., Y. Schlussel, N. von Thun, et al. 2007. Premenopausal overweight women do not lose bone during moderate weight loss with adequate or higher calcium intake. *Am J Clin Nutr* 85:972–80. Erratum in: *Am J Clin Nutr.* Sep;86(3):808.

Rittweger J., G. Beller, J. Ehrig, et al. 2000. Bone-muscle strength indices for the human lower leg. *Bone* 27:319–326.

Rocher E., C. Chappard, C. Jaffre, et al. 2008. Bone mineral density in prepubertal obese and control children: Relation to body weight, lean mass, and fat mass. *J Bone Miner Metab* 26:73–78.

Roemmich J. N., P. A. Clark, C. S. Mantzoros, et al. 2003. Relationship of leptin to bone mineralization in children and adolescents. *J Clin Endocrinol Metab* 88:599–604.

Rosen C. J., M. L. Bouxsein. 2006. Mechanisms of disease: Is osteoporosis the obesity of bone? *Nat Clin Pract Rheumatol* 2:35–43.

Ryan A. S., B. J. Nicklas, K. E. Dennis. 1998. Aerobic exercise maintains regional bone mineral density during weight loss in postmenopausal women. *J Appl Physiol* 84: 305–1310.

Sakarcan A., J. Jerrell. 2007. Population-based examination of the interaction of primary hypertension and obesity in South Carolina. *Am J Hypertens* 20:6–10.

Salamone L. M., N. Glynn, D. Black, et al. 1995. Body composition and bone mineral density in premenopausal and early perimenopausal women. *J Bone Miner Res* 10:1762–1768.

Sayers A., J. H. Tobias. 2009. Fat mass exerts a greater effect on cortical bone mass in girls than boys. *J Clin Endocrinol Metab* DOI:10.1210/jc.2009-1907.

Schoenau E., C. M. Neu, B. Beck, et al. 2002. Bone mineral content per muscle cross-sectional area as an index of the functional muscle–bone unit. *J Bone Miner Res* 17:1095–1101.

Schoenau E., C. M. Neu, E. Mokov, et al. 2000. Influence of puberty on muscle area and cortical bone area of the forearm in boys and girls. *J Clin Endocrinol Metab* 85:1095–1098.

Schoenau E., M. C. Neu, F. Manz. 2004. Muscle mass during childhood—relationship to skeletal development. *J Musculoskelet Neuronal Interact* 4:105–108.

Schoenau E., E. Werhahn, U. Schiedermaier, et al. 1996. Influence of muscle strength on bone strength during childhood and adolescence. *Horm Res* 45 (Suppl 1):63–66.

Shapses S. A., C. S. Riedt. 2006. Bone, body weight, and weight reduction: What are the concerns? *J Nutr* 136:1453–1456.

Shapses S. A., C. S. Riedt, Y. Schlussel, et al. 2007. Body weight and menopausal status influence trabecular and cortical BMD. In: *Nutritional Aspects of Osteoporosis*. Eds. Burckhardt P., Dawson Hughes B., Heaney R. P. pp. 231–240. Elsevier, Amsterdam, The Netherlands.

Shapses S. A., N. L. Von Thun, S. B. Heymsfield, et al. 2001. Bone turnover and density in obese premenopausal women during moderate weight loss and calcium supplementation. *J Bone Miner Res.* 16:1329–1336.

Shapses S.A. In: von Thun Rutgers Univ. dissertation, 2009.

Silverman N. E., B. J. Nicklas, A. S. Ryan. 2009 Addition of aerobic exercise to a weight loss program increases BMD, with an associated reduction in inflammation in overweight postmenopausal women. *Calcif Tissue Int* 84(4):257–265.

Sinha R., G. Fisch, B. Teague, et al. 2002. Prevalence of impaired glucose tolerance among children and adolescents with marked obesity. *N Engl J Med* 346:802–810.

Skaggs D. L., M. L. Loro, P. Pitukcheewanont, et al. 2001. Increased body weight and decreased radial cross-sectional dimensions in girls with forearm fractures. *J Bone Miner Res* 16:1337–1342.

Sowers M. F., A. Kshirsagar, M. M. Crutchfield, et al. 1992. Joint influence of fat and lean body composition compartments on femoral bone mineral density in premenopausal women. *Am J Epidemiol* 136:257–265.

Sowers M. R., M. K. Clark, M. L. Jannausch, et al. 1993. Body size, estrogen use and thiazide diuretic use affect 5-year radial bone loss in postmenopausal women. *Osteoporos Int* 3:314–321.

Specker B., T. Binkley, N. Fahrenwald. 2004. Increased periosteal circumference remains present 12 months after an exercise intervention in preschool children. *Bone* 35:1383–1388.

Sukumar D., Ambia-Sobhan, H., Zurfluh, R., Schlussel, Y., Stahl, T., Gordon, C., Shapses, S. 2010. Areal and volumetric bone mineral density and geometry at two levels of protein intake during caloric restriction: A randomized controlled trial. *J Bone Miner Res* [Epub ahead of print].

Svendsen O. L., C. Hassager, C. Christiansen. 1993. Effect of an energy-restrictive diet, with or without exercise, on lean tissue mass, resting metabolic rate, cardiovascular risk factors, and bone in overweight postmenopausal women. *Am J Med* 95:131–140.

Szulc P., T. J. Beck, F. Marchand, et al. 2005. Low skeletal muscle mass is associated with poor structural parameters of bone and impaired balance in elderly men—the MINOS study. *J Bone Miner Res* 20:721–729.

Taaffe D. R., J. A. Cauley, M. Danielson, et al. 2001. Race and sex effects on the association between muscle strength, soft tissue, and bone mineral density in healthy elders: The Health, Aging, and Body Composition Study. *J Bone Miner Res* 16:1343–1352.

Taaffe D. R., M. L. Villa, L. Holloway, et al. 2000. Bone mineral density in older non-Hispanic Caucasian and Mexican-American women: Relationship to lean and fat mass. *Ann Hum Biol* 27:331–344.

Talbott S. M., M. Cifuentes, M. G. Dunn, S. A. Shapses. 2001. Energy restriction reduces bone density and biomechanical properties in aged female rats. *J Nutr* 131: 2382 -2387.

Takada I., A. P. Kouzmenko, S. Kato. 2009. Wnt and PPARgamma signaling in osteoblastogenesis and adipogenesis. *Nat Rev Rheumatol* 5:442–447.

Takata S., T. Ikata, H. Yonezu. 1999. Characteristics of bone mineral density and soft tissue composition of obese Japanese women: Application of dual-energy X-ray absorptiometry. *J Bone Miner Metab* 17:206–210.

Tarquini B., N. Navari, F. Perfetto, et al. 1997. Evidence for bone mass and body fat distribution relationship in postmenopausal obese women. *Arch Gerontol Geriatr* 24:15–21.

Taylor E. D., K. R. Theim, M. C. Mirch, et al. 2006. Orthopedic complications of overweight in children and adolescents. *Pediatrics* 117:2167–2174.

Timpson N. J., A. Sayers, G. Davey-Smith, et al. 2009. How does body fat influence bone mass in childhood? A Mendelian randomization approach. *J Bone Miner Res* 24:522–533.

Tothill P. 2005 Dual-energy X-ray absorptiometry measurements of total-body bone mineral during weight change. *J Clin Densitom* 8:31–38.

Travison T. G., A. B. Araujo, G. R. Esche, et al. 2008a. Lean mass and not fat mass is associated with male proximal femur strength. *J Bone Miner Res* 23:189–198.

Travison T. G., A. B. Araujo, G. R. Esche, et al. 2008b. The relationship between body composition and bone mineral content: Threshold effects in a racially and ethnically diverse group of men. *Osteoporos Int* 19:29–38.

Tontonoz P., B. M. Spiegelman. 2008. Fat and beyond: The diverse biology of PPAR gamma. *Annu Rev Biochem* 77:289–312.

Tremollieres F. A., J. M. Pouilles, C. Ribot. 1993. Vertebral postmenopausal bone loss is reduced in overweight women: A longitudinal study in 155 early postmenopausal women. *J Clin Endocrinol Metab* 77:683–686.

Turner C. H., D. B. Burr. 1993. Basic biomechanical measurements of bone: A tutorial. *Bone* 14:595–608.

Uusi-Rasi K., A. Rauhio, P. Kannus, et al. 2009a. Three-month weight reduction does not compromise bone strength in obese premenopausal women. *Bone* 46:1286–1293.

Uusi-Rasi K., H. Sievanen, P. Kannus, et al. 2009b Influence of weight reduction on muscle performance and bone mass, structure and metabolism in obese premenopausal women. *J Musculoskelet Neuronal Interact* 9:72–80.

Valdimarsson O., J. O. Kristinsson, S. O. Stefansson, et al. 1999. Lean mass and physical activity as predictors of bone mineral density in 16–20-year old women. *J Intern Med* 245:489–496.

Van der Meulen M. C., K. J. Jepsen, B. Mikic. 2001. Understanding bone strength: Size isn't everything. *Bone* 29:101–104.

Verma S., J. H. Rajaratnam, J. Denton, et al. 2002. Adipocytic proportion of bone marrow is inversely related to bone formation in osteoporosis. *J Clin Pathol* 55:693–698.

Villareal D. T., L. Fontana, E. P. Weiss, et al. 2006. Bone mineral density response to caloric restriction-induced weight loss or exercise-induced weight loss: A randomized controlled trial. *Arch Intern Med* 166:2502–2510.

Villareal D. T., K. Shah, M. R. Banks, et al. 2008. Effect of weight loss and exercise therapy on bone metabolism and mass in obese older adults: A one-year randomized controlled trial. *J Clin Endocrinol Metab* 93:2181–2187.

Von Thun N. 2009. Weight loss and bone loss in postmenopausal women: Follow up at 2 years. Ed, Shapses S.A. Thesis at Rutgers University Press.

Wainwright S. A., W. D. Biggs, J. D. Currey, et al. 1976. *Mechanical Design in Organisms*. London: Edward Arnold.

Wang Y., T. Lobstein. 2006. Worldwide trends in childhood overweight and obesity. *Int J Pediatr Obes* 1:11–25.

Warming L., P. Ravn, C. Christiansen. 2003 .Visceral fat is more important than peripheral fat for endometrial thickness and bone mass in healthy postmenopausal women. *Am J Obstet Gynecol* 188:349–353.

Weiler H. A., L. Janzen, K. Green, et al. 2000. Percent body fat and bone mass in healthy Canadian females 10 to 19 years of age. *Bone* 27:203–207.

Weiss R., J. Dziura, T. S. Burgert, et al. 2004. Obesity and the metabolic syndrome in children and adolescents. *N Engl J Med* 350:2362–2374.

Wetzsteon R. J., M. A. Petit, H. M. Macdonald, et al. 2008. Bone structure and volumetric BMD in overweight children: A longitudinal study. *J Bone Miner Res* 23:1946–1953.

Wisse B. E. 2004. The inflammatory syndrome: The role of adipose tissue cytokines in metabolic disorders linked to obesity. *J Am Soc Nephrol* 15:2792–2800.

Witzke K. A., C. M. Snow. 1999. Lean body mass and leg power best predict bone mineral density in adolescent girls. *Med Sci Sports Exerc* 31:1558–1563.

Wosje K. S., P. R. Khoury, R. P. Claytor, et al. 2009. Adiposity and TV viewing are related to less bone accrual in young children. *J Pediatr* 154:79–85.e72.

Young D., J. L. Hopper, R. J. Macinnis, et al. 2001. Changes in body composition as determinants of longitudinal changes in bone mineral measures in 8 to 26-year-old female twins. *Osteoporos Int* 12:506–515.

Young D., J. L. Hopper, C. A. Nowson, et al. 1995. Determinants of bone mass in 10- to 26-year-old females: A twin study. *J Bone Miner Res* 10:558–567.

Zhao L. J., H. Jiang, C. J. Papasian, et al. 2008. Correlation of obesity and osteoporosis: Effect of fat mass on the determination of osteoporosis. *J Bone Miner Res* 23:17–29.

Zhao L. J., Y. J. Liu, P. Y. Liu, et al. 2007. Relationship of obesity with osteoporosis. *J Clin Endocrinol Metab* 92:1640–1646.

23 Exercise and Skeletal Growth

Adam D.G. Baxter-Jones and R.A. Faulkner

CONTENTS

INTRODUCTION

The principal cause of osteoporotic fractures is reduced bone mass, and the increased risk of fractures later in life is related to a failure of the skeleton to achieve optimal mass and strength during the growing years (Raisz, 2005). Childhood and adolescence are particularly important periods of early life to maximize bone accrual because the skeleton undergoes rapid change to accommodate the processes of growth, modeling, and remodeling (Faulkner and Bailey, 2007). Recent data confirm that peak bone mass likely occurs by the end of the second decade or early in the third decade and that over the circum-pubertal years 33% to 43% (depending on site) of adult bone mineral content (BMC) is accrued (Forwood et al., 2007; Baxter-Jones et al., 2011).

Although bone mineral accrual depends on many factors, especially genetics, modifiable factors such as physical activity and nutrition also are clearly important in affecting skeletal growth and development (Heaney and Weaver, 2005; Bonjour et al., 2007). The skeleton needs calcium for bone gain, and physical activity exerts the mechanical loading on bone to stimulate mineral deposition; thus, it seems logical that adequate calcium intake and physical activity would optimize the genetic potential for bone accrual during growth. Although the physiology is not completely understood, calcium is considered to have a potentiating effect in allowing mechanical loading of bone (through physical activity) to affect bone mineral accrual (Branca et al., 2001). Considerable data have been reported on the effects of physical activity and nutrition on bone accrual during childhood and adolescence; however, relatively few studies have investigated specifically the interactive effects of physical activity and nutrition. Anderson (2000) suggested that one of the reasons for this lack of information is that nutrition scientists have undervalued the importance of physical activity in bone development, especially because physical activity is likely an important mechanism to counter low calcium intakes in children.

In this chapter, we focus on examining the evidence on the interactive effects of physical activity and nutrition (primarily calcium) on bone health. However, to set the context, a brief overview on the role of physical activity and nutrition during childhood and adolescence on bone mineral accrual is included. Then, the evidence on the interactive effects of physical activity and nutrition on bone accrual is summarized, and finally, potential physiological mechanisms explaining interaction effects are discussed.

MEASURING BONE MASS BY DUAL ENERGY X-RAY ABSORPTIOMETRY

Bone has many interesting attributes, including its size, shape, and strength. In humans, these properties, with some limitations, can be measured using various forms of imaging. One of the most commonly used methods of imaging bone mass during growth is by dual-energy X-ray absorptiometry (DXA). DXA measures are based on the decrease in photon energy of a photon beam as it passes through bone and nonmineralized soft tissue. DXA provides a precise evaluation of BMC (g) within a given bone area (cm^2). These values are then used to identify an areal bone mineral density (BMD) (g/cm^2). Although BMD is the most useful measure because it partially corrects for the effect of size, it fails to assess the skeleton in three dimensions. Thus, if two bones are made of precisely the same material, the larger one will be measured to have greater BMD by DXA (Khan et al., 2001). In children, the three-dimensional shape and size of bones change dramatically during growth. Thus, a simple adjustment of BMC based on bone size in two dimensions (BMD) is an inadequate surrogate for bone density during growth (Nelson and Koo, 1999). For these reasons, it is suggested that BMC and not areal BMD be reported for studies of children's bone growth.

PHYSICAL ACTIVITY

The effect of physical activity during growth on bone development is well documented (Bailey et al., 1996; Burrows, 2007; Tobias et al., 2007; Janz et al., 2008), and as summarized by McKay and Smith (2008), level 1 evidence now strongly supports the beneficial effects of weight-bearing physical activity during the growing years on bone mass accrual and skeletal health. For example, data from randomized control studies have shown that a 7-month exercise intervention in normal health active children resulted in a 2.5% greater BMC accrual in the intervention compared with the nonintervention group (MacKelvie et al., 2001, 2002); after 20 months, the difference doubled to about 5% greater accrual in the intervention group (MacKelvie et al., 2003, 2004). Weeks and colleagues (2008) found sex-specific affects after an 8-month randomized control jumping intervention study: Boys increased in total body (TB) bone mass, whereas girls increased in bone mass at the hip and spine compared with controls.

Longitudinal studies that control for the effects of normal growth and development (such as biological maturation) also have shown positive effects of physical activity on bone development. BMC accrual across 6 years of growth was significantly greater in physically active children than that in inactive children, and active children had greater BMC at maturity (Bailey et al., 1999). In a 3-year prospective study over the pubertal period, gymnasts had 24%–51% (depending on site) more BMC than did controls (Nurmi-Lawton et al., 2004). Similarly, Mathews and coworkers (2006) found that female ballet dancers (8 to 11 years at entry) accrued significantly more BMC at multiple skeletal sites over a 3-year period compared with controls. Gunter and coworkers (2008a) showed that skeletal benefits of a high-impact jumping intervention in children 7 to 8 years at baseline persisted from 7 months to 3 years after the interventions.

Bone strength is a factor of material properties, dimensions, quality, architecture, and bone mass. Earlier studies were restricted to the latter; however, there is increasing evidence on other bone strength factors such as cross-sectional area (CSA) and section modulus (Z) of bones. For example, results from studies predicting bone strength parameters from DXA measures have shown positive effects of physical activity (Petit et al., 2002). Prepubertal gymnasts had higher CSAs and section modulus (Z) at the hip compared with controls (Faulkner et al., 2003). MacDonald and coresearchers (2007) reported modest changes in measures of bone strength at the tibia in boys, but not girls, who had at least 80% compliance with a school-based 16-month jumping intervention. A 3-year physical activity intervention program in boys and girls 6 to 8 years of age affected BMC at the forearm and bone width at the calcaneus (Hasselstrom et al., 2008).

Everyday amounts of physical activity also have been associated with greater CSA and Z at the hip in children 4 to 12 years of age (Janz et al., 2007). In a longitudinal study, physical activity was a significant independent predictor of CSA and Z at the femoral neck (FN) after controlling for biological maturity (Forwood et al., 2006). In many of these studies, the effects of physical activity were attenuated when adjusted for lean body mass; that is, the affects were explained by the interdependence between physical activity and lean (muscle) mass. Dowthwaite and coinvestigators (2009) did find gymnastics training remained a significant predictor of skeletal strength parameters after controlling for muscle mass. Nevertheless, the moderating effect of lean mass on the relationship between physical activities on skeletal adaptation makes physiological sense. For example, physical activity has an independent effect on the growth of lean body mass during adolescence (Baxter-Jones et al., 2008), and its the mechanical loading of bone through muscle action that is thought to be osteogenic (Rauch et al., 2004). Thus, the link between muscle and bone is a reflection of the skeleton's ability to elicit an adaptive response to mechanical strains (Frost and Shonau, 2000). Data from longitudinal studies over the growth period illustrate this concept, as peak gains in lean tissue mass (surrogate for muscle) precede gains in peak bone mass during the adolescent growth period (Rauch et al., 2004; Jackowksi et al., 2009).

In summary, considerable evidence exists showing the beneficial effects of physical activity on optimizing skeletal development during the growing years, but the importance of these effects from a clinical perspective depends on their permanence. The argument has been raised that increasing bone acquisition during childhood is transient and thus may not be important clinically (Gafni and Baron, 2007). However, some retrospective data suggest that BMD and bone geometry in adulthood are related to physical activity or sport participation during early life (Nilsson et al., 2008, 2009). Also, structural changes, such as cortical bone size and shape, have been shown to be affected by exercise, and the benefits may be retained with age, despite reduced training (Kontulainen et al., 2003). Increased hip BMC from high-impact exercise in growing children has also been shown to persist following 7 years of detraining (Gunter et al., 2008b). Janz and colleagues (2010) found that children in the highest quartile for moderate and vigorous activity (MPVA) at 5 years of age had 4% to 14% more BMC at ages 8 and 11 years than did those in the lowest quartile for MPVA at the age of 5 years. We reported that the skeletal benefits of physical activity during adolescence are maintained at least into young adulthood. In this prospective study, we found, after adjusting for adult physical activity levels, that subjects who were more active during the adolescent growth period had 8% to 10% greater BMC (depending on site) in young adulthood than did their less active peers (Baxter-Jones et al., 2008). Ultimately, however, these effects only will be meaningful if the benefits continue to persist into the later adult years and thus reduce the risk of fracture (Karlsson, 2007).

NUTRITION (CALCIUM)

Nutritional quality is recognized as an important component in optimizing skeletal health during childhood and adolescent growth (Heaney and Weaver, 2005). In particular, there is considerable evidence that dietary calcium, vitamin D, and protein intakes affect bone mineral accrual and maintenance (Bonjour et al., 2003; Whiting et al., 2004). The importance of all of these various nutrients, including calcium, is described in other chapters of this text; thus, the following section is a very brief summary on the relationship of nutrient intake (primarily calcium) and skeletal health during childhood and adolescence.

In a longitudinal study over the growing years, adequate calcium and fruit and vegetable intake had beneficial effects on TB BMC accrual in both boys and girls (Vatanparast et al., 2005). In another longitudinal study, over a 4-year period, Fiorito and collaborators (2006) reported an association between calcium intake and TB BMC in girls 5–11 years of age, and calcium intake was positively associated with TB BMC. Greater BMC values also have been found in children with high calcium intakes compared with those with low intakes (Prais et al., 2008). Studies in boys in late adolescence have also shown a positive effect of calcium supplementation on bone growth and bone mineral acquisition (Prentice et al., 2005). The effects of calcium supplementation on the skeleton during growth may be site-specific; for example, Chevalley and coinvestigators (2005a) found a positive effect of calcium on BMD at appendicular sites, but not at the lumbar spine. Other nutrients such as protein may interact with calcium; for example, protein intake has been shown to predict BMC during the growing years when calcium intakes are at least 1000 mg/day (Vatanparast et al., 2007).

Results from several other studies, however, suggest that calcium supplementation may affect bone in calcium-deficient children, but only minimally in children with adequate calcium intakes. For example, positive effects on BMD over a 2-year calcium supplementation period were reported in Chinese girls, but all had low dietary calcium intakes at baseline (Zhu et al., 2008). Additional calcium supplementation in healthy children already consuming about 800 mg of daily calcium did not result in any clinical meaningful skeletal benefits (Iuliano-Burns et al., 2006). Lambert and colleagues (2008), in an 18-month randomized control trial of 96 girls, 12 years of age at study entry, with low calcium intakes, followed their subjects for 2 years after withdrawing the supplements. The supplement group had significantly greater BMC and BMD at multiple sites compared with controls after completion of the intervention, but these differences disappeared after the 2-year follow-up. Similar findings were found by Slemenda and colleagues (1997) in a 6-year study of monozygotic twin pairs, aged 6–14 years, enrolled in a calcium supplementation trial. Supplemented children had approximately 3% higher rates of gain in BMD during the 3-year period of supplementation. During the 3-year postsupplement period, follow-up differences in BMD disappeared.

Winzenberg and coworkers (2006), in a review of randomized control trials on calcium supplementation in healthy children, concluded that there was a small effect of supplementation in the upper limbs only, but the effects were not likely of clinical importance. In another recent meta-analysis, Huncharek and coinvestigators (2008) concluded that calcium supplementation with and without vitamin D increases TB and lower spine (LS) BMC in children with low baseline intakes of these nutrients, but the supplements did not affect BMC in those with adequate amounts of calcium and vitamin D in their diets.

Some of the inconsistencies in data from various studies likely result from the difficulties in studying children. For example, the effects of nutrition on bone health are complicated by maturational variability in children (Chevalley et al., 2005b), and some controversy exists regarding accuracy of dietary assessments in children. The exact amount of calcium required for optimal bone health has not been fully confirmed. Calcium requirements over the growing period have previously been estimated to be about 1300 mg/day for both boys and girls over the whole adolescent age range (Institute of Medicine, 1997); however, more recent data suggest that calcium requirements should be gender and age specific: with a mean requirement of 1100 mg/day for boys and girls from 9 to 13 years of age, but from age 14 to18 years of age, the estimated requirement would be 1000 mg for girls and increased to 1200 mg for boys (Vatanparast et al., 2009). Even allowing for potential disagreements on the recommended dietary intakes for calcium, concern is widespread that existing calcium intakes are not adequate to ensure optimal bone health, particularly in adolescent girls (Faulkner and Bailey, 2007). Nevertheless, healthy adult bone mass has been achieved by many children who have calcium intakes below recommended values (Nickols-Richardson et al., 1999); therefore, some adaptations, such as increased retention efficiency, must be occurring during growth to account for the accrual despite inadequate calcium intakes (Anderson, 2001).

INTERACTIVE EFFECTS OF CALCIUM AND PHYSICAL ACTIVITY

As noted previously, in spite of a theoretical basis, limited specific research on the interactive effects of exercise and calcium during the growing years has been reported (Baxter-Jones et al., 2003a);

however, the cumulative data now represent the full growth range, from early childhood to late adolescence.

Specker and coresearchers (1999) investigated the effects of physical activity and calcium intakes on bone mass accrual during the rapid period of growth between 6 and 18 months of age. The infants consuming a low to moderate calcium intake had less bone accretion than did those involved in fine motor activities. No effect of activity on bone mass accretion was found with moderate to high dietary intakes of calcium. The results suggest that increased bone loading during periods of rapid skeletal growth may lead to an increased demand for calcium. In other words, it may not be possible for a child with increased bone loading to maintain comparable bone mass accretion if the increased demand for calcium is not met by dietary intake. In a 12-month intervention study, Specker and Binkley (2003) randomized young children into activity (gross or fine motor) and calcium supplement groups. Multiple BMC sites were measured, as well as bone dimensions using peripheral quantitative computed tomography. No main effect for activity or calcium supplementation was found for BMC measures, but the gross motor activity group receiving calcium supplementation had greater leg BMC and greater periosteal width at the tibia than did the fine motor activity group. A significant calcium/activity interaction between calcium supplementation and activity groups was found in both cortical thickness and cortical area related to increased periosteal width. Based on these results, it was concluded that calcium intake modifies the bone response to physical activity in young children. In a follow-up study, the increased periosteal circumference in the activity groups was still evident 12 months after cessation of the exercise program (Specker et al., 2003).

Results from studies investigating interactive effects in prepubescent or early-pubescent children are mixed. Gunnes and Lehmann (1996) investigated the effects of 1 year of weight-bearing physical activity on forearm BMD. Physical activity predicted bone gain in children under 11 years of age, but the greatest gains were found in those with the highest calcium intakes, suggesting an interactive effect. In a study in pubertal boys and girls 8 to 11 years of age, Rowlands and collaborators (2004) found an interactive effect of vigorous physical activity and calcium intake for TB BMC in both boys and girls, but only in boys at the FN. No interactive effect between total physical activity (by definition lower intensity) and calcium intake was found. Courteix and coauthors (2005) studied the combined skeletal effects of physical activity and calcium supplementation (800 mg/day) in 113 premenarcheal girls. They found that calcium supplementation increased the beneficial effect of physical activity on bone mineral acquisition, but that calcium supplementation without physical activity had no effect. They suggested that exercise that stimulates bone accretion in prepubertal children needs a high calcium intake to produce a maximum effect. In a randomized control trial in prepubertal and early-pubertal boys, Bass and coinvestigators (2007) examined the combined effect of exercise and calcium intake on BMC accrual. The 8.5-month intervention showed that exercise and calcium together resulted in a 2% greater increase in BMC at the femur than either condition alone and a 3% greater increase in BMC at the tibia–fibula compared with controls. They concluded that increasing dietary calcium may be important in optimizing the effects of exercise on bone adaptation. A region-specific interaction of moderate exercise and calcium supplementation was reported in prepubescent girls (Iuliano-Burns et al., 2003). In this randomized control trial, lasting 8.5 months, an exercise–calcium interaction was found at the femur but not at the tibia–fibula. At the tibia, only exercise had a significant effect.

In contrast to the above studies, some investigations have found little or no evidence for an interactive effect of calcium and exercise. Slemenda and colleagues (1994) reported a significant effect of calcium intake combined with physical activity on BMD at the lumbar spine, proximal femur, and distal radius in prepubescent children but found no evidence of an interaction effect. Ward and coworkers (2007) in a 12-month randomized control study hypothesized that calcium supplementation would enhance the effects of gymnastic participation on BMD and geometric properties of the skeleton. A significant interaction of calcium and activity was found in the distal tibia BMD for the controls only, but not in any other sites. The gymnasts in this study were already consuming recommended intakes of calcium (888 mg/day); thus, it was speculated that when calcium intake is sufficient, no added benefits of additional supplementation are likely to be found. Results from a study of 1359 Dutch children, 7 to 11 years of age, showed increased BMC only in those children with high levels of physical activity, whereas calcium intake was not associated with BMC and no interaction effect was reported (Van Den Bergh et al., 1995). However, the calcium intakes in over 80% of the children were high and exceeded 1400 mg/day. In another study, bone mass and size were related to higher levels of physical activity in prepubertal and early-pubertal children at the highest levels of physical activity; however, calcium intake had no effect, and no interactive effect of calcium intake and physical activity was found (McVeigh et al., 2007). In a study in late adolescent boys, no differences in BMD between tennis players and control subjects were revealed in the dominant arm. Furthermore, no interaction of physical activity and calcium was found, although the calcium intakes were below recommended intake levels (Juzwiak et al., 2008). Finally, Chevalley and coinvestigators (2008) found that protein enhanced the effects of physical activity on BMC accrual in prepubertal boys, but no interactive effect of calcium and physical activity existed.

Evidence that physical activity and calcium intake during later childhood and adolescence positively affect adult bone status has not been generated. Kanders and colleagues (1988) reported a positive relationship in females between physical fitness and calcium intakes with vertebral BMD measured in young adulthood (20–29 years of age). Welten and coresearchers (1994) found that weight-bearing physical activity at the age of 13 years predicted adult BMD, whereas calcium intake was not a significant predictor when controlling for physical activity patterns. Higher BMD, however, was found in those boys who were active and had high calcium intakes, suggesting an interaction effect. In a retrospective study, young females who had both adequate calcium intakes and regular physical activity patterns during their high school years had greater bone mass in young adulthood (18 to 22 years of age) than did those with lower calcium intakes and less physical activity (Tylavsky et al., 1992). Exercise exerted a greater overall beneficial effect than did calcium intake, and those with both high calcium and high physical activity levels had greater radial BMD compared with those with low/high combinations, suggesting an interactive effect of calcium and physical activity.

Pure longitudinal data, in which the same subjects are followed through childhood, adolescence, and adulthood are the best designs to study factors affecting outcomes, such as skeletal health. These data are sparse, however, due to the difficulty in planning, coordinating, and funding long-term prospective studies. The most comprehensive longitudinal data are from our own laboratory (Bailey et al., 1999). Results from this ongoing study have demonstrated the importance of controlling for factors, such as biological maturity and growth-related changes in body size, in trying to assess the independent or interactive effects of lifestyle variables on the skeleton (Baxter-Jones et al., 2003b). Using a multilevel random effects modeling procedure, we previously investigated the relationships between measure of growth (height and body mass), maturity (biological age, defined as the chronological age in years minus age of peak height velocity), and environmental exposure, that is, physical activity and calcium intake, on BMC accrual (Baxter-Jones et al., 2003a). We found that TB, FN, and lumbar spine BMC increased with biological age and, as expected, height and body mass were also significant predictors of BMC. After adjusting for these confounders, physical activity was a significant predictor of BMC at the LS and TB, but not at the FN in girls. In boys, physical activity was a significant predictor of BMC at the LS only. In girls, calcium intake did not predict BMC at any site. Calcium intake was a significant predictor of TB BMC only in boys. Although both physical activity and calcium intake had independent effects on BMC accrual, no interactive relationships were found at any BMC site. Calcium intakes for the groups were relatively high (over 1000 mg/day), and average physical activity was fairly homogeneous among the children in this investigation.

MECHANISMS

Physiologically, it makes sense that calcium and physical activity would have an interactive effect on bone accretion during growth in healthy children. Physical activity provides the mechanical loadings necessary to stimulate bone modeling and remodeling, whereas adequate calcium is necessary for bone mineralization (Barr and McKay, 1996; Branca et al., 2001). It is also important to consider the specific skeletal site when assessing the effects of environmental factors on bone. Environmental factors, such as nutrition and physical activity, affect trabecular and cortical bone tissue in different ways. Cortical bone adapts to mechanical loading by increasing BMC or by adapting geometric dimensions to the load. In contrast, trabecular bone responds to the stress of loading by altering the orientation of individual trabeculae (Forwood, 2001).

Based on the existing evidence, however, the effects of nutrition, such as calcium intake, appear to have permissive effects in their actions, whereas the mechanical loading of physical activity provides the actual stimulus for bone mineralization to reach its genetic potential (Specker and Vukovich, 2007). Calcium also affects other actions. For example, calcium levels affect both serum parathyroid hormone (PTH) and vitamin D activity and subsequent metabolic events affecting bone (Juppner et al., 1999). Evidence also suggests that a threshold exists for calcium intake, below which accumulation of bone mass is a function of intake and above which it is not dependent on higher intakes (Matkovic, 1993). However, the level of calcium intake needed to meet this theoretical threshold across age groups remains controversial (Branca et al., 2001). Although as noted previously, longitudinal-based data currently suggest that calcium requirements during growth range from about 1000 to 1200 mg/day, depending on age and gender (Vatanparast et al., 2009).

Another theoretical basis for expecting calcium and mechanical loading to have synergistic effects on bone is that calcium and vitamin D may modify the threshold of the intensity of exercise at which bone formation exceeds bone resorption. In other words, a permissive effect of calcium may make bone more sensitive to the mechanical loading stimulus (Iwamoto et al., 2001). This conjecture is consistent with the mechanostat theory, which theorizes that strain thresholds that control resorption and formation can be influenced by the hormonal and nutritional milieu. As proposed by Frost (1992), muscle and bone form an operational unit, that is, what affects muscle (loading) also affects bone. Furthermore, muscle contraction causes the largest load (strain) on bone, affecting the biological mechanisms that regulate bone strength. Adequate calcium availability is unquestionably required for optimizing bone mineral accrual, and as stated by Frost and Schonau (2000), "trying to increase significantly whole-bone strength in healthy subjects through nutrition (such as calcium supplements) or hormonal interventions (alone) is like trying to make a car go faster by adding petrol to its tank."

As noted previously, other physiological adaptations may occur during the growing period to compensate for low calcium intakes (Anderson, 2001). Increased retention efficiency of dietary calcium is likely to be an important factor in this adaptation (Bailey, 2000). Exercise may play a role in affecting greater calcium retention in the skeleton. For example, in animal models, in the absence of dietary calcium, exercise is associated with an increased skeletal accretion of calcium with transient hypocalcemia and hypophosphatemia, resulting in increased intestinal absorption of calcium and phosphorus (Yeh and Aloia, 1990).

SUMMARY AND CONCLUSIONS

As in any research with humans, many inconsistencies and weaknesses in research designs among the various studies on nutrition and physical activity become apparent. As noted previously, many of the studies involve relatively homogeneous groups in terms of calcium intakes and physical activity, and many have low statistical power. Although increasing information has been reported on calcium requirements (Vatanparast et al., 2009), the amount of calcium needed to optimize skeletal health during growth is not yet defined specifically. Nutritional intervention varies, with some studies using supplements, and others, nutrient enrichment; this variability of source of calcium may result in disparity in the responses and or mechanisms of the responses (French et al., 2000). Considerable variation also occurs in the definition and/or type and intensity of physical activity intervention across studies. Assessing physical activity in children in observational studies also has many potential problems (Crocker et al., 1997). Finally, a paucity of data are available from longitudinal studies over the entire growth period as most of the existing data are based on cross-sectional studies or prospective studies with minimal follow-up. Although more recent studies adjust bone outcome variables for changes in size and also account for biological maturity, many earlier studies did not.

Despite these weaknesses in the reported evidence, the following conclusions are warranted on the role of physical activity and calcium on bone health during the active growing years.

- Adequate calcium intake and regular physical activity are required for optimizing the genetic potential for skeletal health; however, physical activity is quantitatively a more important factor in affecting bone accrual than calcium intake is.
- The greater importance of physical activity is particularly evident when calcium intakes approach recommended calcium requirements.
- Calcium has a permissive effect on bone mineral accrual and maintenance, whereas physical activity has a modifying effect.
- Calcium intake that reaches an apparent threshold is needed to optimize the effects of mechanical loading on bone. Results from several studies suggest that this threshold for adolescent boys and girls is over 1000 mg/day; however, controversy remains as to the exact level.

REFERENCES

Anderson, J.J.B. 2000. The important role of physical activity in skeletal development: How exercise may counter low calcium intake. *Am J Clin Nutr* 71:1384–1386.

Anderson, J.J.B. 2001. Calcium requirements during adolescence to maximize bone health. *J Am Coll Nutr* 20:186S–191S.

Bailey, D.A. 2000. Physical activity and bone mineral acquisition during adolescence. *Osteoporos Int* 11:S2–S3

Bailey, D.A., Faulkner, R.A., and McKay, H.A. 1996. Growth, physical activity, and bone mineral acquisition. *Exerc Sport Sci Rev* 24:233–266.

Bailey, D.A., McKay, H.A., Mirwald, R.L., et al. 1999. Six years longitudinal study of the relationship of physical activity to bone mineral accrual in growing children: The University of Saskatchewan Bone Mineral Accrual Study. *J Bone Miner Res* 14:1672–1676.

Barr, S.I., and McKay, H.A. 1996. Nutrition, exercise, and bone status in youth. *Int J Sport Nutr.* 8:124–142.

Bass, S.L., Naughton, G., Saxon, L., et al. 2007. Exercise and calcium combined result in greater osteogenic effect than either factor alone: A blinded randomized placebo-controlled study in boys. *J Bone Miner Res* 22:458–464.

Baxter-Jones, A.D.G., Eisenmann, J.C., Mirwald, R.L., et al. 2008. The influence of physical activity on lean mass accrual during adolescence: A longitudinal analysis. *J Appl Physiol* 105:734–741.

Baxter-Jones, A.D.G., Faulkner, R.A, Forwood, M., Mirwald, R.L., Bailey, D.A. 2011. Bone mineral accrual from 8 to 30 years of age: An estimation of peak bone mass. *J Bone Min Res* doi: 10.102/jbmr.4.12.

Baxter-Jones, A.D.G., Faulkner, R.A., and Whiting, S.J. 2003a. Interaction between nutrition, physical activity and skeletal health. In *Nutritional Aspects of Bone Health*. New, S., and Bonjour, J.-P., eds. Cambridge: Royal Society of Chemistry, pp. 544–564.

Baxter-Jones, A.D.G., Kontulainen, S.A., Faulkner, R.A., et al. 2008. A longitudinal study of the relationship of physical activity to bone mineral accrual from adolescence to young adulthood. *Bone* 43:1101–1107.

Baxter-Jones, A.D.G., Mirwald, R.L., McKay, H.A., et al. 2003b. A longitudinal analysis of sex differences in bone mineral accrual in healthy 8 to 19 year old boys and girls. *Ann Hum Biol* 30:160–175.

Bonjour, J.-P., Amman, P., Chevalley, T., et al. 2003. Nutritional aspects of bone growth. In *Nutritional Aspects of Bone Health*. New, S. and Bonjour, J.-P., eds. Cambridge: Royal Society of Chemistry, pp. 111–128.

Bonjour, J.-P., Chevalley, T., Rizzoli, R., et al. 2007. Gene–Environment interactions in the skeletal response to nutrition and exercise during growth. Optimizing Bone Mass and Strength: In *The Role of Physical Activity and Nutrition During Growth, Med Sci Sport*. Daley, R.M., and Petit, M.A., eds. Basel: Karger, pp 64–80.

Branca, F., Valtuena, S., and Vatuena, S. 2001. Calcium, physical activity and bone health-building bones for a stronger future. *Pub Health Nutr* 4:117–123.

Burrows, M. 2007. Exercise and bone mineral accrual in children and adolescents. *Sports Sci Med* 6:05–312.

Chevalley, T., Bonjour, J.-P., Ferrari, S., et al. 2005a. Skeletal site selectivity in the effects of calcium supplementation on areal bone mineral density gain: A randomized, double-blind, placebo-controlled trial in prepubertal boys. *J Clin Endocr Metab* 90:3342–3349.

Chevalley, T., Bonjour, J.-P., Ferrari, S., et al. 2008. High-protein intake enhances the positive impact of physical activity on BMC in prepubertal boys. *J Bone Miner Res* 23:131–142.

Chevalley, T., Rizzoli, R.H., Hans, D., et al. 2005b. Interaction between calcium intake and menarcheal age on bone mass gain: An eight-year follow-up study from prepuberty to postmenarche. *J Clin Endocr Metab* 90:44–51.

Courteix, D., Jaffre, C., Lespessailles, E., et al. 2005. Cumulative effects of calcium supplementation and physical activity on bone accretion in premenarcheal children: A double blind randomised placebo-controlled trial. *Int J Sports Med* 26:332–338.

Crocker, P., Bailey, D.A., Faulkner, R.A., et al. 1997. Measuring general levels of physical activity: Preliminary evidence for the Physical Activity Questionnaire for Older Children. *Med Sci Sports Exerc* 29:1344–1349.

Dowthwaite, J.N., Kanaley, J.A., Spadaro, J.A., et al. 2009. Muscle indices do not fully account for enhanced upper extremity bone mass and strength in gymnasts. *J Musculoskelet Neuronal Interact* 9:2–14.

Faulkner, R.A., and Bailey, D.A. 2007. Osteoporosis: A pediatric concern? In *The Role of Physical Activity and Nutrition During Growth, Med Sci Spor.* Daley, R.M., and Petit, M.A., eds. Basel: Karger, pp. 1–12.

Faulkner, R.A., Forwood, M.R., Beck, T.J., et al. 2003. Strength indices of the proximal femur and shaft in prepubertal female gymnasts. *Med Sci Sports Exerc* 35:513–518.

Fiorito, L.M., Mitchell, D.C., Smiciklas-Wright, H., et al. 2006. Girls' calcium intake is associated with bone mineral content during middle childhood. *J Nutr* 136:1281–1286.

Forwood, M. 2001. Physiology. In *Physical Activity and Bone Health.* Khan, K., McKay, H., Kannus, P., et al., eds. Champaign, IL: Human Kinetics Press, pp. 11–19.

Forwood, M.R., Baxter-Jones, A.D., Beck, T.J., et al. 2006. Physical activity and strength of the femoral neck during the adolescent growth spurt: A longitudinal analysis. *Bone* 38:576–583.

Forwood, M.R., Baxter-Jones, A.D.G., Faulkner, R.A., et al. 2007. Tempo and timing of bone mineral accrual during pre, peri and post adolescent growth periods. *J Bone Miner Res*, 22(Suppl. 1):S49.

French, S.A., Fulkerson, J.A., and Story, M. 2000. Increasing weight-bearing physical activity and calcium intake for bone mass growth in children and adolescents: A review of intervention trials. *Prev Med* 31:722–731.

Frost, H.M. 1992. The role of changes in mechanical usage set points in the pathogenesis of osteoporosis. *J Bone Miner Res* 7:253–261.

Frost, H.M., and Schonau, E. 2000. The "muscle–bone unit" in children and adolescents: A 2000 overview. *J Pediatr* 13:571–590.

Gafni, R.I., and Baron, J. 2007. Childhood bone mass acquisition and peak bone mass may not be important determinants of bone mass in late adulthood. *Pediatrics* 119:S131–S136.

Gunnes, M., and Lehmann, E.H. 1996. Physical activity and dietary constituents as predictors of forearm cortical and trabecular bone gain in healthy children and adolescents: A prospective study. *Acta Pediatr* 85:19–25.

Gunter, K., Baxter-Jones, A.D.G., Mirwald, R.L., et al. 2008a. Jump starting skeletal health: A 4-year longitudinal study assessing the effects of jumping on skeletal development in pre and circum pubertal children. *Bone* 42:710–718.

Gunter, K., Baxter-Jones, A.D.G., Mirwald, R.L., et al. 2008b. Impact exercise increases BMC during growth: An 8-year longitudinal study. *J Bone Miner Res* 23:986–993.

Hasselstrom, H.A., Karlsson, M.K., Hansen, S.E., et al. 2008. A 3-year physical intervention program increases the gain in bone mineral and bone width in prepubertal girls but not boys: The prospective Copenhagen School Child Interventions Study. *Calcif Tissue Int* 83:243–250.

Heaney, R.P., and Weaver, C.M. 2005. Newer perspectives on calcium nutrition and bone quality. *J Am Coll Nutr* 24:574S–581S.

Huncharek, M., Muscat, J., and Kupelnick, B. 2008. Impact of dairy products and dietary calcium on bone-mineral content in children: Results of a meta-analysis. *Bone* 43:310–321.

Institute of Medicine. 1997. *Dietary Reference Intakes: Calcium, Magnesium, Phosphorus, Vitamin D, and Fluoride.* Washington: National Academy Press.

Iuliano-Burns, S., Naughton, G., Gibbons, K., et al. 2003. Regional specificity of exercise and calcium during skeletal growth in girls: A randomized control trial. *J Bone Miner Res* 18:156–162.

Iuliano-Burns, S., Want, X.-F., Evans, A., et al. 2006. Skeletal benefits from calcium supplementation are limited in children with calcium intakes near 800 mg daily. *Osteoporos Int* 17:1794–1780.

Iwamoto J., Takeda, T., and Ichimura, S. 2001. Effect of exercise training and detraining on bone mineral density in postmenopausal women with osteoporosis. *J Orthop Sci* 6:128–132.

Jackowksi, S.A, Faulkner, R.A., Farthing, J.P., et al. 2009. Peak lean tissue mass accrual precedes changes in bone strength indices at the proximal femur during the pubertal growth spurt. *Bone* 44:1186–1190.

Janz, K.F., Gilmore, J.M., Eichenberger, L., et al. 2007. Physical activity and femoral neck bone strength during childhood: The Iowa Bone Development Study. *Bone* 41:216–222.

Janz, K.F., Letuchy, E.M., Eichenberger Gilmore, J.M., et al. 2010. Early physical activity provides sustained bone health benefits later in childhood. *Med Sci Sports Exerc* 42:1072–1078.

Janz, K.F., Medema-Johnson, H.C., Letuchy, E.M., et al. 2008. Subjective and objective measures of physical activity in relationship to bone mineral content during late childhood: The Iowa Bone Development Study. *Br J Sports Med* 42:658–663.

Juppner, H., Brown, E.M., and Kronenberg, H.M. 1999. Parathyroid hormone. In *Primer on the Metabolic Bone Diseases and Disorders of Mineral Metabolism*, 4th ed. Favus, M.J., ed. Philadelphia: Lipincott Williams & Wilkins, pp. 80–87.

Juzwiak, C.R., Amancio, O.M., Vitalle, M.S., et al. 2008. Effect of calcium intake, tennis playing, and body composition on bone-mineral density of Brazilian male adolescents. *J Sport Nutr Exerc Metab* 18:524–538.

Kanders, B., Dempster, D.W., and Lindsay, R. 1988. Interaction of calcium nutrition and physical activity on bone mass in young women. *J Bone Miner Res* 3:145–149.

Karlsson, M.K. 2007. Does exercise during growth prevent fractures in later life? *Med Sport Sci* 51:121–136.

Khan, K., McKay, H., Kannus, P., et al. 2001. *Physical Activity and Bone Health*. Champaign, IL: Human Kinetics Press, pp. 35–54.

Kontulainen, S., Sievanen, H., Kannus, P., et al. 2003. Effect of long-term impact-loading on mass, size, and estimated strength of humerus and radius of female racquet-sport players: A peripheral quantitative computed tomography study between young and old starters and controls. *J Bone Miner Res* 18:352–359.

Lambert, H., Eastell, R., Karnik, K., et al. 2008. Calcium supplementation and bone mineral accretion in adolescent girls: An 18-month randomized controlled trial with 2-yr follow-up. *Am J Clin Nutri* 87:455–462.

MacDonald, H.M., Kontulainen, S.A., Petit, M.A., et al. 2008. Does a novel school-based physical activity model benefit femoral neck bone strength in pre-and early pubertal children? *Osteoporos Int* 19:1445–1456.

MacKelvie, K.J., Khan, K.M., Petit, M.A., et al. 2003. A school-based exercise intervention elicits substantial bone health benefits: A 2-year randomized controlled trial in girls. *Pediatrics* 112:e447–e452.

MacKelvie, K.J., McKay, H.A., Khan, K.M., et al. 2001. A school-based exercise intervention augments bone mineral accrual in early pubertal girls. *J Pediatr* 139:501–508.

MacKelvie, K.J., McKay, H.A., Petit, M.A., et al. 2002. Bone mineral response to a 7 month randomized controlled, school-based jumping intervention in 121 prepubertal boys: Associations with ethnicity and body mass index. *J Bone Miner Res* 17:834–844.

MacKelvie, K.J., Petit, M.A., Khan, K.M., et al. 2004. Bone mass and structure are enhanced following a 2-year randomized controlled trial of exercise in prepubertal boys. *Bone* 34:755–764.

Matkovic, V. 1993. Calcium requirements for growth: Are current recommendations adequate? *Nutr Rev* 51:171–180.

Mathews, B.L., Bennell, K.L., McKay, H.A., et al. 2006. Dancing for bone health: A 3-year longitudinal study of bone mineral accrual across puberty in female novice dancers and controls. *Osteoporos Int* 17:1043–1054.

McKay, H., and Smith, E. 2008. Commentary: Winning the battle against childhood physical inactivity: The key to bone strength? *J Bone Miner Res* 23:980–985.

McVeigh, J.A., Norris, S.A., and Pettifor, J.M. 2007. Bone mass accretion rates in pre- and early-pubertal South African black and white children in relation to habitual physical activity and dietary calcium. *Act Paediatr* 96:874–880.

Nelson, D.A., and Koo, W.W. 1999. Interpretation of absorptiometric bone mass measurements in the growing skeleton: Issues and limitations. *Calcif Tissue Int* 65:1–3.

Nickols-Richardson, S.M., O'Conner, P.J., and Shapses, S. 1999. Longitudinal bone mineral density changes in female child artistic gymnasts. *J Bone Miner Res* 14:994–1002.

Nilsson, M., Eriksson, C., Frandin, A.L., et al. 2008. Competitive physical activity early in life is associated with bone mineral density in elderly Swedish men. *Osteoporos Int* 19:1557–1566.

Nilsson, M., Ohlsson, C., Mellstrom, D., et al. 2009. Previous sport activity during childhood and adolescence is associated with increased cortical bone size in young adult men. *J Bone Miner Res* 24:125–133.

Nurmi-Lawton, J.A., Baxter-Jones, A.D.G., Mirwald, R.L., et al. 2004. Evidence of sustained skeletal benefits from impact-loading exercise in young females: A 3-year longitudinal study. *J Bone Miner Res* 19:314–322.

Petit, M.A., McKay, H.A., MacKelive, K.J., et al. 2002. A randomized school-based jumping intervention confers site and maturity-specific benefits on bone structural properties in girls: A hip structural analysis study. *J Bone Miner Res* 17:363–372.

Prais, D., Diamond, G., Kattan, A., et al. 2008. The effect of calcium intake and physical activity on bone quantitative ultrasound measurements in children: A pilot study. *J Bone Miner Metab* 26:248–253.

Prentice, A., Ginty, F., Stear, S.J., et al. 2005. Calcium supplementation increases stature and bone mineral mass of 16–18 year old boys. *J Clin Endocr Metab* 90:3153–3161.

Raisz, L.G. 2005. Pathogenesis of osteoporosis: Concepts, conflicts and prospects. *J Clin Invest* 115:3318–3325.

Rauch, F., Bailey, D.A., Baxter-Jones, A.D.G., et al. 2004. The muscle–bone unit during the pubertal growth spurt. *Bone* 34:771–775.

Rowlands, A.V., Ingledew, D.K., Powell, S.M., et al. 2004. Interactive effects of habitual physical activity and calcium intake on bone density in boys and girls. *J Appl Phsiol* 95:1203–1208.

Slemenda, C.W., Reister, T.K., Hui, S., et al. 1994. Influences on skeletal mineralization in children and adolescents: Evidence for varying effects of sexual maturation and physical activity. *J Pediatr* 125:201–207.

Slemenda, C.W., Peacock, M., Hui, S., et al. 1997. Reduced rates of skeletal remodelling are associated with increased bone mineral density during the development of peak skeletal mass. *J Bone Miner Res* 12:676–682.

Specker, B.L., and Binkley, T. 2003. Randomized trial of physical activity and calcium supplementation on bone mineral content in 3–5 year old children. *J Bone Miner Res* 18:885–892.

Specker, B.L., Mulligan, L., and Ho, M. 1999. Longitudinal study of calcium intake, physical activity, and bone mineral content in infants 6-18 months of age. *J Bone Miner Res* 14:569–576.

Specker, B.L., and Vukovich, M. 2007. Evidence for an interaction between exercise and nutrition for improved bone health during growth. *Med Sport Sci* 51:50–63.

Tobias, J.H., Steer, C.D., Mattocks, C.G., et al. 2007. Habitual levels of physical activity influence bone mass in 11-year old children from the United Kingdom: Findings from a large population-based cohort. *J Bone Miner Res* 22:101–109.

Tylavsky, F.A., Anderson, J.J., Talmage, V.R., et al. 1992. Are calcium intakes and physical activity patterns during adolescence related to radial bone mass of white college-age females? *Osteoporos Int* 2:232–240.

Van Den Bergh, M.F., DeMan, S.A., Witteman, J.C., et al. 1995. Physical activity, calcium intake, and bone mineral content in children in The Netherlands. *J Epidemiol Commun Health* 49:299–304.

Vatanparast, H., Bailey, D.A., Baxter-Jones, A.D.G., et al. 2007. The effects of dietary protein on bone mineral mass in young adults may be modulated by adolescent calcium intake. *J Nutr* 137:2674–2679.

Vatanparast, H., Bailey, D.A., Baxter-Jones, A.D.G., et al. 2009. Calcium requirements for optimal bone growth in Canadian boys and girls during adolescence. *Br J Nutr* 26:1–6.

Vatanparast, H., Baxter-Jones, A.D.G., Faulkner, R.A., et al. 2005. Positive effects of vegetable and fruit consumption and calcium intake on bone mineral accrual in boys during growth from childhood to adolescence: The University of Saskatchewan Pediatric Bone Mineral Accrual Study. *Am J Clin Nutr* 82:700–706.

Ward, K.A., Roberts, S.A., Adams, J.E., et al. 2007. Calcium supplementation and weight bearing physical activity-do they have a combined effect on the bone density of pre-pubertal children? *Bone* 41:496–504.

Weeks, B.K. Young, C.M., and Beck, B.R. 2008. Eight months of regular in-school jumping improves indices of bone strength in adolescent boys and girls: The POWER PE Study. *J Bone Miner Res* 23:1002–1011.

Welten, D.C., Kemper, H.C., Post, G.B., et al. 1994. Weight-bearing activity during youth is a more important factor for peak bone mass than calcium intake. *J Bone Miner Res* 9:1089–1096.

Whiting, S.J., Vatanparast, H., Baxter-Jones, A.D.G., et al. 2004. Factors that affect bone mineral accrual in the adolescent growth spurt. *J Nutr* 134:696S–700S.

Winzenberg, T.M., Shaw, K., Fryer, J., et al. 2006. Calcium supplementation for improving bone mineral density in children. *Cochrane Database Syst Rev 2006 April 19;(2):*CD005119.

Yeh, J.K., and Aloia, J.F. 1990. Effect of physical activity on calciotropic hormones and calcium balance in rats. *Am J Physiol* 258:E263–E268.

Zhu, K., Greenfield, H., Du, X., et al. 2008. Effects of two years' milk supplementation on size-corrected bone mineral density of Chinese girls. *Asia Pacif J Clin Nutr* 17:147–150.

24 Peak Bone Mass
Influence of Nutrition and Lifestyle Variables

Jennifer L. Bedford and Susan I. Barr

CONTENTS

Peak bone mass (PBM), the maximum amount of bone mass achieved at the end of growth, has been suggested to be more important than the amount of adulthood bone loss in the risk of osteoporosis and fractures (Bonjour et al., 2009). As PBM must maintain the skeleton for the remainder of life, it is important to understand what regulates the attainment of PBM and how the amount of bone gained during growth can be optimized, thus offsetting the inevitable bone loss that occurs with age. This chapter describes the attainment of PBM and summarizes what is known about its determinants, focusing on nutrition but also addressing other nonnutritional variables.

PEAK BONE MASS

To understand how lifestyle variables affect PBM attainment, an accurate noninvasive means of measuring the changes in bone mass that occur from infancy to early adulthood is necessary. The most common method is dual-energy X-ray absorptiometry (DXA), a measurement of areal bone mineral density (aBMD, g/cm^2). aBMD is a function of bone volume, mineral density, and estimated bone size. During growth, bone geometry is continuously changing, and therefore, approximated bone size is prone to error. The correction made for soft tissue in the area of bone measured is also a source of error as corrections are based on a homogenous distribution of fat around the bone, which is not always true during growth. Thus, it is suggested that bone mineral content (BMC, g, the actual weight of bone mineral) and bone area be used to determine how lifestyle variables affect bone mineral accretion and skeletal development during growth (Heaney, 2005; Prentice, 2004). Measurements of BMC in a defined volume are obtained by quantitative computed tomography (QCT). Bone measured by QCT can separate cortical and trabecular bone. Volumetric BMD (vBMD, g/cm^3) is independent of surrounding soft tissue and bone size and shape. However, this method currently has limited reference data in children.

The rate of bone mass accumulation varies during childhood based on skeletal site (appendicular vs. axial), type of bone (cortical vs. trabecular), gender, and potentially, race/ethnicity. Overall, bone mass increases from ~75–95 g at birth to ~2400–3300 g in young adulthood (Mora and Gilsanz, 2003). The considerable increase in bone mass that occurs during growth is mainly the result of increases in bone size as vBMD increases by only a small amount (Bonjour et al., 2009). Bone mass increases gradually throughout childhood and accelerates radically during puberty: The rate of accrual increases four- to six-fold over a 3- to 4-year period (Bonjour et al., 2009). Although cortical bone density appears to be relatively stable during puberty, density of trabecular bone is highly responsive to sexual development increasing by 13% during this time (Mora and Gilsanz, 2003).

Almost no gender differences in bone mass exist at birth or during much of childhood before puberty, after adjusting for age, nutrition, and physical activity (Bonjour et al., 2009). In girls, the greatest rate of bone mass accumulation occurs from ages 12 to 15 years (Davies et al., 2005), with no additional accumulation observed at the lumbar spine or femoral neck 2 years after menarche (Bonjour et al., 2009). Boys on the other hand have the highest rate of gain between ages 13 and 17 years, with some continued gains at the lumbar spine until the age of 20 years (Bonjour et al., 2009). Overall, at least 90% of PBM is achieved by the age of 20 years, with possible small gains in the appendicular skeleton until the age of 30 years (Mora and Gilsanz, 2003). Although vBMD does not appear to differ by gender at the end of puberty, boys do have longer and wider long bones and greater vertebral cross-sectional area than do girls (Bonjour et al., 2009; Mora and Gilsanz, 2003).

Most studies have found higher aBMD and BMC and greater calcium retention (Weaver et al., 2008) among Black versus Caucasian children (Mora and Gilsanz, 2003; Walker et al., 2008). American Asian and Hispanic children have bone mass that is more similar to that of Caucasian than Black children, although there is a limited amount of reference data for these two ethnic groups (Mora and Gilsanz, 2003; Walker et al., 2008).

NONNUTRITIONAL DETERMINANTS OF PBM

This section provides an overview of several nonnutritional determinants of PBM, including genetics, hormones, physical activity, and smoking.

GENETICS

Twin studies suggest that 60%–80% of bone mass, particularly at the lumbar spine, is determined by genetic factors (Bonjour et al., 2009). Further evidence of the influence of heredity comes from studies finding reduced aBMD in the daughters of osteoporotic patients versus daughters of parents with normal bone density and lower aBMD among women with a first-degree relative with osteoporosis (Bonjour et al., 2009). The search for gene polymorphisms related to aBMD suggests that the heritability of PBM is polygenic, with each gene accounting for a small percentage of PBM variance (Bonjour et al., 2009).

HORMONES

Attainment of PBM is dependent on several hormones including the sex steroids estrogen and testosterone and the growth hormone (GH) and insulin-like growth factor-1 (IGF-1) system. From childhood to the end of puberty, circulating levels of GH and IGF-1 rise in parallel to bone mass and size increases (Bonjour et al., 2009). IGF-1 directly promotes bone mass accrual via osteoblast activation and stimulates the growth plate chondrocytes promoting growth in length and width (Bonjour et al., 2009). Bone mineralization is affected indirectly by IGF-1 as receptors are present on the renal tubular cells, where it is connected to reabsorption of inorganic phosphate and active vitamin D production.

Estrogen is the most important sex steroid in the growth of the skeleton. At puberty, estrogens cause bone growth to progress more quickly and play a role in growth plate closure (Bonjour et al., 2009). Estrogen inhibits bone resorption resulting in increased cortical thickness (Davies et al., 2005). In adolescent girls, normal menstrual cycle function, an indicator of adequate exposure to estrogen, is crucial for attainment of PBM. Later age of menarche is associated with lower aBMD and a higher risk of adult fracture (Bonjour et al., 2009). Recent work, however, suggests that estrogen exposure may not be the only explanatory variable linking later age of menarche and lower aBMD: Differences in aBMD exist prior to puberty between girls destined to have earlier versus later puberty, and the two groups do not differ in the amount of bone accrued between prepuberty and PBM (Chevalley et al., 2009). The authors suggested that similar genetic factors may influence both bone accrual and pubertal timing (Chevalley et al., 2009). Nevertheless, insufficient energy intake and excessive exercise (often related to eating disorders) among young girls can result in amenorrhea (the absence of menstruation), an indicator of estrogen insufficiency. Teenaged girls with amenorrhea have lower aBMD than do girls with normal menses (Mora and Gilsanz, 2003). Whether bone mass can recover following resumption of menses depends on a number of variables, including the timing and duration of amenorrhea and whether body weight is normal (Weaver, 2002).

PHYSICAL ACTIVITY

The benefit of weight-bearing physical activity on the achievement and maintenance of PBM is well established. The mechanism by which physical activity promotes bone turnover is explained as the mechanostat theory (Frost, 1987): Bone is adaptable and is capable of altering its mass, size, and density in response to the strain that is placed upon it (Daly, 2007). When the physiological load zone is surpassed, there are gains in bone mass or density, and when activity falls below the physiological strain threshold, bone loss can occur (Bonjour et al., 2009). Bone structure and internal architecture may also change in response to increasing load or strain, which may not be detected by DXA, as concurrent changes in bone density do not always occur (Daly, 2007). Bone strength has been suggested to be more important for survival than bone mass from an evolutionary perspective (Schoenau and Fricke, 2008). Therefore, documenting the effect of activity, or any lifestyle variable, on bone structure is important. The increasing use of QCT will allow for exploration of other aspects of bone strength.

Growing bone is more responsive to physical activity and exercise than adult bone is, and the greatest window of opportunity to promote gains in bone mass and size is before puberty (Daly, 2007). When compared with less active controls, children and teenagers involved in competitive sports (such as gymnastics, soccer, and skating) have greater bone mass gains, particularly in the weight-bearing bones (Bonjour et al., 2009; Vicente-Rodriguez, 2006). Moderate physical activity levels have also been shown to be associated with greater bone mass in children and teens: A recent systematic review of randomized and nonrandomized control interventions among children aged 8–17 years examined whether weight-bearing exercise improves bone mineral accumulation during growth (Hind and Burrows, 2007). A positive effect was observed on bone in all eight trials of early-pubertal children, six of nine studies in prepubertal children, and two of five studies in pubertal children (Hind and Burrows, 2007). In the studies for which changes in bone structure were available, increases in bone area were reported among prepubertal and early-pubertal children participating in jumping exercises and increases in femoral cortical thickness in prepubertal and early-pubertal children participating in various weight-bearing activities for three or more times per week (Hind and Burrows, 2007). Evidence from these studies and findings among children in sport suggests that higher generated forces result in larger gains in aBMD and BMC (Hind and Burrows, 2007; Mora and Gilsanz, 2003).

The optimal exercise intervention has not been established. Future studies should include varying exercise frequency and load intensity and address the limitations of previous work including small sample sizes, selection bias, poor compliance rates, and inadequate control of potentially confounding variables (Hind and Burrows, 2007). In a population-based study of prepubertal girls (not included in the Hinds and Burrows review), schools were randomized to physical education for 40 min/day versus the control standard of 60 min/week (Valdimarsson et al., 2006). The intervention group had significantly greater 1-year gains in lumbar spine BMC and aBMD and third lumbar vertebra width versus controls (Valdimarsson et al., 2006). Although not truly randomized, selection bias and compliance issues (physical education is mandatory) were reduced, and both physical activity level outside of school and calcium intake were accounted for.

An interaction between calcium and physical activity resulting in further gains in bone accrual may occur (Vicente-Rodriguez et al., 2008). A meta-analysis of 17 studies found that calcium intakes >1000 mg/day were required for a combined effective benefit with physical activity (Specker, 1996). Since the publication of that analysis, several randomized controlled trials (RCTs) have found greater gains in bone mass at weight-bearing sites when increased calcium and exercise were combined than with manipulation of either factor alone (Bass et al., 2007; Courteix et al., 2005; Iuliano-Burns et al., 2003; Specker and Binkley, 2003; Stear et al., 2003; Ward et al., 2007). This effect has been reported among young children and adolescents, using moderate and intense exercise, with dietary and supplemental sources of calcium. Although the mechanism for the greater osteogenic effect when exercise and adequate calcium are combined is not certain, it seems logical that adequate calcium is required for exercise-induced gains in bone mass to occur (Bass et al., 2007).

Whether a positive effect of exercise on PBM is sustained into adulthood is not clear as no prospective data currently exist. Cross-sectional studies generally find higher aBMD among retired athletes than among controls (Karlsson et al., 2008). However, this may be related to their continued higher activity levels versus sedentary adults (Karlsson, 2004). Longitudinal studies suggest that athletes have more rapid bone loss after cessation of sport, although the positive changes in bone structure may be maintained (Karlsson et al., 2008). A small number of studies have also found reduced fracture rates after the age of 50 years in former athletes versus controls (Gustavsson et al., 2003; Karlsson et al., 2002; Nordstrom et al., 2005). These studies must be interpreted with caution due to sampling bias and the positive effects of sport on strength, coordination, and balance (Karlsson, 2004). Further evidence that bone mass gains from activity during growth are sustained comes from retrospective studies: Activity during adolescence was a significant independent predictor of current aBMD in postmenopausal women (Rideout et al., 2006), and older men who participated in high impact activity during adolescence and young adulthood had higher cortical BMC and femur total and cortical area than did men who did not (Daly and Bass, 2006).

In summary, both exercise related to sport and habitual moderate physical activity, particularly prior to puberty, result in gains in bone mass accrual. The positive influence of activity on bone appears to be sustained into adulthood, although it is unclear if this is related to bone density or changes in structure and whether this infers protection against fracture.

Smoking

Very little research has specifically addressed smoking and PBM. A large meta-analysis of studies conducted in older adults found an association between smoking, primarily cigarette smoking, reduced aBMD, and increased fracture risk (Kanis et al., 2005). As research indicates that smoking starts during teenaged years and continues and/or becomes heavier, the effect of smoking on PBM may not be apparent until later in life, when a gradual reduction in aBMD is likely over time relative to nonsmokers (Heaney et al., 2000). A small number of studies have examined smoking among teenagers and young adults, and a small adverse effect on aBMD has been found (Heaney et al., 2000; Mora and Gilsanz, 2003). A recent population-based study of male siblings aged 25–45 years found that those who started smoking before the age of 16 years had a higher risk of fracture, lower aBMD, lower tibial cortical bone area, and lower radial trabecular and cortical bone area (Taes et al., 2009). These findings were less profound among those who started smoking after puberty (Taes et al., 2009). The authors suggested that bone structure may be influenced by smoking during the growth period and that smoking during growth may interfere with the skeletal effects of estrogens (Taes et al., 2009). Furthermore, smoking is associated with other behaviors that have a negative influence on PBM, including lower physical activity levels and poor dietary intake (Heaney et al., 2000).

NUTRITIONAL DETERMINANTS OF PBM

Nutrition plays a key role in skeletal development. This section discusses what is known about the effects of calcium, phosphorus, magnesium, and vitamins A, D, and K on attaining PBM and also discusses a number of whole-diet considerations.

NUTRIENTS

Many nutrients are essential for normal skeletal development. Therefore, a generally healthy diet with sufficient but not excess calories, protein, and all vitamins and minerals is important in the attainment of PBM. Energy balance is important as both overweight/obese and underweight children are at a greater risk of low aBMD and fracture (Davies et al., 2005). Sufficient protein with the proper balance of amino acids is essential as amino acids are necessary for the production of hormones, which are critically important to both the growth and mineralization of the skeleton as described above. Protein and carbohydrates are required for the production of glycoproteins and proteoglycans, which along with the protein collagen, make up the ground substance in which the mineralized portion of bone, hydroxyapatite, is embedded. As described elsewhere, the crystals of hydroxyapatite are composed of calcium and phosphorus. Many other vitamins (C, D, and K) and minerals (magnesium, zinc, copper, and manganese) are also involved in the processes described above. Highlighting the most important nutrients, we will discuss calcium, phosphorus, magnesium, and vitamins A, D, and K and their role in PBM in more detail.

Calcium

Calcium is the most important bone mineral, as part of the crystal hydroxyapatite, making up ~39% of BMC in the skeleton. The importance of calcium to bone is reviewed in more detail in Chapter 8. Although the importance of calcium in the accumulation of bone mass during growth is well established, the optimal intake for maximizing PBM and whether this intake leads to increased bone strength and reduced fracture risk later in life remain controversial.

A recent meta-analysis examined 19 RCTs that provided calcium supplementation (300–1200 mg) for at least 3 months to 2859 healthy children over 0.7–7 years with a follow-up of 0.7–8 years (Winzenberg et al., 2006). The authors concluded that calcium supplementation had no effect on BMC or aBMD at the lumbar spine or femoral neck (Winzenberg et al., 2006). Small effects, which are likely not clinically significant, were observed for total body BMC (standardized mean difference = 0.14, 95% confidence interval (CI) 0.01–0.27) and for upper limb aBMD (standardized mean difference = 0.14, 95% CI 0.04–0.24). The effect was not modified by sex, puberty, ethnicity, physical activity, or baseline calcium intake. Limitations of the RCTs include no information on changes in bone size or structure and a lack of data among children with very low calcium intakes. As the general population of children and adolescents has low calcium intakes (Looker, 2006; Prentice et al., 2006), examining the effect of calcium supplement on PBM in this group is necessary.

A more recent meta-analysis of 21 calcium and dairy supplemental RCTs among 3821 children found a nonsignificant increase in total body BMC (~2 g) among the intervention groups (Huncharek et al., 2008). Sensitivity analyses revealed three studies with substantially lower calcium intakes and higher calcium supplementation. When pooled, a significant increase in total body BMC (50 g) was found with intervention (Huncharek et al., 2008). These findings support the hypothesis that the effect of calcium on bone may only be apparent when intake is inadequate. When the two RCTs that provided dairy products to their experimental group were pooled, a nonsignificant increase of 35 g total body BMC was observed versus controls (Huncharek et al., 2008).

Since publication of the meta-analyses described above, an 18-month calcium supplemental RCT was conducted among 11- to 12-year-old girls with calcium intakes of <650 mg/day (Lambert et al., 2008). The supplemental group had significantly greater gains in total body and lumbar spine BMC and aBMD and lower concentrations of bone resorption markers and parathyroid hormone (PTH). Interestingly, significantly more girls in the supplemented group reached menarche than did the placebo group at the end of the trial (84% vs. 57%). Similar findings were observed in a 1-year double-blind RCT of calcium-enriched versus placebo foods (similar in energy and macronutrient composition) given to prepubertal girls (Chevalley et al., 2005). Eight years after supplementation had ceased, the intervention group had a significantly lower age of menarche than did placebo (Chevalley et al., 2005). When the girls were examined by median split of menarcheal age, the benefit in aBMD that was observed in the entire sample remained significant only for those below the median age of menarche. The authors hypothesized that calcium may have an interactive affect with hormones: Higher calcium intakes lead to earlier menarche and therefore longer exposure to estrogen. As noted previously, however, these authors have subsequently reported data indicating that estrogen exposure may not be the only determinant of the link between early menarche and increased aBMD (Chevalley et al., 2009).

Whether the small gains in bone mass that are achieved with calcium supplementation are maintained is also a relevant question for which insufficient data exist to make conclusions. Three studies have found the gains in bone mass to be maintained 2–3.5 years after removal of calcium supplementation (Chevalley et al., 2005; Dibba et al., 2002; Dodiuk-Gad et al., 2005). On the other hand, four studies found no long-term benefit 1–3 years after supplementation had ceased (Lambert et al., 2008; Lee et al., 1996, 1997; Slemenda et al., 1997).

In summary, calcium appears to promote modest additional gains in BMC, particularly before puberty and when dietary intake is insufficient. Calcium may promote bone accrual both directly and indirectly by interacting with physical activity and hormones. Further research is required to establish whether the sources of calcium (i.e., dairy products, nondairy foods or supplements) are equivalent and whether bone structural changes occur with calcium supplementation that are maintained in the long term.

Vitamin D

Rickets in children has long been known to result from vitamin D deficiency, and dietary intakes of 200–400 IU/day effectively prevent the condition (Wagner et al., 2008). Perhaps of greater current interest than the association between vitamin D and rickets, however, is the question of the extent to which vitamin D status contributes to bone accrual in growing infants and children (see also Chapter 10). This topic was assessed in a comprehensive review of the literature through 2005 (Cranney et al., 2007). The authors concluded that, in infants, there was inconsistent evidence of an association between vitamin D status (assessed using serum 25(OH)D) and BMC: In two randomized trials, supplementation with 400 IU/day vitamin D_2 significantly increased infants' 25 (OH) D concentrations, but BMC did not differ between the supplemented and placebo groups. In three case–control studies, serum 25(OH)D was positively, negatively, or unrelated to whole body or lumbar spine BMC. In older children and adolescents, fair evidence of an association between serum 25(OH)D and increased bone accrual was found in observational studies, but the results of two RCTs did not confirm a consistent benefit of vitamin D supplementation on gain in bone mass.

Data from two recent RCTs also fail to show a consistent benefit of vitamin D supplementation on bone accrual during growth. In one study, 228 Finnish girls, initially aged 11–12 years were randomly assigned to receive placebo, 5 μg, or 10 μg vitamin D per day for 1 year (Viljakainen et al., 2006). Vitamin D supplementation significantly increased serum 25(OH)D in a dose–response manner, but differential changes in bone accrual were not observed when an intent-to-treat analysis was conducted. However, when subgroups with >80% compliance were assessed, those receiving vitamin D had greater accrual of femoral and spinal BMC. A second RCT was conducted in 168 Lebanese girls aged 10–17 years who received weekly doses of placebo, 1400 IU vitamin D (equivalent to 5 μg/day), or 14,000 IU vitamin D (equivalent to 50 μg/day) for 1 year (El-Hajj Fuleihan et al., 2006). Serum 25(OH)D did not change in those receiving the lower vitamin D dose but increased in those on the high dose. When the data were analyzed by menarcheal status, vitamin D supplementation had no effects on aBMD or BMC at any measured site among the 134 postmenarcheal girls. In the 34 premenarcheal girls, findings were inconsistent: Girls in the low dose group (among whom serum 25(OH)D did not increase) gained more trochanteric BMC than did those in the placebo group, but BMC gains in the high dose group did not differ from those receiving the placebo. A parallel study conducted by these authors with boys did not detect any effects of vitamin D supplementation.

Although serum 25(OH)D at or above ~75–80 nmol/L has been suggested as optimal for prevention of bone loss in adults (Dawson-Hughes et al., 2005), very little data have been reported on whether this range applies to children and adolescents. The lack of consistent data from randomized trials referred to above suggests that it may not. Additional evidence in this regard is available from calcium balance studies: Among 105 girls aged 11–15 years, there was no association between serum 25(OH)D (over the range of ~25–125 nmol/L) and calcium absorption or retention (Weaver et al., 2008). In contrast, calcium intake was positively related to balance. The authors concluded that "to date, there is no evidence related to calcium absorption or retention to support a cut-off for vitamin D insufficiency for children and adolescents."

In summary, further studies are required before the amount of vitamin D required to optimize bone acquisition during growth can be ascertained.

Phosphorus

Phosphorus is part of the bone crystal hydroxyapatite, as reviewed in Chapter 9. In contrast to other nutrients, an excess of dietary phosphorus in the modern diet is a concern for bone development and bone health. The ratio of serum phosphorus to calcium affects secretion of PTH, and therefore a high ratio may potentially lead to bone loss. A review of available evidence suggests that excess phosphorus is likely only to affect PTH secretion in combination with very low calcium intakes in children and adolescents (Heaney et al., 2000). This may be a concern in the adolescent diet as caffeinated carbonated soft drinks (colas) contain phosphoric acid, and carbonated drink consumption has been found to be associated with lower aBMD, particularly among teenaged girls (Prentice et al., 2006). However, high soft drink consumption may be associated with other lifestyle factors that affect bone, including a more sedentary lifestyle, higher caffeine intake, and lower milk intake (Prentice et al., 2006). More recently, a study of 228 German children found caffeinated soft drink consumption to be associated with lower radial polar strength index and periosteal circumference after adjustment for confounders (Libuda et al., 2008). The relationship continued after the individual addition of potential renal acid load (PRAL), or intakes of milk, calcium, or protein (Libuda et al., 2008). However, it was observed in this study that increasing soft drink consumption was associated with lower milk consumption and protein intake (Libuda et al., 2008).

Another mechanism whereby excess phosphorus may be negatively associated with bone is through its impact on acid–base balance, and this is discussed below under the section "Whole-Diet Considerations."

In summary, whether excess phosphorus intake has the potential to influence bone mass during growth either by affecting calcium, PTH, or acid–base balance is unclear. The dietary reference intake (DRI) review committee recently called for research on phosphorus in order "to define the intake needed to optimize bone accretion in children 1 to 18 years" (Bergman et al., 2009).

Magnesium

Approximately 60% of body magnesium is found in the skeleton where magnesium is thought to prevent the development of brittle bones by decreasing the size of the crystal hydroxyapatite. Chapter 14 discusses the role of magnesium in bone in more detail, including the lack of a reliable body magnesium indicator.

Few studies have examined magnesium and bone growth. In the 10-year longitudinal National Heart, Lung, and Blood Institute Growth and Health Study, magnesium intake of girls aged 9–11 years was associated with speed of sound and ultrasound velocity at the age of 18–19 years (Wang et al., 1999). Only one magnesium RCT has been conducted: Among 44 premenarcheal girls aged 8–14 years with dietary magnesium intake <220 mg/day (the Recommended Dietary Allowance for this group is 240 mg/day), those supplemented with 300 mg/day of magnesium for 1 year had significantly greater hip BMC gains (3%) versus controls (Carpenter et al., 2006). No significant differences were found in lumbar spine BMC gain or in markers of bone turnover (Carpenter et al., 2006). However, the small sample size limited statistical power to observe differences by treatment. In summary, research examining the role of magnesium in attainment of PBM is extremely limited. Hence, the DRI review committee has identified the need to determine a "valid and accurate assessment protocol for magnesium" and suggests that "future research is needed to identify the magnesium intake for optimal accretion of bone in children" (Bergman et al., 2009).

Vitamin A

As reviewed elsewhere in this volume (Chapter 11), excessive vitamin A intakes lead to adverse skeletal effects in animals, and excessive vitamin A has been associated with increased fracture risk in some studies of human adults. We were not able to locate studies relating vitamin A intake to bone health in children.

Vitamin K

Vitamin K participates in the γ-carboxylation of osteocalcin, a noncollagenous protein produced by osteoblasts during bone formation. The ability of osteocalcin to bind calcium requires the vitamin-K-dependent γ-carboxylation and is thought to underlie the possible beneficial effect of vitamin K on bone (see Chapter 12 for more information).

To date, evidence suggesting that vitamin K has the potential to influence children's skeletal health is derived primarily from cross-sectional studies. A recent review by Shea and Booth (2008) concluded that outcomes of pediatric studies are inconsistent, as some studies found no associations and others "report an inverse association between vitamin K status and BMC in children aged 8–14 years of age". This wording appears to be unfortunate because in these studies, the inverse associations were between BMC and either the percent undercarboxylated osteocalcin (%ucOC) or the ratio of ucOC to carboxylated osteocalcin (UCR). For both %ucOC and UCR, higher values reflect poorer vitamin K status, and thus, an inverse association suggests that vitamin K status is positively associated with BMC. In this regard, a cross-sectional study of 223 healthy Danish girls aged 11–12 years found that higher %ucOC was associated with lower values for both total body and lumbar spine BMC, but the higher %ucOC was not associated with markers of bone turnover (O'Connor et al., 2007). A study of 307 healthy Dutch children aged 8–14 years also reported that poorer vitamin K status (in this case, higher UCR values) was associated with lower total body BMC (van Summeren et al., 2008). This study also included a prospective component: Over a 2-year period, the changes in total body and femoral neck BMC were negatively associated with changes in UCR, meaning greater gains in BMC were observed in children whose vitamin K status improved over time, as reflected by a decrease in UCR. Other evidence supporting a relationship between vitamin K status and bone is provided by studies reporting low BMC in groups of children with clinical conditions characterized by suboptimal vitamin K status. For example, low BMC is reported in children with cystic fibrosis, who malabsorb vitamin K (Fewtrell et al., 2008), and in those on long-term anticoagulant therapy, which antagonizes vitamin K (Avgeri et al., 2008).

Only one small, nonrandomized intervention trial of vitamin K supplementation could be located in the literature. Twenty children with cystic fibrosis received 10 mg of vitamin K per week for 1 year; no unsupplemented patient control group was included in the study (Nicolaidou et al., 2006). At the end of the supplementation period, vitamin K status had improved and bone formation markers increased substantially, whereas no changes were seen in markers of bone resorption. Despite these apparently positive changes in bone turnover, no differences in aBMD Z score at the lumbar spine were observed after 1 year (total body BMD was not assessed) (Nicolaidou et al. 2006). The dose of vitamin K used in this study was very large, which should be noted, equivalent to a daily intake of 1400 µg. In contrast, the Adequate Intake for vitamin K in children ranges from 55 to 75 µg/day, depending on age.

Thus, although cross-sectional and observational studies provide suggestive evidence of positive associations between vitamin K status and bone mass accrual in children, no data have been reported from RCTs. Evidence from RCTs is critical to understanding the relationship between vitamin K and bone in children and adolescents, particularly given RCT data in adults indicating that vitamin K supplementation may not protect against bone loss (Shea and Booth, 2008).

WHOLE-DIET CONSIDERATIONS

In addition to continuing to assess the role of individual nutrients in bone mass accretion, research is increasingly focusing on the importance of the whole diet, including topics such as infant feeding method, acid–base balance, and the effects of vegetarian diets. Growing interest is emerging in the concept that osteoporosis may have developmental origins. Summaries of these topics conclude the chapter.

Infant Feeding

How feeding practices among infants and toddlers affect bone mass development has received some attention in recent years. A narrative review (Specker, 2004) noted that the majority of research suggests that total body BMC is lower among infants fed human milk versus formula, although these differences are no longer apparent at the age of 1 year after the introduction of solid foods. Regarding the type of formula, Specker (2004) noted that evidence suggesting that infants on soy-based formulas have lower radial aBMD than do those fed cow's milk-based formula was conducted before calcium and phosphate fortification of soy formula was the norm. More recent studies have found no differences. Palm olein oil is added to formula to mimic the fatty acid profile of human milk; however, evidence suggests that it may inhibit the absorption of calcium, which may impact bone (Koo et al., 2006). In a double-blind RCT of 128 infants aged 2 weeks to 6 months, those on a palm olein fortified formula had less bone gain than did infants fed formula without palm olein (Koo et al., 2003). Yet, the differences in bone mass accrual may not be lasting: In a retrospective analysis of feeding practices, bone mass at the age of 4 years was not different among infants fed human milk, a palm olein formula, or a nonsupplemented formula during the first 4 months of life (Young et al., 2005). Finally, most studies indicate that the timing of the introduction of solids foods does not appear to affect total body BMC (Specker, 2004). A recent study of ~600 mother–child pairs provides further support, finding no correlation between bone size or aBMD at 4 years of age and breast-feeding duration or adherence to "infant guidelines" regarding the introduction of foods (Harvey et al., 2009). In summary, although the evidence is limited, the method of infant feeding does not appear to have an important influence on PBM.

Dietary Acid–Base Balance

Many prominent bone researchers have emphasized the value of considering overall diet patterns and bone mass development rather than individual nutrients, allowing for examination of energy sufficiency, dietary factors affecting nutrient absorption or excretion, and acid–base balance (Lanham-New, 2008; Prentice et al., 2006; Weaver, 2002; Weaver et al., 2008). In a narrative review of studies linking a high intake of fruits and vegetables (or potassium- and bicarbonate-rich foods or dietary alkali) in relation to bone health, five large observational studies were cited that noted a positive relationship between fruit and vegetable intake and bone mass accrual in children and adolescents (Lanham-New, 2008).

The possible mechanism linking fruit and vegetable intake and improved indicators of bone health relates to the acid–base balance hypothesis, discussed in more detail in Chapter 18. Components of the diet contribute to dietary acidity by either generating or consuming protons. Evidence suggests that the typical Western diet results in chronic low-grade metabolic acidosis, which has been shown to stimulate bone resorption (Lanham-New, 2008). Acid contributors include phosphorus, sulfur-containing amino acids, and chloride, which are found in meat, grains, dairy, and processed foods. Alkaline salts include potassium and magnesium and are found in fruits, vegetables, and dairy foods. Dietary PRAL is estimated by an equation that balances the intake of protein and phosphorus to calcium, magnesium, and potassium. Among children, one study found an association between lower indicators of dietary acidosis and higher aBMD (Alexy et al., 2005). In the Cambridge Bone Study of teenagers, fruit and vegetable intake was associated with higher size-adjusted BMC, although there was no association between bone mass and PRAL (Prentice et al., 2006). It could be that other components found in fruits and vegetables promote bone health (Lanham-New, 2008). The authors of the Cambridge Bone Study highlighted the complexities when considering whole diet and PBM: In their sample of adolescents, cheese and yogurt were the greatest contributors to dietary acid load whereas potatoes and beverages were the greatest alkaline contributors, meaning that lower net endogenous acid production was observed in diets that were high in fruits and vegetables as well as in French fries, potato chips, baked beans, chocolate, and beer (Prentice et al., 2006).

VEGETARIAN AND VEGAN DIETS

Vegetarians follow a diet that excludes meat, fish, and poultry, whereas vegans consume no animal products, including dairy and eggs. This distinction is important to consider when examining the effect of these dietary patterns on bone. A recent Bayesian meta-analysis of nine studies pooling data from 2749 adults found vegetarians to have ~4% lower aBMD at the femoral neck and lumbar spine than do omnivores, and this effect was more pronounced among vegans (Ho-Pham et al., 2009). Although significant, the difference in aBMD was assessed by the authors as not clinically relevant. A recent point–counterpoint published in the *American Journal of Clinical Nutrition* (Lanou, 2009; Weaver, 2009) debated whether vegetarian diets should include dairy products. Although the data presented mainly related to adults, some of the evidence pertained to children: Higher rates of fracture were reported in milk avoiders from New Zealand (Goulding et al., 2004), and an association between lumbar spine BMC and perceived milk intolerance exists among white, Hispanic, and Asian children from the United States (Matlik et al., 2007).

Dairy products contain many nutrients that are important for bone health other than calcium such as phosphorus, magnesium, and vitamin D. The dairy protein whey has been shown to affect bone turnover, and milk consumption (but not other sources of protein) has been linked to increases in IGF-1 (Prentice et al., 2006). A recent study of 192 healthy girls and young women found associations between milk intake (not vitamin D fortified) and lumbar spine BMC, aBMD, and serum IGF-1 and PTH in the postmenarcheal but not premenarcheal girls (Esterle et al., 2009). Other calcium sources and total intake of calcium, phosphorus, magnesium, protein, and energy from milk were not associated with bone health indicators (Esterle et al., 2009). Also in this study, those with milk intakes in the lowest tertile had lower aBMD, BMC, and IGF-1 and higher PTH than did girls with milk intake in the highest tertile, although milk consumption was not associated with height, bone length, or area (Esterle et al., 2009).

No studies have prospectively examined aBMD or BMC and vegetarianism during growth. A small Polish study of 49 healthy children aged 2–10 years found that compared with omnivores, vegetarians had significantly lower levels of serum osteocalcin (Ambroszkiewicz et al., 2003), and lower levels of serum 25(OH)D and bone turnover markers (Ambroszkiewicz et al., 2007). In this study, body mass index, energy, and macronutrient intakes were similar by diet and were within the recommended range, although calcium and vitamin D intakes were significantly lower among vegetarian children (Ambroszkiewicz et al., 2003, 2007). As no long-term studies of bone mass accrual comparing vegetarians and/or vegans and omnivore children have been reported, no conclusions can be made.

DEVELOPMENTAL ORIGINS OF OSTEOPOROSIS

The hypothesis that chronic disease may have developmental origins arose from studies showing that low birthweight was associated with increased coronary heart disease mortality (Barker, 2004) and that the relationship did not result from confounding variables. Because low birthweight can occur as a result of maternal nutritional deprivation, a nutritional basis for the relationship is apparent. The hypothesis, now known as the fetal (or developmental) origins hypothesis, has since been extended to other chronic diseases, including osteoporosis (Cooper et al., 2009). The primary concept is that developmental plasticity in response to adverse conditions in utero may lead to lifelong alterations in metabolism and hormones, as well as in the number of cells in key organs, thereby affecting chronic disease risk.

As summarized by Cooper and colleagues (2009), evidence for the developmental origins of osteoporosis is based on four types of studies: (1) population studies linking adult bone mass to birthweight or weight in early infancy; (2) physiologic studies of endocrine systems that might be programmed in early life and their association with birthweight and age-related bone loss; (3) studies characterizing women during pregnancy with regard to nutrition and lifestyle and relating these factors to the bone mass of their children; and (4) studies relating birth size and early childhood growth patterns to risk of adult hip fracture. Examples of compelling findings include the observation that even among monozygotic twin pairs, differences in birthweight were found to be related to differences in adult bone mass, that maternal vitamin D status during pregnancy is related to a child's BMC at the age of 9 years, and that birthweight modulates the relationship between vitamin D receptor genotype and adult spinal aBMD.

Intervention studies designed to directly explore these relationships are needed. In the meantime, however, the accumulating body of knowledge of initiation of early-life diet–bone relationships points to the importance of ensuring that pregnant women are well nourished to support intrauterine growth.

SUMMARY

Although genetics appears to be the primary determinant of PBM, diet and exercise are two important factors contributing to skeletal development and PBM attainment. Developing bone may benefit greatly from repeated activities whereas the skeleton remains plastic, and this may be potentiated by calcium intake. For nutrients other than calcium, relatively little research has been conducted in children and adolescents: Such research, along with a greater understanding of whole-diet considerations, is urgently needed to maximize the potential contribution of nutrition to PBM.

REFERENCES

Alexy, U., Remer, T., Manz, F., et al. 2005. Long-term protein intake and dietary potential renal acid load are associated with bone modeling and remodeling at the proximal radius in healthy children. *Am J Clin Nutr* 82: 1107–1114.

Ambroszkiewicz, J., Klemarczyk, W., Gajewska, J., et al. 2007. Serum concentration of biochemical bone turnover markers in vegetarian children. *Adv Med Sci* 52: 279–282.

Ambroszkiewicz, J., Laskowska-Klita, T., and Klemarczyk, W. 2003. Low levels of osteocalcin and leptin in serum of vegetarian prepubertal children. *Med Wieku Rozwoj* 7: 587–591.

Avgeri, M., Papadopoulou, A., Platokouki, H., et al. 2008. Assessment of bone mineral density and markers of bone turnover in children under long-term oral anticoagulant therapy. *J Pediatr Hemato Oncol* 30: 592–597.

Barker, D.J. 2004. The developmental origins of adult disease. *J Am Coll Nutr* 23: 588S–595S.

Bass, S.L., Naughton, G., Saxon, L., et al. 2007. Exercise and calcium combined results in a greater osteogenic effect than either factor alone: A blinded randomized placebo-controlled trial in boys. *J Bone Miner Res* 22: 458–464.

Bergman, C., Gray-Scott, D., Chen, J.J., et al. 2009. What is next for the Dietary Reference Intakes for bone metabolism related nutrients beyond calcium: Phosphorus, magnesium, vitamin D, and fluoride? *Crit Rev Food Sci Nutr* 49: 136–144.

Bonjour, J.P., Chevalley, T., Ferrari, S., et al. 2009. The importance and relevance of peak bone mass in the prevalence of osteoporosis. *Salud Publica Mex* 51: S5–S17.

Carpenter, T.O., DeLucia, M.C., Zhang, J.H., et al. 2006. A randomized controlled study of effects of dietary magnesium oxide supplementation on bone mineral content in healthy girls. *J Clin Endocrinol Metab* 91: 4866–4872.

Chevalley, T., Bonjour, J.P., Ferrari, S., et al. 2009. The influence of pubertal timing on bone mass acquisition: A predetermined trajectory detectable five years before menarche. *J Clin Endocrinol Metab* 94: 3424–3431.

Chevalley, T., Rizzoli, R., Hans, D., et al. 2005. Interaction between calcium intake and menarcheal age on bone mass gain: An eight-year follow-up study from prepuberty to postmenarche. *J Clin Endocrinol Metab* 90: 44–51.

Cooper, C., Westlake, S., Harvey, N., et al. 2009. Developmental origins of osteoporotic fracture. *Adv Exp Med Biol* 639: 217–236.

Courteix, D., Jaffre, C., Lespessailles, E., et al. 2005. Cumulative effects of calcium supplementation and physical activity on bone accretion in premenarcheal children: A double-blind randomised placebo-controlled trial. *Int J Sport Med* 26: 332–338.

Cranney, A., Horsley, T., O'Donnell, S., et al. 2007. Effectiveness and safety of vitamin D in relation to bone health. *Evid Rep Technol Assess* 158: 1–235.

Daly, R.M. 2007. The effect of exercise on bone mass and structural geometry during growth. *Med Sport Sci* 51: 33–49.

Daly, R.M., and Bass, S.L. 2006. Lifetime sport and leisure activity participation is associated with greater bone size, quality and strength in older men. *Osteoporos Int* 17: 1258–1267.

Davies, J.H., Evans B.A., and Gregory, J.W. 2005. Bone mass acquisition in healthy children. *Arch Dis Child* 90: 373–378.

Dawson-Hughes, B., Heaney, R.P., Holick, M.F., et al. 2005. Estimates of optimal vitamin D status. *Osteoporos Int* 16: 713–716.

Dibba, B., Prentice, A., Ceesay, M., et al. 2002. Bone mineral contents and plasma osteocalcin concentrations of Gambian children 12 and 24 mo after the withdrawal of a calcium supplement. *Am J Clin Nutr* 76: 681–686.

Dodiuk-Gad, R.P., Rozen, G.S., Rennert, G., et al. 2005. Sustained effect of short-term calcium supplementation on bone mass in adolescent girls with low calcium intake. *Am J Clin Nutr* 81: 168–174.

El-Hajj Fuleihan, G., Nabulsi, M., Tamim, H., et al. 2006. Effect of vitamin D replacement on musculoskeletal parameters in school children: A randomized controlled trial. *J Clin Endocrinol Metab* 91: 405–412.

Esterle, L., Sabatier, J.P., Guillon-Metz, F., et al. 2009. Milk, rather than other foods, is associated with vertebral bone mass and circulating IGF-1 in female adolescents. *Osteoporos Int* 20: 567–575.

Fewtrell, M.S., Benden, C., Williams, J.E., et al. 2008. Undercarboxylated osteocalcin and bone mass in 8-12 year old children with cystic fibrosis. *J Cystic Fibros* 7: 307–312.

Frost, H.M. 1987. Bone "mass" and the "mechanostat": A proposal. *Anat Rec* 219: 1–9.

Goulding, A., Rockell, J.E., Black, R.E., et al. 2004. Children who avoid drinking cow's milk are at increased risk for prepubertal bone fractures. *J Am Diet Assoc* 104: 250–253.

Gustavsson, A., Olsson, T., and Nordstrom, P. 2003. Rapid loss of bone mineral density of the femoral neck after cessation of ice hockey training: A 6-year longitudinal study in males. *J Bone Miner Res* 18: 1964–1969.

Harvey, N.C., Robinson, S.M., Crozier, S.R., et al. 2009. Breast-feeding and adherence to infant feeding guidelines do not influence bone mass at age 4 years. *Br J Nutr* 102: 915–920.

Heaney, R.P. 2005. BMD: The problem. *Osteoporos Int* 16: 1013–1015.

Heaney, R.P., Abrams, S., Dawson-Hughes, B., et al. 2000. Peak bone mass. *Osteoporos Int* 11: 985–1009.

Hind, K., and Burrows, M. 2007. Weight-bearing exercise and bone mineral accrual in children and adolescents: A review of controlled trials. *Bone* 40: 14–27.

Ho-Pham, L.T., Nguyen, N.D., and Nguyen, T.V. 2009. Effect of vegetarian diets on bone mineral density: A Bayesian meta-analysis. *Am J Clin Nutr* 90: 943–950.

Huncharek, M., Muscat, J., and Kupelnick, B. 2008. Impact of dairy products and dietary calcium on bone-mineral content in children: Results of a meta-analysis. *Bone* 43: 312–321.

Iuliano-Burns, S., Saxon, L., Naughton, G., et al. 2003. Regional specificity of exercise and calcium during skeletal growth in girls: A randomized controlled trial. *J Bone Miner Res* 18: 156–162.

Kanis, J.A., Johnell, O., Oden, A., et al. 2005. Smoking and fracture risk: A meta-analysis. *Osteoporos Int* 16: 155–162.

Karlsson, M.K. 2004. Physical activity, skeletal health and fractures in a long term perspective. *J Musculoskelet Neuronal Interact* 4: 12–21.

Karlsson, M.K., Alborg, H.G., Obrant, K., et al. 2002. Exercise during growth and young adulthood is associated with reduced fracture risk in old ages. *J Bone Miner Res* 17: S297. [Abstract]

Karlsson, M.K., Nordqvist, A., Karlsson, C. 2008. Sustainability of exercise-induced increases in bone density and skeletal structure. *Food Nutr Res* 2008. DOI 10.3402/fnr.v52i0.1872.

Koo, W.W., Hammami, M., Margeson, D.P., et al. 2003. Reduced bone mineralization in infants fed palm olein-containing formula: A randomized, double-blinded, prospective trial. *Pediatrics* 111: 1017–1023.

Koo, W.W., Hockman, E.M., and Dow, M. 2006. Palm olein in the fat blend of infant formulas: Effect on the intestinal absorption of calcium and fat, and bone mineralization. *J Am Coll Nutr* 25: 117–122.

Lambert, H.L., Eastell, R., Karnik, K., et al. 2008. Calcium supplementation and bone mineral accretion in adolescent girls: An 18-mo randomized controlled trial with 2-y follow-up. *Am J Clin Nutr* 87: 455–462.

Lanham-New, S.A. 2008. The balance of bone health: Tipping the scales in favour of potassium-rich, bicarbonate-rich foods. *J Nutr* 138: 172S–177S.

Lanou, A.J. 2009. Should dairy be recommended as part of a healthy vegetarian diet? Counterpoint. *Am J Clin Nutr* 89: 1638S–1642S.

Lee, W.T., Leung, S.S., Leung, D.M., et al. 1996. A follow-up study on the effects of calcium-supplement withdrawal and puberty on bone acquisition of children. *Am J Clin Nutr* 64: 71–77.

Lee, W.T., Leung, S.S., Leung, D.M., et al. 1997. Bone mineral acquisition in low calcium intake children following the withdrawal of calcium supplement. *Acta Paediatr* 86: 570–576.

Libuda, L., Alexy, U., Remer, T., et al. 2008. Association between long-term consumption of soft drinks and variables of bone modeling and remodeling in a sample of healthy German children and adolescents. *Am J Clin Nutr* 88: 1670–1677.

Looker, A.C. 2006. Dietary calcium: Recommendations and intakes around the world. In *Calcium in Human Health*, Weaver, C.M., and Heaney, R.P., eds. Totowa, New Jersey, Humana Press, pp. 105–127.

Matlik, L., Savaiano, D., McCabe, G., et al. 2007. Perceived milk intolerance is related to bone mineral content in 10- to 13-year-old female adolescents. *Pediatrics* 120: e669–e677.

Mora, S., and Gilsanz, V. 2003. Establishment of peak bone mass. *Endocrinol Metab Clin North America* 32: 39–63.

Nicolaidou, P., Stavrinadis, I., Loukou, I., et al. 2006. The effect of vitamin K supplementation on biochemical markers of bone formation in children and adolescents with cystic fibrosis. *Eur J Pediatr* 165: 540–545.

Nordstrom, A., Karlsson, C., Nyquist, F., et al. 2005. Bone loss and fracture risk after reduced physical activity. *J Bone Miner Res* 20: 202–207.

O'Connor, E., Molgaard, C., Michaelsen, K.F., et al. 2007. Serum percentage undercarboxylated osteocalcin, a sensitive measure of vitamin K status, and its relationship to bone health indices in Danish girls. *Br J Nutr* 97: 661–666.

Prentice, A. 2004. Diet, nutrition and the prevention of osteoporosis. *Public Health Nutr* 7: 227–243.

Prentice, A., Schoenmakers, I., Laskey, M.A., et al. 2006. Nutrition and bone growth and development. *Proc Nutr Soc* 65: 348–360.

Rideout, C.A., McKay, H.A., and Barr, S.I. 2006. Self-reported lifetime physical activity and areal bone mineral density in healthy postmenopausal women: The importance of teenage activity. *Calcif Tissue Int* 79: 214–222.

Schoenau, E., and Fricke, O. 2008. Mechanical influences on bone development in children. *Eur J Endocrinol* 159: S27–S31.

Shea, M.K., and Booth, S.L. 2008. Update on the role of vitamin K in skeletal health. *Nutr Rev* 66: 549–557.

Slemenda, C.W., Peacock, M., Hui, S., et al. 1997. Reduced rates of skeletal remodeling are associated with increased bone mineral density during the development of peak skeletal mass. *J Bone Miner Res* 12: 676–682.

Specker, B. 2004. Nutrition influences bone development from infancy through toddler years. *J Nutr* 134: 691S–695S.

Specker, B.L. 1996. Evidence for an interaction between calcium intake and physical activity on changes in bone mineral density. *J Bone Miner Res* 11: 1539–1544.

Specker, B., and Binkley, T. 2003. Randomized trial of physical activity and calcium supplementation on bone mineral content in 3- to 5-year-old children. *J Bone Miner Res* 18: 885–892.

Stear, S.J., Prentice, A., Jones, S.C., et al. 2003. Effect of a calcium and exercise intervention on the bone mineral status of 16–18-y-old adolescent girls. *Am J Clin Nutr* 77: 985–992.

Taes, Y., Lapauw, B., Vanbillemont, G., et al. 2009. Early smoking is associated with peak bone mass and prevalent fractures in young healthy men. *J Bone Miner Res* 25: 379–387.

Valdimarsson, O., Linden, C., Johnell, O., et al. 2006. Daily physical education in the school curriculum in prepubertal girls during 1 year is followed by an increase in bone mineral accrual and bone width—data from the prospective controlled Malmo Pediatric Osteoporosis Prevention study. *Calcif Tissue Int* 78: 65–71.

van Summeren, M.J., van Coeverden, S.C., Schurgers, L.J., et al. 2008. Vitamin K status is associated with childhood bone mineral content. *Br J Nutr* 100: 852–858.

Vicente-Rodriguez, G. 2006. How does exercise affect bone development during growth? *Sport Med* 36: 561–569.

Vicente-Rodriguez, G., Urzanqui, A., Mesana, M.I., et al. 2008. Physical fitness effect on bone mass is mediated by the independent association between lean mass and bone mass through adolescence: A cross-sectional study. *J Bone Miner Metab* 26: 288–294.

Viljakainen, H.T., Natri, A.M., Karkkainen, M., et al. 2006. A positive dose–response effect of vitamin D supplementation on site-specific bone mineral augmentation in adolescent girls: A double-blinded randomized placebo-controlled 1-year intervention. *J Bone Miner Res* 21: 836–844.

Wagner, C.L., Greer, F.R., and American Academy of Pediatrics Section on Breastfeeding, and American Academy of Pediatrics Committee on Nutrition. 2008. Prevention of rickets and vitamin D deficiency in infants, children, and adolescents. *Pediatrics* 122: 1142–1152.

Walker, M.D., Novotny, R., Bilezikian, J.P., et al. 2008. Race and diet interactions in the acquisition, maintenance, and loss of bone. *J Nutr* 138: 1256S–1260S.

Wang, M.C., Moore, E.C., Crawford, P.B., et al. 1999. Influence of pre-adolescent diet on quantitative ultrasound measurements of the calcaneus in young adult women. *Osteoporos Int* 9: 532–535.

Ward, K.A., Roberts, S.A., Adams, J.E., et al. 2007. Calcium supplementation and weight bearing physical activity—do they have a combined effect on the bone density of pre-pubertal children? *Bone* 41: 496–504.

Weaver, C.M. 2002. Adolescence: The period of dramatic bone growth. *Endocrine* 17: 43–48.

Weaver, C.M. 2009. Should dairy be recommended as part of a healthy vegetarian diet? Point. *Am J Clin Nutr* 89: 1634S–1637S.

Weaver, C.M., McCabe, L.D., McCabe, G.P., et al. 2008. Vitamin D status and calcium metabolism in adolescent black and white girls on a range of controlled calcium intakes. *J Clin Endocrinol Metab* 93: 3907–3914.

Winzenberg, T., Shaw, K., Fryer, J., et al. 2006. Effects of calcium supplementation on bone density in healthy children: Meta-analysis of randomised controlled trials. *BMJ* 333: 775–778.

Young, R.J., Antonson, D.L., Ferguson, P.W., et al. 2005. Neonatal and infant feeding: Effect on bone density at 4 years. *J Pediatr Gastroenterol Nutr* 41: 88–93.

25 Calcium, Other Nutrients, Exercise, and Bone Health in Twins

John D. Wark

CONTENTS

INTRODUCTION

Genetic and environmental factors impact on bone development early in life and on maintenance of bone health later in life. Between 50% and 85% of the variation in bone mineral density (BMD) measurements may be explained by additive genetic determinants (Ralston and Uitterlinden, 2010). Using identical (monozygotic) twins as study models reduces within-pair variability greatly as does examining fraternal (dizygotic) twins, although less than for identical twins. Controlling for the genetic contributions to bone mineral measures in this way permits modeling to obtain better estimates of the contributions of environmental factors, such as diet and exercise, to variation in bone mineral measures. Research using various twin approaches has revealed several interesting findings regarding skeletal growth and maturation as well as the maintenance of bone mass and density during adulthood, particularly in females.

One powerful factor associated with changes in bone measures is the change in body composition during growth and maturation, as demonstrated in 8- to 26-year-old female twins (Young et al., 2001). For example, lean mass increases correlate strongly with bone mass changes during linear growth, that is, up to approximately 16 years of age in females, and variations in fat mass become a biologically significant determinant of variation in bone mass after the age of 16 years.

This chapter reviews some highlights of our studies of bone mineral measurements in twins and compares our findings with data from other reports in the literature on the linkages between environmental factors and bone mineral measures of twins.

GENETIC AND ENVIRONMENTAL SOURCES OF VARIATION IN BONE MINERAL MEASUREMENTS

The contributions of genetic and environmental determinants of bone mineral measures, that is, BMD, usually measured by dual-energy x-ray absorptiometry, are more complex than originally recognized (Pollitzer and Anderson, 1989; Hopper et al., 1998), particularly because the strength of various contributions to variance may vary according to the stage in life. Differences in the genetic and environmental contributions to BMD variation are evident even during the growth years as additive genetic variance and environmental variance shared within pairs of twins (the common environmental variance component) fluctuate inversely up to the age of 18 years, following which additive genetic variance increases and common environmental variance drops considerably (Figure 25.1) (Hopper et al., 1998). These authors concluded that the genetic and environmental contributions to BMD variance are complex. They found that adjustment for lean mass substantially reduced genetic variance at peak growth in adolescence, during which time genetic variances peaked (Figure 25.2). This effect was in keeping with the shared determinants of variation in lean mass and bone mineral measures (see below). Genetic variances in bone measures then fell in the late teenaged years and increased with early adulthood. The latter may reflect gene–environment interactions or covariable effects. Rapid skeletal and soft tissue changes associated with puberty and maturation are likely to contribute to these variations. Evidence exists that environmental effects shared by twins (common environmental effect) impact on lumbar spine and femoral neck BMD, even after adjusting for lean mass and age. We found that common environmental variance was greatest during the late teenaged years, diminished as pairs started to live apart, and appeared to be independent of lean mass during adolescence but not in early adulthood (Hopper et al., 1998).

In elderly twins aged 60 to 89 years, genetic factors maintain a substantial role in explaining variation in areal BMD at the hip and other sites (except the forearm) (Flicker et al., 1995), but the persistence of predominant genetic effects on hip strength, as measured by hip structural analysis, in older age groups is less clear (Paton et al., 2004). The reasons for these age-related differences are probably several fold. Although genetic–environmental modeling of twin data suggests strong additive genetic sources of variation in BMD at all ages beyond infancy, the actual genes involved may differ at various life stages. One recent twin study (Makovey et al., 2007) demonstrated a significant genetic contribution to changes in BMD around the age of menopause, and it is likely, for example, that the genes mediating this association are different from those determining peak bone mass. The nature and relative strength of environmental determinants of bone mineral measures also vary through life, as does the extent to which these influences are shared within pairs of twins.

Evidence suggests that shared environmental factors are significant during childhood and adolescence when most twin pairs live together and that individual environmental factors (unique to each twin within a pair) begin to emerge in early adult life as twins begin to live separately and develop more individualized lifestyles (Figure 25.3). The strength of individual environmental covariance increases through life, whereas shared environmental covariance diminishes for most measured variables. The emergence of significant individual environmental influences on bone means that the proportion of variance attributable to additive genetic effects will decrease with aging. Moreover, these effects may well vary between skeletal sites. For example, effects of estrogen exposure may be more evident at the spine than the hip, whereas the reverse may be true with respect to effects of weight-bearing exercise.

The sharing of genetic and environmental influences affecting bone mineral measures and other traits also appears to be an important determinant of bone measures. For example, twin studies have shown such sharing of determinants between non-bone lean body mass (LBM) and bone mineral measures (Seeman et al., 1996). LBM itself tends to be highly similar in identical twins. This was demonstrated by Seeman and coauthors (1996) who concluded that genetic factors accounted for 60%–80% of the individual variances of both femoral neck BMD and lean mass and greater than 50% of their covariance. These authors proposed that the association between greater muscle mass

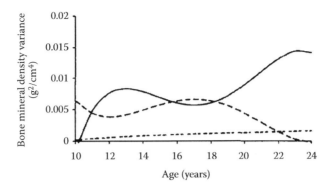

FIGURE 25.1 The best-fitting curves for additive genetic variance (solid line), common environment variance (dashed line), and individual specific variance (dotted line) for bone mineral density at the lumbar spine adjusted for age alone in female twins aged 10 to 26 years. (From Hopper, J.L., et al., Genetic common environment, and individual specific components. *Am. J. Epidemiol.*, 147, 17–29, 1998, by permission of Oxford University Press.)

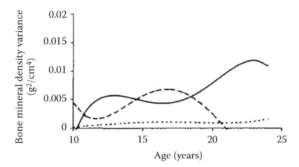

FIGURE 25.2 The best-fitting curves for additive genetic variance (solid line), common environment variance (dashed line), and individual specific variance (dotted line) for bone mineral density at the lumbar spine adjusted for age and lean mass in female twins aged 10 to 26 years. (From Hopper, J.L., et al., Genetic common environment, and individual specific components. *Am. J. Epidemiol.*, 147, 17–29, 1998, by permission of Oxford University Press.)

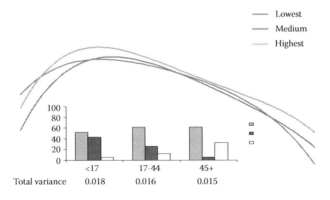

FIGURE 25.3 Distribution of total hip BMD with age by height tertile (lowest, medium, highest) and variance components [additive genetic (G), common environment (C), unique environment (E)] by age groups (<17, 17–44, 45 years and older) in female twins. %G: additive genetic variance as a proportion of total variance. %C: common environment variance as a proportion of total variance. %E: unique environment variance as a proportion of total variance.

and greater BMD was likely to be determined by genes regulating body size. However, non-twin exercise intervention studies in children suggest that environmental influences, such as physical activity, also contribute appreciably to covariation in BMD and LBM (Morris et al., 1997).

Interactions between environmental factors and genes, the new field of epigenetics, are considered to be major actors in the development and maintenance of bone, including bone mass or density and microarchitectural or quality measurements. Hip structural analysis helps in approaching the possible interactions occurring during different stages of the life cycle (see below). Calcium supplementation trials using the co-twin approach have been especially helpful in assessing these interactions.

CALCIUM AND BONE HEALTH IN TWINS: STUDIES IN CHILDHOOD AND ADOLESCENCE

Calcium and vitamin D rank highly among the major nutritional factors contributing to bone development in children and adolescents. In our studies, a calcium supplement has typically been given to one twin and a similarly-appearing placebo has been administered to the other twin. Observational, intervention, and other studies are detailed in this section.

OBSERVATIONAL STUDIES IN 8- TO 26-YEAR-OLD FEMALE TWINS

Our cross-sectional (and longitudinal) observational studies of 8- to 26-year-old female twins have revealed only modest associations between dietary calcium intake and BMD. Some possible reasons for this weak association include that calcium intake across a broad range is not a key determinant of bone accrual, that dietary calcium intake in this sample generally was relatively high, and that twins living together did not differ much in usual dietary calcium intake. Therefore, any significant associations between diet and bone measures were difficult to detect (Young et al., 1995, 2001).

CALCIUM INTERVENTION TRIALS IN YOUNG FEMALE TWINS

A randomized, placebo-controlled, single-blind intervention trial measured the responses of several skeletal variables to calcium supplementation in premenarcheal female twins who were on average 10.4 years of age at baseline (Cameron et al., 2004). Within-pair differences in bone mineral measures in fifty-one 8- to 13-year-olds were followed from baseline for 18 months. The supplements contained 1200 mg of calcium as calcium carbonate, and they were taken as one 600 mg tablet twice daily. The placebo tablets were identical in appearance and also taken in split doses. Usual calcium intakes, assessed by a 4-day food record, including 3 weekdays and 1 weekend day, were approximately 715 mg/day in each pair. Bone density measurements were made at baseline and at 6, 12, 18, and 24 months. Hip structural analysis of physical properties of the proximal femur also was performed on each of the four hip measurements. Calcium supplementation was associated with increased areal BMD compared with placebo ($p < .05$), adjusted for age, height, and weight at the following time points from baseline: total hip: 6 months (1.9%), 12 months (1.6%), and 18 months (2.4%); lumbar spine: 12 months (1.0%); and femoral neck: 6 months (1.9%). Adjusted total body bone mineral content was higher in the calcium group at 6 months (2.0%), 12 months (2.5%), 18 months (4.6%), and 24 months (3.7%), respectively (all $p < .001$).

Calcium supplementation was effective in increasing BMD at regional sites over the first 12–18 months and total body BMC from 6 to 24 months, but the gains were not maintained at regional sites by 24 months. These findings were generally in accord with an earlier twin study in which 70 pairs of monozygotic twins were randomized to calcium (1000 mg calcium citrate malate per day) or placebo for 3 years (Johnston et al., 1992). Notably, in the latter study, the positive effects of calcium supplementation on BMD were seen only in twin pairs who were prepubertal throughout the study. In contrast, in our randomized trial of female twin pairs aged 10–17 years with a mean age of 14 years (Nowson et al., 1997), there was no evidence of a pubertal effect on the response to calcium. At the end of the first 6 months, there was a significant within-pair difference of 1.5% at the lumbar spine and 1.3% at the hip in favor of calcium. However, there were no significant differences in the changes in BMD after the initial effect over the first 6 months. Moreover, in the study by Johnston and colleagues, 2-year follow-up data of twins no longer receiving calcium supplements showed that bone measurements, that is, BMC and BMD, became similar, if not identical, to the control twins (Slemenda et al., 1994). This regression to the same bone values 2 years later during pubertal growth in boys and girls may indicate that the consumption of higher calcium intake needs to be continued for several years during this important period of skeletal growth to achieve a sustained effect on bone measures.

In our co-twin calcium supplementation trials, using hip structural analysis of the acquired hip densitometry scans, significant differences between the calcium-supplemented and placebo-administered twins were found by 18 months for the femoral shaft, but not for the narrow femoral neck or the intertrochanteric region. Cortical bone was significantly thicker in the treated twins, which reflected both relative increases in periosteal bone formation and declines in endosteal resorption, that is, cortical cross-sectional area was increased, and consequently, the cortical shaft sites had significantly greater areal BMD. However, indices of bending strength in the cortical shaft were not increased by calcium over the 18-month period. The calcium-mediated increases in the cross-sectional area of the femoral shaft suggest that, at least in premenarcheal girls, additional calcium intake increases bone mass at the midshaft regions in a manner similar to exercise alone (Petit et al., 2002). The earlier twin calcium intervention trial by Johnston et al. (1992) showed a similar positive effect of calcium at the midshaft of radius, that is, 5.1% greater gain.

DIETARY CALCIUM AS A DETERMINANT OF BONE HEALTH IN ADULT FEMALE TWINS

Adult female twins also have been investigated in an effort to identify dietary and other factors that influence bone mineral measures after peak bone mass has been achieved, that is, those female twin pairs over 30 years of age. These twin studies have not revealed a major influence of usual dietary calcium intake on bone mineral measures in adult women.

In a cross-sectional co-twin study involving 146 female twin pairs aged 30–65 years, calcium intake was related to total body bone mineral content and forearm BMD (both 1.4% ± 0.7% increase for every 1000 mg consumed daily), but not to BMD at the lumbar spine and hip (MacInnis et al., 2003). This association with calcium intake was modest compared with the positive effect observed for the hip in relation to regular recreational physical activity and the negative relationship seen with smoking.

In another twin study of 69 volunteer female twin pairs aged 60–89 years, age, body composition, and lifestyle factors accounted for 20%–33% of variation in BMD, whereas about 75% of residual variation in BMD at the non-forearm sites was determined by genetic factors (Flicker et al., 1995). Lifetime smoking was the most significant lifestyle determinant of lower bone mineral measures, whereas lifetime alcohol consumption was another possible adverse influence. Of interest, daily calcium intake was not significantly associated with either regional or total body bone mineral, despite mean calcium intake measured by short food frequency questionnaire being less than 600 mg daily.

PHYSICAL ACTIVITY AND BONE HEALTH IN TWINS FROM CHILDHOOD TO OLD AGE

In addition to dietary intake, physical activity is a major factor that influences skeletal development in prepubertal children and, to a lesser degree, in postpubertal children. Twin studies do not lend themselves well to exercise intervention studies unless twins within a pair are separated early in life and raised under different circumstances. Identical twins typically have similar changes in body weight in adulthood, and possibly in bone variables, even when raised and separated shortly after birth and raised under differing environmental conditions (Price and Gottesman, 1991).

Observational studies in adult female twins have identified important associations between recreational physical activity and bone mineral measures. MacInnis et al. (2003) in their study of 30- to 65-year-old twins reported that in all women, a 0.8% (SE, 0.3) difference in hip BMD was associated with each hour per week of difference in recreational physical activity, with effects more evident in premenopausal women. This association is in keeping with the magnitude of effect seen in exercise intervention trials in adult women and supports a clinically significant benefit from regular sporting activity. In contrast, among postmenopausal pairs, time spent walking was inversely associated with forearm BMD and with total body BMC.

In another study involving healthy adult female twins, measures of gait, balance, and lower limb muscle strength were obtained and the data subjected to linear and nonlinear modeling to examine the associations of these measures with age (El Haber et al., 2008). Performance was maintained until 45–55 years of age, with some variation between the outcome measures. Beyond that age range, performance in all measures declined with increasing age. A significant nonlinear relationship with age was demonstrated for lower limb strength measures, velocity, and double support duration of gait and in a range of clinical and laboratory balance tests. Thus, aspects of balance, lower limb muscle strength, and gait may decline nonlinearly with age, with differing age thresholds for some of these changes. Further research into these threshold effects may have implications for the optimal timing of exercise and other interventions to reduce the risk of falls and fractures in older women.

IMPACT OF SMOKING AND OTHER FACTORS ON BONE HEALTH IN FEMALE TWINS

SMOKING

Cigarette smoking has been found to be an adverse factor in practically all studies of BMD in adults. Many population-based studies also have shown an increase in osteoporotic fracture risk associated with smoking (Wong et al., 2007). Twin studies have been few, but they also support this negative effect of smoking on bone (Hopper and Seeman, 1994; Flicker et al., 1995; MacInnis et al., 2003). Smoking was found to be independently negatively related to bone mineral measures at all sites (MacInnis et al., 2003). Moreover, a within-pair discordance of 10 pack-years was associated with bone deficits of 3.3%, 2.7%, and 2.3% at the lumbar spine, total hip, and total body, respectively. Hepatic clearance of circulating estrogens may occur in female smokers, but the mechanisms underlying these smoking-associated bone deficits are not well understood and warrant further research.

VITAMIN D STATUS

Many reports have shown that vitamin D deficiency during the period of skeletal growth is associated with poor development of both peripheral and axial bones, and these effects are worse when calcium intake is also deficient. Reports on vitamin D and bone in twins have been few. A Swedish study of same-sex twins revealed evidence of a genetic influence on summer season vitamin D status, which the authors attributed to a possible genetic influence on cutaneous synthesis of vitamin D (Snellman et al., 2009). Another study reported a strong genetic influence on 25-hydroxyvitamin D levels among male but not female rural Chinese adolescent twins (Arguelles et al., 2009).

Interestingly, a study conducted in healthy, older female twins demonstrated that within-pair differences in aspects of gait and balance performance were related significantly to within-pair differences in serum 25-hydroxyvitamin D levels (El Haber et al., 2006). These gait and balance measures are validated predictors of falls risk, suggesting that vitamin D status may explain in part the within-pair similarities in performance in these tests.

SUMMARY

Twin studies have yielded important findings about additive genetic influences and environmental variables, especially calcium intake, that influence skeletal development early in life and help maintain bone health in midlife and later adult life. Hip structural analysis applied to twin data has provided important qualitative information about determinants of bone architectural changes in the hip that potentially may reduce the risk of hip fractures and resultant mortality during later life. Based on the available evidence, high calcium consumption increases bone mass and quality in growing children, but evidence is not yet convincing that the early life gains from high calcium consumption alone carry over into adulthood and late life. Although twin studies have not been able to address whether physical activity early in life helps to assure optimal peak bone mass development, observational studies in adult female twins have lent strong support to and have helped to quantify the beneficial effect of moderate levels of physical activity in maintenance of bone mass. In contrast, twin studies have also been valuable in quantifying adverse lifestyle influences on bone, such as bone loss associated with smoking and excessive alcohol consumption.

REFERENCES

Arguelles, L.M., Langman, C.B., Ariza, A.J., et al. 2009. Heritability and environmental factors affecting vitamin D status in rural Chinese adolescent twins. *J Clin Endocrinol Metab* 94:3273–3281.

Cameron, M.A., Paton, L.M., Nowson, C.A., et al. 2004. The effect of calcium supplementation on bone density in premenarcheal females—a co-twin approach. *J Clin Endocrinol Metab* 89:4916–4922.

El Haber, N., Erbas, B., Hill, K., et al. 2008. The relationship between age and measures of balance, strength and gait: Linear and non-linear analyses. *Clin Sci (Lond)* 114: 719–727.

El Haber, N., Hill, K., and Wark, J.D. 2006. Vitamin D status, parathyroid hormone levels and predictors of falls risk in well women aged 47–80 years. 3rd IOF Asia-Pacific Regional Conference on Osteoporosis and 16th Annual Meeting of the Australian & New Zealand Bone & Mineral Society. [Abstract]

Flicker, L., Hopper, J.L., Rodgers, L, et al. 1995. Bone density determinants in elderly women: A twin study. *J Bone Miner Res* 10:1607–1613.

Hopper, J.L., Green, R., Nowson, C., et al. 1998. Genetic, common environment, and individual specific components of variance for bone mineral density in 10- to 26-year-old females: a twin study. *Am J Epidemiol* 147:17–29.

Hopper, J.L., and Seeman, E. 1994. The bone density of female twins discordant for tobacco use. *New Engl J Med* 330:387–392.

Johnston, C.C., Jr., Miller, J.Z., Slemenda, C.W., et al. 1992. Calcium supplementation and increases in bone mineral density in children. *New Engl J Med* 327:82–87.

MacInnis, R.J., Cassar, C., Nowson, C.A., et al. 2003. The impact of smoking and other factors on bone mineral measures in adult female twins: Determinants of bone density in 30 to 65 year old women: A twin study. *J Bone Miner Res* 18:1650–1656.

Makovey, J., Nguyen, T.V., Naganathan, V., et al. 2007. Genetic effects on bone loss in peri- and postmenopausal women: A longitudinal twin study. *J Bone Miner Res* 22:1773–1780.

Morris, F.L., Naughton, G.A., Gibbs, J.L., et al. 1997. Prospective ten-month exercise intervention in premenarcheal girls: Positive effects on bone and lean mass. *J Bone Miner Res* 12:1453–1462.

Nowson, C.A., Green, R.M., Hopper, J.L., et al. 1997. A co-twin study of the effect of calcium supplementation on bone density during adolescence. *Osteoporos Int* 7:219–225.

Paton, L.M., Beck, T.J., Semanick L. et al. 2004. Genetic and environmental contributions to hip strength: In female twins aged 18 and Over. *J Bone Miner Res* 19(1): S48.

Petit, M.A., McKay, H.A., MacKelvie, K.J., et al. 2002. A randomized school-based intervention confers site and maturity-specific benefits on bone structural properties in girls: Hip structural analysis. *J Bone Miner Res* 17:363–372.

Pollitzer, W.S., and Anderson, J.J.B. 1989. Ethnic and genetic differences in bone mass: A review with an hereditary vs. environmental perspective. *Am J Clin Nutr* 50:1244–1259.

Price, R.A., and Gottesman, I.I. 1991. Body fat in identical twins reared apart: Roles of genes and environment. *Behav Genet* 21:1–7.

Ralston, S.H., and Uitterlinden, A.G. 2010. Genetics of osteoporosis. *Endocr Rev* 31(5 October): (Apr 29, 2010. doi:10.1210/er.2009-0044). [Epub ahead of print]

Seeman, E., Hopper, J.L., Young, N.R., et al. 1996. Do genetic factors explain associations between muscle strength, lean mass, and bone density? A twin study. *Am J Physiol* 270(2 Pt 1):E320–E327.

Slemenda, C.W., Reister, T.K., Hui, S.L., et al. 1994. Influences on skeletal mineralization in children and adolescents: Evidence for varying effects of sexual maturation and physical activity. *J Pediatr* 125:201–207.

Snellman, G., Melhus, H., Gedeborg, R., et al. 2009. Seasonal genetic influence on serum 25-hydroxyvitamin D levels: A twin study. *PLoS One* 4(11):e7747.

Wark, J.D., Paton, L.M., Beck, T.J., et al. 2003. A co-twin calcium intervention trial in young females: Effects measured by hip structural analysis. *J Bone Miner Res* 18(2): S12.

Wong, P.K., Christie, J.J., and Wark, J.D. 2007. The effects of smoking on bone health. *Clin Sci (Lond)* 113:233–241.

Young, D., Hopper, J.L., MacInnis, R.J., et al. 2001. Changes in body composition as determinants of longitudinal changes in bone mineral measures in 8 to 26-year-pol female twins. *Osteoporos Int* 12:506–515.

Young, D., Hopper, J.L., Nowson, C.A., et al. 1995. Determinants of bone mass in 10 to 26 year old females: A twin study. *J Bone Miner Res* 10:558–567.

26 Nutrition and Bone in Young Adults

Christel Lamberg-Allardt and Merja Kärkkäinen

CONTENTS

INTRODUCTION

Studies on nutrition and bone health have principally focused on postmenopausal women and the elderly and to some extent on children and adolescents, whereas young adults have not received very much attention. In this review, we focus on the effects of nutritional factors on the skeleton during the period between the time after peak bone mass (PBM) is reached in men and women and well before menopause in women. Many nutritional factors influence bone tissue directly or through calcium (Ca) metabolism. Studies have mostly focused on vitamin D and Ca. Yet, many other nutritional factors have an influence on the adult bone such as phosphorus (P), protein, vitamin K, vitamin C, magnesium, and fatty acids.

A large increase in bone mass occurs during the growth period in childhood and in adolescence. A consensus exists now that PBM is reached at the age of approximately 20 years in men and 18 years in women, but the bone mass can increase until around age 30 years. After reaching PBM, bone mass starts to decline slowly. At menopause, the bone mass of women decreases faster, but the decrease levels off after a few years. In men, the loss in bone mass is not as rapid as that in women.

VITAMIN D

The role of vitamin D for bone health has been studied intensively during the last decades in adults, focusing, however, mainly on the prevention on fractures in the elderly. Vitamin D status is best reflected by the serum 25-hydroxyvitamin D concentration (S-25OHD). Vitamin D, as the biologically active form, 1,25-dihydroxyvitamin D ($1,25(OH)_2D$), is essential for active intestinal Ca absorption. It is bound in the cells to the vitamin D receptor, which acts as a transcription factor for many proteins participating in the transport of Ca across the intestinal cell.

Overt vitamin D deficiency leads to osteomalacia in adults. It is characterized by deficient mineralization of the osteoid. Osteomalacia is seldom definitely diagnosed as the osteomalacia can only be confirmed by histomorphometry. However, low S-25OHD, low urinary Ca (U-Ca) excretion, and high serum alkaline phosphate activity and elevated parathyroid hormone (PTH) suggest osteomalacia. Only a bone biopsy with non-decalcified preparation can confirm diagnosis.

Serum PTH (S-PTH) typically plays an important role in the relation between skeletal health and vitamin D status. An increase in S-PTH leads to an increased bone resorption. Low serum 25OHD has been shown to be associated with increased concentrations of S-PTH, and supplementation with vitamin D decreases S-PTH in vitamin-D-deficient elderly subjects (for review, see Lips, 2001). Low 25OHD and vitamin D insufficiency have been shown to be associated with both low bone mineral density (BMD) and an increased fracture risk especially in the elderly (Lips, 2001). Intervention studies with vitamin D supplementation together with Ca supplementation have shown both an effect on BMD as well as a decreased fracture risk in the elderly (Bischoff-Ferrari et al., 2009a, 2009b; Lips et al., 2009; DiPART Group, 2010).

Is vitamin D deficiency or insufficiency common in young adults in the Western world and does it influence bone health? Vitamin D in relation to bone has been studied mostly in elderly postmenopausal women. Studies in children and adolescents are few.

It has been assumed that healthy adults get enough vitamin D through the synthesis in the skin, in addition to what is supplied through dietary sources. However, some reports indicate that low vitamin D status is a problem in countries where sunshine is not abundant and that this has may adversely affect skeletal health. Low vitamin D status, however, is also a problem in sunny countries. Skin pigmentation and use of sun screens are also risk factors for vitamin D deficiency.

Cross-Sectional Studies

In a study in 30- to 45-year-old persons in Finland, it was found that vitamin D status was low, and it was also reflected in low BMD at the radius and ulna (Lamberg-Allardt et al., 2001). In 200 young women aged 18–36 years in Bangladesh, low vitamin D status was associated with low BMD in the lumbar spine and the hip in women (Islam et al., 2008). In Norway, 869 subjects born in Norway and 177 Pakistani were studied in a cross-sectional study (Meyer et al., 2004). Vitamin D deficiency was prevalent among the Pakistani immigrants, and in great contrast to the vitamin D replete status of Norwegians. Whereas BMD at the forearm site (measured with single-energy x-ray absorptiometry) was significantly lower in Norwegian women with secondary hyperparathyroidism compared with those without, no difference in BMD was found, however, between Pakistani women with and without secondary hyperparathyroidism. In a cross-sectional study of 201 Gujarati and white female and male volunteers aged 20–40 years living in the United Kingdom, Gujarati females had significantly lower BMD both at the spine and hip than did white females. A trend suggested that Gujarati males have a lower BMD at the hip and spine than do their white counterparts, but these differences did not reach statistical significance. A significantly higher proportion of the Gujarati men and women had S-25OHD concentrations below the lower limit of the laboratory range of normal. Of those who had lower mean S-25OHD concentrations, greater frequencies were found in Gujarati men and women (Hamson et al., 2003).

Fractures have not been studied in a larger extent in this age group. Nevertheless, in a study of male healthy military recruits (mean age 19 years) in Finland, an association between stress fractures and low S-25OHD concentration was found (Ruohola et al., 2006).

INTERVENTION STUDIES

The effect of relatively low dosages of supplemental vitamin D on vitamin D and bone status in Pakistani immigrants was studied in Denmark (Andersen et al., 2008). The 1-year-long randomized double-blind placebo-controlled intervention with vitamin D_3 of girls (10.1–14.7 years), women (18.1–52.7 years), and men (17.9–63.5 years) of Pakistani origin living in Denmark was undertaken. Mean Ca intake was below recommendations, and no Ca supplementation was provided. The study showed that daily supplementation with 10 µg (400 IU) and 20 µg (800IU) of vitamin D_3 increased S-25OHD concentrations four-fold in both vitamin-D-deficient Pakistani women and girls and that 10 µg (400 IU) increased S-25OHD concentrations two-fold and 20 µg (800 IU) three-fold in Pakistani men. S-PTH concentrations decreased at 6 months, but no significant effect of the intervention was observed on bone turnover markers and dual-energy x-ray absorptiometry measurements of the whole body and lumbar spine (Andersen et al., 2008). A randomized controlled study in 200 women (aged 16–36 years) in Bangladesh with initial low vitamin D status BMD demonstrated improved status during a 1-year supplementation trial with vitamin D (10 µg [400 IU]) and Ca or a multivitamin D preparation, but not with vitamin D alone (Islam et al., 2010); Institute of Medicine, 1997. Viljakainen et al. (2009) gave different doses of vitamin D supplementation to men aged 21–49 years during 6 months. The mean habitual Ca intake (about 1200–1500 mg/day) was sufficient. The authors found that a daily intake of vitamin D in the range of 17.5–20 µg (700–800 IU) was required to prevent winter seasonal increases in S-PTH and maintain stable bone turnover in young, healthy white men. Supplementation inhibited the winter elevation of S-PTH and decreased the bone formation as measured by bone alkaline phosphatase activity, but its benefit on cortical BMD was not significant.

SUMMARY

In summary, studies have shown that vitamin D deficiency is common especially among certain dark-skinned ethnic groups in this age group. In addition, diets, for example, vegan diet, may predispose to vitamin D deficiency. Furthermore, both cross-sectional studies and intervention studies showed that there is a response to vitamin D in bone in young adults. Ca intake should probably be optimal. Some of the studies also indicated that ethnic differences in the response to vitamin D may exist, but the studies are not comparable as all of them have not been adequately controlled, for example, for Ca intake. This issue of Ca intake points out that proper vitamin D intake is important also in this age group, when Ca intake is ensured.

CALCIUM

Ca is essential for skeletal health as a part of Ca phosphate crystals, primarily hydroxyapatite, which gives the skeleton its strength and rigidity together with collagen. Thus, optimal Ca intake during growth is important for the development of the skeleton and PBM. Because of inbound and outbound fluxes of Ca to and from the skeleton as a result of continuous bone remodeling in adulthood, the daily intake of Ca is needed to maintain the mineral homeostasis in the skeleton. Furthermore, the skeleton is an important part of Ca metabolism as Ca is mobilized from the bone in response to a low serum Ca concentration (S-Ca). A decrease in S-Ca increases the secretion of S-PTH from the parathyroid glands, which in turn increases bone resorption. Consequently, acute fluctuations in S-PTH result from changes in serum ionic Ca (S-iCa), resulting from fluctuations in Ca intake which may influence bone metabolism.

ACUTE EFFECTS

Does dietary Ca intake influence S-PTH concentrations in adults and does it have an effect on bone resorption markers? In a few acute studies, a clear dose–response to Ca supplementation has been shown (Guillemant and Guillemant, 1993; Kärkkäinen et al., 2001). Even single intakes as low as 250 mg decrease the S-PTH concentration acutely. Ca-containing foodstuff have different acute effects on the S–S-PTH concentration; for example, fermented cheese has a more pronounced lowering effect on S-PTH than does fluid milk, whereas spinach and sesame seeds do not affect S-PTH concentration when given in amounts of 400 mg (Kärkkäinen et al., 1997). In summary, following ingestion and absorption, dietary Ca has an acute effect on serum S-PTH concentration, but the absence of changes in S-PTH following the ingestion of spinach and sesame seeds suggests that low Ca bioavailability and low intestinal absorption of Ca ions explain the absence of a PTH response.

In some studies (Blumsohn et al., 1994; Guillemant et al., 2000, 2003), supplemental Ca in doses ranging from 170 to 1000 mg has been shown to decrease bone resorption markers in young men when the subjects have fasted the entire study period. However, in a study (Kärkkäinen et al., 2001) in which the subjects followed a normal meal pattern, Ca supplementation had no effect on bone formation and resorption markers in young females. These studies used different bone markers, subject genders differed, and meal patterns varied, any of which could affect the results.

CROSS-SECTIONAL, LONGITUDINAL, AND INTERVENTION STUDIES

Does a relationship exist between S-PTH and habitual Ca intake? In a cross-sectional study, Kärkkäinen et al. (1998) found an inverse relationship between fasting S-PTH concentrations and habitual Ca intake in postmenopausal women, indicating that habitual Ca intake per se has an effect on S-PTH concentration. Recently, this finding was given support by a study in 30- to 40-year-old healthy subjects in Lebanon (Gannagé-Yared et al., 2005).

A few cross-sectional and longitudinal studies have focused on the association between Ca intake and BMD in young adults, and a few additional long-term intervention studies have been conducted. A meta-analysis was performed in 1995 to study the relation between Ca intake and BMD in premenopausal women and adult men between the ages of 18 and 50 years (Welten et al., 1995). The studies published between 1966 and 1994 offered evidence that Ca intake is positively associated with bone mass in premenopausal females. The intervention studies found that Ca supplementation of ~1000 mg/day in premenopausal women can prevent the loss of ~1% of bone/year at all bone sites except the ulna. In males, too few studies (only three) were published to draw firm conclusions. It is noteworthy that the methods used for measuring BMD differed significantly between these studies, and only a few investigations measured BMD in the proximal femur and the lumbar spine. Ca intake alone in relation to BMD has been examined only in a few studies during recent years in young adults. Barger-Lux et al. (2005) did not find an effect of Ca supplementation (average intake 800 mg/day) in 121 young women (mean age 23 years) for 12 months on BMD. Nevertheless, in one study, 354 females were followed for 7 years from puberty to young adulthood in a randomized controlled trial, in which the study subjects were supplemented with 670 mg Ca/day, on average, with a mean dietary intake of 830 mg/day over 7 years (Matkovic et al., 2005). The study showed that Ca supplementation in excess of a habitual Ca intake of about 830 mg/day affects BMD during the pubertal growth spurt, but a diminishing effect was found thereafter that may be related to the catch-up phenomenon in bone mineral accretion. By young adulthood, significant effects of Ca supplementation were evident at the metacarpals and at the proximal forearm in subjects who had better Ca intake compliance and in subjects who developed larger body frames. The authors concluded that their results imply that standards for dietary Ca intake in adolescence should be based on growth rate and body and bone size development (Matkovic et al., 2005).

Because they are rare, fractures have not been studied as an outcome variable in relation to Ca intake or supplementation in this age group. Furthermore, long-term dose–response studies of Ca on bone variables have not been performed; hence, no definite conclusions can be made on the optimal intake needed for growth and maintenance.

PHOSPHORUS

A few studies have shown that high P intake is harmful for bones in animal models (Koshihara et al., 2005; Huttunen et al., 2007). A diet high in P may result in an increase in S-PTH secretion and affect bone metabolism in humans as well. Thus, in the long run, high dietary P intake may lead to secondary hyperparathyroidism, increased bone resorption, and poorer bone quality, especially if the dietary Ca intake is inadequate. Almost all studies on dietary P and bone in healthy humans have been done in young adults.

ACUTE EFFECTS

In a randomized controlled study in 10 young females, an oral phosphate dose either as a single 1500 mg or divided to three 500 mg doses given with standardized meals increased S-P and –S-PTH and decreased U-Ca excretion. S-iCa decreased only when phosphate was given as a single dose. Bone formation markers serum carboxy-terminal propeptide of type I collagen and bone-specific alkaline phosphatase (BALP) decreased after phosphate load, whereas there were no significant changes in serum osteocalcin or in bone resorption markers serum carboxy-terminal telopeptide of type I collagen or urinary deoxypyridinoline (U-DPD) (Kärkkäinen and Lamberg-Allardt, 1996). In 14 young females, oral phosphate supplements of 250, 750, and 1500 mg given with meals increased serum S-PTH dose dependently as compared with placebo. The highest dose also decreased S-iCa concentration. The bone formation marker, BALP, decreased and the bone resorption marker, urinary N-terminal telopeptide of collagen type I (NTX), increased in response to supplemental phosphate. The meals provided 500 mg P and 250 mg Ca (Kemi et al., 2008). The effects of phosphate-containing foods (meat, whole-grain cereals, cheese, and P supplement) containing 1000 mg P with control meal providing altogether 1500 mg P were compared with those of plain control meal (500 mg P) in 16 young females. S-PTH increased only after phosphate-supplement-containing meal, whereas it decreased after cheese consumption compared with the control meal. Bone metabolism was unaffected by the foods except for meat, which increased both bone formation and resorption markers (Karp et al., 2007). In conclusion, an acutely high P intake adversely affects bone metabolism by decreasing bone formation and increasing bone resorption, as indicated by changes in the bone metabolism markers and by an elevated S-PTH concentration.

SHORT-TERM STUDIES

Some early studies exist in which the effect of high P intake on S-PTH and bone markers has been studied for periods between 5 days and 8 weeks. Two grams of oral phosphate daily for 5 days (Silverberg et al., 1986; Calvo et al., 1988) caused a 26% increase in S-P, a 50% increase in S-PTH, and a decrease in S-Ca. A persistent phosphaturia and a 69% fall in U-Ca were also observed. $S-1,25(OH)_2D$ and urinary hydroxyproline excretion, a marker of bone resorption, did not change appreciably. The serum osteocalcin concentration (S-OC) rose 41%. S-OC has been considered to be a marker of bone formation, but it could also be considered a marker of bone turnover, that is, a marker of an increase in bone formation or an increase in bone turnover. The effects of diet with high P (1660 mg) and moderately low Ca (420 mg) intakes typical of U.S. teenagers and young adults were compared with those of a diet with Ca (820 mg) and P (930 mg) contents near the recommended daily intakes in 16 young adults. Both diets were based on common grocery store foods. In 8 days, the 24-h mean S-PTH levels increased in men by 11% and in women by 22% during the test diet. In both sexes, the test diet significantly increased S-P, plasma $1,25(OH)_2D$, and urinary hydroxyproline excretion. In a study lasting 56 days with almost similar test diets, the increase in

S-PTH was shown to persist (Calvo et al., 1990). Thus, short-term ingestion of a diet with typical Ca and P intakes (~400 mg Ca and ~1700 mg P) resulted in elevated S-PTH levels, changes in mineral metabolism, and bone resorption in young adults.

The studies by Calvo et al. (1988, 1990) did not indeed show that it was high P per se that induced the effect on S-PTH. Their study diets were also low in Ca, and the effect could have been due to the low Ca intake and could possibly be corrected by an increase in Ca intake. The fact, however, remains that their study diets were typical for a Western diet. Consequently, Barger-Lux and Heaney (1993) studied 28 healthy premenopausal women before and after manipulating their Ca intake. None of the subjects had high P diets. Women with low Ca intakes at entry were restricted to about 200 mg/day (low Ca), and those with higher self-selected intakes were supplemented to about 2800 mg/day (high Ca). After 8 weeks, the low Ca women had higher S-PTH and urine hydroxyproline excretion than did the women on the high Ca diet. The investigators' findings showed that Ca restriction supports a persistent S-PTH response in the absence of a high P intake.

Could an increase in Ca intake counteract the effects of increased P intake on bone markers, that is, is the effect of P only due to a low Ca intake, as indicated by Barger-Lux and Heaney (1993)? The effect of increasing doses of Ca on markers of Ca and bone metabolism was studied when the diet was high in P (1850 mg) and low in Ca (480 mg) (Kemi et al., 2006). Each of the 12 healthy female subjects aged 21–40 years attended three 24-h study sessions, which were randomized with regard to a Ca dose of 0 (control day), 600, or 1200 mg, and each subject served as her own control. S-PTH concentration decreased and serum ionized Ca concentration increased with increasing Ca doses. The bone formation marker, S-BALP, did not differ significantly between sessions, indicating that Ca could not counteract the effect of P. By contrast, the bone resorption marker, urinary NTX, decreased significantly with both Ca doses. When P intake was above current recommendations, increased Ca intake was beneficial for bone, as indicated by decreased PTH concentration and the marker of bone resorption (urinary NTX). Not even a high Ca intake, however, could change the effect of P intake on the bone formation markers.

The short-term effect of phosphate supplements (0–2000 mg) with Ca intake above 800 mg on Ca homeostasis and bone turnover was studied in men (Whybro et al., 1998). In 10 young men, 1000 mg phosphate supplement with meals providing 800 mg Ca for 1 week increased S-PTH but had no effect on bone markers, S-OC, and urinary NTX excretion. In the second part of the study, the doses were 0, 1000, 1500, and 2000 mg/day phosphate, each given for 1 week, with a similar diet of 1000 mg/day each of Ca and phosphate to 12 young men. Although differences did exist in S-Ca and S-P between the highest and the lowest P diet, the researchers did not find any difference in S-PTH or U-DPD secretion. The authors concluded that phosphate supplementation of the diet did not affect bone turnover in young men (Whybro et al., 1998). The study may, however, have been underpowered so that it was not able to detect changes in bone markers; also, the diet was not controlled in this study, and the blood samples were not taken after an overnight fast, which could increase the measurement variation.

All studies have shown that increased or high P intakes elevate S-PTH concentrations when Ca intake is low. Some studies also showed that bone turnover was increased, as indicated by changes in S-OC concentration, and a few others also have demonstrated an increase in bone resorption. However, the bone markers used in these investigations were not very specific and sufficiently sensitive. The effectiveness of new bone markers developed during the last decades show that they are more sensitive and improves our knowledge of bone metabolism. Finally, the power of these high P studies may also have been too low to detect differences in bone markers.

HABITUAL P INTAKE AND CA AND BONE METABOLISM

The effect of habitual P intake either from sources containing either natural P (NP) food items or food additives (AP) on morning fasting S-PTH was investigated in a cross-sectional study of 140 premenopausal women (Kemi et al., 2009). The investigators focused on the consumption on milk and cheese as natural P sources and cheese containing AP, for example, spreadable cheese, as sources of P AP. Higher habitual total dietary P intakes were associated with higher mean S-PTH and lower mean S-iCa concentrations. AP might affect bone more negatively than other P sources, as indicated by higher mean S-PTH concentrations among participants consuming AP-containing foods. The intakes of AP and total P have been shown to have risen because of the increasing consumption of fast, snack, and convenience foods. High dietary P intake may no longer be a problem only in patients with impaired renal function, but it may also affect healthy individuals whose diet contains excessive P derived from AP.

IS THE DIETARY CA:P RATIO IMPORTANT?

The recommended optimal Ca:P ratio in the diet is 1.0 on a molar basis (Whybro et al., 1998; Männistö et al., 2003), which corresponds to 1.3 on a mass basis. The imbalance between P intake and Ca intake results in a low Ca:P-ratio in many Western nations. The overall trend in food consumption in Europe (Comité de Nutrición de la Asociación Española de Pediatría, 2003; Urho and Hasunen, 2003) as well as in the United States (Calvo et al., 1996; Harnack et al., 1999) is the drinking of less milk but more phosphoric-acid-containing soft drinks. In fact, it was reported that consumption of cola beverages may predict a higher risk of fracture in girls (Wyshak and Frisch, 1994) and result in development of higher S-PTH concentration and hypocalcemia in postmenopausal women (Fernando et al., 1999). These two dietary habits may lead to the lower dietary Ca:P ratios that have been recently observed in many countries (Brot et al., 1999; Chwojnowska et al., 2002; Takeda et al., 2002; Männistö et al., 2003). Furthermore, recent evidence from Poland revealed that, for 10% of young girls and boys, the dietary Ca:P ratio was lower than 0.25 (Chwojnowska et al., 2002). Criticism (Sax, 2001) has been raised regarding the American dietary reference intakes because the report excluded several studies whose results supported the importance of the role played by the dietary Ca:P ratio in bone health.

The effect of different Ca:P ratios has not gained much attention and has not been studied sufficiently. In a cross-sectional study of 147 premenopausal healthy women (Kemi et al., 2010), none of the participants achieved the suggested Ca:P molar ratio of 1 in their diets. This lack was mainly a result of the excessive P content in their habitual diets, rather than low dietary Ca intake, as even the lowest quartile with a Ca:P ratio <0.50 had a mean Ca intake of 750 mg. In the lowest (first) quartile, mean S-PTH concentration and mean U-Ca excretion were higher than in all other quartiles. The higher 24-h U-Ca excretion in the first quartile was unexpected because the mean dietary Ca intake and Ca:P ratio in the first quartile were the lowest and the mean S–S-PTH concentration in this quartile was the highest. Thus, a low U-Ca would be expected. Elevated U-Ca excretion in subjects with low Ca:P ratio in diet might reflect an increase in bone resorption due to increased serum S-PTH. Because low habitual dietary Ca:P ratios are so common in Western diets, more attention should be focused on both decreasing excessively high dietary P intakes and increasing low Ca intakes to the recommended levels.

OTHER NUTRITIONAL FACTORS

Besides vitamin D, two other fat-soluble vitamins, vitamin K and vitamin A, have been associated with bone health. Protein intake has also been linked with bone.

In elderly people some studies have shown an association between low vitamin K intake and fracture risk (Feskanich et al., 1999; Booth et al., 2000). However, only a few studies have concentrated on the effects of vitamin K on bone in healthy younger adults. In Japan, natto (fermented soybean product rich in vitamin K) intake was not associated with BMD in premenopausal women. Furthermore, no association between natto intake and the change of BMD was found at the 3-year follow-up (Ikeda et al., 2006). A placebo-controlled 2-year clinical trial with a high dose (10 mg/day) of supplemental vitamin K, as phylloquinone, showed no effects of supplementation in femoral neck or lumbar spinal BMD of 115 female endurance athletes (15–50 years). In conclusion, vitamin K may have a protective effect of preventing fractures in elderly people, but studies in young adults have shown no association between vitamin K and BMD.

High vitamin A intake has been suggested to increase fracture risk in women (Melhus et al., 1998; Feskanich et al., 2002; Promislow et al., 2002). The results of observational studies on vitamin A intake and bone on young adults have been conflicting. In a small longitudinal study of 66 premenopausal women (28–39 years), vitamin A and carotene were associated with a decreased total body bone mineral loss (Houtkooper et al., 1995). MacDonald et al. (2004) found that dietary vitamin A was associated with increased bone loss in 891 women (45–55 years, mostly premenopausal in the beginning of the study) during a 7-year follow-up. A 6-week placebo-controlled clinical trial with 25,000-IU retinyl palmitate in 80 healthy 18- to 58-year-old men showed no effect on bone formation markers, BALP and osteocalcin, or on the bone resorption marker, urinary NTX (Kawahara et al., 2002). To date, not enough evidence has been produced to conclude that vitamin A has a negative, positive, or no effect on the maintenance of bone mass in adulthood.

A high protein intake has been postulated to be harmful to bone because of an increased Ca excretion, but little evidence supports this claim. Kerstetter and coworkers (1999) showed that although high dietary protein increases U-Ca excretion, low protein intake leads to an elevation in PTH. In fact, Kerstetter et al. (2005) showed later that high protein intake increased Ca absorption and caused a reduction in the bone-derived fraction of U-Ca. Some studies have shown a negative association between high protein intake and bone health. In a small (38 subjects) cross-sectional study in premenopausal women, high protein intake was negatively associated with radial BMD (Metz et al., 1993). Feskanich et al. (1996) found that dietary protein intake was associated with an increased risk of forearm fracture in 85,900 adult (35–59 years) women. In another cohort study of 19,700 women (Meyer et al., 1997), the increase in relative risk of fracture was found in the highest protein intake quartile, but only in the women with lowest Ca intake. However, many other studies have shown beneficial effect of protein on bone health. In cross-sectional studies by Cooper et al. (1996) and Lacey et al. (1991), dietary protein intake was positively associated with bone mineral content in premenopausal women. Michaëlsson et al. (1995) and Teegarden et al. (1998) found a positive association between protein intake and BMD at some measurement sites in cross-sectional studies of ~200 women. The positive association of protein on BMD has also been shown in men (Whiting et al., 2002). Aoe et al. (2001) found a positive effect of a daily 40-g milk-protein supplement (6 months) on BMD of the calcaneus in a placebo-controlled clinical trial in premenopausal women.

CONCLUSIONS

Vitamin D and Ca have been shown to have beneficial effects on bone health in young adults. P seems to have negative effects, but epidemiological as well as intervention studies are lacking. Although the effect of different Ca:P ratios has not been studied sufficiently, some evidence has shown that a low Ca:P ratio maybe harmful to bone. Because a diet with low Ca:P ratio is common in many countries around the world, this issue should be thoroughly investigated. Although many other nutritional factors affect bone, evidence on the optimal intake that may have beneficial effects in this age group is missing.

REFERENCES

Andersen, R., Mølgaard, C., Skovgaard, L.T., et al. 2008. Effect of vitamin D supplementation on bone and vitamin D status among Pakistani immigrants in Denmark: A randomized double-blinded placebo-controlled intervention study. *Br J Nutr* 100:197–207.

Aoe, S., Toba, Y., Yamamura, J., et al. 2001. Controlled trial of the effects of milk basic protein (MBP) supplementation on bone metabolism in healthy adult women. *Biosci Biotechnol Biochem* 65:913–918.

Barger-Lux, M.J., Davies, K.M., and Heaney, R.P. 2005. Calcium supplementation does not augment bone gain in young women consuming diets moderately low in calcium. *J Nutr* 135:2362–2366.

Barger-Lux, M.J., and Heaney, R.P. 1993. Effects of calcium restriction on metabolic characteristics of premenopausal women. *J Clin Endocr Metab* 76:103–107.

Bischoff-Ferrari, H.A., Dawson-Hughes, B., Staehelin, H.B., et al. 2009a. Fall prevention with supplemental and active forms of vitamin D: A meta-analysis of randomised controlled trials. *BMJ* 339:b3692.

Bischoff-Ferrari, H.A, Willett, W.C., Wong, J.B., et al. 2009b.Prevention of nonvertebral fractures with oral vitamin d and dose dependency a meta-analysis of randomized controlled trials. *Arch Intern Med* 169:551–561.

Blumsohn, A., Herrington, K., Hannon, R.A., et al. 1994. The effect of calcium supplementation on the circadian rhythm of bone resorption. *J Clin Endocrinol Metab* 79:730–735.

Booth, S.L. Tucker, K.L. Chen, H. et al., 2000. Dietary vitamin K intakes are associated with hip fracture but not with bone mineral density in elderly men and women. *Am J Clin Nutr* 71(5):1201–1208.

Brot, C., Jorgensen, N., Madsen, O.R., et al. (1999). Relationships between bone mineral density, serum vitamin D metabolites and calcium:phosphorus intake in healthy perimenopausal women. *J Intern Med* 245: 509–516.

Calvo, M.S. and Park, Y.K. 1996. Changing phosphorus content of the U.S. diet: Potential for adverse effects on bone. *J Nutr* 126(4):1168S–1180S.

Calvo, M.S., Kumar, R., and Heath, H., 3rd. 1988. Elevated secretion and action of serum parathyroid hormone in young adults consuming high phosphorus, low calcium diets assembled from common foods. *J Clin Endocrinol Metab* 66:823–829.

Calvo, M.-S., Kumar, R. and Heath, H., 3rd. 1990. Persistently elevated parathyroid hormone secretion and action in young women after four weeks of ingesting high phosphorus, low calcium diets. *J Clin Endocrinol Metab* 70:1334–1340.

Chwojnowska, Z., Charzewska, J., Chabros, E., et al. 2002. Contents of calcium and phosphorus in the diet of youth from Warsaw elementary schools. *Rocz Panstw Zakl Hig* 53: 157–165.

Comité de Nutrición de la Asociación Española de Pediatría. 2003. Consumption of fruit juices and beverages by Spanish children and teenagers: Health implications of their poor use and abuse. *An Pediatr (Barc)* 58:584–593.

Cooper, C., Atkinson, E.J., Hensrud, D.D., et al. 1996. Dietary protein intake and bone mass in women. *Calcif Tissue Int* 58:320–325.

DiPART (Vitamin D Individual Patient Analysis of Randomized Trials) Group. 2010. Patient level pooled analysis of 68 500 patients from seven major vitamin D fracture trials in US and Europe. *BMJ* 340:b5463.

Fernando, G.R., Martha, R.M., and Evangelina, R. 1999. Consumption of soft drinks with phosphoric acid as a risk factor for the development of hypocalcemia in postmenopausal women. *J Clin Epidemiol* 52:1007–1010.

Feskanich, D., Singh, V., Willett, W.C., et al. 2002.Vitamin A intake and hip fractures among postmenopausal women. *JAMA* 287:47–54.

Feskanich, D., Weber, P., and Willett, W.C., et al. 1999. Vitamin K intake and hip fractures in women: A prospective study.

Feskanich, D., Willett, W.C., Stampfer, M.J., et al. 1996. Protein consumption and bone fractures in women. *Am J Epidemiol* 143:472–479.

Gannagé-Yared, M.H., Chemali, R., Sfeir, C., et al..2005. Dietary calcium and vitamin D intake in an adult Middle Eastern population: Food sources and relation to lifestyle and S-PTH. *Int J Vitam Nutr Res* 75:281–289.

Guillemant, J.A., Accarie, C.M., de la Gueronniere, V., et al. 2003. Different acute responses of serum type I collagen telopeptides, CTX, NTX and ICTP, after repeated ingestion of calcium. *Clin Chim Acta* 337:35–41.

Guillemant, J., and Guillemant, S. 1993. Comparison of the suppressive effect of two doses (500 mg vs 1500 mg) of oral calcium on parathyroid hormone secretion and on urinary cyclic AMP. *Calcif Tissue Int* 53:304–306.

Guillemant, J., Le, H., Maria, A., et al. 2000. Acute effects of oral calcium load on parathyroid function and on bone resorption in young men. *Am J Nephrol* 20:48–52.

Hamson, C., Goh, L., Sheldon, P., et al. 2003. Comparative study of bone mineral density, calcium, and vitamin D status in the Gujarati and white populations of Leicester. *Postgrad Med J* 79:279–283.

Harnack, L., Stang, J., and Story, M. 1999. Soft drink consumption among US children and adolescents: Nutritional consequences. *J Am Diet Assoc* 99:436–441.

Houtkooper, L.B., Ritenbaugh, C., Aickin, M., et al. 1995.Nutrients, body composition and exercise are related to change in bone mineral density in premenopausal women. *J Nutr* 125:1229–1237.

Huttunen, M.M., Tillman, I., Viljakainen, H.T., et al. 2007. High dietary phosphate intake reduces bone strength in the growing rat skeleton. *J Bone Miner Res* 22:83–92.

Ikeda, Y., Iki, M., Morita, A., et al. 2006. Intake of fermented soybeans, natto, is associated with reduced bone loss in postmenopausal women: Japanese Population-Based Osteoporosis (JPOS) Study. *J Nutr* 136:1323–1328.

Institute of Medicine, National Research Council, Standing Committee on the Scientific Evaluation of Dietary Reference Intakes, Food and Nutrition Board. 1997. *Dietary Reference Intakes: Calcium, Phosphorus, Magnesium, Vitamin D, and Fluoride.* Washington, DC, National Academy Press.

Islam, M.Z., Shamim, A.-A., Kemi, V., et al. 2008. Vitamin D deficiency and low bone status: Grave concern in normal adult female garment factory workers in Bangladesh. *Br J Nutr* 99:1322–1329.

Islam, M.Z., Shamim, A.-A., Viljakainen, H.T., et al. 2010. Effect of supplementation of vitamin D, calcium and multiple micronutrients on vitamin D and bone status in Bangladeshi premenopausal female garment factory workers with hypovitaminosis D: A double-blinded, randomized, placebo-controlled 1-year intervention, *Br J Nutr* 2010 Mar 1:1–7. [Epub ahead of print]

Kärkkäinen, M.U.M., and Lamberg-Allardt, C. 1996. An acute intake of phosphate increases parathyroid hormone secretion and inhibits bone formation in young women. *J Bone Miner Res* 11:1905–1912.

Kärkkäinen, M.U.M., Lamberg-Allardt, C.J., Ahonen, S., et al. 2001. Does it make a difference how and when you take your calcium? The acute effects of calcium on calcium and bone metabolism. *Am J Clin Nutr* 74:335–342.

Kärkkäinen, M.U.M., Outila, T., and Lamberg-Allardt, C. 1998. Habitual dietary calcium intake affects serum parathyroid hormone concentration in postmenopausal women with a normal vitamin D status. *Scand J Nutr* 3:104–107.

Kärkkäinen, M.U.M., Wiersma, J.W., and Lamberg-Allardt, C.J. 1997. Postprandial parathyroid hormone response to four calcium-rich foodstuffs. *Am J Clin Nutr* 65:1726–1730.

Karp, H., Vaihia, K.P., Kärkkäinen, M.U.M., et al. 2007. Acute effects of different phosphorus sources on calcium and bone metabolism in young women: A whole-foods approach. *Calcif Tissue Int* 80:251–258.

Kawahara, T.N., Krueger, D.C., Engelke, J.A., et al. 2002. Short-term vitamin A supplementation does not affect bone turnover in men. *J Nutr* 132:1169–1172.

Kemi, V., Kärkkäinen, M.U.M., and Lamberg-Allardt, C. 2006. Low dietary calcium-to-phosphorus ratios negatively affects calcium and bone metabolism in a dose-dependent manner in healthy young females. *Br J Nutr* 96:545–552.

Kemi, V., Rita, H., Kärkkäinen, M.U.M., et al. 2009. Habitual high phosphorus intakes and foods with phosphate additives negatively affect serum parathyroid hormone concentration: A cross-sectional study on healthy pre-menopausal women. *Public Health Nutr* 12:1885–1892.

Kemi, V.E., Kärkkäinen, M.U.M., Karp, H.J., et al. 2008. Increased calcium intake does not completely counteract the adverse effects of high phosphorus intake on bone: A dose–response study in healthy females. *Br J Nutr* 99:832–839.

Kemi, V.E., Kärkkäinen, M.U.M., Rita, H.J., et al. 2010. Low calcium-to-phosphorus ratio in habitual diets affects serum parathyroid hormone concentration and calcium metabolism in healthy women with adequate calcium intake. *Br J Nutr* 103:561–568.

Kerstetter, J., Caseria, D., Mitnick, N., et al.1999. Bone turnover in response to dietary protein intake. *J Clin Endocrinol Metab* 84:1052–1055.

Kerstetter, J.E., O'Brien, K.O., Caseria, D.M., et al. 2005. The impact of dietary protein on calcium absorption and kinetic measures of bone turnover in women. *J Clin Endocrinol Metab* 90:26–31.

Koshihara, M., Katsumata, S., Uehara, M., et al. 2005. Effects of dietary phosphorus intake on bone mineralization and calcium absorption in adult female rats. *Biosci Biotechnol Biochem* 69:1025–1028.

Lacey, J.M., Anderson, J.J., Fujita, T., et al. 1991. Correlates of cortical bone mass among premenopausal and postmenopausal Japanese women. *J Bone Miner Res* 6:651–659.

Lamberg-Allardt, C., Outila, T., Kärkkäinen, M.U.M., et al. 2001. Vitamin D deficiency and bone health in Northern Europe—could this be a concern in other parts of Europe? *J Bone Mineral Res* 16:2066–2073.

Lips, P. 2001. Vitamin D deficiency and secondary hyperparathyroidism in the elderly: Consequences for bone loss and fractures and therapeutic implications. *Endocr Rev* 22:477–501.

Lips, P., Bouillon, R., van Schoor, N.M., et al.2009. Reducing fracture risk with calcium and vitamin D. *Clin Endocrinol (Oxf)* Sep 10. [Epub ahead of print]

MacDonald, H.M., New, S.A., Golden, M.H., et al. 2004. Nutritional associations with bone loss during the menopausal transition: Evidence of a beneficial effect of calcium, alcohol, and fruit and vegetable nutrients and of a detrimental effect of fatty acids. *Am J Clin Nutr* 79:155–165.

Matkovic, V., Goel, P.K., Badenhop-Stevens, N.E., et al. 2005. Calcium supplementation and bone mineral density in females from childhood to young adulthood: A randomized controlled trial. *Am J Clin Nutr* 81:175–188.

Melhus, H., Michaëlsson, K., Kindmark, A., et al. 1998. Excessive dietary intake of vitamin A is associated with reduced bone mineral density and increased risk for hip fracture. *Ann Intern Med* 129:770–778.

Metz, J.A., Anderson, J.J., and Gallagher, P.N., Jr. 1993. Intakes of calcium, phosphorus, and protein, and physical-activity level are related to radial bone mass in young adult women. *Am J Clin Nutr* 58:537–542.

Meyer, H.E., Falch, J.A., Søgaard, A.J., et al. 2004. Vitamin D deficiency and secondary hyperparathyroidism and the association with bone mineral density in persons with Pakistani and Norwegian background living in Oslo, Norway, The Oslo Health Study. *Bone* 35:412–417.

Meyer, H.E., Pedersen, J.I., Loken, E.B., et al. 1997. Dietary factors and the incidence of hip fracture in middle-aged Norwegians. A prospective study. *Am J Epidemiol* 145:117–123.

Michaëlsson, K., Holmberg, L., Mallmin, H., et al. 1995. Diet, bone mass, and osteocalcin: A cross-sectional study. *Calcif Tissue Int* 57:86–93.

Promislow, J.H., Goodman-Gruen, D., Slymen, D.J., et al. 2002. Retinol intake and bone mineral density in the elderly: The Rancho Bernardo Study. *J Bone Miner Res* 17:1349–1358.

Ruohola, J.P., Laaksi, I., Ylikomi, T., et al. 2006. Association between serum 25(OH)D concentrations and bone stress fractures in Finnish young men. *J Bone Miner Res* 21:1483–1488.

Sax, L. 2001. The Institute of Medicine's 'dietary reference intake' for phosphorus: A critical perspective. *J Am Coll Nutr* 20:271–278.

Silverberg, S.J., Shane, E., Clemens, T.L., et al. 1986. The effect of oral phosphate administration on major indices of skeletal metabolism in normal subjects. *J Bone Miner Res* 1:383–388.

Takeda, E., Sakamoto, K., Yokota, K., et al. 2002. Phosphorus supply per capita from food in Japan between 1960 and 1995. *J Nutr Sci Vitaminol* 48:102–108.

Teegarden, D., Lyle, R.M., McCabe, G.P., et al. 1998. Dietary calcium, protein, and phosphorus are related to bone mineral density and content in young women. *Am J Clin Nutr* 68:749–754.

Urho, U.-M., and Hasunen, K. 2003. School catering in the upper level of the comprehensive school in 2003. Reports of the Ministry of Social Affairs and Health Helsinki, Finland 2004 (ISSN 1236–2115: 2003:17). English summary.

Viljakainen, H.T., Väisänen, M., Kemi, V., et al. 2009. Wintertime vitamin D supplementation inhibits seasonal variation of calcitropic hormones and maintains bone turnover in healthy men. *J Bone Miner Res* 24:346–352.

Welten, D.C., Kemper, H.C., Post, G.B., et al. 1995. A meta-analysis of the effect of calcium intake on bone mass in young and middle aged females and males. *J Nutr* 125:2802–2813.

Whiting, S.J., Boyle, J.L., Thompson, A., et al. 2002. Dietary protein, phosphorus and potassium are beneficial to bone mineral density in adult men consuming adequate dietary calcium. *J Am Coll Nutr* 21:402–409.

Whybro, A., Jagger, H., Barker, M., et al. 1998. Phosphate supplementation in young men: Lack of effect on calcium homeostasis and bone turnover. *Eur J Clin Nutr* 52:29–33.

Wyshak, G. and Frisch, R.E. 1994. Carbonated beverages, dietary calcium, the dietary calcium/phosphorus ratio, and bone fractures in girls and boys. *J Adolesc Health* 15(3): 210–215.

27 Nutrition and Bone Health in Older Adults

Connie W. Bales, Kenlyn R. Young, and John J.B. Anderson

CONTENTS

INTRODUCTION

Whereas the development and maintenance of adequate bone mineralization and strength are critically important throughout the life cycle, the later years of adulthood are when problems with bone health can be most devastating. Osteoporosis and associated fractures constitute a major health concern in terms of both prevalence and impact on health, function, and quality of life (QOL) in older adults. The impact of this disabling disease increases dramatically with age, and women aged 80 years or more are at great risk for fracture (Gehlbach et al., 2007). Moreover, the increasing rates of fracture exceed those explained by demographic changes alone (Boonen et al., 2008),

415

emphasizing the importance of beneficial nutrients as modifiable determinants of bone health in later life.

In this chapter, we focus on the nutritional factors most relevant for the prevention and management of bone health problems in middle-aged and older adults. In addition, intervention trials using calcium (Ca) and vitamin D supplements are reviewed, and specialty topics in geriatrics, including frailty, sarcopenia, sarcopenic obesity, and medical comorbidities, are discussed.

BONE HEALTH OF OLDER ADULTS: BACKGROUND AND IMPACT

As has been well described in earlier chapters, peak bone mineral density (BMD) is achieved during early adulthood, generally between the ages of 20 and 29 years. Following a period of relative stability, a slow but steady loss of BMD begins around the age of 50 years. Men lose bone at a relatively constant rate of about 1% per year. The rate of bone loss in women accelerates during the postmenopausal period (being around 2%–3% for about 5 years) and then resumes a rate comparable with that of men (Sanders et al., 2009). Individuals with risk factors for bone loss (risk factors include being a postmenopausal female, of small build, and/or having a history of smoking, heavy alcohol use, or taking corticosteroids) should have an assessment of their BMD level. This measurement is ideally conducted using dual-energy x-ray absorptiometry (DXA). The term *osteopenia* refers to a BMD that is lower than normal for a given age. With aging and continued gradual loss, high-risk individuals will reach a level of BMD that is characterized as "osteoporosis." Osteoporosis is the most common metabolic bone disease in humans, characterized by low bone mass, deterioration of bone tissue, and disruption of bone architecture that becomes progressively worse with age.

The World Health Organization defines osteoporosis as a BMD *T* score at either spine or hip that is at least 2.5 standard deviations below the normal mean BMD for the young reference population (20- to 29-year-old healthy adults). Because it leads to compromised bone strength, osteoporosis signals a greatly increased likelihood of sustaining a nontraumatic fracture. Sometimes, the BMD is said to have "fallen below the fracture threshold." However, in elderly persons, the risk of fracture at any given *T* score is higher than that of a younger individual because of other risk factors such as a tendency to fall, poor vision, cognitive impairment, and other poorly understood factors. Thus, older adults with nontraumatic fractures should be treated regardless of BMD level, and those with DXA-defined osteoporosis should be treated whether or not of if they have sustained a fracture (Boonen et al., 2008).

OSTEOPOROSIS: PREVALENCE AND HEALTH IMPACT

Osteoporosis affects 44 million Americans, accounting for more than 1.5 million fractures/year. Exponential increases in rates of osteoporosis and related fractures are projected for the coming decades. Whereas the greater prevalence of osteoporosis is related in part to increased testing of bone mass and to programs that enhance awareness of the disease, other factors such as greater life expectancies, the aging of the "baby boom" cohort, and, we can suspect, detrimental lifestyle factors such as physical inactivity and poor dietary choices also drive this trend. In fact, osteoporosis-related fracture rates are anticipated to rise to over 3 million per year by 2025 (American Academy of Orthopaedic Surgeons [AAOS], 2008; National Osteoporosis Foundation [NOF], 2008).

Osteoporosis brings serious health consequences to those aged 65 years and older; it affects individuals of all ethnicities and is particularly prevalent in older women. Women are more likely to develop the disease because of a smaller skeletal stature. Furthermore, they have a lower peak bone mass and density than men, and a dramatic loss of BMD that occurs during the postmenopause years. Current statistics suggest that 1 in 2 women over the age of 50 years will experience a fracture of some type in their lifetime. However, men are also at risk for osteoporosis, and about

1 in 4 will experience a fracture in their lifetime (AAOS, 2008; NOF, 2008). Moreover, men who do experience fractures have a greater mortality rate than that observed for women (Surgeon General Report [SGR], 2004).

An increased likelihood of falling occurs with advancing age, and those who sustain a fall-related fracture remain at risk for additional falls and related fractures. These patients require more intensive medical resources, and the older the patient, the more likely it is that he or she will be transferred to short-, intermediate-, or long-term nursing care. Osteoporotic hip fractures are the most serious type of fracture in the later years of life, as well as commonly affecting almost 300,000 elderly Americans in 2005 (Burge et al., 2007). Hip fractures have the highest mortality rates of any fracture type (20%–25% in the first year), and of those who survive, 33% continue to be totally dependent and/or require long-term care (International Osteoporosis Foundation, 2009). Fractures of the hip typically lead to nursing home admission, but fractures of the pelvis, ribs, upper and lower limbs, ankles, and feet are also common causes for admission in those aged 75 years and greater (AAOS, 2008). Individuals who experience fractures are also at risk of other medical complications, including pneumonia, urinary tract infections, and pressure sores (SGR, 2004).

The current economic cost associated with treating osteoporosis and related fractures is staggering. The estimated cost for incident fracture care (outpatient, inpatient, and long-term care) was nearly $17 billion in 2005. Moreover, osteoporosis is likely to bring an overwhelming medical and financial burden for older adults in the future. Costs for care of osteoporosis and nontraumatic fractures over the next two decades are projected to be $474 billion (NOF, 2008).

OSTEOPOROSIS: IMPACT ON QUALITY OF LIFE

In addition to the obvious economic costs, osteoporosis-related fractures have profound effects on the QOL of older adults, often leading to a downward spiral in physical and mental health that may ultimately result in death. Vertebral fractures contribute to loss of height, reduced mobility, impaired pulmonary function, and physical deformity. Other adverse effects of vertebral fractures include chronic pain, distorted body image, and loss of self-esteem (Lips and van Schoor, 2005). The most serious hip fractures often necessitate lengthy hospital stays and are frequently followed by painful disability, dependence upon others, and decreased physical function (Hallberg et al., 2004). Profound negative effects on general QOL factors (depression, cognitive decline, social interactions) often follow, including deterioration of health-related quality of life (HRQOL) indicators such as pain, physical function, and morbidities (SGR, 2004).

In a study of HRQOL impact 2 years after a hip fracture, Hallberg and colleagues (2004) showed that individuals with osteoporotic fractures had lower HRQOL scores and demonstrated declines in physical function as well as in social and mental function. Because of the loss of physical function and of the challenges associated with physical and emotional pain, older individuals with osteoporosis may lose the ability to conduct their activities of daily living, that is, dress, bathe, move freely in their environment, and even stand. They may also be immobilized by the fear of falling and sustaining additional fractures, and thus they may become increasingly socially isolated and experience feelings of loneliness and helplessness (Prince et al., 2008).

NUTRITIONAL DETERMINANTS OF BONE HEALTH IN LATE LIFE

Whereas overall good nutrition is important for skeletal integrity, a small group of key nutrients, namely, Ca, vitamin D, vitamin K, phosphorus, vitamin A, sodium, and protein, are recognized to be important modifiable determinants of bone health of the elderly (Earl et al., 2010). In this section, the most important nutrients needed for bone maintenance, in our estimation, are emphasized. Fundamental nutritional information, discussion of new diet-related findings, and recommendations for promoting bone health in the later years are presented.

VITAMIN D AND CA

As illustrated in Figure 27.1, the critical role of these two micronutrients in bone health has been well recognized for decades, and many of the mechanisms of action are well delineated. Vitamin D plays an essential role in bone health via beneficial effects on skeletal mineralization, serum Ca and phosphorus concentrations, and also by regulation of parathyroid growth and parathyroid hormone (PTH) production (Boonen et al., 2008). Vitamin D also likely plays a role in preventing falls (Bischoff-Ferrari et al., 2009), which is an important determinant of fracture risk, as discussed further in a later section. Ca is also an obligatory nutrient for bone health. When dietary Ca is deficient, a reduction in bone mass occurs because of the increase in bone resorption that follows the elevation of serum PTH, which acts to preserve the level of ionized Ca in the extracellular fluid.

A lifelong adequacy of both vitamin D and Ca status serves to support skeletal health. Even in the later years of life, adequate dietary intakes of Ca and vitamin D attenuate secondary hyperparathyroidism, help maintain bone mass and strength, improve skeletal muscle strength, and reduce fracture risk (Holick and Chen 2008; Wortsman et al., 2000). Thus, age-related changes in nutrient requirements need to be recognized and addressed by implementing ongoing monitoring of nutrient intakes of elderly individuals.

Changes in Status and Requirements with Age

A number of important age-related changes contribute to increased requirements for vitamin D and Ca. For vitamin D, these changes include reduced rates of skin photosynthesis, impaired renal conversion of 25-hydroxyvitamin D (calcidiol) to the active form, and lowered gut responsiveness to $1,25(OH)_2D$ (calcitriol) (Suter et al., 1991). Older adults also have decreased skin exposure to the sun due to limited time outside and/or concerns about skin cancer. Medications such as glucocorticoids may also adversely affect vitamin D status. In obesity, fat tissue sequesters vitamin D in the large cellular fat pools, and therefore this harboring may contribute to vitamin D insufficiency or even deficiency (Greenspan et al., 2005; Souberbielle et al., 2001). Absorption of dietary Ca from the gut typically decreases with aging due to atrophic gastritis, which occurs in about one of three adults over the age of 50 years (Kiebzak et al., 2007). Reduced Ca absorption, along with other factors, accounts mainly for the age-associated increase in the requirement for Ca in those beyond 50 years.

Based on serum levels of calcidiol (25-hydroxyvitamin D), mild vitamin D deficiency is fairly common in otherwise healthy older adults (Malik, 2007), as well as in hospitalized older adults (Ervin and Kennedy-Stephenson, 2002) and nursing home residents (Bischoff-Ferrari et al., 2006). Ca intakes are marginal in almost all population groups; in the National Health and Nutrition Examination Survey (NHANES) III study (1988–1994), mean Ca intake levels for adults over

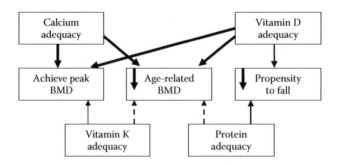

FIGURE 27.1 Nutritional factors with potential bone health benefits in older adults: The width of the line for each arrow indicates the strength of the association. Hashed lines represent relationships that are potentially possible, but yet established.

TABLE 27.1
New Recommended Dietary Allowances (RDAs) for Calcium and Vitamin D Intakes by Older Adults

Life Stage Group	RDAs for Calcium, mg/day	RDAs for Vitamin D, IU/day
31–50 years	1000	600
51–70 years males	1000	600
51–70 years females	1200	600
71 years plus	1200	800

Source: Institute of Medicine. 2011. *Dietary Reference Intakes for Calcium and Vitamin D.* Washington, DC: National Academies.

60 years were below the adequate intake for 87% of women and up to 75% of men (Moore et al., 2004). The high relative risk of deficiency of both Ca and vitamin D is a particular concern for the older population. Moreover, with the recent recognition that vitamin D of 10 μg (or 400 IU/day) for 51–70 years and 15 μg (or 600 IU/day) for ≥71 years may not be sufficient, even more concern exists about a low vitamin D status, particularly in the latter age group (Lichtenstein et al., 2008). Newly released Institute of Medicine (2011) dietary reference intakes for Ca and vitamin D include slight increases in recommended vitamin D intakes for older adults, but little change was recommended for Ca intakes (Table 27.1).

Dietary and Supplemental Sources

Because only a few common foods, such as oily fish, egg yolk, and a couple of fortified foods, contain good sources of vitamin D, achieving vitamin D adequacy from dietary sources alone is a challenge that is even more difficult with advancing age. As reported in 2005, no more than an estimated 2% of adults aged 70 years or more met the recommended level for vitamin D from food sources (Grant et al., 2005). Ca is generally more widely distributed in the diet than is vitamin D. The best sources of Ca, taking into account both composition and bioavailability, tend to be dairy foods. However, the dairy group is often avoided by older adults because of personal preferences, lactose intolerance, or concerns about consuming saturated fat.

Because dietary intakes of both Ca and vitamin D are commonly substandard in older adults, the authors of the Modified Food Guide Pyramid for Older Adults recommended that supplements of both nutrients be considered for adults over the age of 70 years (Lichtenstein et al., 2008). Whenever possible, supplement doses should be based on an assessment of the dietary intake. The amount of supplemental Ca prescribed should be just enough to bring the total nutrient intake into the recommended range. Such guidance is particularly true for Ca so that the number of pills taken daily may be minimized; this will enhance compliance and reduce the likelihood of side effects, such as constipation and arterial calcification (Bolland et al., 2008). With regard to antiosteoporosis agents such as bisphosphonates, assurances of adequacy of both vitamin D and Ca become important for the benefits of these medications to be realized. Also, separating the ingestion of oral bisphosphonates and Ca by several hours is recommended because of concerns that Ca may bind with the bisphosphonates in the gut lumen and reduce the absorption of both the drug and Ca (Booth, 2009).

OTHER DIETARY FACTORS THAT AFFECT BONE HEALTH

In addition to the recognized importance of vitamin D and Ca, recent studies have begun to clarify the importance of a number of other nutrients and food components for bone health. Several nutrients found in vegetables and fruits are known to be beneficial, including vitamin K, magnesium, potassium, carotenoids, and vitamin C. Some dietary constituents are almost certainly detrimental, like foods/beverages high in phosphorus and/or sodium. A few constituents like protein, vitamin A, and alcoholic beverages seem to have variable influences depending on the intake level (Tucker, 2009). These and many other diet-related factors are covered in Chapter 1 of this text. Here, we briefly summarize the available information on some of the factors most relevant for older adults.

Vitamin K

Phylloquinone, or vitamin K_1, is the predominant form found in green leafy vegetables and vegetable oils, some of the most important dietary sources of this nutrient. Although older adults tend to eat more vegetables than do younger individuals, intakes of dark green and cruciferous vegetables are typically very low in all adults, with a total consumption of only six servings per month (Johnston et al., 2000). Vitamin K status in older adults is of particular concern because of the recently recognized role of the vitamin in bone health. Vitamin K supports posttranslational modification of osteocalcin and possibly other matrix proteins synthesized by osteoblasts by promoting the insertion of a carboxyl group at the gamma position of the amino acid glutamic acid (Gla). Studies of vitamin K supplementation suggest that it promotes more complete carboxylation of osteocalcin and other matrix Gla proteins, and it may be associated with a reduced risk of osteoporotic fractures. The majority of observational studies, summarized by Booth et al. (2008), associated vitamin K_1 intake with lower risk of hip fractures. However, conflicting evidence has resulted from the randomized controlled trials (RCTs) of vitamin K supplementation regarding effects on BMD and risk of fractures. A 2-year RCT of vitamin K_1 plus vitamin D and Ca showed a beneficial effect on BMD of the distal radius that was independent of the effects of vitamin D/Ca (Booth, 2009). A number of RCTs in Japan have tested a different form of vitamin K, menaquinone-4 (also known as MK-4) at pharmacologic levels (Binkley et al., 2009; Promislow et al., 2002), showing some skeletal benefits. However, a 3-year controlled trial showed no effect of phylloquione on BMD apart from vitamin D and Ca (Cockayne et al., 2006).

Based on these and other trials that also have shown no effect of vitamin K supplements (Binkley et al., 2009; Tucker, 2009), the efficacy of vitamin K supplementation in preventing age-associated bone loss and fractures remains debatable. Additional well-designed trials using dose-finding experiments of different vitamin K molecules are needed before a recommendation concerning the use of vitamin K in fracture prevention can be made (Devine et al., 2005). In addition, the efficacy and safety of dietary and supplemental vitamin K need to be considered, as well as interactions with anticoagulant medications—a commonly used therapy in older adults (Rohde et al., 2007).

Protein

Until recently, dietary protein was thought to negatively impact BMD (Darling et al., 2009). This was based on the acid–base hypothesis, which proposes that during the metabolism of amino acids from animal proteins, the increased production of acids (e.g. phosphoric, sulfuric) results in bone resorption to maintain acid–base balance (Ginty, 2003). The net effect of this acidic shift is an increased loss of Ca ions in urine; indeed, excess protein intake has been shown to contribute to negative Ca balance (Kerstetter and Allen, 1990). Recent evidence, however, has challenged the assumption that protein is a negative factor for bone, especially in those of advanced age. For example, a low protein intake has been shown to be a predictor of lower limb BMD in elderly women (Devine et al., 2005). In addition, low protein intake has also been linked with greater bone loss at the femur and spine in men and women in the Framingham Osteoporosis Study (Hannan et al., 2000). Also, for those who have already sustained a fracture, protein supplementation may provide benefits (Schurch et al., 1998; Tkatch et al., 1992). Further studies are needed to establish the optimal protein intake that best preserves BMD and prevents fractures by supporting muscle mass and strength. Protein is particularly needed in adequate amounts by frail older adults, who need high-quality protein to maintain lean body mass and prevent sarcopenia (Paddon and Rasmussen, 2009; Symons et al., 2009).

Vitamin A

Recent concerns about the potential negative effects of high doses of vitamin A on BMD have been prompted by reports that high intakes of vitamin A were associated with an increased risk of hip fracture (Feskanich et al., 2002; Melhus et al., 1998). However, other trials have not confirmed this observation. In the Women's Health Initiative, vitamin A and retinol intake were not related to the risk of hip or total fractures in the postmenopausal women being studied. However, a modest increase in total fracture risk with high vitamin A and retinol intakes was observed when vitamin D intake was low (Caire-Juvera et al., 2009). Further studies are needed to confirm or refute concerns about detrimental bone effects of excessive vitamin A (Ribaya-Mercado and Blumberg, 2007); in the meantime, moderation on the intake of such supplements in high-risk elderly is advised.

Phosphorus

Frequently, Western diets are not only low in Ca but also high in the amount of phosphate (P) being consumed, due to the ingestion of naturally occurring P in foods, especially animal proteins, and in processed foods to which P salts have been added. Thus, concerns exist about the unfavorable ratio of P:Ca in the Western diet (Anderson et al., 2006; Kemi et al., 2008). Although cola-type beverages contribute to high intakes of P more commonly in children and young adults than in the elderly, the high intake of processed and convenience foods in the older population could lead to high intakes of both P and sodium.

Sodium

Excessive sodium increases renal losses of Ca because the kidneys favor sodium reabsorption at the expense of Ca ions; thus, a high sodium intake may contribute to negative Ca balance (Teucher et al., 2008).

Alcoholic Beverages

Alcohol is not a nutrient, but the consumption of alcohol remains an important factor that increases the risk of bone loss and osteoporotic fractures when in excessive amounts. As is true for protein, recent thinking about the impact of alcohol on bone health has been revised based on the recent studies. Although alcoholism is associated with negative skeletal effects, it appears that moderate intakes of alcoholic beverages may be beneficial to bone in both men and postmenopausal women (Tucker et al., 2009). However, these authors also found that men with high liquor intakes (>2 drinks/day) had significantly lower BMD. Similar findings have been reported in a number of other studies. In the third NHANES, BMD at the total hip and femoral neck was higher in men who had ≥5 drinking occasions/month, relative to fewer occasions or none (Wosje and Kalkwarf, 2007). In the Cardiovascular Health Study, there was a positive relation between BMD at the hip and alcohol intake, but a U-shaped association between alcohol intake and the risk of hip fracture in those over the age of 65 years (Mukamal et al., 2007). Further studies are needed to explore the bone/alcohol relationship, potential age and gender differences in responses, and variations in the effects of different types of alcoholic beverages. For example, wine, a good source of flavonoids, and beer, a good source of silicon, may be more beneficial than liquor (Tucker et al., 2009).

NUTRITIONAL INTERVENTIONS TO PRESERVE BMD AND PREVENT FRACTURES

Trials of Vitamin D and/or Ca Supplementation

Although vitamin D and Ca are clearly important for bone health and adequate status for these nutrients is positively associated with BMD, there continues to be a debate concerning their role in improving skeletal outcomes, that is, the lowering of actual fracture rates, because of contradictory findings in the literature (Tang et al., 2007). As presented in Table 27.2, a number of very recent, well-conducted meta-analyses have summarized scores of studies of interventions with

TABLE 27.2
Summary of Recent Meta-Analyses and Reviews of Trials of Bone-Related Outcomes with Interventional Calcium and Vitamin D Supplementation

Study	Populations/Trials/ Outcomes	Supplement(s) and Dose	Findings and Conclusions
Boonen et al., 2007	Population: both genders, mean age = 62–85 years Trials: 9 RCTs; 53,260 ppts Primary outcome: hip fx	Range of doses: Vitamin D 400 to 800 IU Ca 500 to 1200 mg Duration of doses: Vitamin D 24 to 62 months Vitamin D + Ca 24 to 84 months.	Vitamin D reduces risk of hip fractures only when given with Ca. Ca alone does not prevent fx. Recommend vitamin D 700–800 IU/day + Ca 1000–1200 mg/day
Tang et al., 2007	Population: both genders, mean age = 52–85 years Trials: 29 RCTs, 63,897 ppts Primary outcome: fx of hip, vertebra, and wrist—17 trials, 52,625 ppts Secondary outcomes: BMD—23 trials, 41,419 ppts	Range of doses: Vitamin D 200 to 800 IU Ca 200 to 1200 mg Duration of doses: Average treatment duration 3.5 years	Ca supplementation alone or in combination with vitamin D best for preventative treatment of osteoporosis; recommend 1200 mg Ca + 800 IU of vitamin D
Avenell et al., 2009 (Cochrane Review)	Population: men >65 years, postmenopausal women Trials: 45 RCTs, 84,585 ppts Primary outcome: hip fx—17 trials, 71,407 ppts Secondary outcomes: vertebral fx, new fx	Range of doses: Vitamin D: 400 to 1100 IU Ca: 1000 mg	Supplementation with vitamin D + Ca reduces hip fx. Supplementation with Vitamin D alone is unlikely to be effective in preventing fx.
Nordin, 2009	Population: postmenopausal women, age = 50–83 years Trials: 32 RCTs; 3169 ppts Primary outcome: BMD change	Range of doses: Ca only 700–2000 mg Duration of dose: 1–5 years, mean 2 years	Ca supplementation of about 1000 mg daily has significant preventative effect on bone loss.
The DIPART (vitamin D Individual Patient Analysis of Randomized Trials) Group, 2010	Population: men and women, age = 47–107 years Trials: 7 RCTs, 68,517 ppts Primary outcome: all fxs	Range of doses: Vitamin D 10–20 μg and/ or 100,000–300,000 IU Ca—1000 mg Duration of dose: 8–62 months	Vitamin D in combination with Ca showed a reduced risk of fracture. Vitamin D alone is not effective.

Notes: RCTs = randomized controlled trials; ppts = participants; fx = fractures; Ca = calcium; BMD = bone mineral density.

vitamin D and/or Ca with regard to fracture rate as a primary outcome. The reviews listed in Table 27.2 concern studies of vitamin D plus Ca, Ca alone, and vitamin D alone. Fracture rates serve as the primary outcomes for most of these studies, but the site(s) of fracture varies.

A recent meta-analysis (Boonen et al., 2007) examined studies of the effects of supplementation with vitamin D in conjunction with Ca and Ca alone on hip fractures. The overall conclusions were (1) that vitamin D along with Ca reduces the risk of hip fractures but that (2) Ca alone provides little or no benefit. Another report (Tang et al., 2007) included all available trials in a systematic review and meta-analysis and examined vitamin D in combination with Ca, as well as Ca alone, with respect to the outcome of all fracture types. This analysis also indicated a strong role of vitamin D plus Ca supplements in reducing fracture risks. In contrast to the findings of Boonen et al. (2007) noted above, however, Tang et al., (2007) showed a benefit of Ca alone for preventing fractures. A comprehensive analysis of 45 RCTs focusing on all fracture types confirmed that vitamin D and Ca reduce fracture rates (Avenell et al., 2009) but found that vitamin D alone is unlikely to be beneficial, a position supported by Reid and colleagues (2010). The Vitamin D Individual Patient Analysis of Randomized Trials (DIPART) considered studies assessing vitamin D plus Ca and vitamin D supplementation alone. In full agreement with the analysis of Avenell and coauthors (2009), the DIPART reviewers concluded that vitamin D in conjunction with Ca provided beneficial effects regarding fracture risks but that vitamin D alone did not provide these same benefits.

A recent meta-analysis differed from the others in that it considered only trials of Ca supplementation and used changes in BMD as the primary outcome (Nordin, 2009). The findings of this review indicated a strong benefit for Ca in preventing BMD loss.

SUMMARY OF EVIDENCE AND IMPLICATIONS FOR CLINICAL PRACTICE

Table 27.3 summarizes some of the most important dietary guidelines for maximizing BMD and reducing fracture risk in older adults. As illustrated in the previous section, strong evidence has accumulated in support of the beneficial effects of a combined supplement of vitamin D and Ca for fracture prevention. For a variety of reasons, including differences in baseline status, supplement dose and duration, study population, and target skeletal site, controversy remains regarding the benefits of either nutrient alone. From a practical standpoint, Ca and vitamin D have low potential for toxicity so that older adults at risk for osteoporosis-related fractures may consume modest amounts of supplements of these complementary nutrients to achieve recommended intakes. This usage is in agreement with clinical guidelines published in July 2008 by the National Osteoporosis Committee, and it also takes advantage of the recently demonstrated benefits to muscle and falls reduction relating to higher intakes of vitamin D (Bischoff-Ferrari et al., 2009).

TABLE 27.3
Practical Dietary Recommendations to Promote Bone Health in Later Life

Nutrient or Dietary Factor	Recommendation
Vitamin D	• When possible, there should be exposure to full sun without sunscreen for 15 minutes at least twice weekly. • A supplement of approximately 800 IU (20 mcg) of vitamin D is recommended. Higher amounts may be needed in the case of documented deficiency. • Ideally, the response to supplementation should be assessed by monitoring serum 25-hydroxyvitamin D.
Calcium	• Complement dietary calcium with supplemental calcium to bring total intake to the adequate intake for women and men aged ≥50 years of 1200 mg/day.
Protein	• Consume generous amounts of high-quality protein, 25 to 30 g at each meal.
Vegetables and fruits	• Consume generous amounts of a wide variety, especially dark green leafy vegetables.
Alcohol	• Although bone benefits have been shown with moderate intake, cognitive status and tendency for falling should be carefully evaluated before alcohol intake is endorsed.
Potential detrimental diet/ drug interactions	• Calcium and bisphosphonates (do not take at same time) • Vitamin K and anticoagulant medications
Moderate potentially negative factors	• Avoid excessive supplemental vitamin A. • Limit high-phosphate-containing foods. • Limit sodium. • Keep caffeine intakes to moderate levels.

Whereas many reasons exist to encourage generous intakes of fruits and vegetables for general health benefits, more research on specific plant nutrients is needed before specific amounts of several other bone-active components can be recommended. For example, although theoretical and some experimental support exists for a positive role of vitamin K in bone tissue, the potential for a clinically adverse effect with anticoagulant therapy in elderly adults must be taken into consideration (Rohde et al., 2007). Negative dietary factors, including phosphorus and sodium, should be kept at moderate intake levels, and ample servings of high-quality protein (25–30 g) at each meal should be encouraged.

If alcohol is being consumed in moderate amounts without problems, this would be acceptable. However, in the geriatric population, the benefits of alcoholic beverages need to be weighed against concerns about deleterious effects on balance, that is, potentially increased risks of falls, and cognitive status.

SPECIAL CONSIDERATIONS RELATED TO BONE HEALTH IN OLDER ADULTS

Two important changes in the QOL of the elderly relate to their skeletal frailty and to the loss of lean body mass, primarily skeletal muscle, a condition referred to as sarcopenia. Sarcopenia is often accompanied by excessive body fat, that is, fat mass. So, the three major body mass compartments typically undergo major shifts in late life: losses of bone mass and muscle mass but gains in fat mass.

FRAILTY, INACTIVITY, AND LOW BONE MASS

One of the hallmark changes that occurs in many, although not all, adults in late life is the phenomenon of "frailty," classically defined as the presence of three or more of the following: unintentional weight loss, self-reported exhaustion, weakness, slow gait speed, and low physical activity (Fried et al., 2001). A complex syndrome estimated to occur in 30% of the population aged 60 years and older, frailty develops due to a number of important changes, including (1) the shift in body composition resulting in a loss of lean muscle mass (sarcopenia) and an increase in adipose tissue; (2) nutritional frailty, which is weight loss resulting almost entirely from a reduced intake of energy-yielding nutrients (Bales and Ritchie, 2009); and (3) physical inactivity. The loss of muscle mass and strength that occurs with frailty is an important physiological contributor to falls and age-related increases in fracture risk (Tang et al., 2007). Moreover, reduced lean body mass has been linked to a reduction in BMD (Douchi et al., 2003; Genaro et al., 2010). Thus, the frailty syndrome leads to a high risk of fracture because it contributes to both a reduced BMD and an increased risk of falling due to loss of muscle strength.

Although the etiology of frailty is poorly understood and likely multifactorial, the importance of nutrition in delaying/reducing its ultimate impact is well established. Protein intake is particularly important because requirements for protein are thought to increase slightly with age (Campbell et al., 2001), but older adults have the lowest intake of protein per kilogram of body weight (Fulgoni, 2008). Low energy intake may also increase protein needs (Pellet and Young, 1992). A deficient protein intake is linked with reductions in lean muscle mass (Bopp et al., 2008) and can set up a cycle of frailty and nutritional decline. Poor appetite and fatigue may thus combine to further reduce intakes of calories and other nutrients, contributing to wasting, weakness, cognitive effects, and other manifestations of nutrient deficiencies. Thus, although counteracting the loss of appetite and restoring fully adequate the intake of essential nutrients may not be possible, a concerted effort to do so should be instituted as soon as the trend toward increasing frailty is detected (Bales and Ritchie, 2009).

OBESITY AND SARCOPENIC OBESITY

The effects of the global epidemic of obesity are being seen in all age groups, including older adults (Flegal et al., 2002; Mokdad et al., 2001). The obesity epidemic is occurring in parallel with the aging of the baby boomer age cohort (Jarosz and Bellar, 2009). When the NHANES survey was conducted in 2005–2006, 68.6% of adults aged 60 years and older were found to be overweight or obese (OB), with 30.5% in the OB category (Federal Interagency Forum on Aging-Related Statistics, 2008). Until recently, this condition might have been viewed as a positive for bone health because a heavier body mass has been thought to be associated with a higher BMD (Ribot et al., 1987). However, the negative effects of being OB on bone health, via functional and metabolic effects, are becoming increasingly recognized (Davison et al., 2002; Rolland et al., 2009). OB may contribute to inflammatory changes that promote cartilage degradation and loss of lean muscle mass (Evans, 2010; Schrager et al., 2007). In addition, the chronic diseases associated with OB contribute to increased functional impairment, reducing the ability to continue regular weight-bearing exercises needed to help sustain BMD (Houston et al., 2009).

OB is particularly problematic when coupled with age-related loss of skeletal muscle mass (sarcopenia), a condition referred to as sarcopenic obesity. The prevalence of sarcopenic obesity, also referred to as a syndrome of obese frailty (Roubenoff, 2004), increases with age (Baumgartner, 2000) and leads to a level of disability that may exceed that occurring with sarcopenia alone (Baumgartner et al., 2004; Villareal et al., 2004). Functional limitations occur due to the combination of weakened muscles with a greater amount of body weight to be supported (Jarosz and Bellar, 2009). Sarcopenic obesity, thus, increases the likelihood of falling and sustaining a fracture. Moreover, its presence increases concerns about the risks of weight reduction to alleviate the detrimental effects of OB, that is, to improve glucose tolerance and relieve osteoarthritis, in these individuals. Unless accompanied by physical exercise, weight reduction consistently leads to loss of both BMD and lean body mass, as well as body fat (Ensrud et al., 2003; Knoke and Barrett-Connor, 2003; Langlois et al., 1998). The loss of lean body mass has been shown in adults of all ages, including those aged 60 years and older (Bales and Buhr, 2008, 2009). Thus, caution is advised when considering weight reduction to improve bone health in OB older adults.

AGE-RELATED COMPLEXITIES OF THERAPEUTIC INTERVENTIONS

A number of age-related factors make therapeutic interventions for osteoporosis more problematic. A group of established factors, such as the combination of inactivity, sarcopenia, and low BMD, may complicate physical therapy and/or exercises needed to help relieve pain associated with vertebral fractures from spinal deformity, improve flexibility and balance, and regain/maintain BMD and muscle strength. It is essential that the exercise/treatment program be carefully supervised and appropriate for patients at increased risk for fractures and falling (Shipp, 2006). Another major concern about drug therapy relates to poor tolerance and failure to comply with antiosteoporosis drug regimens. Common agents like the bisphosphonates require individuals to sit upright for at least 30 minutes following administration and may lead to a variety of troublesome side effects, including gastrointestinal problems, headaches, and swelling in the extremities and joints. In an international study of postmenopausal women with osteoporosis, side effects were second only to therapeutic effectiveness as determinants of preferences for osteoporosis medications (Duarte et al., 2007). Problems associated with long-term compliance with these antiresorptive agents are thus common (Gehlbach et al., 2007).

In a recent survey of women enrolled in the Health ABC trial, it was found that 70% of those prescribed an antiresorptive drug either did not ever start the medication or did not remain on the therapy (Ryder et al., 2006). Another aspect of this problem, drug–drug interactions, exists in the nursing home setting. In a 10-year study, it was found that, on average, only 11.5% of residents who had sustained osteoporosis-related fractures received any type of antiosteoporosis medication (Parikh et al., 2008). Finally, with the high use of multiple medications in this age group, an increased likelihood exists for multiple drug interactions that adversely contribute to bone loss, which is recently summarized (Goodman et al., 2007). One important example of a drug with detrimental effects on bone includes corticosteroids, which have strong bone resorptive activities and are more commonly taken with advancing age (van Staa et al., 2002). Another example of an agent with adverse skeletal effects results from long-term therapy with proton pump inhibitors (PPIs). These medications, commonly taken by older adults, may interfere with Ca absorption, and they have been associated with increased risk of hip fracture, especially when Ca intake is low (Yu et al., 2008) or the PPI dose is high (Yang et al., 2006).

SUMMARY

The important contributions to bone health of a number of key nutrients in older adults have been described. The beneficial effects of combined vitamin D and Ca for the preservation of bone mass during the aging process have been confirmed by scientific evidence. Both vitamin D and Ca act to preserve BMD, prevent falls, and optimize fracture risk reduction. Ca supplementation alone may provide as much benefit to the skeleton as the combination, but only when vitamin D status is sufficient. The roles of other nutrients appear to be more subtle and thus continue to be the subject of active study. Although osteoporosis remains an incurable disease, adequate nutrient intakes help support the efficacy of drug treatment and, hence, prevent further bone loss. The importance of primary and secondary prevention of aged-related bone loss with a general healthy diet and other prudent health behaviors, including physical exercise and lifelong adequacy of vitamin D and Ca, needs to be strongly emphasized to young and middle-aged adults so that their risks of osteoporosis and related nontraumatic fractures in old age are minimized. Special care as well as pharmacological interventions may be warranted for high-risk individuals, such as those with low bone mass, that is, <2.5 standard deviations below mean DXA scores of healthy young adults (WHO), or those on long-term corticosteroid therapy.

REFERENCES

American Academy of Orthopaedic Surgeons. 2008. Osteoporosis and bone health. In *The Burden of Musculoskeletal Diseases in the United States*. Bone and Joint Decade, publisher. Rosemont, IL, pp. 1–9.

Anderson, J.J.B., Klemmer, P.J., Watts, M.L.S., et al. 2006. Phosphorus. In *Present Knowledge in Nutrition*. Bowman, B.A., and Russell, R.M., eds, pp 383–399. Washington, DC: ILSI Press.

Avenell, A., Gillespie, W, Gillespie, L., et al. 2009. Vitamin D and vitamin D analogues for preventing fractures associated with involutional and post-menopausal osteoporosis. *Cochrane Database Syst Rev* 15:2.

Bales, C., and Buhr, G. 2008. Is obesity bad for older persons? A systematic review of the pros and cons of weight reduction in later life. *J Am Med Dir Assoc* 9: 302–312.

Bales, C., and Buhr, G. 2009. Body mass trajectory, energy balance, and weight loss as determinants of health and mortality in older adults. *Obes Facts* 2: 171–178.

Bales, C., and Ritchie, C. 2009. Redefining nutritional fraility: Interventions for weight loss due to undernutrition. In *Handbook of Clinical Nutrition and Aging*, pp. 157–182. New York: Humana Press.

Baumgartner, R. 2000. Body composition in healthy aging. *Ann N Y Acad Sc* 904: 437–448.

Baumgartner, R., Wayne, S., Waters, D., et al. 2004. Sarcopenic obesity predicts instrumental activities of daily living disability in the elderly. *Obes Res* 12: 1995–2004.

Binkley, N., Harke, J., Krueger, D., et al. 2009. Vitamin K treatment reduces undercarboxylated osteocalcin but does not alter bone turnover, density, or geometry in healthy postmenopausal North American women. *J Bone Miner Res* 24: 983–991.

Bischoff-Ferrari, H., Dawson-Hughes, B., Staehelin, H., et al. 2009. Fall prevention with supplemental and active forms of vitamin D: A meta-analysis of randomised controlled trials. *BMJ* 339: B3692.

Bischoff-Ferrari, H., Giovannucci, E., Willett, W., et al. 2006. Estimation of optimal serum concentrations of 25-hydroxyvitamin D for multiple health outcomes. *Am J Clin Nutr* 84: 18–28.

Bolland, M., Barber, P., Doughty, R., et al. 2008. Vascular events in healthy older women receiving calcium supplementation: Randomised controlled trial. *BMJ*, 336: 262–266.

Boonen, S., Dejaeger, E., Vanderschueren, D., et al. 2008. Osteoporosis and osteoporotic fracture occurrence and prevention in the elderly: A geriatric perspective. *Best Pract Res Clin Endocrinol Metab* 22: 765–785.

Boonen, S., Lips, P., Bouillon, R., et al. 2007. Need for additional calcium to reduce the risk of hip fracture with vitamin d supplementation: Evidence from a comparative metaanalysis of randomized controlled trials. *J Clin Endocrinol Metab* 92: 1415–1423.

Booth, S. 2009. Roles for vitamin K beyond coagulation. *Annu Rev Nutr* 29: 89–110.

Booth, S., Dallal, G., Shea, M., et al. 2008. Effect of vitamin K supplementation on bone loss in elderly men and women. *J Clin Endocrinol Metab* 93: 1217–1223.

Bopp, M., Houston, D., Lenchik, L., et al. 2008. Lean mass loss is associated with low protein intake during dietary-induced weight loss in postmenopausal women. *J Am Diet Assoc* 108: 1216–1220.

Burge, R., Dawson-Hughes, B., Solomon, D., et al. 2007. Incidence and economic burden of osteoporosis-related fractures in the United States. *J Bone Miner Res* 22: 465–475.

Caire-Juvera, G., Ritenbaugh, C., Wactawski-Wende, J., et al. 2009. Vitamin A and retinol intakes and the risk of fractures among participants of the Women's Health Initiative Observational Study. *Am J Clin Nutr* 89: 323–330.

Campbell, W., Trappe, T., Wolfe, R., et al. 2001. The recommended dietary allowance for protein may not be adequate for older people to maintain skeletal muscle. *J Gerontol A Biol Sci Med Sc* 56: M373–M380.

Cockayne, S., Adamson, J., Lanham-New, S., et al. 2006. Vitamin K and the prevention of fractures: Systematic review and meta-analysis of randomized controlled trials. *Arch Intern Med* 166: 1256–1261.

Darling, A., Millward, D., Torgerson, D., et al. 2009. Dietary protein and bone health: A systematic review and meta-analysis. *Am J Clin Nutr* 90: 1674–1692.

Davison, K., Ford, E., Cogswell, M., et al. 2002. Percentage of body fat and body mass index are associated with mobility limitations in people aged 70 and older from NHANES III. *J Am Geriatr Soc* 50: 1802–1809.

Devine, A., Dick, I., Islam, A., et al. 2005. Protein consumption is an important predictor of lower limb bone mass in elderly women. *Am J Clin Nut* 81: 1423–1428.

Douchi, T., Kuwahata, R., Matsuo, T., et al. 2003. Relative contribution of lean and fat mass component to bone mineral density in males. *J Bone Miner Metab* 21: 17–21.

Duarte, J., Bolge, S., Sen, S. 2007. An evaluation of patients' preferences for osteoporosis medications and their attributes: The PREFER-International study. *Clin Ther* 29: 488–503.

Earl, S., Cole, Z.A., Holroyd, C., et al. 2010. Dietary management of osteoporosis throughout the life course. *Br J Nutr* 69: 25–33.

Ensrud, K., Ewing, S., Stone, K., et al. 2003. Intentional and unintentional weight loss increase bone loss and hip fracture risk in older women. *J Am Geriatr Soc* 51: 1740–1747.

Ervin, R., and Kennedy-Stephenson, J. 2002. Mineral intakes of elderly adult supplement and non-supplement users in the third national health and nutrition examination survey. *J Nutr* 132: 3422–3427.

Evans, W. 2010. Skeletal muscle loss: Cachexia, sarcopenia, and inactivity. *Am J Clin Nutr* 91: 1123S–1127S.

Federal Interagency Forum on Aging-Related Statistics. 2008. *Older Americans 2008: Key Indicators of Well-being*. National Center for Health Statistics. Retrieved January 15, 2010, from www.agingstats.gov/agingstatsdotnet/main_site

Feskanich, D., Singh, V., Willett, W., et al. 2002. Vitamin A intake and hip fractures among postmenopausal women. *JAMA* 287: 47–54.

Flegal, K., Carroll, M., Ogden, C., et al. 2002. Prevalence and trends in obesity among US adults 1999–2000. *JAMA* 288: 1723–1727.

Fried, L., Tangen, C., Walston, J., et al. 2001. Frailty in older adults: Evidence for a phenotype. *J Gerontol A Biol Sci Med Sci* 56: M146–M156.

Fulgoni, V., 2008. Current protein intake in America: Analysis of the National Health and Nutrition Examination Survey, 2003–2004. *Am J Clin Nutr* 87: 1554S–1557S.

Gehlbach, S., Avrunin, J., Puleo, E., et al. 2007. Fracture risk and antiresorptive medication use in older women in the USA. *Osteoporos Int* 18: 805–810.

Genaro, P.S. Pereira, G.A. Pinheiro, M.M., et al. 2010. Influence of body composition on bone mass in post-menopausal osteoporotic women. *Arch Gerontol Geriatr.* Epub

Ginty, F. 2003. Dietary protein and bone health. *Proc Nutr Soc* 62: 867–876.

Goodman, S., Jiranek, W., Petrow, E., et al. 2007. The effects of medications on bone. *J Am Acad Orthop Surg* 15: 450–460.

Grant, A., Avenell, A., Campbell, M., et al. 2005. Oral vitamin D3 and calcium for secondary prevention of low-trauma fractures in elderly people (Randomised Evaluation of Calcium Or vitamin D, RECORD): A randomised placebo-controlled trial. *Lanct*, 365: 1621–1628.

Greenspan, S., Resnick, N., Parker, R. 2005. Vitamin D supplementation in older women. *J Gerontol A Biol Sci Med Sci* 60: 754–759.

Hallberg, I., Rosenqvist, A., Kartous, L., et al. 2004. Health-related quality of life after osteoporotic fractures. *Osteoporos Int* 15: 834–841.

Hannan, M., Tucker, K., Dawson-Hughes, B., et al. 2000. Effect of dietary protein on bone loss in elderly men and women: The Framingham Osteoporosis Study. *J Bone Miner Res* 15: 2504–2512.

Holick, M., and Chen, T. 2008. Vitamin D deficiency: A worldwide problem with health consequences. *Am J Clin Nutr* 87: 1080S–1086S.

Houston, D., Nicklas, B., Zizza, C. 2009. Weighty concerns: The growing prevalence of obesity among older adults. *J Am Diet Assoc* 109: 1886–1895.

Institute of Medicine. 2011. *Dietary Reference Intakes for Calcium and Vitamin D*. Washington, DC: National Academies.

International Osteoporosis Foundation. 2009. *Facts and Statistics About Osteoporosis and its Impact in 2007*. Retrieved January 13, 2010, from www.iofbonehealth.org/facts-and-statistics.html

Jarosz, P., and Bellar, A. 2009. Sarcopenic obesity: An emerging cause of frailty in older adults. *Geriatr Nurs* 30: 64–70.

Johnston, C., Taylor, C., Hampl, J. 2000. More Americans are eating "5 a day" but intakes of dark green and cruciferous vegetables remain low. *J Nutr* 130: 3063–3067.

Kemi, V., Karkkainen, M., Karp, H., et al. 2008. Increased calcium intake does not completely counteract the effects of increased phosphorus intake on bone: An acute dose–response study in healthy females. *Br J Nutr* 99: 832–839.

Kerstetter, J., and Allen, L.1990. Dietary protein increases urinary calcium. *J Nutr* 120: 134–136.

Kiebzak, G., Moore, N., Margolis, S., et al. 2007. Vitamin D status of patients admitted to a hospital rehabilitation unit: Relationship to function and progress. *Am J Phys Med Rehabil* 86: 435–445.

Knoke, J., and Barrett-Connor, E. 2003. Weight loss: A determinant of hip bone loss in older men and women. The Rancho Bernardo Study. *Am J Epidemiol* 158: 1132–1138.

Langlois, J., Visser, M., Davidovic, L., et al. 1998. Hip fracture risk in older white men is associated with change in body weight from age 50 years to old age. *Arch Intern Med* 158: 990–996.

Lichtenstein, A., Rasmussen, H.,Yu, W., et al. 2008. Modified mypyramid for older adults. *J Nutr* 138: 5–11.

Lips, P., and van Schoor, N. 2005. Quality of life in patients with osteoporosis. *Osteoporos Int* 16: 447–455.

Malik, R. 2007. Vitamin D and secondary hyperparathyroidism in the institutionalized elderly: A literature review. *J Nutr Elderly* 26: 119–138.

Melhus, H., Michaelsson, K., Kindmark, A., et al. 1998. Excessive dietary intake of vitamin A is associated with reduced bone mineral density and increased risk for hip fracture. *Ann Intern Med* 129: 770–778.

Mokdad, A., Bowman, B., Ford, E., et al. 2001. The continuing epidemics of obesity and diabetes in the United States. *JAMA* 286: 1195–1200.

Moore, C., Murphy, M., Keast, D., et al. 2004. Vitamin D intake in the United States. *J Am Diet Assoc* 104: 980–983.

Mukamal, K., Robbins, J., Cauley, J., et al. 2007. Alcohol consumption, bone density, and hip fracture among older adults: The Cardiovascular Health Study. *Osteoporos Int* 18: 593–602.

National Osteoporosis Foundation. 2008. *National Osteoporosis Foundation Fast Facts*. Retrieved January 13, 2010, from http://www.nof.org/osteoporosis/diseasefacts.htm

Nordin, B., 2009. The effect of calcium supplementation on bone loss in 32 controlled trials in postmenopausal women. *Osteoporos Int* 12: 2135–2143.

Paddon-Jones, D., and Rasmussen, B. 2009. Dietary protein recommendations and the prevention of sarcopenia. *Curr Opin Clin Nutr Metab Care* 12: 86–90.

Parikh, S., Mogun, H., Avorn, J., et al. 2008. Osteoporosis medication use in nursing home patients with fractures in 1 US state. *Arch Intern Med* 168: 1111–1115.

Pellet, P.L. 1990. Protein requirements in humans. *Am J Clin Nutr* 51: 723–737.

Prince, R., Austin, N., Devine, A., et al. 2008. Effects of ergocalciferol added to calcium on the risk of falls in elderly high-risk women. *Arch Intern Med* 168: 103–108.

Promislow, J., Goodman-Gruen, D., Slymen, D., et al. 2002. Protein consumption and bone mineral density in the elderly: The Rancho Bernardo Study. *Am J Epidemiol* 155: 636–644.

Reid, I., Bolland, M., Grey, A. 2010. Vitamin D—let's get back to the evidence base. *IBMS BoneKEy* 7: 249–253.

Ribaya-Mercado, J., and Blumberg, J. 2007. Vitamin A: Is it a risk factor for osteoporosis and bone fracture? *Nutr Rev* 65: 425–438.

Ribot, C., Tremollieres, F., Pouilles, J., et al. 1987. Obesity and postmenopausal bone loss: The influence of obesity on vertebral density and bone turnover in postmenopausal women. *Bone* 8: 327–331.

Rohde, L., de Assis, M., Rabelo, E. 2007. Dietary vitamin K intake and anticoagulation in elderly patients. *Curr Opin Clin Nutr Metab Care* 10: 1–5.

Rolland, Y., Lauwers-Cances, V., Cristini, C., et al. 2009. Difficulties with physical function associated with obesity, sarcopenia, and sarcopenic-obesity in community-dwelling elderly women: The EPIDOS (EPIDemiologie de l'OSteoporose) Study. *Am J Clin Nutr* 89: 1895–1900.

Roubenoff, R. 2004. Sarcopenic obesity: The confluence of two epidemics. *Obes Res* 12: 887–888.

Ryder, K., Shorr, R., Tylavsky, F., et al. 2006. Correlates of use of antifracture therapy in older women with low bone mineral density. *J Gen Intern Med* 21: 636–641.

Sanders, K., Nowson, C., Kotowicz, M., et al. 2009. Calcium and bone health: Position statement for the Australian and New Zealand Bone and Mineral Society, Osteoporosis Australia and the Endocrine Society of Australia. *Med J Aust* 190: 316–320.

Schrager, M., Metter, E., Simonsick, E., et al. 2007. Sarcopenic obesity and inflammation in the InCHIANTI study. *J Appl Physiol* 102: 919–925.

Schurch, M., Rizzoli, R., Slosman, D., et al. 1998.Protein supplements increase serum insulin-like growth factor-I levels and attenuate proximal femur bone loss in patients with recent hip fracture: A randomized, double-blind, placebo-controlled trial. *Ann Intern Med* 128: 801–809.

Shipp, K. 2006. Exercise for people with osteoporosis: Translating the science into clinical practice. *Curr Osteoporos Rep* 4: 129–133.

Souberbielle, J., Cormier, C., Kindermans, C., et al. 2001. Vitamin D status and redefining serum parathyroid hormone reference range in the elderly. *J Clin Endocrinol Metab* 86: 3086–3090.

Surgeon General Report. 2004. *Bone Health and Osteoporosis: A Report of the Surgeon General 2004.* Retrieved from www.surgeongeneral.gov/library/bonehealth/content.html

Suter, P., Golner, B., Goldin, B., et al. 1991. Reversal of protein-bound vitamin B12 malabsorption with antibiotics in atrophic gastritis. *Gastroenterology* 101: 1039–1045.

Symons, T., Sheffield-Moore, M., Wolfe, R., et al. 2009. A moderate serving of high-quality protein maximally stimulates skeletal muscle protein synthesis in young and elderly subjects. *J Am Diet Assoc* 109: 1582–1586.

Tang, B., Eslick, G., Nowson, C., et al. 2007. Use of calcium or calcium in combination with vitamin D supplementation to prevent fractures and bone loss in people aged 50 years and older: A meta-analysis. *Lancet* 370: 657–666.

Teucher, B., Dainty, J., Spinks, C., et al. 2008. Sodium and bone health: Impact of moderately high and low salt intakes on calcium metabolism in postmenopausal women. *J Bone Miner Res* 23: 1477–1485.

Tkatch, L., Rapin, C., Rizzoli, R., et al. 1992. Benefits of oral protein supplementation in elderly patients with fracture of the proximal femur. *J Am Coll Nutr* 11: 519–525.

Tucker, K., Jugdaohsingh, R., Powell, J., et al. 2009. Effects of beer, wine, and liquor intakes on bone mineral density in older men and women. *Am J Clin Nutr* 89: 1188–1196.

Tucker, K. 2009. Osteoporosis prevention and nutrition. *Curr Osteoporos Rep* 7: 111–117.

van Staa, T., Leufkens, H., Cooper, C. 2002. The epidemiology of corticosteroid-induced osteoporosis: A meta-analysis. *Osteoporos Int* 13: 777–787.

Villareal, D., Banks, M., Siener, C., et al. 2004. Physical frailty and body composition in obese elderly men and women. *Obes Res* 12: 913–920.

Wortsman, J., Matsuoka, L., Chen, T., et al. 2000. Decreased bioavailability of vitamin D in obesity. *Am J Clin Nutr* 72: 690–693.

Wosje, K., and Kalkwarf, H. 2007. Bone density in relation to alcohol intake among men and women in the United States. *Osteoporos Int* 18: 391–400.

Yang, Y., Lewis, J., Epstein, S., et al. 2006. Long-term proton pump inhibitor therapy and risk of hip fracture. *JAMA* 296: 2947–2953.

Yu, E., Blackwell, T., Ensrud, K., et al. 2008. Acid-suppressive medications and risk of bone loss and fracture in older adults. *Calcif Tissue Int* 83: 251–259.

Part IV

Race, Ethnicity, and Bone

28 Bone Growth in African Children and Adolescents

Ann Prentice, Kate A. Ward, Inez Schoenmakers,
and Gail R. Goldberg

CONTENTS

INTRODUCTION

The continent of Africa occupies an area of approximately 30 million km². It stretches 8000 km from north (Tunisia, 37°N) to south (South Africa 34°S) and 7400 km from west (Cape Verde, 17°W) to east (Somalia, 51°E). Thus, the continent encompasses temperate and tropical countries and has geographical features ranging from desert to tropical rain forest and altitudes from below sea level to mountainous regions. Consequently, the climatic, soil, and other environmental conditions vary widely across Africa, affecting farming, food and water sources, land use, and cultural aspects such as subsistence patterns, housing, and customary clothing (Campbell and Tishkoff, 2008; Prentice et al., 2009). The population of Africa, at 900 million people, is equally heterogeneous, for example, the Bantu people migrated from West Africa throughout sub-Saharan Africa within the past 4000 years, and more recently, Arab, Indian, and European peoples have migrated into Africa (Campbell and Tishkoff, 2008). Africa has the highest levels of human genetic diversity both within and between populations (Reed and Tishkoff, 2006). Despite this heterogeneity, there are many similarities in the problems experienced across Africa with respect to maternal and child health, food security, and prevalence of infectious and chronic diseases, all of which may affect bone growth in children and adolescents and have short- and long-term effects on optimal skeletal function and integrity.

This chapter describes the burden of nutrition-related skeletal disorders in the African continent, the pattern of normal skeletal growth in the African context, the constraints on normal growth for African children and adolescents, and the impact of nutrition on bone health in Africa. The methodological considerations required for interpreting the limited evidence and the need for further research are also discussed.

BURDEN OF NUTRITION-RELATED SKELETAL DISORDERS IN AFRICA

INTRAUTERINE GROWTH RETARDATION AND STUNTING

Many nutrients are essential for the growth and development of the skeleton. Bone formation requires adequate dietary supplies of energy, amino acids, and the main bone-forming minerals (Ca, P, Mg, and Zn). It also requires sources of other ions (e.g., Cu, Mn, carbonate, and citrate) and vitamins (e.g., vitamins C, D, and K) that are involved in hydroxyapatite and collagen formation, cartilage and bone metabolism, and/or calcium and phosphate homeostasis.

An inadequate dietary supply during both fetal and postnatal life from whatever cause may result in negative effects on growth and development (Prentice et al., 2006). Intrauterine growth retardation, primarily due to maternal dietary restriction, malarial placental infection, and high energy expenditure relative to energy intake, is common in many African countries as evidenced by the incidence of low birth weight (<2.5 kg) (World Health Organization [WHO] Technical Consultation, 2006; WHO, 2009). The percentage of infants in the WHO Africa Region born with low birth weight is ~14%, and in some African countries, it is >20% (WHO, 2009).

Maternal nutrition may have long-lasting effects on the growth and development of the child in utero because fetal life is a critical period for organogenesis and development of metabolic systems, including the skeleton (Cooper et al., 2006; Davies et al., 2005; Langley-Evans, 2006). Studies in Caucasian populations of growth in fetal and early life and its relationship to later skeletal outcomes have shown that birth weight and postnatal weight are predictors of adult bone mass and skeletal size (Cooper et al., 1995, 1997; Dennison et al., 2005) and that shortness at birth and slow childhood growth predict adult hip fracture incidence (Cooper et al., 2001). Other effects of early growth restriction may be particularly evident if a child undergoes catch-up growth, an acceleration of growth beyond the normal rate for age, commonly seen after periods of nutritional deprivation or illness.

Chronic undernutrition during infancy, childhood, and adolescence leads to linear growth retardation and eventually, when severe, to stunting (de Onis and Blossner, 2003). Stunting is defined as a height or length for age that is less than 2 standard deviations below the mean for reference children and affects both skeletal and somatic growth (de Onis and Blossner, 2003). Stunting is associated with increased mortality in childhood and adulthood, delayed physical and mental development, and poor educational attainment and thus may have many lifelong implications (Lunn, 2002; Prentice et al., 2006; WHO, 2009), including possible adverse effects on skeletal health in adulthood and old age. Recent estimates suggest that the percentage of children in sub-Saharan

African countries who are stunted and/or underweight for their age is higher than in other WHO regions. In some African countries, the prevalence of stunting and underweight is >50% and >30% respectively (WHO, 2009).

The prevalence of nutritional deficiencies among children remains high in many African countries (Allen et al., 2009; Gross et al., 2005). In addition to generalized poor nutrition, well-characterized deficiency diseases that have resulted from an inadequate supply of specific micronutrients are generally associated with impaired growth, including skeletal development. These diseases include deficiencies of vitamin A, thiamin, vitamin C, vitamin K, Fe, folate, vitamin D, and calcium (Prentice et al., 2006). Some micronutrients are directly involved in cartilage and bone production, and deficiencies cause characteristic skeletal abnormalities (e.g., copper, calcium, vitamin C, and vitamin D).

RICKETS AND OSTEOMALACIA

Rickets and osteomalacia are abnormalities of the skeleton caused by undermineralization, that is, where the ratio of mineral to collagen is low (Pettifor, 2003). Rickets is a failure of calcification in the growth plates of the long bones, which occurs only in children before the growth plates fuse. In children, this disease results in characteristic bone deformities, most notably genu varum (bow legs), genu valgum (knock knees), tibiae sabre (windswept deformities) of the lower limbs, beading of the ribs (rachitic rosary), and widening of the distal forearm. Osteomalacia is a failure of mineralization on the trabecular and cortical surfaces of all bones and can occur in both children and adults. Children with rickets frequently have histological features of osteomalacia. Rickets and osteomalacia are associated with pain, difficulties in walking and other activities of daily living, and although they can be corrected at a young age by therapy and surgery, the deformities often persist into adulthood.

Few data have been reported on the prevalence of rickets and osteomalacia in Africa, but isolated reports from many countries suggest that this is a relatively common and widespread problem, often identified when children present at clinics with other diseases (Pettifor, 2008). It commonly first presents during infancy.

Vitamin D deficiency is the most common cause of rickets and osteomalacia worldwide (Prentice, 2008), and it is present in African regions where vitamin D supply is poor (Prentice et al., 2009). Rickets in the absence of frank vitamin D deficiency has also been reported from a number of African countries, most notably Nigeria, The Gambia, and South Africa, and although the etiology is still to be fully identified, it is associated with low calcium intake and abnormalities of phosphate metabolism (Okonofua et al., 1991; Pettifor, 2003; Prentice et al., 2008a; Thacher et al., 2000, 2006). This type of rickets is most commonly seen in young children 3–4 years of age and in adolescents. Vitamin D and calcium deficiency rickets are often found where more general malnutrition is prevalent (Pettifor, 2008).

FLUOROSIS

When present in drinking water at low concentrations, fluoride contributes to the formation of strong teeth and increases resistance to tooth decay. However, excessive exposure to fluoride in drinking water, or combined with exposure from other sources, can have adverse effects ranging from mild dental fluorosis (mottling and pitting of teeth) to crippling skeletal fluorosis, depending on the level and period of exposure. Skeletal fluorosis is a condition whereby fluoride may accumulate in the bone progressively over many years. Early symptoms include stiffness and pain in the joints, and, in severe cases, the bone structure may change and ligaments may calcify, with resulting impairment of muscles and pain (www. WHO_Water-related diseases.htm). The dental effects of fluorosis develop much earlier than do the skeletal effects, and it is often considered that an individual needs many years of exposure before signs and symptoms of skeletal fluorosis become apparent. However, skeletal changes have been observed in children (Greef, 1997).

Skeletal fluorosis is a significant cause of morbidity in some African countries where high concentrations of fluoride are present in ground water and thus consumed regularly as part of the local diet. This disease is most notable in the East African Rift Valley systems, and regions with volcanic soils, such as West Africa and South Africa (Fawell et al., 2006; Prentice et al., 2009). Detailed nationally representative prevalence data of fluorosis in Africa remain to be established, but where information from African countries has been reported (Fawell et al., 2006), estimates of dental fluorosis in children and adolescents suggest prevalence rates of between 30% and 100%. Dental and skeletal fluorosis is associated with fluoride concentrations in drinking water above 1.5 and 10 mg/L, respectively. A guideline concentration of 1.5 mg/L has been recommended by WHO at or below which dental fluorosis should be minimal. In naturally-low-fluoride areas, the estimated total daily fluoride exposure would be ~0.6 mg per adult per day where no fluoride is added to the drinking water and 2 mg per adult per day where water is fluoridated. Marked contrast exists in some areas in Africa where concentrations of fluoride in drinking water of 7.4 and 14 mg/L have been measured (Malde et al., 2003), and intakes in children have been reported as high as 8.8 mg/day from beverages and 4.8 mg/day from foods (Malde et al., 2003, 2004).

Osteoporosis

Osteoporosis describes a lack of bone within the skeletal envelope where the bone tissue that is present has a normal composition (Marcus et al., 1996; WHO, 2003). In postmenopausal women and in old age, when a net loss of bone tissue occurs, osteoporosis is associated with deterioration of the skeletal trabecular architecture and thinning and increased porosity of the bone cortices. In growing individuals, when they have a net accretion of bone tissue, osteoporosis generally refers to a low bone mass for achieved size coupled with high porosity. Osteoporosis is associated with an increased risk of fragility fracture, that is, fracture caused with minimal trauma, such as a fall from a standing position. In children and adolescents, particularly around puberty, such fractures are most common in the distal forearm (Ferrari et al., 2006; Goulding et al., 2001; Heaney et al., 2000; Khosla et al., 2003).

Global data on adults suggest that compared with age-matched Caucasians, other ethnic groups have a lower incidence of hip fracture. The incidence of hip fracture is predicted to increase six-fold to about 6 million in Africa and Asia by 2050 (Cooper et al., 1992) because of increases in longevity in developing countries. It is also possible that the transition toward a Westernized lifestyle may increase the propensity to osteoporotic fracture (Prentice, 2004). Few reliable data have been reported on the prevalence of osteoporosis and the incidence of fragility fractures on the African continent. Again, in contrast to Caucasian populations where incidence is high and women are more affected than men, Asian studies suggest that males and females are equally affected (Yan et al., 1999). In South Africa, the differences between white and Bantu populations in adult fracture incidence are similar to those reported in North America between African Americans and white Americans (Solomon, 1968). Data from Cameroon suggest that, as with Caucasian populations, women in Africa have a higher incidence than do men of low trauma factures to the hip and wrist (Zebaze and Seeman, 2003), but further data are required to confirm the generalizability of this observation.

In developed countries, childhood fractures are common, and children appear to be most susceptible during periods of rapid growth, that is, infancy and adolescence. No prospective fracture data exist for children in African countries. From data collected from the prospective Birth to Twenty (Bt20) longitudinal cohort in South Africa involving children of all races resident in Soweto, the pattern and timing of fractures appear to be similar to those seen in developed countries. The most prevalent fractures were those of the upper limbs, and peak incidence occurred in toddlers and adolescences in both sexes (Khosla et al., 2003; Thandrayen et al., 2009). However, unlike the white South African children, no peak in fracture incidence during infancy was observed in the black or mixed-race children, and overall, the white children experienced three times as many fractures than did those in the other two ethnic groups. In all three ethnic groups, males were at greater risk than were females.

BONE GROWTH AND DEVELOPMENT

LINEAR GROWTH

Linear growth, that is, increases in body length or height, during childhood is an important yardstick of skeletal growth and development. Growth during infancy and childhood predicts adult stature in low- and middle-income countries, including those in Africa (Coly et al., 2006; Stein et al., 2009). In many African countries, as discussed earlier, stunting is common, and linear growth velocities are generally slower than those in Western countries (Lo et al., 1991). This may be a marker of social deprivation and other environmental factors. Data from the African continent included in the WHO Multicentre Growth Reference Study collected among children exclusively or predominantly breastfed for at least 4 months and with no health, environmental, or economic constraints to their growth demonstrated only small differences in attained height for age between African children (Ghana) and those in other parts of the world (de Onis et al., 2006).

The slower linear growth trajectories common in African countries parallel delays in other aspects of physical development, such as age at menarche in girls (Prentice et al., 2010). Secular trends toward increased adult stature and earlier puberty have been reported from some African countries (Cameron, 2007; Prentice et al., 2006).

OTHER SKELETAL DIMENSIONS

Differences in the relative skeletal dimensions of adults in African populations, which are well recognized compared with those in Western countries, imply differences in skeletal growth and development during childhood and adolescence. Commonly, African populations are characterized by having longer arms and legs relative to the torso than do Caucasians (Aspray et al., 1995; Eveleth and Tanner, 1991; Prentice et al., 1991; Nyati et al., 2006). Other skeletal dimensions may also differ; for example, rural Gambian women have shorter hip axis length relative to their height than do British women (Dibba et al., 1999). The reasons for these differences in skeletal growth are not clear and may be genetically determined or be a reflection of the differences in tempo of development during childhood and puberty. The extent to which such observations account for lower fracture rates in black Africans is also unclear (Adebajo et al., 1991; Aspray et al., 1995; Prentice et al., 1990).

SKELETAL MATURATION AND BONE AGE

Bone age gives a more accurate prediction of skeletal maturity than chronological age does by comparing hand and/or forearm radiographs to a reference atlas and assigning a skeletal age. No specific bone age atlases are available for sub-Saharan Africa, and studies have used the Greulich Pyle, Tanner Whitehouse, or the Fels methods, which consist of reference data from North American or U.K. populations (Greulich and Pyle, 1959; Roche et al., 1988; Tanner et al., 1983). Most studies indicate delayed skeletal maturation in African populations, which is consistent with observations of delayed puberty and growth. However, results generated using Caucasian reference data may overestimate the delay in skeletal maturity in African countries (Agossou-Voyeme et al., 2005; Lewis et al., 2002). Secular trend data from South Africa suggest that skeletal maturity is "catching up" with reference populations, particularly within black children and adolescents (Hawley et al., 2009) in whom discordance with reference populations was previously greatest.

BONE MINERAL ACCRETION, CONTENT AND DENSITY, PEAK BONE MASS, AND STRENGTH

Childhood and adolescence are critical periods for skeletal growth and development. A female accrues up to 40% of her total mineral content during the pubertal growth spurt. The end of longitudinal growth and subsequent fusing of epiphyses signals skeletal maturity (Parfitt, 2002), but growth in bone width (BW) continues throughout life. In general, skeletal mineral accretion continues into early adulthood, with loss at older ages. Peak bone mass is predominantly determined by genetic factors, but environmental factors such as nutritional status, hormones, and physical activity contribute 20%–40% of the variation between individuals (Heaney et al., 2000; Prentice, 2001).

Skeletal strength is determined by bone shape, size, mineral content, turnover, and internal architecture. Bone densitometry techniques have been developed to provide measures of bone mineral content, density, and size. The techniques on which most of the studies discussed in this chapter are based use radiogrammetry, dual-energy X-ray absorptiometry (DXA), and single-photon absorptiometry (SPA). Radiogrammetry is one of the oldest quantitative techniques that used hand radiographs to assess skeletal status by using various measures of metacarpal cortical bone (Barnett and Nordin, 1960; Garn et al., 1971; Meema, 1962). DXA is based on the attenuation of X-rays of two different frequencies and is used predominantly for whole-body, spine, and hip measurements; SPA was the predecessor to DXA, which used a radioactive iodine source (I^{125}) and was able to scan forearm sites. DXA is the most commonly used technique for human studies at the present time. The mineral data from DXA are generally expressed as bone mineral content (BMC) or areal bone mineral density (aBMD) and size as scanned bone area (BA) or BW. DXA measurements of BMC and aBMD serve as proxies for bone strength and predict fracture risk in adults (Marshall et al., 1996) and children (Clark et al., 2006; Goulding et al., 2000). The definitions of outputs from other techniques differ from those of DXA, and they cannot be directly compared (Crabtree and Ward, 2009).

Bone densitometry techniques were developed for use in adults and thus have limitations when measuring the skeleton in childhood because it is constantly changing in size, shape, and mass. The most critical limitation is that DXA derives BMC and aBMD measurements from a two-dimensional image and cannot account for the depth of the bone, making the measurements size dependent. As a consequence, differences in growth rates and size of children will be reflected in differences in these variables, leading to difficulties in interpretation. Several methods have been developed to overcome the size dependency of the technique (Crabtree and Ward, 2009; Mølgaard et al., 1998; Prentice et al., 1994). The different growth rates of the axial and appendicular skeleton between black and white African children, as discussed earlier, and between males and females, may complicate the interpretation of bone mineral accretion unless appropriate size corrections are applied (Nyati et al., 2006; Prentice et al., 1994). Differences or changes in body composition (including extremes in absolute amount or proportions of lean and fat tissues) should also be taken into account. In addition, the use of BMC or aBMD from DXA as markers of fracture risk, using data derived from older Caucasian populations, does not apply to other ethnic groups' populations' or at different times of life (Prentice, 2004; Prentice et al., 2003, 2006).

The use of alternative techniques that are independent of size and encompass other aspects of bone strength (size, shape, geometry, and turnover) may be more appropriate when studying skeletal development and fracture risk in Africa. These techniques may become particularly pertinent as the populations move toward a more Westernized lifestyle, with possible consequences of alterations in porosity and bone remodeling rates. Techniques such as quantitative computed tomography (QCT) allow the study of cortical and trabecular bone separately and measure bone size, geometry, in vivo bone strength, and muscle area and volume. Peripheral QCT is increasingly being incorporated into research studies as a size-independent technique that measures volumetric BMD, bone geometry, and other markers of bone strength of the radius and tibia. High-resolution techniques based on QCT can also quantify trabecular microarchitecture and cortical porosity in vivo.

Very few bone densitometry studies of children in Africa have been conducted; studies have been published from The Gambia and from South Africa. The Gambian studies have been based on a series of small cohorts of children who are being followed longitudinally during childhood and adolescence (Prentice, 2007). In South Africa, the Bt20 study is the largest and longest running study of child and adolescent health and development in Africa. More than 3200 children born between

March and June 1990 in the metropolitan area of Johannesburg-Soweto were enrolled into a long-term birth cohort study and they and their families are being followed for 20 years (http://web.wits.ac.za/Academic/Health/Research/BirthTo20/Home.htm).

In studies in The Gambia using SPA of the forearm, rural children were shown to have lower BMC compared with a group of age-matched British children. However, this was mostly accounted for by differences in bone and body size, the Gambian children being smaller at each age (Prentice et al., 1990). This difference was also demonstrated among adult women in the two populations (Prentice et al., 1991). During adolescence, despite peak height velocity and puberty occurring later, Gambian girls were found to have lower BMC and aBMD at all ages but at least the same BMC as North American children after size correction (Lo et al., 1991).

In Gambian females, BMC accrual in the forearm was shown to lag behind U.S. and U.K. populations but to eventually reach similar levels by the age of 19 years; a similar pattern was observed in males who reached equivalent levels at the age of 25 years (Lo et al., 1991). In the Bt20 study, histomorphometry has shown that growth in width of the iliac crest of the South African children ceased at the age of 15 years and was the same in both white and black individuals (males and females combined), but cortical thickness continued to increase in the black children until 23 years of age. Black individuals had greater osteoid thickness, endocortical wall thickness, and lower porosity (Schnitzler et al., 2009).

In the Bt20 study, using DXA, after appropriate adjustment for differences in body size, black South African children were shown to have higher BMC in the total hip, femoral neck, and radius. They also had shorter vertebral bodies than did white South African children (McVeigh et al., 2007; Vidulich et al., 2007). No differences were found in lumbar spine, whole-body, or distal radius BMC or BA at most other sites except that the radius was wider in black males. Mixed-race South African children had greater size-adjusted whole-body BMC than did black or white children (Micklesfield et al., 2007).

From the limited data available, gender differences in African children appear to be similar to those observed in developed countries, with males having greater BMC and/or aBMD than do females at the hip, ulna, and radius in both black and white children (Lo et al., 1991; Nyati et al., 2006; Patel et al., 1993). In the Bt20 study, BA was greater at the spine and ulna, and the radius was wider, in males compared with females in both black and white South African children (Nyati et al., 2006).

Data from Bt20 suggest that the effects of environment on skeletal growth in Africa appear to be similar to those in developed countries. Early-life environment and its effects on intrauterine and fetal growth was shown to be an independent determinant of size-adjusted whole-body BMC and BA and femoral neck BMC in prepubertal and early-pubertal South African children. Being of lower birth weight was associated with smaller and/or less mineralized bones at the age of 10 years (Norris et al., 2008).

Other environmental determinants of skeletal health are nutrition, physical activity, and socioeconomic status. In the Bt20 study, despite lower birth weight, growth rates (including mineral accumulation rate), physical activity, and calcium intake, the black males had greater hip BMC than did white males (McVeigh et al., 2007). Physical activity and calcium intake were not linked to gain in BMC or BA in black children between the ages of 9 and 10 years. However, in white South African children, there was a positive relationship between physical activity, calcium intake, and gain in BA and BMC (McVeigh et al., 2007). Lower current socioeconomic status was negatively related to BMC, and this was attributed to its effects on BA rather than on mineralization directly, that is, smaller bones (Norris et al., 2008).

Differences and similarities in bone growth exist among African children. Whether the differences between Gambian and South African studies reflect differences in the ethnic origins and/or environment of the children or result from differences in the techniques used remains to be resolved. The limited studies in African children have demonstrated differences and similarities in skeletal growth and development compared with children living in Western countries. How these translate into peak bone strength and later fracture risk is not clear. More research is needed to determine genetic and environmental influences on skeletal health in African children.

BIOCHEMICAL MARKERS OF BONE TURNOVER

Information about bone growth and remodeling can be obtained through measuring biochemical markers in blood or urine (Levine, 2003; Prentice et al., 2003; Szulc et al., 2000). These include markers of osteoblast activity (e.g., osteocalcin, bone alkaline phosphatase), osteoclast activity (e.g., tartrate-resistant acid phosphatase), various collagen propeptides (e.g., P1NP and P1CP), and collagen breakdown products (e.g., hydroxyproline, deoxypyridinoline, and N- and C-terminal telopeptides of collagen [NTX, CTX]). Further insight into mechanisms can be obtained by measuring biochemical markers of bone metabolism, calcium homeostasis, and growth modulators, such as PTH, vitamin D metabolites, cortisol, growth hormone, insulin-like growth factors I and II (American Society for Bone and Mineral Research, 2006; Glorieux et al., 2003; Juul et al., 1994).

The concentrations or outputs of these markers are highly dependent on age, skeletal and sexual maturity, growth velocity, mineral accrual, sex, and ethnicity (Bryant et al., 2003; Szulc et al., 2000). Further sources of variability include circadian periodicity, season, diet, exercise, kidney function, and, in older girls, the phase of the menstrual cycle, use of oral contraceptives, and/or pregnancy. Interpretation of bone markers is further complicated because nutritional and therapeutic interventions are likely to induce different short- and long-term changes as a result, for example, catch-up growth, healing of rachitic lesions, and different phases of the bone remodeling transient (Doherty et al., 2002; Munday et al., 2006; Scariano et al., 1998). The use of reference data derived in Western countries may, therefore, not be appropriate in African settings.

No representative bone marker data are available for children on the African continent, although representative data for children in developed countries, mainly of Caucasian origin, have been reported (Rauchenzauner et al., 2007; Yang and Grey, 2006). Examples of data derived from small, nonrepresentative groups and case-control studies in Africa indicate that bone markers are influenced by rickets, stunting, and poor nutritional status and respond to nutritional intervention (Daniels et al., 2000; Dibba et al., 2000; Munday et al., 2006; Scariano et al., 1998). In comparison with Caucasians, Gambian children have been reported to have lower values of P1NP and comparable values of CTXβ (Munday et al., 2006), These results are similar to findings in children in Bangladesh, where severe malnutrition was associated with low rates of bone collagen synthesis and high rates of collagen degradation (Doherty et al., 2002). However, more research is required to determine patterns of bone remodeling in African children.

ENVIRONMENTAL FACTORS AND SKELETAL GROWTH IN AFRICA

DIET AND NUTRITION

Nutritional Adequacy

The African diet is very heterogeneous and varies from region to region. Assessments of dietary intakes and nutritional status in children and adolescents are difficult to compare between populations because of the use of different assessment techniques and food composition databases, as well as the use of different dietary reference values (Prentice et al., 2006). These variations are particularly acute at certain ages in childhood because of differences in the definition of boundaries between different stages of life, the data used to denote average or desirable growth, and the methods selected for interpolation and extrapolation. All these issues are described in depth elsewhere (Prentice et al., 2004, 2006).

Many dietary assessment studies have been conducted in Africa in adults, for example, in South Africa, Cote d'Ivoire, Kenya, Cameroon, Malawi, and The Gambia (Bah et al., 2001; Bourne et al., 1994; Hallund et al., 2008; Hess et al., 1999; Mennen et al., 2000; van't Riet et al., 2002), and children and adolescents, for example, in Cote d'Ivoire, Kenya, Nigeria, Zimbabwe, The Gambia, and South Africa (Bah et al., 2001; Cooper and Chifamba, 2009; Ene-Obong et al., 2003; Grillenberger et al., 2006; Hess et al., 1999; van't Riet et al., 2002; Walingo and Musamali, 2008). These assessments have been conducted to determine intakes of specific nutrients or foods, despite a lack of nationally representative nutritional survey information from different African countries. The general view, however, is that the nutritional status, as indicated by macronutrient and/or micronutrient intakes, the poor growth, and stunting of many African children, is associated with poverty.

Calcium Intake

The calcium intake of many African children is much lower than that in Europe, Australasia, and the Americas because of the relative scarcity of milk and milk products in the diet (Clemens et al., 2011; Prentice and Bates, 1994; Prentice, 2004): Calcium intakes of 200–300 mg/day have been reported from Egypt, Kenya, Nigeria, The Gambia, and South Africa (Thacher et al., 2006). Such intakes are considerably below international recommendations. The main sources of calcium in Africa, other than animal milks, include leaves and fruits from indigenous plants and bones from small fish consumed whole or dried and added to sauces (Prentice and Bates, 1994). Plant-based diets also contain high amounts of phytates, oxalates, and tannins that are likely to reduce the absorption of calcium. Considerable variation occurs, however, both within and between different regions of Africa, where pastoral communities have greater access to animal milks than do those engaged in subsistence farming, and affluent communities with greater purchasing power have greater access to manufactured milk-based products and calcium-fortified foods than do those in deprived communities.

The effects of habitually low calcium intakes among African children on skeletal growth and development have been studied in some detail by research groups working most notably in The Gambia and South Africa. In The Gambia, observational and supplementation studies of pregnant and lactating women suggest that increasing maternal calcium intake is of no significant benefit to the offspring in terms of an increase in bone mineral accretion or linear growth in utero or the first months of life (Jarjou et al., 2006; Prentice, 2007; Prentice and Bates, 1994; Prentice et al., 1995). In addition, there is little to suggest that the low calcium intake of African infants is, of itself, a limiting factor in infant growth (Prentice et al., 1999). In contrast, intervention studies in older children and adolescents have reported increases in bone mineral accretion, but not skeletal size, in association with increases in calcium intake. Such effects, however, may reflect transient changes in bone remodeling and may not translate into long-term increases in bone mineral mass (Eastell and Hannon, 2008; Eastell and Lambert, 2002; Heaney, 2001; Slemenda et al., 1997). Also, the possibility exists that such increases may disrupt the metabolic process underpinning adaptation to a low calcium intake (Prentice, 2007).

Although little evidence is available to suggest that the low calcium intake of African children limits their skeletal growth, dietary calcium deficiency has been implicated in African rickets among children without overt vitamin D deficiency, as reported from South Africa, The Gambia, and Nigeria (Pettifor, 2008; Prentice et al., 2006; Thacher et al., 2006). Chronic calcium deficiency has effects on the metabolism of phosphate and vitamin D (Prentice et al., 2008a), and calcium has been shown to be an effective treatment for some, but not all, of these children (Pettifor, 2008; Prentice et al., 2006; Thacher et al., 2006).

Vitamin D Status

Vitamin D status and supply are influenced by sunshine exposure, diet, and underlying health conditions. People acquire vitamin D by cutaneous synthesis following exposure to ultraviolet B (UVB) radiation from sunlight, and from the diet. The endogenous supply of vitamin D_3 (cholecalciferol) depends on the skin's exposure to UVB radiation at wavelengths of 290–315 nm, the efficiency of cutaneous vitamin D synthesis, and the extent to which vitamin D is degraded within the skin

(Holick, 2005; Norman, 2008; Webb, 2006). The quantity of UVB radiation of the relevant wavelengths that reaches the skin depends on many factors including time of day and, at latitudes north of 30°N and south of 30°S, month of the year (Jablonski and Chaplin, 2000). In tropical regions, sunlight contains UVB radiation all year round, although this may be affected by differences in cloud cover at different times of the year. Even where abundant sunshine occurs, the extent of UVB skin exposure also depends on climate, clothing, living and working environments, and sunscreen use (Schoenmakers et al., 2008).

In addition, the efficiency of cutaneous synthesis depends on skin pigmentation and age (MacLaughlin and Holick, 1985; Malvy et al., 2000). Many gradations of skin pigmentation are found in African populations, and the lower rates of cutaneous synthesis with darker skin tones may affect vitamin D status if UVB exposure is limited. No studies in the literature have investigated cutaneous synthesis in African people (Prentice et al., 2009). Studies of African Americans and of Indians suggest that no difference in the total capacity for endogenous vitamin D synthesis exists between individuals with different skin types. In lighter skin types, the plateau of maximal synthesis is reached after a shorter duration of UVB exposure compared with darker skin tones, and therefore, in darker skins, a longer period of exposure is required to synthesize the same amount of vitamin D (Brazerol et al., 1988; Holick, 1981; Lo et al., 1986).

When UVB skin exposure is abundant, endogenous synthesis is the primary source of vitamin D for most individuals (Holick, 2004; Willett, 2005). Dietary sources are important during the winter in temperate latitudes and for individuals with restricted exposure to UVB sunlight or reduced capacity for skin synthesis. Little representative information about dietary vitamin D intakes in Africa, or about the consumption of supplements and fortified foods containing vitamin D_2 or D_3, for example, as part of food aid programs has been published. Few naturally occurring food sources are rich in vitamin D (meat, offal, egg yolk, and oily fish), and generally, these are not eaten at all or only rarely by many African peoples (Bwibo and Neumann, 2003; MacKeown et al., 1998; Murphy et al., 1995).

The adequacy of vitamin D supply in African children and adolescents from predictions based on ambient UVB sunshine exposure or dietary intakes is, therefore, almost impossible to predict, in common with other populations in the world (Prentice et al., 2008b). In consequence, plasma 25-hydroxyvitamin concentration (calcidiol, 25OHD) is widely used as a marker of vitamin D status because of its long biological half-life and its relationship to supply of vitamin D from cutaneous and dietary sources (Horst et al., 2005; Prentice et al., 2008b). As summarized elsewhere (Prentice et al., 2009), very few nationally representative data of plasma 25OHD are currently available for African countries; data in the literature have been derived from studies predominantly in The Gambia, Nigeria, and South Africa or from investigations in groups with underlying illness. With these caveats, the plasma 25OHD concentrations recorded in African countries are generally higher than national annualized data from the U.K. and U.S. and show the expected range of values in relation to latitude, seasonality, and dress customs. Mean values from the studies reviewed (Prentice et al., 2009) ranged from 7 to 150 nmol/L (2.8–60 ng/mL) and were mostly above 25 nmol/L (10 ng/mL).

Well-established skeletal consequences of vitamin D deficiency are rickets and osteomalacia, as described earlier. Although vitamin D deficiency rickets is reported in Africa, very few data exist on the burden of disease this imposes or on associations with malnutrition, poverty, and other factors. Therefore, the extent to which primary vitamin D deficiency alone is a cause of poor bone growth and rickets in African children and adolescents is difficult to judge. Low vitamin D status <25 nmol/L (10 ng/mL) is associated with an increased risk of vitamin-D-deficiency rickets and osteomalacia (Scientific Advisory Committee on Nutrition, 2007). Thus, although regions and subgroups, especially in North Africa, where the prevalence of low vitamin D status is high, the majority of Africans, including children and adolescents, appear to have 25OHD values above the upper limit of the rachitic/osteomalacic range. Nevertheless, African children with rickets, where primary vitamin D deficiency is not suspected, often have plasma 25OHD concentrations below those of their African peers, which suggest an increased utilization related to other factors, such as a very low calcium intake (Pettifor, 2008; Prentice et al., 2006; Thacher et al., 2006).

INFECTIOUS DISEASES

Many countries in sub-Saharan Africa have a high prevalence of infectious diseases. The burden of diarrheal diseases, malaria, tuberculosis (TB), and HIV/AIDS in children and adolescents affects growth and development and also has more direct adverse effects on bone health.

Tropical Enteropathy

Tropical enteropathy (tropical sprue), common in many parts of Africa, is characterized by intestinal permeability and poor absorption and abnormal villus structure and function in adults and children. This tropical form is thought to be caused by many factors, including repeated episodes of infection and diarrhea (Anon, 1972; Falaiye, 1971; Lunn, 2002; Mayoral et al., 1967; Menzies et al., 1999). Poor nutrient absorption of calcium and other factors that affect vitamin D metabolism may impact on vitamin D status.

Diarrheal Diseases

Children with poor health and nutritional status are more vulnerable to acute diarrhea and suffer multiple episodes every year. Prolonged diarrhea seriously exacerbates poor health and malnutrition in children, creating a vicious cycle. It is estimated that 696 million cases of diarrhea occur annually in children younger than 5 years old in Africa, and of the 1.5 million under-5 deaths every year from diarrheal diseases, 46% are in Africa (UNICEF/WHO, 2009).

Malaria

Annually, 60% of cases and 90% of deaths occur in sub-Saharan Africa with 75% of these in children under 5 years of age. Malaria contributes to health problems and deaths in many ways, especially in younger children. These health problems include frequent acute infections, anemia as a result of repeated or chronic malaria infection; malaria in pregnancy resulting in low birth weight in infants, and increased susceptibility to other diseases such as respiratory infections and diarrhea (Breman, 2001; WHO Regional Offices for Africa and Eastern Mediterranean, 2006).

Tuberculosis

TB is a major public health problem in many African countries. In 2006, children less than 15 years of age accounted for 3% of new pulmonary cases (Division of AIDS Tuberculosis and Malaria WHO Office for the African Region, 2007). A child with TB disease may present as failure-to-gain weight with loss of energy and a cough lasting for more than 3 weeks. Thus, TB and malnutrition often go together, with consequences for growth and development.

HIV/AIDS

In 2008, sub-Saharan Africa accounted for 67% of HIV infections worldwide, 68% of new HIV infections among adults, and 91% of new HIV infections among children (http://www.unaids.org/en/CountryResponses/Regions/SubSaharanAfrica.asp). Antiretroviral therapy (ART) is associated with an increased prevalence of osteoporosis (Brown and Qaqish, 2006). In South African HIV-positive infants, mortality decreased by 75% in those infants started on ART early compared with those whose treatment was dependent on a decline in CD4 (Violari et al., 2008). Thus, not only would such therapy potentially improve infant survival, but it would also increase the time that individuals are exposed to ART by decades with potential bone sequelae. This therapy, combined with an aging cohort of HIV-positive individuals globally, suggests that an epidemic of HIV-associated bone disease may be evolving and which may emerge in Africa.

CHANGES IN LIFESTYLE AND COUNTRIES IN TRANSITION

Many countries in Africa are undergoing economic and nutrition transitions. Concerns have arisen that as well as many potential benefits, many adverse consequences may also be anticipated. Historically, the climate, geography, and history largely dictated where populations became pastoralists, agriculturalists, and hunter-gatherers and therefore determined local availability and ability to store fresh and saltwater fish, meat, poultry, and milk and the kinds of crops that could be grown and traditionally consumed (Campbell and Tishkoff, 2008; Prentice et al., 2009).

Secular changes in diet and food composition have taken place relatively slowly over hundreds of years. More recently, rapid increases have occurred in Westernized populations in most African countries. Africa is the last continent to experience the nutrition transition, which affects dietary patterns, the sorts of foods consumed, nutrient intakes, and sources of nutrients, for example, the increasing affordability of highly refined oils and carbohydrates, and the risk of chronic diseases of affluence (BeLue et al., 2009; Burlingame, 2003; van Wesenbeeck et al., 2009; Wolmarans, 2009). In Africa, as elsewhere, the nutrition transition is characterized by the paradoxical coexistence of malnutrition and obesity (Prentice, 2009). Although diseases such as malaria and HIV/AIDS remain the major unresolved health problems in many African countries, emerging noncommunicable diseases relating to diet and lifestyle have been increasing, thus creating a double burden of disease. For example, type 2 diabetes mellitus and cardiovascular disease in sub-Saharan Africa have increased 10-fold in the last 20 years (Amuna and Zotor, 2008). African obesity is an adult syndrome, and most of Africa currently has very low rates of obesity in children (Prentice, 2009). However, the move away from subsistence farm work toward sedentary lifestyles and associated decreases in physical activity levels, weight-bearing activities, and loading on the skeleton, has contributed to increased overweight/obesity and adiposity, and reduced exposure to sunshine. Adoption of Western diets and food habits, eating disorders, and inappropriate concerns about bodyweight and image, are all factors with the potential to have a negative impact on bone health of African children and adolescents and in later life.

SUMMARY

Osteoporosis and rickets/osteomalacia are major public health concerns for children and adults in Africa. The prevalence of these skeletal conditions is likely to worsen as life expectancy increases, traditional diets and lifestyles disappear, and individuals reduce their skin UVB exposure through new work practices, migration, changes in dress, and concerns over melanoma risk. In addition, stunting and its associated adverse effects on health and development affect many millions of African children. Population-based strategies are required to promote optimal child growth and optimize bone health at all stages of life. The loading conditions to which the bone is subjected early in life also have an important role in bone strength and should be considered when studying skeletal development and differences between populations. Therefore, a need exists for a greater understanding of healthy bone growth in the African context and the effects of the ongoing transition to Western lifestyles, and the importance of dietary calcium, vitamin D status, and other environmental factors in childhood and adolescence on the etiology and prevention of stunting, rickets/osteomalacia, and osteoporosis in Africa.

REFERENCES

Adebajo, A.O., Cooper, C., and Evans, J.G. 1991. Fractures of the hip and distal forearm in West Africa and the United Kingdom. *Age Ageing* 20: 435–438.

Agossou-Voyeme, A.K., Fachehoun, C.R., Boco, V., et al. 2005. Osseus age of the black children of Benin. A population study of 600 children aged from 9 to 18 years and living in Cotonou. *Morphologie* 89: 64–70.

Allen, L.H., Peerson, J.M. and Olney, D.K. 2009. Provision of multiple rather than two or fewer micronutrients more effectively improves growth and other outcomes in micronutrient-deficient children and adults. *J Nutr* 139: 1022–1030.

American Society for Bone and Mineral Research. 2006. *Primer of the Metabolic Bone Diseases and Disorders of Mineral Metabolism.* Washington, DC: The American Society for Bone and Mineral Research.

Amuna, P. and Zotor, F.B. 2008. Epidemiological and nutrition transition in developing countries: Impact on human health and development. *Proc Nutr Soc* 67: 82–90.

Anon. 1972. The tropical intestine. *Br Med J* 1: 2–3.

Aspray, T.J., Prentice, A. and Cole, T.J. 1995. The bone mineral content of weight-bearing bones is influenced by the ratio of sitting to standing height in elderly Gambian women. *Bone* 17: 261–263.

Bah, A., Semegah-Janneh, I., Prentice, A.M., et al. 2001. *Nationwide Survey on the Prevalence of Vitamin A and Iron Deficiency in Women and Children in The Gambia.* National Nutrition Agency and Medical Research Council, Banjul, The Gambia.

Barnett, E. and Nordin, B.E. 1960. The radiological diagnosis of osteoporosis: A new approach. *Clin Radiol* 11: 166–174.

BeLue, R., Okoror, T.A., Iwelunmor, J., et al. 2009. An overview of cardiovascular risk factor burden in sub-Saharan African countries: A socio-cultural perspective. *Glob Health* 5: 10.

Bourne, L.T., Langenhoven, M.L., Steyn, K., et al. 1994. The food and meal pattern in the urban African population of the Cape Peninsula, South Africa: The BRISK Study. *Cent Afr J Med* 40: 140–148.

Brazerol, W.F., McPhee, A.J., Mimouni, F., et al. 1988. Serial ultraviolet B exposure and serum 25 hydroxyvitamin D response in young adult American blacks and whites: No racial differences. *J Am Coll Nutr* 7: 111–118.

Breman, J.G. 2001. The ears of the hippopotamus: Manifestations, determinants, and estimates of the malaria burden. *Am J Trop Med Hyg* 64: 1–11.

Brown, T.T. and Qaqish, R.B. 2006. Antiretroviral therapy and the prevalence of osteopenia and osteoporosis: A meta-analytic review. *AIDS* 20: 2165–2174.

Bryant, R.J., Wastney, M.E., Martin, B.R., et al. 2003. Racial differences in bone turnover and calcium metabolism in adolescent females. *J Clin Endocrinol Metab* 88: 1043–1047.

Burlingame, B. 2003. The food of Near East, North West and Western African regions. *Asia Pac J Clin Nutr* 12: 309–312.

Bwibo, N.O. and Neumann, C.G. 2003. The need for animal source foods by Kenyan children. *J Nutr* 133(Suppl 2): 3936S–3940S.

Cameron, N. 2007. Growth patterns in adverse environments. *Am J Hum Biol* 19: 615–621.

Campbell, M.C. and Tishkoff, S.A. 2008. African genetic diversity: Implications for human demographic history, modern human origins and complex disease mapping. *Ann Rev Gen Hum Genet* 9: 403–433.

Clark, E.M., Ness, A.R., Bishop, N.J., et al. 2006. Association between bone mass and fractures in children: A prospective cohort study. *J Bone Miner Res* 21: 1489–1495.

Clemens R.A., Hernell O., Michaelsen K.F. (eds). 2011. Milk and milk products in human nutrition. Karger, Basel, Switzerland.

Coly, A.N., Milet, J., Diallo, A., et al. 2006. Preschool stunting, adolescent migration, catch-up growth, and adult height in young Senegalese men and women of rural origin. *J Nutr* 136: 2412–2420.

Cooper, C., Campion, G. and Melton LJ 3rd. 1992. Hip fractures in the elderly: A world-wide projection. *Osteoporos Int* 2: 285–289.

Cooper, C., Cawley, M., Bhalla, A., et al. 1995. Childhood growth, physical activity, and peak bone mass in women. *J Bone Miner Res* 10: 940–947.

Cooper, C., Fall, C., Egger, P., et al. 1997. Growth in infancy and bone mass in later life. *Ann Rheum Dis* 56: 17–21.

Cooper, C., Eriksson, J.G., Forsen, T., et al. 2001. Maternal height, childhood growth and risk of hip fracture in later life: A longitudinal study. *Osteoporos Int* 12: 623–629.

Cooper, C., Westlake, S., Harvey, N., et al. 2006. Review: Developmental origins of osteoporotic fracture. *Osteoporos Int* 17: 337–347.

Cooper, R.G. and Chifamba, J. 2009. The nutritional intake of undergraduates at the University of Zimbabwe College of Health Sciences. *Tanzan J Health Res* 11: 35–39.

Crabtree, N. and Ward, K. 2009. Bone densitometry: Current status and future perspectives. *Endocr Dev* 16: 58–72.

Daniels, E.D., Pettifor, J.M. and Moodley, G.P. 2000. Serum osteocalcin has limited usefulness as a diagnostic marker for rickets. *Eur J Pediatr* 159: 730–733.

Davies, J.H., Evans, B.A. and Gregory, J.W. 2005. Bone mass acquisition in healthy children. *Arch Dis Child* 90: 373–378.

de Onis, M. and Blossner, M. 2003. The World Health Organization global database on child growth and malnutrition: Methodology and applications. *Int J Epidemiol* 32: 518–526.

de Onis, M., Onyango, A.W., Borghi, E., et al. 2006. Comparison of the World Health Organization (WHO) Child Growth Standards and the National Centre for Health Statistics/WHO International Growth Reference: Implications for child health programmes. *Pub Health Nutr* 9: 942–947.

Dennison, E.M., Syddall, H.E., Sayer, A.A., et al. 2005. Birth weight and weight at 1 year are independent determinants of bone mass in the seventh decade: The Hertfordshire cohort study. *Pediatr Res* 57: 582–586.

Dibba, B., Prentice, A., Laskey, M.A., et al. 1999. An investigation of ethnic differences in bone mineral, hip axis length, calcium metabolism and bone turnover between West African and Caucasian adults living in the United Kingdom. *Ann Hum Biol* 26: 229–242.

Dibba, B., Prentice, A., Ceesay, M., et al. 2000. Effect of calcium supplementation on bone mineral accretion in Gambian children accustomed to a low-calcium diet. *Am J Clin Nutr* 71: 544–549.

Division of AIDS Tuberculosis and Malaria WHO Office for the African Region. 2007. *Annual Tuberculosis Surveillance Report, WHO African Region 2007.* WHO Regional Office for Africa, Republic of Congo, Africa.

Doherty, C.P., Crofton, P.M., Sarkar, M.A., et al. 2002. Malnutrition, zinc supplementation and catch-up growth: Changes in insulin-like growth factor I, its binding proteins, bone formation and collagen turnover. *Clin Endocrinol (Oxf)* 57: 391–399.

Eastell, E.R. and Hannon, R.A. 2008. Biomarkers of bone health and osteoporosis risk. *Proc Nutr Soc* 67: 157–162.

Eastell, R. and Lambert, H. 2002. Diet and healthy bones. *Calcif Tiss Int* 70: 400–404.

Ene-Obong, H.N., Odoh, I.F. and Ikwuagwu, O.E. 2003 Plasma vitamin A and C status of in-school adolescents and associated factors in Enugu State, Nigeria. *J Health Pop Nutr* 21: 18–25.

Eveleth, P.B. and Tanner, J.M. 1991. *Worldwide Variation in Human Growth. 2nd edition*, Cambridge: Cambridge University Press. Stanford CA.

Falaiye, J.M. 1971. Present status of subclinical intestinal malabsorption in the tropics. *Br Med J* 4: 454–458.

Fawell, J., Bailey, K., Chilton, J., et al. 2006. *Fluoride in drinking-water*, London: World Health Organization and IWA Publishing.

Ferrari, S.L., Chevalley, T., Bonjour, J.P., et al. 2006. Childhood fractures are associated with decreased bone mass gain during puberty: An early marker of persistent bone fragility? *J Bone Miner Res* 21: 501–507.

Garn, S.M., Poznanski, A.K. and Nagy, J.M. 1971. Bone measurement in the differential diagnosis of osteopenia and osteoporosis. *Radiology* 100: 509–518.

Glorieux, F., Jueppner, H. and Pettifor, J.M. 2003. *Pediatric Bone—Biology and Disease.* San Diego, CA: Elsevier Science.

Goulding, A., Jones, I.E., Taylor, R.W., et al. 2000. More broken bones: A 4-year double cohort study of young girls with and without distal forearm fractures. *J Bone Miner Res* 15: 2011–2018.

Goulding, A., Jones, I.E., Taylor, R.W., et al. 2001. Bone mineral density and body composition in boys with distal forearm fractures: A dual energy x-ray absorptiometry study. *J Pediatr* 139: 509–515.

Greef, R.M. 1997. *The Effects of High Fluoride Intake on Schoolchildren in Kwandebele, South Africa.* Johannesburg, South Africa: University of the Witwatersrand. PhD thesis.

Greulich, W.W. and Pyle, S.I. 1959. *Radiographic Atlas of Skeletal Development of Hand and Wrist 2nd revised edition*. Stanford University Press. Stanford CA.

Grillenberger, M., Neumann, C.G., Murphy, S.P., et al. 2006. Intake of micronutrients high in animal-source foods is associated with better growth in rural Kenyan school children. *Br J Nutr* 95: 379–390.

Gross, R., Benade, S. and Lopez, G. 2005. The International Research on Infant Supplementation Initiative. *J Nutr* 135: 628S–630S.

Hallund, J., Hatløy, A., Benesi, I., et al. 2008. Snacks are important for fat and vitamin intakes among rural African women: A cross-sectional study from Malawi. *Eur J Clin Nutr* 62: 866–871.

Hawley, N.L., Rousham, E.K., Norris, S.A., et al. 2009. Secular trends in skeletal maturity in South Africa: 1962–2001. *Ann Hum Biol* 36: 584–594.

Heaney, R.P. 2001. The bone remodeling transient: Interpreting interventions involving bone-related nutrients. *Nut Revs* 59: 327–334.

Heaney, R.P., Abrams, S., Dawson-Hughes, B., et al. 2000. Peak bone mass. *Osteoporos Int* 11: 985–1009.

Hess, S.Y., Zimmermann, M.B., Staubli-Asobayire, F., et al. 1999. An evaluation of salt intake and iodine nutrition in a rural and urban area of the Côte d'Ivoire. *Eur J Clin Nutr* 53: 680–686.

Holick, M.F. 1981. The cutaneous photosynthesis of previtamin D3: A unique photoendocrine system. *J Invest Dermatol* 77: 51–58.

Holick, M.F. 2004. Sunlight and vitamin D for bone health and prevention of autoimmune diseases, cancers, and cardiovascular disease. *Am J Clin Nutr* 80 (Suppl 6): 1678S–1688S.

Holick, M.F. 2005. Photobiology of vitamin D. In *Vitamin D, 2nd edition.* Feldman, D., Pike, J.W. and Glorieux, F.H., eds., pp. 37–46. Burlington, MA: Elsevier Academic Press.

Horst, R.L., Reinhardt, T.A. and Reddy, G.S. 2005. Vitamin D metabolism. In *Vitamin D. 2nd edition*, Feldman, D., Pike, J.W. and Glorieux, F.H., eds., pp. 15–36. Burlington, MA: Elsevier Academic Press.

Jablonski, N.G. and Chaplin, G. 2000. The evolution of human skin coloration. *J Hum Evol* 39: 57–106.

Jarjou, L.M., Prentice, A., Sawo, Y., et al. 2006. Randomized, placebo-controlled, calcium supplementation study in pregnant Gambian women: Effects on breast-milk calcium concentrations and infant birth weight, growth, and bone mineral accretion in the first year of life. *Am J Clin Nutr* 83: 657–666.

Juul, A., Bang, P., Hertel, N.T., et al. 1994. Serum insulin-like growth factor-I in 1030 healthy children, adolescents, and adults: Relation to age, sex, stage of puberty, testicular size, and body mass index. *J Clin Endocrinol Metab* 78: 744–752.

Khosla, S., Melton III, L.J., Dekutoski, M.B., et al. 2003. Incidence of childhood distal forearm fractures over 30 years. A population based study. *J Am Med Assoc* 290: 1479–1485.

Langley-Evans, S.C. 2006. Developmental programming of health and disease. *Proc Nutr Soc* 65: 97–105.

Levine, R.A. 2003. Biochemical markers of bone metabolism: Application to understanding bone remodeling in children and adolescents. *J Pediatr Endocrinol Metab* 16 (Suppl 3): 661–672.

Lewis, C.P., Lavy, C.B.D. and Harrison, W.J. 2002. Delay in skeletal maturity in Malawian children. *J Bone Joint Surg* 84-B: 732–734.

Lo, C.W., Jarjou, L.M.A., Poppitt, S., et al. 1991. Delayed development of bone mass in West African Adolescents. In *Osteoporosis 1990*, Christiansen, C. and Overgaard, H., eds, pp. 73–77. Aalborg, Denmark: Handelstrykveriat.

Lo, C.W., Paris, P.W. and Holick, M.F. 1986. Indian and Pakistani immigrants have the same capacity as Caucasians to produce vitamin D in response to ultraviolet irradiation. *Am J Clin Nutr* 44: 683–685.

Lunn, P.G. 2002. Growth retardation and stunting of children in developing countries. *Br J Nutr* 88: 109–110.

MacKeown, J.M., Cleaton-Jones, P.E., Edwards, A.W., et al. 1998. Energy, macro- and micronutrient intake of 5-year old urban black South African children in 1984 and 1995. *Pediatr Perinatal Epidemiol* 12: 297–312.

MacLaughlin, J. and Holick, M.F. 1985. Aging decreases the capacity of human skin to produce vitamin D3. *J Clin Invest* 76: 1536–1538.

Malde, M.K., Zerihun, L., Julshamn, K., et al. 2003. Fluoride intake in children living in a high-fluoride area in Ethiopia—intake through beverages. *Int J Ped Dent* 13: 27–34.

Malde, M.K., Zerihun, L., Julshamn, K., et al. 2004. Fluoride, calcium and magnesium intake in children living in a high-fluoride area in Ethiopia. Intake through food. *Int J Ped Dent* 14: 167–174.

Malvy, D.J., Guinot, C., Preziosi, P., et al. 2000. Relationship between vitamin D status and skin phototype in general adult population. *Photochem Photobiol* 71: 466–469.

Marcus, R., Feldman, D. and Kelsey, J., eds. 1996. *Osteoporosis.* San Diego: Academic Press.

Marshall, D., Johnell, O. and Wedel, H. 1996. Meta-analysis of how well measures of bone mineral density predict occurrence of osteoporotic fractures. *Br Med J* 312: 1254–1259.

Mayoral, L.G., Tripathy, K., Garcia, F.T., et al. 1967. Malabsorption in the tropics: A second look. *Am J Clin Nutr* 20: 866–883.

McVeigh, J.A., Norris, S.A. and Pettifor, J.M. 2007. Bone mass accretion rates in pre- and early-pubertal South African black and white children in relation to habitual physical activity and dietary calcium intakes. *Acta Paediatr* 96: 874–880.

Meema, M.E. 1962. The occurrence of cortical bone atrophy in old age and in osteoporosis. *J Can Med Assoc* 13: 27–32.

Mennen, L.I., Mbanya, J.C., Cade, J., et al. 2000. The habitual diet in rural and urban Cameroon. *Eur J Clin Nutr* 54: 150–154.

Menzies, I.S., Zuckerman, M.J., Nukajam, W.S., et al. 1999. Geography of intestinal permeability and absorption. *Gut* 44: 483–489.

Micklesfield, L.K., Norris, S.A., Nelson, D.A., et al. 2007. Comparisons of body size, composition, and whole body bone mass between North American and South African children. *J Bone Miner Res* 22: 1869–1877.

Mølgaard, C., Thomsen, B.L. and Michaelsen, K.F. 1998. Influence of weight, age and puberty on bone size and bone mineral content in healthy children and adolescents. *Acta Paediatr* 87: 494–499.

Munday, K., Ginty, F., Fulford, A., et al. 2006. Relationships between biochemical bone turnover markers, season, and inflammatory status indices in prepubertal Gambian boys. *Calcif Tiss Int* 79: 15–21.

Murphy, S.P., Calloway, D.H. and Beaton, G.H. 1995. Schoolchildren have similar predicted prevalences of inadequate intakes as toddlers in village populations in Egypt, Kenya and Mexico. *Eur J Clin Nutr* 49: 647–657.

Norman, A.W. 2008. From vitamin D to hormone D: Fundamentals of the vitamin D endocrine system essential for good health. *Am J Clin Nutr* 88: 491S–499S.

Norris, S.A., Sheppard, Z.A., Griffiths, P.L., et al. 2008. Current socio-economic measures, and not those measured during infancy, affect bone mass in poor urban South African children. *J Bone Miner Res* 23: 1409–1416.

Nyati, H.L., Norris, S.A., Cameron, N., et al. 2006. Effect of ethnicity and sex on the growth of the axial and appendicular skeleton of children living in a developing country. *Am J Phys Anthropol* 130: 135–141.

Okonofua, F., Gill, D.S., Alabi, Z.O., et al. 1991. Rickets in Nigerian children: A consequence of calcium malnutrition. *Metabolism* 40: 209–213.

Parfitt, A.M. 2002. Misconceptions (1): Epiphyseal fusion causes cessation of growth. *Bone* 30: 337–339.

Patel, D.N., Pettifor, J.M. and Becker, P.J. 1993. The effect of ethnicity on appendicular bone mass in white, coloured and Indian schoolchildren. *South Afr Med J* 83: 847–853.

Pettifor, J.M. 2003. Nutritional rickets. In *Pediatric Bone—Biology and Disease*, Glorieux, F., Jueppner, H. and Pettifor, J.M., eds., pp. 541–566. San Diego, CA: Elsevier Science.

Pettifor, J.M. 2008. Vitamin D and/or calcium deficiency rickets in infants and children: A global perspective. *Ind J Med Res* 127: 245–249.

Prentice, A. 2001. The relative contribution of diet and genotype to bone development. *Proc Nutr Soc* 60: 1–8.

Prentice, A. 2004. Diet, nutrition and osteoporosis. *Pub Health Nutr* 7: 237–254.

Prentice, A. 2007. Studies of Gambian and UK children and adolescents: Insights into calcium requirements and adaptation to a low calcium intake. *Int Cong Ser* 1297: 15–24.

Prentice, A. 2008. Vitamin D deficiency: A global perspective. *Nut Revs* 66: S153–S164.

Prentice, A. and Bates, C.J. 1994. Adequacy of dietary mineral supply for human bone growth and mineralisation. *Eur J Clin Nutr* 48(Suppl 1): S161–S176.

Prentice, A., Bonjour, J.-P., Branca, F., et al. 2003. PASSCLAIM—Bone health and osteoporosis. *Eur J Nutr* 42 (Suppl 1): I/28–I/49.

Prentice, A., Branca, F., Decsi, T., et al. 2004. Energy and nutrient dietary reference values for children in Europe: Methodological approaches and current nutritional recommendations. *Br J Nutr* 92 (Suppl 2): S83–S146.

Prentice, A., Ceesay, M., Nigdikar, S., et al. 2008a. FGF23 is elevated in Gambian children with rickets. *Bone* 42: 788–797.

Prentice, A., Goldberg, G.R. and Schoenmakers, I. 2008b. Vitamin D across the lifecycle: Physiology and biomarkers. *Am J Clin Nutr* 88: 500S–506S.

Prentice, A., Jarjou, L.M., Cole, T.J., et al. 1995. Calcium requirements of lactating Gambian mothers: Effects of a calcium supplement on breast-milk calcium concentration, maternal bone mineral content, and urinary calcium excretion. *Am J Clin Nutr* 62: 58–67.

Prentice, A., Laskey, M.A. and Jarjou, L.M.A. 1999. Lactation and bone development: Implications for the calcium requirements of infants and lactating mothers. In *Nutrition and Bone Development*, Bonjour, J.P. and Tsang, R.C., eds., pp. 127–145. Philadelphia: Vestey/Lippincott-Raven Publishers.

Prentice, A., Laskey, M.A., Shaw, J., et al. 1990. Bone mineral content of Gambian and British children aged 0–36 months. *Bone Miner* 10: 211–224.

Prentice, A., Parsons, T.J. and Cole, T.J. 1994. Uncritical use of bone mineral density in absorptiometry may lead to size-related artifacts in the identification of bone mineral determinants. *Am J Clin Nutr* 60: 837–842.

Prentice, A., Schoenmakers, I., Jones, K.S., et al. 2009. Vitamin D deficiency and its health consequences in Africa. *Clin Rev Bone Miner Metab* 94–106.

Prentice, A., Schoenmakers, I., Laskey, M.A., et al. 2006. Nutrition and bone growth and development. *Proc Nutr Soc* 65: 348–360.

Prentice, A., Shaw, J., Laskey, M.A., et al. 1991. Bone mineral content of British and rural Gambian women aged 18–80+ years. *Bone Miner* 12: 201–214.

Prentice, A.M. 2009. Regional case studies—Africa. In *Emerging Societies—Coexistence of Childhood Malnutrition and Obesity, Nestlé Nutr Inst Workshop Ser Pediatr Program, vol 63*, Kalhan, S.C., Prentice, A.M. and Yajnik, C.S., eds., pp. 33–46. Basel, Switzerland: Nestec Ltd., Vevey/S. Karger AG.

Prentice, S., Fulford, A.J., Jarjou, L.M.A., et al. 2010. Evidence for a downward secular trend in age of menarche in a rural Gambian population. *Ann Hum Biol* in press.

Rauchenzauner, M., Schmid, A., Heinz-Erian, P., et al. 2007. Sex- and age-specific reference curves for serum markers of bone turnover in healthy children from 2 months to 18 years. *J Clin Endocrinol Metab* 92: 443–449.

Reed, F.A. and Tishkoff, S.A. 2006. African human diversity, origins and migrations. *Curr Opin Genet Dev* 16: 597–605.

Roche, A.F., Chumlea, W., Thissen, D. 1988. Assessing the skeletal maturity of the hand-wrist: FELS method. Springfield IL: Charles C Thomas Publisher Ltd.

Scariano, J.K., Vanderjagt, D.J., Thacher, T., et al. 1998. Calcium supplements increase the serum levels of crosslinked N-telopeptides of bone collagen and parathyroid hormone in rachitic Nigerian children. *Clin Biochem* 31: 421–427.

Schnitzler, C.M., Mesquita, J.M. and Pettifor, J.M. 2009. Cortical bone development in black and white South African children: Iliac crest histomorphometry. *Bone Miner* 44: 603–611.

Schoenmakers, I., Goldberg, G.R. and Prentice, A. 2008. Abundant sunshine and vitamin D deficiency. *Br J Nutr* 99: 1171–1173.

Scientific Advisory Committee on Nutrition. 2007. *Update on Vitamin D*, London: The Stationery Office.

Slemenda, C.W., Peacock, M., Hui, S., et al. 1997. Reduced rates of skeletal remodeling are associated with increased bone mineral density during the development of peak skeletal mass. *J Bone Miner Res* 12: 676–682.

Solomon, L. 1968. Osteoporosis and fracture of the femoral neck in the South African Bantu. *J Bone Joint Surg* 50: 2–13.

Stein, A.D., Wang, M., Martorell, R., et al. 2009. Growth patterns in early childhood and final attained stature: Data from five birth cohorts from low- and middle-income countries. *Am J Hum Biol* 22: 353–359.

Szulc, P., Seeman, E. and Delmas, P.D. 2000. Biochemical measurements of bone turnover in children and adolescents. *Osteoporos Int* 11: 281–294.

Tanner, J.M., Whitehouse, R.H., Cameron, N., et al. 1983. *The Assessment of Skeletal Maturity and the Prediction of Adult Height (TW2 Method), Second Ed.* London: Academic Press.

Thacher, T.D., Fischer, P.R., Pettifor, J.M., et al. 2000. Case–Control study of factors associated with nutritional rickets in Nigerian children. *J Pediatr* 137: 367–373.

Thacher, T.D., Fischer, P.R., Strand, M.A., et al. 2006. Nutritional rickets around the world: Causes and future directions. *Ann Trop Paediatr* 26: 1–16.

Thandrayen, K., Norris, S.A. and Pettifor, J.M. 2009. Fracture rates in urban South African children of different ethnic origins: The Birth to Twenty cohort. *Osteoporos Int* 20: 47–52.

UNICEF/WHO. 2009. *Diarrhoea: Why Children Are Still Dying and What Can Be Done*, Geneva, Switzerland: World Health Organization.

van't Riet, H., den Hartog, A.P. and van Staveren, W.A. 2002. Non-home prepared foods: Contribution to energy and nutrient intake of consumers living in two low-income areas in Nairobi. *Pub Health Nutr* 5: 515–522.

van Wesenbeeck, C., Keyzer, M.A. and Nube, M. 2009. Estimation of undernutrition and mean calorie intake in Africa: Methodology, findings and implications. *Int J Health Geograph* 8: 37.

Vidulich, L., Norris, S.A., Cameron, N., et al. 2007. Infant programming of bone size and bone mass in 10-year-old black and white South African children. *Pediatr Perinatal Epidemiol* 21: 354–362.

Violari, A., Cotton, M.F., Gibb, D.M., et al. 2008. Early antiretroviral therapy and mortality among HIV-infected infants. *New Eng J Med* 359: 2233–2244.

Walingo, M.K. and Musamali, B. 2008. Nutrient intake and nutritional status indicators of participant and non-participant pupils of a parent-supported school lunch program in Kenya. *J Nut Ed Behav* 40: 298–304.

Webb, A.R. 2006. Who, what, where and when—influences on cutaneous vitamin D synthesis. *Prog Biophys Mol Biol* 92: 17–25.

Willett, A.M. 2005. Vitamin D status and its relationship with parathyroid hormone and bone mineral status in older adolescents. *Proc Nutr Soc* 64: 193–203.

Wolmarans, P. 2009. Background paper on global trends in food production, intake and composition. *Ann Nutr Metab* 55: 244–272.

World Health Organization. 2003. *Prevention and Management of Osteoporosis. Report of a WHO Scientific Group. WHO Technical Report Series 921*, Geneva, Switzerland: WHO.

World Health Organization. 2009. *World Health Statistics 2009*, Geneva, Switzerland: WHO.

World Health Organization Regional Offices for Africa and Eastern Mediterranean. 2006. *The Africa Malaria Report 2006*, Geneva, Switzerland: WHO.

World Health Organization Technical Consultation. 2006. *Towards the Development of a Strategy for Promoting Optimal Fetal Development*, Geneva, Switzerland: WHO.

Yan, L., Zhou, B., Prentice, A., et al. 1999. Epidemiological study of hip fracture in Shenyang, People's Republic of China. *Bone* 24: 151–155.

Yang, L. and Grey, V. 2006. Pediatric reference intervals for bone markers. *Clin Biochem* 39: 561–568.

Zebaze, R.M.D. and Seeman, E. 2003. Epidemiology of hip and wrist fractures in Cameroon, Africa. *Osteoporos Int* 14: 301–305.

29 Skeletal Racial Differences

Felicia Cosman and Jeri W. Nieves

CONTENTS

INTRODUCTION

Fracture rates and bone density levels differ in people of different racial groups. Previous investigations have revealed potential racial differences in body composition and skeletal size and structure, which may play a role in determining fracture risk. In addition, racial differences in calcium intake, vitamin D status, and bone metabolism have been reported. This chapter provides an overview of the racial differences that can have an impact on the skeleton. In this chapter, the terms *African American* and *black*, and *Caucasian* and *white*, are used interchangeably.

FRACTURE RATES

Epidemiologic data from several U.S. population studies confirm that Caucasian women have consistently higher fracture rates in the hip (Cauley et al., 2005b; Cummings and Melton, 2002; Fang et al., 2004; Karagas et al., 1996; Silverman and Madison, 1988) and the rest of the skeleton compared with African American women (Baron et al., 1996; Barrett et al., 1999; Cummings and Melton, 2002; Griffin et al., 1992). A sample of 1.4 million people from a large Medicare database was used to calculate the actuarial risk of hip fracture for a 65-year-old having a hip fracture before the age of 90 years. Resulting lifetime fracture risks were 16% for a white woman and 5.3% for a black woman (Barrett et al., 1999). In the same sample, the actuarial risk of a 65-year-old having a fracture by the age of 90 years at other skeletal sites for Caucasian and African Americans, respectively, was 9.1% and 2.4% for the distal forearm, 5.0% and 1.1 % for the proximal humerus, and 3.9% and 2.4% for the ankle. Therefore, white women will have actuarial fracture risks between 1.5- and 4-fold higher than will black females depending on the skeletal site (Barrett et al., 1999). In the National Osteoporosis Risk Factor Assessment (NORA) database (total cohort of 197,848 women above the age of 50 years), the 1-year incidence of any fracture was 1.5% for white women and 0.8% for black women (Barrett-Connor et al., 2005). Other studies have confirmed that Asian (Xu et al., 1996) and Asian American (Lauderdale et al., 1997; Silverman and Madison, 1988) individuals have relatively low rates of hip fracture, whereas vertebral fracture rates in most studies have been reported to be similar to that of American white populations (Lau et al., 1996; Ling et al., 2000).

In a recent study, the comparison of African Americans and Hispanics versus whites led to adjusted hazard ratios for fracture (0.37 and 0.46, respectively), indicating a considerably lower fracture rate in not only African Americans but also Hispanics (Cummings et al., 1994; Mikhail et al., 1996; Nelson et al., 2000; Theobald et al., 1998; Wolinsky et al., 2009). In the recently published FRAX model, the ratio of hip fracture incidence rates for the following races as compared with white women was black females, 0.43; Hispanics, 0.53; and Asian women, 0.50 (Dawson-Hughes et al., 2008). In a multivariate logistic regression model of hip fracture risk in the Women's Health Initiative observational study, the odds ratio (OR) for each race/ethnicity for Asian, Hispanic, and Blacks were 0.26, 0.32, and 0.41, respectively (Robbins et al., 2007). Among 911,327 beneficiaries with 6 or 7 years of Medicare coverage, the overall prevalence of osteoporosis was lowest for African American women (22.2%) then Caucasian (44.1%) and highest (52.9%) for Asian American women (Cheng et al., 2009).

Racial differences in fracture risk have been ascribed, in part, to differences in body composition, body size, bone mass, and bone size (Aloia, 2008; Aloia et al., 1997; Cauley et al., 1994; Gilsanz et al., 1998; Kleerekoper et al., 1994b; Liel et al., 1988; Nelson et al., 2006; Seeman, 1998). Differences in hip and pelvic geometry, including shorter hip–axis length, thicker cortical bone in the hip, and smaller endocortical diameter in the femoral neck of black individuals as compared with whites, may also contribute to a lower fracture risk in black women (Cummings et al., 1994; Mikhail et al., 1996; Nelson et al., 2000; Theobald et al., 1998). However, in the NORA study, after adjusting for BMD, weight, and other covariates, white and Hispanic women had the highest risk for fracture, followed by Native Americans, blacks, and Asian Americans (Barrett-Connor et al., 2005).

BONE MINERAL DENSITY

The racial difference in fracture rates is consistent with the differences in bone mineral density (BMD) observed among racial groups (Barrett-Connor et al., 2005; Cauley et al., 2005b; Finkelstein et al., 2002a; Kleerekoper et al., 1994b; Looker et al., 1995; Pollitzer and Anderson, 1989). African American women also have higher BMD at peripheral sites than do other racial groups, including Caucasian, Asian, Hispanic, and Native Americans (Barrett-Connor et al., 2005). Results from the National Health and Nutrition Examination Survey (NHANES) III indicated an 11% to 17% difference in BMD at the hip between blacks and whites of both males and females at different ages, results that are similar to numerous other studies (Barrett-Connor et al., 2005; Cauley et al., 2005b; Finkelstein et al., 2002b; Kleerekoper et al., 1994b; Liel et al., 1988; Looker et al., 1995; Luckey et al., 1989, 1996; Meier et al., 1992).

Racial differences in the skeleton begin early in life. BMD is higher in African American than in American white, Asian, or Hispanic children (Bachrach et al., 1999; Kalkwarf et al., 2007). Bone accrual was reported to be lower in Asian compared with Caucasian children from a very young age (Burrows et al., 2009). Most, but not all, (Barrett-Connor et al., 2005) studies in adults indicate that Hispanic Americans have similar (Cauley et al., 2005a; Looker et al., 1998; Morton et al., 2003) or slightly higher (Marcus et al., 1994) BMD compared with American whites. Studies in Asians have consistently shown lower BMD than that in whites (Walker et al., 2006; Woo et al., 2001; Xiaoge et al., 2000), although correction for weight or bone size minimizes these differences (Bhudhikanok et al., 1996; Duan et al., 2005; Finkelstein et al., 2002a; Weaver et al., 2007). Bone mass in the proximal femur of native Chinese women was significantly lower, and the rate of bone loss greater, than those of non-Asian women in the United States(Hou et al., 2007). In addition, rates of bone loss may vary by race. Significantly lower rates of postmenopausal bone loss were seen in blacks versus whites at both the total hip and femoral neck in the Study of Osteoporotic Fracture cohort (age range 65 to 99 years) (Cauley et al., 2005b). In a much smaller cohort, however, slower bone loss rates in black women versus white women in the spine and forearm were seen only in early postmenopausal women (Luckey et al., 1996). Different regions of the skeleton may show varying differences in bone mass; the difference between bone density of African Americans and women of other ethnicities seems most apparent at the more trabecular skeletal sites (Cohn et al., 1977; Gilsanz et al., 1991; Kleerekoper et al., 1994a; Li et al., 1989; Liel et al., 1988; Luckey et al., 1989; Nelson et al., 1995; Prentice et al., 1991; Specker et al., 1987). Differences in BMD between races persist but are slightly reduced when BMD is adjusted for weight, bone size, and other lifestyle variables (Cauley et al., 2005a; Finkelstein et al., 2002b). Data from the Study of Women's Health Across the Nation indicate that apparent ethnic differences in rates of BMD loss during the menopause transition are largely due to ethnic differences in body weight (Finkelstein et al., 2008).

Factors other than BMD that may account for racial differences in fracture incidence include variability in hip–axis length, bone size, and rates of bone loss. At the femoral neck, the volumetric BMD (vBMD) of Chinese women was similar to that of non-Hispanic white women (Hou et al., 2007). Black and Asian men have features in the proximal femur that may confer advantages for bone strength. Specifically, greater cortical thickness and higher trabecular vBMD among black and Asian men could help explain the lower hip fracture rates in these populations over the age of 65 years (Marshall et al., 2008). Newer technology in the imaging of bone has led to an increased understanding of these differences. vBMD and microarchitectural properties were assessed using high-resolution peripheral quantitative computed tomography (HRpQCT). Mean areal BMD was similar between 31 Chinese American and 32 Caucasian premenopausal women. However, HRpQCT at the radius and tibia indicated greater trabecular and cortical density, trabecular bone volume, and trabecular and cortical thickness, with lower total bone area in the Chinese versus white women (Walker et al., 2009). HRpQCT was also used to evaluate 61 healthy premenopausal Chinese and 111 white women 18–45 years of age, and the data indicate that the Chinese had thicker cortices and trabeculae within a smaller bone than did whites. These differences in macrostructure and microstructure of the distal radius and tibia may account for the lower fracture rates in Asians than in whites (Wang et al., 2009). Asian adolescents were reported to have higher "speed of sound" ultrasound values at the heel compared with white adolescents living in Hawaii (Novotny et al., 2004).

Several other factors including differences in body composition and lifestyle factors may relate to BMD differences. Hip, but not spine BMD, was higher in Mexican Americans than in Asian Americans after adjustment for age, body mass index, income, and physical activity index. Lean body mass was a significant predictor of hip BMD for both groups, and this relationship was stronger for the Asian group, indicating that lean body mass may explain some of the ethnic differences in BMD (Crespo et al., 2009). In a recent Canadian study of bone accrual over 7 years in Asian and Caucasian women; physical activity, dietary calcium, and lean mass positively influenced bone accrual, and all of these were lower in Asian compared with Caucasian children beginning at a very young age (Burrows et al., 2009). In another study, skeletal differences in bone mineral content (BMC) at the total body, distal radius, lumbar spine, and total hip among white, Asian, and Hispanic groups during growth were explained by differences in bone area, sexual maturity, physical activity, and dairy calcium intake. Bone size explained most of the racial/ethnic differences in BMC, although physical activity and diet were also significant predictors of BMC (Weaver et al., 2007).

Differences in bone mass among racial groups may also be affected by cultural, historical, and geographical traits that are determined by ethnicity, in addition to genetic traits (Burchard et al., 2003). Examples of ethnic behaviors that may impact on the skeleton include cultural differences in dietary intake, physical activity, and limiting exposure to sunlight (Walker et al., 2008).

VITAMIN D, CALCIUM, AND BONE METABOLISM

Differences in BMD among ethnic groups have been investigated to determine if variability in vitamin D and calcium metabolism, or racial differences in skeletal metabolism may account for the racial differences in BMD, and potentially fracture risk.

BLACKS

The findings, regarding lower fracture risk and higher BMD in blacks versus whites, are surprising in light of what is known about vitamin D status in blacks. Mean serum 25-hydroxyvitamin D (25OHD or calcidiol) concentrations are lower in blacks versus whites at all stages of life, and a greater proportion of blacks meet criteria for vitamin D deficiency or insufficiency with any of the multiple cut points used (Bell et al., 1985; Bikle et al., 1999; Dawson-Hughes et al., 1995; Ettinger et al., 1997; Harris et al., 2000; Henry and Eastell, 2000; Kleerekoper et al., 1994a; Looker et al., 2002; Meier et al., 1991; Nesby-O'dell et al., 2002; Wigertz et al., 2005), with only one exception (Meier et al., 1991). For example, winter measurements from southern latitude populations from NHANES III indicate that 13%–33% of white men and women above the age of 60 years versus 33%–69% of black men and women of similar age have 25OHD levels below 50 nmol/L (Looker et al., 2002). The racial difference in serum 25OHD level primarily results from increased pigmentation that reduces vitamin D production in the skin (Clemens et al., 1982; Matsuoka et al., 1991). Seasonal differences in 25OHD levels are correspondingly blunted in blacks (Harris and Dawson-Hughes, 1998; Webb et al., 1988). Vitamin D intakes are also lower in blacks than those in whites, in part related to reduced consumption of D-fortified milk, milk products, and cereals (Harris et al., 2000; Moore et al., 2005).

In African Americans, vitamin D deficiency, assessed by serum 25OHD, generally exists across the life cycle. So how can the black skeleton remain strong in the face of vitamin D deficiency? Norman Bell proposed, in 1985, that although blacks had the expected secondary hyperparathyroidism in response to vitamin D deficiency, the fact that bone turnover markers were lower in blacks (assessed both biochemically and histomorphometrically) indicated that the skeleton was resistant to the effects of parathyroid hormone (PTH) (Bell et al., 1985; Weinstein and Bell, 1988). In contrast, renal conservation of calcium in response to PTH, with respect to urinary calcium excretion, is preserved in blacks. In both cases, the skeleton would be protected against the effects of low 25OHD.

In response to lower serum 25OHD levels, in addition to lower average calcium intake (Bell et al., 2002; Bronner et al., 2006; Harris et al., 2000; Heaney, 2006), black women have relative secondary hyperparathyroidism (average PTH levels in the upper normal range that are significantly higher than those of white women). The resultant higher levels of 1,25-dihydroxyvitamin D [1,25(OH)$_2$D] and lower urinary calcium excretion helped to conserve bone. Populations demonstrating these elevations in PTH levels include premenopausal and postmenopausal black women and men (Bikle et al., 1999; Bryant et al., 2003; Dawson-Hughes et al., 1995; Moore et al., 2005; Weinstein and Bell, 1988). For example, in the Boston Low Income Elderly Osteoporosis study (Harris et al., 2000), in women and men, mean serum PTH levels were elevated in blacks versus whites, and the prevalence of relative secondary hyperparathyroidism in black women and men was almost twice that of whites in both genders. Serum 1,25(OH)$_2$D levels were higher in blacks versus whites in studies involving children, adolescents, young, and older adult men and women in most studies (Bikle et al., 1999; Kleerekoper et al., 1994a), but not all (Meier et al., 1991). Higher serum PTH concentrations in African Americans are an appropriate response to lower dietary intakes of calcium and vitamin D, as well as to lower rates of biosynthesis of vitamin D in melanin-rich skin. However, African Americans seem to avoid the skeletal catabolic effects of PTH.

A deficiency of 25OHD is common in all ethnic groups in the United States; in fact, 9% of the pediatric population was 25OHD deficient, and 61% were 25OHD insufficient. Vitamin D deficiency, even in children, was associated with elevated PTH levels (OR = 3.6; 1.8 to 7.1), compared with those with 25OHD levels ≥30 ng/mL (Kumar et al., 2009). Also consistent with a state of mild relative secondary hyperparathyroidism, urinary calcium excretion is typically lower in blacks versus whites across age groups from children to older adults (Bell et al., 1993; Bryant et al., 2003; Dawson-Hughes et al., 1995; Ettinger et al., 1997; Kleerekoper et al., 1994a; Meier et al., 1992; Wigertz et al., 2005). The average urinary calcium excretion in black children was reported to be about half that in white children (84 vs. 165 mg/day) (Bell et al., 1993). In one study, urinary calcium excretion was 46% lower in black compared with white adolescent girls (Bryant et al., 2003), and another study confirmed that black adolescent girls had greater renal calcium retention at both low and high sodium intake diets (Wigertz et al., 2005). Lower urinary calcium excretion in adult black women and men has also been reported (Bikle et al., 1999; Ettinger et al., 1997). Black women were reported to have lower urinary calcium excretion in response to 1,25(OH)$_2$D administration compared with white women (Dawson-Hughes et al., 1995). In postmenopausal women, a racial difference in urinary calcium excretion was also demonstrated (Kleerekoper et al., 1994a).

Whereas the data are consistent for renal calcium handling, whether racial differences exist in intestinal calcium absorption is not clear. In one study, no racial differences were found in calcium absorption efficiency in children (Bell et al., 1993), but in two other studies, greater calcium absorption occurred in black compared with white adolescents (Abrams et al., 1995; Bryant et al., 2003). In another study, there were no racial differences in calcium absorption in premenopausal women (Dawson-Hughes et al., 1993), and furthermore, the increment in calcium absorption to provocative testing with 1,25(OH)$_2$D was actually blunted in black women (Dawson-Hughes et al., 1995). In a calcium balance study in African American and white adolescent girls, African Americans had greater calcium retention with higher rates of calcium and a higher bone formation rate. African American girls also had higher calcium absorption efficiency, when serum 25OHD levels were similar, perhaps as a result of higher concentrations of serum 1,25(OH)$_2$D. These girls also had lower urinary calcium excretion, indicating superior renal conservation (Bryant et al., 2003). In a pooled sample of 182 balance studies in American white and black adolescent girls, calcium intake explained 12.3% and race explained 13.7% of the variance in calcium retention (Braun et al., 2007). Whether Hispanics or Asians have any difference in calcium absorption as compared with whites is not known.

Despite the relative secondary hyperparathyroidism, biochemical measurements of bone turnover levels are, in general, lower in blacks compared with whites. Although not all data are consistent, the expected finding in a population with relative secondary hyperparathyroidism would be an increase in bone turnover, not a decrease, as most studies report. Some inconsistencies in studies may relate to differences among the bone turnover markers chosen, analytical issues, methods of sample collection, assays used, differential effects in different populations, population sizes, diurnal variation, and effects of exercise and other biological variables. Lower levels of osteocalcin in blacks as compared with whites have been shown quite consistently in young women, men, and perimenopausal or postmenopausal women (Bikle et al., 1999; Finkelstein et al., 2002b; Han et al., 1997; Meier et al., 1992). Lower levels of bone resorption markers have been shown in black compared with white premenopausal and perimenopausal women (Meier et al., 1992) and postmenopausal women (Aloia et al., 1998; Kleerekoper et al., 1994a; Meier et al., 1992), although not all studies were consistent (Harris et al., 2001). Slower rates of age-related bone loss (Cauley et al., 2005c; Tracy et al., 2005) or remodeling (Leder et al., 2007) might be protective as shown in comparisons between white American and African American adults.

In one calcium balance study, net calcium retention was higher in black versus white girls (greater formation vs. resorption) (Bryant et al., 2003). Clearly, African American adolescents had a higher rate of modeling than did white American adolescents, consistent with high rates of skeletal acquisition during growth.

Racial differences in skeletal and renal responses to (1-34)PTH administration by intravenous infusion over 24 hours were evaluated (Cosman et al., 1997). This study provided direct confirmation that the black skeleton is resistant to the bone-resorbing effects of PTH, whereas osteoblastic sensitivity to PTH is maintained and the renal response to PTH is heightened in blacks. The black skeleton seems to be protected against high ambient PTH levels by skeletal resistance to the bone-resorbing effects of PTH.

Histomorphometric assessments of racial differences comparing black and white premenopausal women are consistent with the biochemical bone turnover data (Han et al., 1997; Parfitt et al., 2000; Parisien et al., 1997). In one major study, 142 women, including 31 blacks and 108 whites, were enrolled. Of the total, 61 were premenopausal and 81 were postmenopausal. Expected estrogen-deficiency-related changes were seen in both races. Racial comparisons showed that mean bone formation rate and mineralizing surface were 25% lower in blacks compared with whites. In another study (Parisien et al., 1997), 21 black and 34 white premenopausal women, matched for education and socioeconomic class, as well as body size and weight, were enrolled. This study showed no racial difference in activation frequency of bone remodeling. Two studies (Han et al., 1997; Parfitt et al., 2000) found lower mineralizing surface and lower apposition rate and also adjusted mineral apposition rate (bone formation rate per osteoid surface) in black women, and the total formation period was longer. Rather than being detrimental to bone maintenance, a slower rate of bone formation may facilitate the development of bone of greater mass and greater strength. Furthermore, wall thickness was maintained in black women so that the ultimate amount of bone formed within each remodeling unit was not different between blacks and whites. Filling in the remodeling cavity simply appears to take longer in black women than in whites. A study performed in South Africa confirmed greater cancellous bone volume and trabecular thickness in blacks versus whites, but in sharp contrast to the U.S. studies, bone turnover was apparently higher in blacks than in whites. However, turnover in that study was only assessed by static variables (osteoid volume, surface and thickness, and eroded surface), which may account for the discrepancy (Schnitzler and Mesquita, 1998).

ASIANS

In Asian women, higher serum 25OHD concentrations are associated with higher BMD of the femoral neck. Serum 25OHD concentration of at least 50 nmol/L was needed to achieve normal PTH levels and prevent low BMD in home-dwelling postmenopausal Japanese women (Nakamura et al., 2008). South Asian women were found to be at high risk of hypovitaminosis D due in part to deliberate sun avoidance and an indoor lifestyle, with lowest vitamin D levels in winter and spring (von Hurst et al., 2009). A significant positive correlation has been found between serum vitamin D levels and BMD in South Asian women living in Britain (Roy et al., 2007), India (Arya et al., 2004), and Bangladesh (Islam et al., 2008).

In a study of Japanese college-aged women, the proportions of the subjects with low 25OHD (<30 nmol/L) and high intact PTH (≥6.9 pmol/L) concentrations were 32.4% and 15.7%, respectively. Serum 25OHD concentrations and calcium intake were inversely associated with serum intact PTH. In addition to weight and physical activity, the presence of mild hyperparathyroidism was associated with a low BMD of the lumbar spine and the femoral neck (Nakamura et al., 2005).

In a study of nine ethnic groups of Asian postmenopausal women participating in the Pan-Asia Menopause study, bone turnover markers were all significantly associated with ethnicity, independent of age and body mass index (Ausmanas et al., 2007; Holinka et al., 2008). The clinical significance of these findings remains to be established.

Calcidiol levels appear to be low in Asians, and there is some evidence that this relates to elevations in PTH levels and bone turnover and ultimately lower BMD.

ETHNIC DIFFERENCES IN LIFESTYLE FACTORS

Prior to puberty, differences in bone become associated with ethnicity, but differences in diet and physical activity also become apparent. In a cohort of sixth graders recruited from six geographical locations in the United States, composed of 326 American white, 234 Hispanic, and 188 Asian girls, bone size explained most differences in BMC based on race or ethnicity, although lifestyle factors such as dairy calcium intake and physical activity were also significant predictors of BMC (Weaver et al., 2007). In these children, models including race/ethnicity predicted BMC better than BMD, which in this age group is a more meaningful measure. Longitudinal studies have shown that calcium intake is a small but significant predictor of total body bone mass in Asian girls (Zhu et al., 2007) and Canadian boys, but not girls (Bailey et al., 2000).

A significant interaction between race and diet on bone has been observed with dietary salt in black and white adolescent girls (Wigertz et al., 2005). In balance studies where subjects were crossed over on high- and low-salt intakes, white girls excreted more sodium in urine on high-salt diets than did black girls, perhaps the result of higher urinary calcium excretion via shared Na/Ca transporters in the proximal tubule of the kidney. Calcium retention was lower with high-salt diets in both races, but the detrimental effect of salt was greater in white subjects. Calcium retention was higher in black girls consuming high-salt diets than that in white girls consuming low-salt diets.

Whether diet contributes to racial differences in rates of bone loss is not clear. Calcium intake within a number of racial groups is associated with higher BMD or slower rates of bone loss (Cauley et al., 2005a; Ho et al., 2004; Jackson et al., 2006). The beneficial effect of soy, likely due to phytoestrogens, which have been investigated particularly in Asian postmenopausal women, may result from a small effect on minimizing bone loss (Chen et al., 2003). Soy consumption was related to reduced fracture risk in a cohort of >75,000 Asian women living in Shanghai (Zhang et al., 2005). Research to determine whether this dietary effect on fracture risk is specific to race (Asian) or ethnicity (habitual soy consumption, for example) is needed. Protein intake may also influence bone loss (Hannan et al., 2000), although the effect may be dependent on adequate calcium intake (Dawson-Hughes and Harris, 2002). Nutritional and other lifestyle factors appear to explain only minimal differences in rates of bone loss among races.

Dairy products provide approximately three fourths of calcium consumed in the diet and are the most concentrated sources of calcium. The NHANES II results (Looker et al., 1993) showed that mean calcium intakes of white and Hispanic-American women were similar, within 60 mg for each age group. Asian Americans have been found to consume less dietary calcium when compared with the Caucasian population (Hirota et al., 1992; Kim et al., 1993; Wu-Tso et al., 1995). Approximately 50 million people in the United States are lactose intolerant (Bannan and Levitt, 1996; Srinivasan and Minocha, 1998), and the prevalence of lactose intolerance varies widely among ethnic groups. In the United States, some degree of primary lactose maldigestion occurs in an estimated 15% (6% to 19%) of whites, 53% of Mexican Americans, 62% to 100% of Native Americans, 80% of African Americans, and 90% of Asian Americans (Sahi, 1994). Clearly calcium consumption among many ethnic groups is reduced because of lactose intolerance. Several dietary management strategies exist for lactose maldigesters to increase calcium consumption including (1) consuming dairy foods with meals, (2) increasing intake of yogurts, (3) adding calcium-fortified foods, (4) using lactose-digestive aids, and (5) including dairy foods daily in the diet to enhance the colonic metabolism of lactose by bacteria.

VITAMIN D SUPPLEMENTATION

BLACKS

Aloia and colleagues enrolled 208 healthy postmenopausal women (age range 50 to 75 years) and randomly assigned them to receive 800 IU vitamin D_3 daily for 2 years and 2000 IU vitamin D_3 daily for 1 year or placebo (Aloia et al., 2005). Mean serum 25OHD levels increased as expected from baseline level of 18 to 28 ng/mL during the 800 IU daily dose and to 35 ng/mL during the 2000 IU daily dose. Nevertheless, over the 3-year trial, no significant differences in BMD change were found in the vitamin-D-supplemented compared with the placebo group. A second vitamin D supplementation study was composed of 79 postmenopausal women who received either 1000 IU vitamin D_3 daily or placebo for 2 years (Nieves et al., 2007). Expected increments in 25OHD were seen in the vitamin-D-supplemented group, although mean levels did not exceed 25 ng/mL at any time point. Over the 2-year trial, rates of bone loss were similar in the two groups at the spine, total hip, and greater trochanter but were slower in the femoral neck of the D-treated group. When BMD responses were evaluated as a function of the FOK-1 domain of the vitamin D receptor gene, the homozygous FF group showed more dramatic losses at all skeletal sites, and losses were blunted by vitamin D supplementation.

Lack of a consistent effect on rates of bone loss, particularly in African Americans, may be a function of inadequate vitamin D dose in relation to adipose stores, calcium supplementation in both active and control groups obfuscating treatment effects of vitamin D, or genetic variability of response in subgroups of black women. The skeletal and renal adaptations to vitamin D deficiency may be so effective that vitamin D supplementation might not confer any further benefit to the black skeleton. These findings, however, should not be extrapolated to de-emphasize the potential pluripotent benefits of vitamin D supplementation in nonskeletal tissues.

ASIANS

The effect of supplementing with a high calcium milk drink containing added vitamin D, magnesium and zinc versus a placebo drink on serum PTH concentration and vitamin D status as well as markers of bone formation/resorption in postmenopausal women living in South East Asia were studied over a period of 4 months. Fortified milk supplementation significantly improved vitamin D status, lowered PTH levels, and reduced bone turnover in two groups of Southeast Asian women (Kruger et al., 2010). The effectiveness of calcium (1000 mg/day) and vitamin D (400 IU) therapy in Indo-Asians with low serum vitamin D and secondary hyperparathyroidism produced increased serum calcium and 25OHD levels and PTH suppression, but no change in bone mass (Serhan and Holland, 2005).

SUMMARY

Compared with whites, black individuals have a lower risk of all fractures and higher BMD at all ages, despite the high prevalence of vitamin D deficiency. Asians have an intermediate risk of fracture. BMD differences cannot account for the fracture differences among ethnic groups. Relative secondary hyperparathyroidism, as a response to vitamin D deficiency and low calcium intake, produces a corresponding elevation in serum $1,25(OH)_2D$ and a lower urinary calcium excretion. An expected increase in bone turnover has been found in most races, but not in blacks. The black skeleton is resistant to the acute bone-resorbing effects of PTH, with maintenance or perhaps even particularly high renal sensitivity to PTH. Although paradoxical, these elegant adaptive responses to vitamin D deficiency allow the black skeleton to remain strong while still providing a means for maintenance of calcium homeostasis. No notable biochemical differences exist between Asians or Hispanics and whites; the ethnic fracture differences may be more related to skeletal structure than simply BMD. Vitamin D supplementation in most racial groups improves serum 25OHD concentrations, reduces PTH, and may minimize bone loss. Whether vitamin D supplementation may be effective in improving the skeleton of blacks remains unclear.

REFERENCES

Abrams, S.A., O'Brien, K.O., Liang, L.K., et al. 1995. Differences in calcium absorption and kinetics between black and white girls aged 5-16 years. *J Bone Miner Res* 10:829–833.
Aloia, J.F. 2008. African Americans, 25-hydroxyvitamin D, and osteoporosis: A paradox. *Am J Clin Nutr* 88:545S–550S.

Aloia, J.F., Mikhail, M., Pagan, C.D., et al. 1998. Biochemical and hormonal variables in black and white women matched for age and weight. *J Lab Clin Med* 132:383–389.

Aloia, J.F., Talwar, S.A., Pollack, S., et al. 2005. A randomized controlled trial of vitamin D3 supplementation in African American women. *Arch Intern Med* 165:1618–1623.

Aloia, J.F., Vaswani, A., Ma, R., et al. 1997. Comparison of body composition in black and white premenopausal women. *J Lab Clin Med* 129:294–299.

Arya, V., Bhambri, R., Godbole, M., et al. 2004. Vitamin D status and its relationship with bone mineral density in healthy Asian Indians. *Osteoporos Int* 15:56–61.

Ausmanas, M.K., Holinka, C.F., Ling, Y.S., et al. 2007. Effect of three doses of conjugated estrogens/medroxy-progesterone acetate on biomarkers of bone turnover and cartilage degradation in postmenopausal women: The Pan-Asia Menopause PAM Study. *Climacteric* 104:306–313.

Bachrach, L.K., Hastie, T., Wang, M.C., et al. 1999. Bone mineral acquisition in healthy Asian, Hispanic, black, and Caucasian youth: A longitudinal study. *J Clin Endocrinol Metab* 8:4702–4712.

Bailey, D.A., Martin, A.D., Mckay, H.A., et al. 2000. Calcium accretion in girls and boys during puberty: A longitudinal analysis. *J Bone Miner Res* 15:2245–2250.

Bannan, P.M., and Levitt, M.D. 1996 Calcium, dairy products, and osteoporosis: Implications of lactose intolerance. *Prim Care Update Ob/Gyn* 3:146–151.

Baron, J.A., Karagas, M., Barrett, J., et al. 1996. Basic epidemiology of fractures of the upper and lower limb among Americans over 65 years of age. *Epidemiology* 7:612–618.

Barrett, J.A., Baron, J.A., Karagas, M.R., et al. 1999. Fracture risk in the U.S. Medicare population. *J Clin Epidemiol* 52:243–249.

Barrett-Connor, E., Siris, E.S., Wehren, L.E., et al. 2005. Osteoporosis and fracture risk in women of different ethnic groups. *J Bone Miner Res* 20:185–194.

Bell, N.H., Greene, A., Epstein, S., et al. 1985. Evidence for alteration of the vitamin D–endocrine system in blacks. *J Clin Invest* 76:470–473.

Bell, R.A., Quandt, S.A., Spangler, J.G., et al. 2002. Dietary calcium intake and supplement use among older African American, white, and Native American women in a rural southeastern community. *J Am Diet Assoc* 102:844–847.

Bell, N.H., Yergey, A.L., Vieira, N.E., et al. 1993. Demonstration of a difference in urinary calcium, not calcium absorption, in black and white adolescents. *J Bone Miner Res* 8:111–115.

Bhudhikanok, G.S., Wang, M.C., Eckert, K., et al. 1996. Differences in bone mineral in young Asian and Caucasian Americans may reflect differences in bone size. *J Bone Miner Res* 11:1545–1556.

Bikle, D.D., Ettinger, B., Sidney, S., et al. 1999. Differences in calcium metabolism between black and white men and women. *Miner Electrolyte Metab* 25:178–184.

Braun, M., Palacios, C., Wigertz, K., et al. 2007. Racial differences in skeletal calcium retention in adolescent girls with varied controlled calcium intakes. *Am J Clin Nutr* 85:1657–1663.

Bronner, Y.L., Hawkins, A.S., Holt, M.L., et al. 2006. Models for nutrition education to increase consumption of calcium and dairy products among African Americans. *J Nutr* 136:1103–1106.

Bryant, R.J., Wastney, M.E., Martin, B.R., et al. 2003. Racial differences in bone turnover and calcium metabolism in adolescent females. *J Clin Endocrinol Metab* 88:1043–1047.

Burchard, E.G., Ziv, E., Coyle, N., et al. 2003. The importance of race and ethnic background in biomedical research and clinical practice. *New Engl J Med* 348:1170–1175.

Burrows, M., Baxter-Jones, A., Mirwald, R., et al. 2009. Bone mineral accrual across growth in a mixed-ethnic group of children: Are Asian children disadvantaged from an early age? *Calcif Tissue Int* 84:366–378.

Cauley, J.A., Fullman, R.L., Stone, K.L., et al. 2005a. Factors associated with the lumbar spine and proximal femur bone mineral density in older men. *Osteoporos Int* 16:1525–1537.

Cauley, J.A., Gutai, J.P., Kuller, L.H., et al. 1994. Black-white differences in serum sex hormones and bone mineral density. *Am J Epidemiol* 139:1035–1046.

Cauley, J.A., Lui, L.Y., Ensrud, K.E., et al. 2005b. Bone mineral density and the risk of incident nonspinal fractures in black and white women. *JAMA* 293:2102–2108.

Cauley, J.A., Lui, L.Y., Stone, K.L., et al. 2005c. Longitudinal study of changes in hip bone mineral density in Caucasian and African-American women. *J Am Geriatr Soc* 53:183–189.

Chen, Y.M., Ho, S.C., Lam, S.S., et al. 2003. Soy isoflavones have a favorable effect on bone loss in Chinese postmenopausal women with lower bone mass: A double-blind, randomized, controlled trial. *J Clin Endocrinol Metab* 88:4740–4747.

Cheng, H., Gary, L.C., Curtis, J.R., et al. 2009. Estimated prevalence and patterns of presumed osteoporosis among older Americans based on Medicare data. *Osteoporos Int* 20:1507–1515.

Clemens, T.L., Adams, J.S., Henderson, S.L., et al. 1982. Increased skin pigment reduces the capacity of skin to synthesise vitamin D3. *Lancet* 1:74–76.

Cohn, S.H., Abesamis, C., Yasumura, S., et al. 1977. Comparative skeletal mass and radial bone mineral content in black and white women. *Metabolism* 26:171–178.

Cosman, F., Morgan, D.C., Nieves, J.W., et al. 1997. Resistance to bone resorbing effects of PTH in black women. *J Bone Miner Res* 12:958–966.

Crespo, N.C., Yoo, E.J., and Hawkins, S.A. 2009. Anthropometric and lifestyle associations of bone mass in healthy pre-menopausal Mexican and Asian American women. *J Immigr Minor Health.* DOI 10.1007/s10903-009-9259-2.

Cummings, S.R., Cauley, J.A., Palermo, L., et al. 1994. Racial differences in hip axis lengths might explain racial differences in rates of hip fracture. Study of Osteoporotic Fractures Research Group. *Osteoporos Int* 4:226–229.

Cummings, S.R., and Melton, L.J. 2002. Epidemiology and outcomes of osteoporotic fractures. *Lancet* 359:1761–1767.

Dawson-Hughes, B., and Harris, S.S. 2002. Calcium intake influences the association of protein intake with rates of bone loss in elderly men and women. *Am J Clin Nutr* 75:773–779.

Dawson-Hughes, B., Harris, S.S., Finneran, S., et al. 1995. Calcium absorption responses to calcitriol in black and white premenopausal women. *J Clin Endocrinol Metab* 80:3068–3072.

Dawson-Hughes, B., Harris, S., Kramich, C., et al. 1993. Calcium retention and hormone levels in black and white women on high- and low-calcium diets. *J Bone Miner Res* 8:779–787.

Dawson-Hughes, B., Tosteson, A.N., Melton, L.J., et al. 2008. Implications of absolute fracture risk assessment for osteoporosis practice guidelines in the USA. *Osteoporos Int* 19:449–458.

Duan, Y., Wang, X.F., Evans, A., et al. 2005. Structural and biomechanical basis of racial and sex differences in vertebral fragility in Chinese and Caucasians. *Bone* 36:987–998.

Ettinger, B., Sidney, S., Cummings, S.R., et al. 1997. Racial differences in bone density between young adult black and white subjects persist after adjustment for anthropometric, lifestyle, and biochemical differences. *J Clin Endocrinol Metab* 82:429–434.

Fang, J., Freeman, R., Jeganathan, R., et al. 2004. Variations in hip fracture hospitalization rates among different race/ethnicity groups in New York City. *Ethn Dis* 14:280–284.

Finkelstein, J.S., Brockwell, S.E., Mehta, V., et al. 2008. Bone mineral density changes during the menopause transition in a multiethnic cohort of women. *J Clin Endocrinol Metab* 93:861–868.

Finkelstein, J.S., Lee, M.L., Sowers, M., et al. 2002a. Ethnic variation in bone density in premenopausal and early perimenopausal women: Effects of anthropometric and lifestyle factors. *J Clin Endocrinol Metab* 87:3057–3067.

Finkelstein, J.S., Sowers, M., Greendale, G.A., et al. 2002b. Ethnic variation in bone turnover in pre- and early perimenopausal women: Effects of anthropometric and lifestyle factors. *J Clin Endocrinol Metab* 87:3051–3056.

Gilsanz, V., Roe, T.F., Mora, S., et al. 1991. Changes in vertebral bone density in black girls and white girls during childhood and puberty. *New Engl J Med* 325:1597–1600.

Gilsanz, V., Skaggs, D.L., Kovanlikaya, A., et al. 1998. Differential effect of race on the axial and appendicular skeletons of children. *J Clin Endocrinol Metab* 83:1420–1427.

Griffin, M.R., Ray, W.A., Fought, R.L., et al. 1992. Black–White differences in fracture rates. *Am J Epidemiol* 136:1378–1385.

Han, Z.H., Palnitkar, S., Rao, D.S., et al. 1997. Effects of ethnicity and age or menopause on the remodeling and turnover of iliac bone: Implications for mechanisms of bone loss. *J Bone Miner Res* 12:498–508.

Hannan, M.T., Tucker, K.L., Dawson-Hughes, B., et al. 2000. Effect of dietary protein on bone loss in elderly men and women: The Framingham Osteoporosis Study. *J Bone Miner Res* 15:2504–2512.

Harris, S.S., and Dawson-Hughes, B. 1998. Seasonal changes in plasma 25-hydroxyvitamin D concentrations of young American black and white women. *Am J Clin Nutr* 67:1232–1236.

Harris, S.S., Soteriades, E., Coolidge, J.A., et al. 2000. Vitamin D insufficiency and hyperparathyroidism in a low income, multiracial, elderly population. *J Clin Endocrinol Metab* 85:4125–4130.

Harris, S.S., Soteriades, E., and Dawson-Hughes, B. 2001. Secondary hyperparathyroidism and bone turnover in elderly blacks and whites. *J Clin Endocrinol Metab* 86:3801–3804.

Heaney, R.P. 2006. Low calcium intake among African Americans: Effects on bones and body weight. *J Nutr* 136:1095–1098.

Henry, Y.M., and Eastell, R. 2000. Ethnic and gender differences in bone mineral density and bone turnover in young adults: Effect of bone size. *Osteoporos Int* 11:512–517.

Hirota, T., Nara, M., Ohguri, M., et al. 1992. Effect of diet and lifestyle on bone mass in Asian young women. *Am J Clin Nutr* 55:1168–1173.

Ho, S.C., Chen, Y.M., Woo, J.L., et al. 2004. High habitual calcium intake attenuates bone loss in early post-menopausal Chinese women: An 18-month follow-up study. *J Clin Endocrinol Metab* 89:2166–2170.

Holinka, C.F., Christiansen, C., Tian, X.W., et al. 2008. Ethnic differences in levels of bone and cartilage bio-markers and hormonal responsiveness in nine groups of postmenopausal Asian women: The Pan-Asia Menopause PAM Study. *Climacteric* 11:44–54.

Hou, Y.L., Wu, X.P., Luo, X.H., et al. 2007. Differences in age-related bone mass of proximal femur between Chinese women and different ethnic women in the United States. *J Bone Miner Metab* 25:243–252.

Islam, M.Z., Shamim, A.A., Kemi, V., et al. 2008. Vitamin D deficiency and low bone status in adult female garment factory workers in Bangladesh. *Br J Nutr* 99:1322–1329.

Jackson, R.D., Lacroix, A.Z., Gass, M., et al. 2006. Calcium plus vitamin D supplementation and the risk of fractures. *New Engl J Med* 354:669–683.

Kalkwarf, H.J., Zemel, B.S., Gilsanz, V., et al. 2007. The bone mineral density in childhood study: Bone mineral content and density according to age, sex, and race. *J Clin Endocrinol Metab* 92:2087–2099.

Karagas, M.R., Lu-Yao, G.L., Barrett, J.A., et al. 1996. Heterogeneity of hip fracture: Age, race, sex, and geographic patterns of femoral neck and trochanteric fractures among the US elderly. *Am J Epidemiol* 143:677–682.

Kim, K.K., Yu, E.S., Liu, W.T., et al. 1993. Nutritional status of Chinese-, Korean-, and Japanese-American elderly. *J Am Diet Assoc* 93:1416–1422.

Kleerekoper, M., Nelson, D.A., Peterson, E.L., et al. 1994a. Reference data for bone mass, calciotropic hormones, and biochemical markers of bone remodeling in older 55–75 postmenopausal white and black women. *J Bone Miner Res* 9:1267–1276.

Kleerekoper, M., Nelson, D.A., Peterson, E.L., et al. 1994b. Body composition and gonadal steroids in older white and black women. *J Clin Endocrinol Metab* 79:775–779.

Kruger, M.C., Schollum, L.M., Kuhn-Sherlock, B., et al. 2010. The effect of a fortified milk drink on vitamin D status and bone turnover in post-menopausal women from Southeast Asia. *Bone* 46:759–767.

Kumar, J., Muntner, P., Kaskel, F.J., et al. 2009. Prevalence and associations of 25-hydroxyvitamin D deficiency in us children: NHANES 2001–2004. *Pediatrics* 124:e362–e370.

Lau, E.M., Chan, H.H., Woo, J., et al. 1996. Normal ranges for vertebral height ratios and prevalence of vertebral fracture in Hong Kong Chinese: A comparison with American Caucasians. *J Bone Miner Res* 11:1364–1368.

Lauderdale, D.S., Jacobsen, S.J., Furner, S.E., et al. 1997. Hip fracture incidence among elderly Asian-American populations. *Am J Epidemiol* 146:502–509.

Leder, B.Z., Araujo, A.B., Travison, T.G., et al. 2007. Racial and ethnic differences in bone turnover markers in men. *J Clin Endocrinol Meta* 92:3453–3457.

Li, J.Y., Specker, B.L., Ho, M.L., et al. 1989. Bone mineral content in black and white children 1 to 6 years of age. Early appearance of race and sex differences. *Am J Dis Child* 143:1346–1349.

Liel, Y., Edwards, J., Shary, J., et al.1988. The effects of race and body habitus on bone mineral density of the radius, hip, and spine in premenopausal women. *J Clin Endocrinol Metab* 66:1247–12450.

Ling, X., Cummings, S.R., Mingwei, Q., et al. 2000. Vertebral fractures in Beijing, China: The Beijing Osteoporosis Project. *J Bone Miner Res* 15:2019–2025.

Looker, A.C., Dawson-Hughes, B., Calvo, M.S., et al. 2002. Serum 25-hydroxyvitamin D status of adolescents and adults in two seasonal subpopulations from NHANES III. *Bone* 30:771–777.

Looker, A.C., Loria, C.M., Carroll, M.D., et al. 1993. Calcium intakes of Mexican Americans, Cubans, Puerto Ricans, non-Hispanic whites, and non-Hispanic blacks in the United States. *J Am Diet Assoc* 93:1274–1279.

Looker, A.C., Wahner, H.W., Dunn, W.L., et al. 1995. Proximal femur bone mineral levels of US adults. *Osteoporos Int* 5:389–409.

Looker, A.C., Wahner, H.W., Dunn, W.L., et al. 1998. Updated data on proximal femur bone mineral levels of us adults. *Osteoporos Int* 8:468–489.

Luckey, M.M., Meier, D.E., Mandeli, J.P., et al. 1989. Radial and vertebral bone density in white and black women: Evidence for racial differences in premenopausal bone homeostasis. *J Clin Endocrinol Metab* 69:762–770.

Luckey, M.M., Wallenstein, S., Lapinski, R., et al. 1996. A prospective study of bone loss in African-American and white women—a clinical research center study. *J Clin Endocrinol Metab* 81:2948–2956.

Marcus, R., Greendale, G., Blunt, B.A., et al. 1994. Correlates of bone mineral density in the postmenopausal estrogen/progestin interventions trial. *J Bone Miner Res* 9:1467–1476.

Marshall, L.M., Zmuda, J.M., Chan, B.K., et al. 2008. Race and ethnic variation in proximal femur structure and BMD among older men. *J Bone Miner Res* 23:121–130.

Matsuoka, L.Y., Wortsman, J., Haddad, J.G., et al.1991. Racial pigmentation and the cutaneous synthesis of vitamin D. *Arch Dermatol* 127:536–538.

Meier, D.E., Luckey, M.M., Wallenstein, S., et al. 1991. Calcium, vitamin D, and parathyroid hormone status in young white and black women: Association with racial differences in bone mass. *J Clin Endocrinol Metab* 72:703–710.

Meier, D.E., Luckey, M.M., Wallenstein, S., et al. 1992. Racial differences in pre- and postmenopausal bone homeostasis: Association with bone density. *J Bone Miner Res* 7:1181–1189.

Mikhail, M.B., Vaswani, A.N., and Aloia, J.F. 1996. Racial differences in femoral dimensions and their relation to hip fracture. *Osteoporos Int* 6:22–24.

Moore, C.E., Murphy, M.M., and Holick, M.F. 2005 Vitamin D intakes by children and adults in the united states differ among ethnic groups. *J Nutr* 135:2478–2485.

Morton, D.J., Barrett-Connor, E., Kritz-Silverstein, D., et al. 2003. Bone mineral density in postmenopausal Caucasian, Filipina, and Hispanic women. *Int J Epidemiol* 32:150–156.

Nakamura, K., Tsugawa, N., Saito, T., et al. 2008. Vitamin D status, bone mass, and bone metabolism in home-dwelling postmenopausal Japanese women: Yokogoshi Study. *Bone* 42:271–277.

Nakamura, K., Ueno, K., Nishiwaki, T., et al. 2005. Nutrition, mild hyperparathyroidism, and bone mineral density in young Japanese women. *Am J Clin Nutr* 82:1127–1133.

Nelson, D.A., Barondess, D.A., Hendrix, S.L., et al. 2000. Cross-sectional geometry, bone strength, and bone mass in the proximal femur in black and white postmenopausal women. *J Bone Miner Res* 15:1992–1997.

Nelson, D.A., Jacobsen, G., Barondess, D.A., et al. 1995. Ethnic differences in regional bone density, hip axis length, and lifestyle variables among healthy black and white men. *J Bone Miner Res* 10:782–787.

Nelson, H.D., Vesco, K.K., Haney, E., et al. 2006. Nonhormonal therapies for menopausal hot flashes: Systematic review and meta-analysis. *JAMA* 295:2057–2071.

Nesby-O'dell, S., Scanlon, K.S., Cogswell, M.E., et al. 2002. Hypovitaminosis D prevalence and determinants among African American and white women of reproductive age: Third National Health and Nutrition Examination Survey, 1988–1994. *Am J Clin Nutr* 76:187–192.

Nieves, J., Ralston, S.H., Vasquez, E., Ambrose, B., Cosman, F., and Lindsay, R. 2007. Vitamin D receptor Fok1 polymorphism influences response to vitamin D supplementation in postmenopausal African American women. In *Nutritional Aspects of Osteoporosis*, Burckhardt, P., Heaney, R., and Dawson-Hughes, B., eds. Academic Press, San Diego, pp. 126–132.

Novotny, R., Daida, Y.G., Grove, J.S., et al. 2004. Adolescent dairy consumption and physical activity associated with bone mass. *Prev Med* 39:355–360.

Parfitt, A.M., Travers, R., Rauch, F., et al. 2000. Structural and cellular changes during bone growth in healthy children. *Bone* 27:487–494.

Parisien, M., Cosman, F., Morgan, D., et al. 1997. Histomorphometric assessment of bone mass, structure, and remodeling: A comparison between healthy black and white premenopausal women. *J Bone Miner Res* 12:948–957.

Pollitzer, W.S., and Anderson, J.J. 1989. Ethnic and genetic differences in bone mass: A review with a hereditary vs environmental perspective. *Am J Clin Nutr* 50:1244–1259.

Prentice, A., Shaw, J., Laskey, M.A., et al. 1991. Bone mineral content of British and rural Gambian women aged 18–80+ years. *Bone Miner* 12:201–214.

Robbins, J., Aragaki, A.K., Kooperberg, C., et al. 2007. Factors associated with 5-year risk of hip fracture in postmenopausal women. *JAMA* 298:2389–2398.

Roy, D.K., Berry, J.L., Pye, S.R., et al. 2007. Vitamin D status and bone mass in UK south Asian women. *Bone* 40:200–204.

Sahi, T. 1994. Hypolactasia and lactase persistence. Historical review and the terminology. *Scand J Gastroenterol Suppl* 202:1–6.

Schnitzler, C.M., and Mesquita, J. 1998. Bone marrow composition and bone microarchitecture and turnover in blacks and whites. *J Bone Miner Res* 13:1300–1307.

Seeman, E. 1998. Growth in bone mass and size—are racial and gender differences in bone mineral density more apparent than real? *J Clin Endocrinol Metab* 83:1414–1419.

Serhan, E., and Holland, M.R. 2005. Calcium and vitamin d supplementation failed to improve bone mineral density in Indo-Asians suffering from hypovitaminosis D and secondary hyperparathyroidism. *Rheumatol Int* 25:276–279.

Silverman, S.L., and Madison, R.E. 1988. Decreased incidence of hip fracture in Hispanics, Asians, and Blacks: California hospital discharge data. *Am J Public Health* 78:1482–1483.

Specker, B.L., Brazerol, W., Tsang, R.C., et al. 1987. Bone mineral content in children 1 to 6 years of age. Detectable sex differences after 4 years of age. *Am J Dis Child* 141:343–344.

Srinivasan, R., and Minocha, A. 1998. When to suspect lactose intolerance. Symptomatic, ethnic, and laboratory clues. *Postgrad Med* 104:109–111, 115–116, 122–123.

Theobald, T.M., Cauley, J.A., Gluer, C.C., et al. 1998. Black–White differences in hip geometry. Study of Osteoporotic Fractures research group. *Osteoporos Int* 8:61–67.

Tracy, J.K., Meyer, W.A., Flores, R.H., et al. 2005. Racial differences in rate of decline in bone mass in older men: The Baltimore Men's Osteoporosis Study. *J Bone Miner Res* 20:1228–1234.

von Hurst, P.R., Stonehouse, W., and Coad, J. 2009. Vitamin D status and attitudes towards sun exposure in South Asian women living in Auckland, New Zealand. *Public Health Nutr* 13:1–6.

Walker, M.D., Babbar, R., Opotowsky, A.R., et al. 2006. A referent bone mineral density database for Chinese American women. *Osteoporos Int* 17:878–887.

Walker, M.D., Mcmahon, D.J., Udesky, J., et al. 2009. Application of high-resolution skeletal imaging to measurements of volumetric BMD and skeletal microarchitecture in Chinese-American and white women: Explanation of a paradox. *J Bone Miner Res* 24:1953–1959.

Walker, M.D., Novotny, R., Bilezikian, J.P., et al. 2008. Race and diet interactions in the acquisition, maintenance, and loss of bone. *J Nutr* 138:1256S–1260S.

Wang, X.F., Wang, Q., Ghasem-Zadeh, A., et al. 2009. Differences in macro- and microarchitecture of the appendicular skeleton in young Chinese and white women. *J Bone Miner Res* 24:1946–1952.

Weaver, C.M., McCabe, L.D., McCabe, G.P., et al. 2007. Bone mineral and predictors of bone mass in white, Hispanic, and Asian early pubertal girls. *Calcif Tissue Int* 81:352–363.

Webb, A.R., Kline, L., and Holick, M.F. 1988. Influence of season and latitude on the cutaneous synthesis of vitamin d3: Exposure to winter sunlight in Boston and Edmonton will not promote vitamin D3 synthesis in human skin. *J Clin Endocrinol Metab* 67:373–378.

Weinstein, R.S., and Bell, N.H. 1988. Diminished rates of bone formation in normal black adults. *New Engl J Med* 319:1698–1701.

Wigertz, K., Palacios, C., Jackman, L.A., et al. 2005. Racial differences in calcium retention in response to dietary salt in adolescent girls. *Am J Clin Nutr* 81:845–850.

Wolinsky, F.D., Bentler, S.E., Liu, L., et al. 2009. Recent hospitalization and the risk of hip fracture among older Americans. *J Gerontol A Biol Sci Med Sc* 64:249–255.

Woo, J., Li, M., and Lau, E. 2001. Population bone mineral density measurements for Chinese women and men in Hong Kong. *Osteoporos Int* 12:289–295.

Wu-Tso, P., Yeh, I.L., and Tam, C.F. 1995. Comparisons of dietary intake in young and old Asian Americans: A two-generation study. *Nutr Res* 15:1445–1462.

Xiaoge, D., Eryuan, L., Xianping, W., et al. 2000. Bone mineral density differences at the femoral neck and Ward's triangle: A comparison study on the reference data between Chinese and caucasian women. *Calcif Tissue Int* 67:195–198.

Xu, L., Lu, A., Zhao, X., et al. 1996. Very low rates of hip fracture in Beijing, People's Republic of China: The Beijing Osteoporosis Project. *Am J Epidemiol* 144:901–907.

Zhang, X., Shu, X.O., Li, H., et al. 2005. Prospective cohort study of soy food consumption and risk of bone fracture among postmenopausal women. *Arch Intern Med* 165:1890–1895.

Zhu, K., Greenfield, H., Zhang, Q., et al. 2007. Growth and bone mineral accretion during puberty in Chinese girls: A five-year longitudinal study. *J Bone Miner* Res 23:167–172.

30 Nutrition and Bone Health of the Japanese

Takuo Fujita

CONTENTS

INTRODUCTION

Osteoporosis is one of the most prevalent diseases of mankind. Although ethnic, nutritional, and lifestyle factors of nations differ, osteoporosis remains a universal disorder, despite having a wide variety of incidence rates and health manifestations that impact a population. Because osteoporosis increases with age, its prevalence is expected to rise as the life expectancy of a nation increases. In developed nations, life expectancy in females may exceed 80 years, as in Japan, and each population might be called an "osteoporotic nation"; osteoporosis in economically developed nation is a far more serious health threat than in a developing country. In a developing country, a "preosteoporotic nation," the corresponding life expectancy is as short as the 50s, when osteoporosis scarcely exists. In the former, increasing numbers of osteoporotic fractures require extensive nursing care, which increases the need for health support mechanisms for the elderly. No nation, however, achieves its longevity and high health indices without having long-term healthy lifestyle behaviors, including good nutrition. Japan represents one of the few nations that have undergone the transition from preosteoporotic to osteoporotic stage quite rapidly, within a period as short as the last 50 years.

This chapter explores the positive nutritional and lifestyle factors that promote health, especially skeletal health, and at the same time prevent osteoporosis among elderly Japanese citizens, against confronting negative factors. From a worldwide health perspective, the model of Japan in promoting bone health and preventing osteoporosis may serve other nations as well in the future.

NUTRITIONAL AND LIFESTYLE CHARACTERISTICS OF JAPANESE

GEOGRAPHIC AND NUTRITIONAL BACKGROUND

Japan, located on the eastern end of the Eurasian Continent (once connected to it), is no doubt an Asian nation, but it is also an Oceanic nation, as part of a group of volcanic islands on the Pacific rim. The Japanese people have essentially an Asiatic eating pattern, favoring cereals, soybean products, and vegetables, on one hand, and oceanic eating habit, mainly depending on fish, shellfish, and seaweeds, on the other hand. Enough space on the small islands for dairy farms has never existed so that animal meat and milk have never occupied a major part of the nutritional intake of the Japanese population.

The Japanese diet is low in calcium (Ca), based on these geographic and historical backgrounds and possibly because of other characteristics, such as soft drinking water with low mineral content from the volcanic soil. As one of the Asian countries exposed early to Western civilization and with rapid subsequent industrialization, the traditional diet of Japan has partly been replaced by rich Western style food such as animal meat and fat, milk, and dairy products.

LOW CA INTAKE OF JAPANESE

Dietary Reference Intakes for Japanese

Low Ca intakes by Japanese across the life cycle exist according to the recommended intake for Ca published by the Ministry of Health, Welfare and Labor, based on the results of national nutritional survey over many years by the duplicate portion sampling method (Ministry of Health, Welfare and Labor Committee for Dietary Reference Intakes for Japanese, 2009). Recommended Dietary Allowances (RDAs) for Japanese citizens are based on Estimated Average Requirement (EAR), which represent daily Ca intake needed to meet the requirements of 50% of the members of the group in each stage of the life cycle. In Japan, Ca RDAs correspond to 1.2 times the EAR, taking into consideration the amount of Ca stored in bone, urinary excretion, transdermal loss, and apparent absorption rate. EARs and RDAs for Ca in the age groups ~18 to 70 years are listed in Table 30.1, along with EAR and RDA of protein in these age groups. Compared with recommendations for these two nutrients in the United States and many other Western nations, the Japanese recommendations tend to be low.

The safe upper limit (UL) of Ca, which is set uniformly at 2500 mg/day, has recently been added to the list of recommendations; the Ca UL permits the use of intakes up to the UL to ensure bone health. Such high intakes as the UL are not recommended, but the Japanese elderly may need higher Ca intakes to counteract a more severe deficiency. When the milk–alkali syndrome was described a few decades ago, 13 patients were reported to have taken between 2800 and 16,500 mg of Ca per day with an alkali salt, considerably higher than the UL level considered safe in the United States, that is, 2500 mg/day. This amount of Ca is also close to the level reported to be capable of suppressing parathyroid gland secretion of parathyroid hormone (PTH) and hence lowering elevated serum PTH concentrations in elderly patients (McKane et al., 1996).

TABLE 30.1
Estimated Average Requirement (EAR) and Recommended Dietary Allowance (RDA) for Calcium and Protein in the Age Groups 18 to 70 Years and Older

Age Group, Years	Calcium, mg/day				Protein, mg/day			
	EAR		RDA		EAR		RDA	
	Male	Female	Male	Female	Male	Female	Male	Female
18–29	650	550	800	650	50	40	60	50
30–49	550	550	650	650	50	40	60	50
50–69	600	550	700	650	50	40	60	50
70 and over	600	500	700	600	50	40	60	50

Source: From Ministry of Health, Welfare and Labor Committee for Dietary Reference Intakes for Japanese, 2009. *Dietary Reference Intakes for Japanese, 2010.* Daiichi Shuppan Publishing Co., Ltd., Tokyo.

Ca Balance Studies

Balance studies of Japanese postmenopausal women (62 to 77 years) suggested that a lower amount of Ca is required to achieve metabolic equilibrium compared with the Western requirement. Balance studies of Japanese women placed on low Ca (250 mg/day) to high Ca intakes (850 mg/day) revealed that zero balance was achieved at 702 mg/day in males and 788 mg/day for females (Uenishi et al., 2001). In Ca balance studies of young Japanese adults on Ca intakes ranging from 294 to 1131 mg/day, however, zero balance was achieved at 550 to 759 mg/day (Nishimuta et al., 2004).

Measured Ca intakes of Japanese women typically are lower than the amounts of Ca consumed in Western nations. For example, a group of postmenopausal women (mean age of 64.5 years) had a mean Ca intake of 527 mg/day (Nakamura et al., 2009). In the lowest quartile of Ca intake (less than 417mg/day), bone resorption was augmented, as indicated by the elevated bone marker of resorption, urinary N-telopeptide (NTx) (Nakamura et al., 2009). Among 106 female college students (19 to 23 years), Ca intake was 380 ± 209 mg/day and protein intake, 41.7 ± 12.6 g/day (Ueno et al., 2005). In 43 postmenopausal women (mean age of 68.2 years), Ca intake by the duplicate portion sampling method was 660 ± 195 mg/day, a level significantly associated with urinary NTx and one other marker of bone resorption. Protein intake was 63.9 ± 15.5 g/day (Nakamura et al., 2004).

In 53 postmenopausal women (aged 68.2 years), duplicate portion sampling method revealed Ca intake of 670 ± 219 mg/day and protein intake of 65.2 ± 18.3 g/day. Dietary phosphorus, potassium, and protein (65.2 g) intakes were significantly correlated with dietary Ca intake (Nakamura et al., 2003). According to Lacey et al. (1991), Ca intake in 89 premenopausal Japanese women, 458 ± 171 (SD) mg/day, was even lower than 601 ± 209 in the postmenopausal counterpart, whereas protein intake of 70.9 ± 19.6 g/day and 72.6 ± 15.6, respectively, was similar between the two groups.

These data suggest that consumption of the typical Japanese diet provides too little Ca and protein. The inadequate Ca intake stimulates PTH secretion, which increases bone resorption, and the inadequate protein intake does not permit sufficient synthesis of collagen and other bone proteins needed for new bone formation. How the Japanese people are able to develop and maintain their skeletal tissues with such low Ca and protein intakes remains an enigma.

As was pointed out by Anderson (2000), exercise and physical load on the bone are quite important to develop healthy skeleton in the growing period as well as during and after maturity. Japanese had to be hardworking and physically active especially prior to the current era of motorization. It appears possible that adequate routine exercise may cover up low Ca intake by augmenting its absorption or by having a direct effect on the bone to increase Ca utilization. Thus, a regular pattern of physical activities may have contributed to the maintenance of relatively normal bone despite low Ca and protein intakes in hardworking Japanese people.

CHARACTERISTICS OF OSTEOPOROSIS OF JAPANESE

Vertebral and Hip Fracture

In view of the geographical, historical, nutritional, and lifestyle characteristics of Japanese described above, Japanese no doubt must be classified as an extremely osteoporotic nation. When Professor BEC Nordin visited Japan for the first time in the 1960s under WHO traveling fellowship to survey osteoporosis problem in Japan, he was quite impressed by the frequent sight of "doubled-up" women with marked kyphosis, surprisingly active and freely walking around the street (Nordin, 1966). Subsequent epidemiological studies indeed revealed a high prevalence of spinal fracture and kyphosis among elderly Japanese (Ross et al., 1995). Compared with Japanese Americans living in Hawaii, the prevalent vertebral fracture was 1.8 times greater for native Japanese. Hip fracture incidence, however, was unexpectedly low among Japanese (Fujiwara and Ross, 1997) until recent years when incidence rates have been increasing (Orimo et al., 1997).

The low hip fracture incidence rate has been explained by the geometrical structure of the proximal femur, specifically a short hip–axis length (Cummings et al., 1994). Tall Scandinavian women with long legs are known to suffer from hip fracture more frequently than do shorter Asian women including Japanese, in part because of a longer hip–axis length. Such apparent discrepancy in the site preference of osteoporotic fracture, that is, hip versus spine, may also depend on environmental and lifestyle factors. The working environment may also have contributed to the frequent occurrence of kyphosis and hip fracture. For example, a narrow living space, especially a narrow kitchen space, may force women to stoop for cooking, and farm work such as seeding and harvesting may aggravate kyphosis. Frequent needs for squatting and sitting directly on the floor with knees completely flexed in a Japanese manner may strengthen the hips and increase postural stability and, therefore, to decrease the risk of hip fracture.

Kii Peninsula Studies

In the mountain district of the Kii Peninsula located on the Pacific side of the Japan Mainland (Honshu), Ca intake was traditionally low because of low Ca content of river water, and vitamin D insufficiency has been common because of insufficient solar exposure. Among the Kii inhabitants, bone density was traditionally lower and spinal compression fractures were more frequent than were those in the residents of the adjacent seacoast area, who enjoyed abundant sunshine and fish, shellfish, and seaweed (Fujita et al., 1977, 1984).

The prevalence of amyotrophic lateral sclerosis was once quite high in this mountain area but decreased along with improvement of nutritional intake. A role for Ca deficiency has been suggested as one of the contributing etiological factors of amyotrophic lateral sclerosis in this area, like other areas along the Mariana Volcano Belt, Guam, and New Guinea (Tsubaki and Yase, 1988). Differences between inhabitants of mountain versus seacoast areas are summarized in Table 30.2. The geographical and climatic backgrounds of the Kii Peninsula contribute to the mountain residents the following abnormalities: vitamin D insufficiency, low serum 25-OH vitamin D, low serum phosphorus, high alkaline phosphatase, and high serum PTH. These findings suggested insufficient dietary consumption of vitamin D, total protein, and cholesterol, all representative of poor general nutrition. Such dietary inadequacies of the Kii mountain citizens might have contributed to the short stature and common osteoporosis, which presents with thin cortical thickness, frequent backaches, and spinal fractures, especially in females after menopause. Aortic calcification was also more frequent in postmenopausal women in the mountain area than in the seacoast area.

Table 30.3 provides impressive difference in the morbidity and mortality rates of these two Kii communities. In the mountain region in which mineral and general nutritional intake and solar

TABLE 30.2

Parameters of Bone and Mineral Metabolism in Mountain and Seacoast Inhabitants Tested in 1975–1977

Parameters	Seacoast	Mountain
Height	Normal	Short
Backache	Rare	Frequent
Cortical thickness	Normal	Thin
Compression fracture	Rare	Frequent
Aortic calcification	Rare	Frequent
Solar exposure	Abundant	Poor
Serum 25 (OH) vitamin D	Normal	Low
Serum PTH	Norma	High
Serum calcium	Normal	Low
Serum phosphate	Normal	Low
Serum alkaline phosphatase	Normal	High
Serum total protein	Normal	Low
Serum cholesterol	Normal	Low

Note: PTH = parathyroid hormone.

Source: Summarized by the author from Fujita et al., 1977. *J Am Geriat Soc* 24: 254–257; Fujita et al., 1984. *J Am Geriat Soc* 32: 124–128; and Report on the Joint Epidemiological Survey on the Health of the Elderly in Shichikawa and Oshima Districts, Wakayama Prefecture, 1975, 1976 and 1977, by the Wakayama Medical College.

TABLE 30.3

Differences in Causes of Death between Mountain and Seacoast Inhabitants (1965–1975) per 100,000

Cause of Death	Seacoast	Mountain
Malignancy	182	243
Cerebrovascular disease	143	215
Cardiovascular disease	78	154
Infection	34	83
Suicide	0	44
Senescence with no specific disease causing death	304	88

Source: From Report on the Joint Epidemiological Survey on the Health of the Elderly in Shichikawa and Oshima Districts, Wakayama Prefecture, 1975, by the Wakayama Medical College.

exposure have been either insufficient or deficient, the causes of death from cerebrovascular disease, cardiovascular disease, cancer, and infection, mainly pneumonia, were much higher compared with the seacoast area with a generally more favorable nutritional pattern and general nutritional intake and solar exposure. The incidence of suicide, 44 per 100,000 population in the mountain area compared with 0 in the seacoast area over the period of 10 years, is hardly due to chance alone, reminding us of a possible role of insufficient intakes of Ca and vitamin D on depressive episodes (Hoogendijk et al., 2008). The nutritional status of the mountain people has improved in Japan so that such tragic difference no longer exists among various districts in Japan, let alone the mountain and seacoast districts in and around the Kii Peninsula. The importance of Ca and vitamin D nutrition not only for bone health but also for general health and welfare of the nation is clearly indicated by the results of this survey conducted more than 30 years ago.

THE CALCIUM PARADOX

The human body, despite its complexity, may be regarded as a pool of its constituents such as metal ions. After entrance of a substance into the human body, it is distributed uniformly. The more substance enters the body, the higher is its concentration expected to become. This actually occurs in the case of iron. For example, iron concentration rises on a high iron intake and falls on a low iron intake in blood and many tissues. This is an orthodox or straightforward sequence of event.

Not so in the case of Ca; higher Ca intake does not raise serum Ca concentration; neither does deficient Ca intake brings down serum Ca. Strangely enough, Ca concentration in the blood vessel wall, cartilage, and other tissues increases despite a decrease of Ca in the bone presenting with osteoporosis, whereas serum Ca concentration is maintained constant in Ca deficiency. This paradox, coexistence of Ca deficiency in the bone and Ca excess in other tissues, is called *the calcium paradox*.

The secret of the Ca paradox is hidden in the bone, which acts as a huge and unlimited Ca bank but refuses to be a bank for iron and other substances. Whatever Ca comes into the body, the bone simply stores it, preventing a sudden rise of serum Ca. When Ca income is insufficient and serum Ca starts to drop, the bone releases Ca to prevent further fall, restoring it to the constant normal level. Because the bone has 10^4 times as much Ca as blood and 108 times as much as cytosol or intracellular fluid, Ca released from bone readily enters various tissues and even inside of the cells like flood, causing all kinds of troubles associated with aging, such as arteriosclerosis, hypertension, and degenerative diseases of the brain and joints, through disturbance of cellular signal transduction due to increased cytosolic Ca concentration.

LOW CA INTAKE AND HIGH SERUM PTH

A low Ca intake in combination with low vitamin D status from both dietary intake and seasonal sunlight exposure is considered the major cause of osteoporosis in Japan. Postmenopausal osteoporosis, although traditionally considered a manifestation of estrogen withdrawal, is also influenced in a major way by inadequate intake of Ca and/or vitamin D. Estrogen deficiency, it should be recalled, also contributes to Ca deficiency through increased urinary Ca loss (Nordin, 1997), and a decrease of intestinal Ca absorption induces Ca deficiency (Caniggia et al., 1963). Fujita et al. (1972) were the first to report an increase of serum PTH in Japanese women with postmenopausal osteoporosis, and this observation was followed by similar reports in other parts of the world (Roof et al., 1976; Wiske et al., 1979; Insogna et al., 1981). Hiroshima atomic bomb survivors also showed a high serum PTH (Fujiwara et al., 1994). Chapuy et al. (1983) in France found a high prevalence of osteoporosis and fracture, with elevated serum PTH concentration, in homes for the elderly, and they reported a favorable effect, that is, reduction of nonvertebral fractures, with Ca and vitamin D treatment for over 1 year. McKane et al. (1996) were able to suppress the elevated serum PTH concentration in elderly subjects by simple Ca supplementation, up to as much as 2400 mg/day.

The Kii Peninsula mountain inhabitants, who had high prevalence of osteoporosis and spinal compression fracture, presumably resulting from low Ca and vitamin D intakes, also showed a high prevalence of aortic calcification and mortality due to cardiovascular diseases. Such contrasting bone and cardiovascular comorbidities, that is, osteoporosis with decreased Ca content in bone and arterial calcification with increased Ca content in the arteries, were first recognized as early as 1957 by a radiologist, who advanced a theory on the shift of Ca from bone to blood vessel as a typical manifestation of aging (Elkeles, 1957). Many reports on bone–blood vessel comorbidity have followed, until an association of low bone mass with carotid atherosclerosis in postmenopausal women was recently published in Japan (Tamaki et al., 2009).

Parathyroid cells respond to a low serum Ca concentration via a membrane Ca-sensing receptor (Brown, 1991). Because Ca-sensing receptors also detect low serum amino acid concentration resulting from a low protein intake, insufficient protein consumption may also contribute to secondary hyperparathyroidism and osteoporosis (Conigrave et al., 2000; Kerstetter et al., 2003).

PHYSIOLOGICAL AND CLINICAL CA PARADOX

Myocardial cells placed in Ca-deficient medium followed by a Ca-rich solution caused a marked increase of myocardial cytosolic Ca and eventually cell death (Goshima et al., 1980). The physiological concept of the Ca paradox was apparently derived from this experiment in which perfusion with a solution low in Ca concentration paradoxically caused a high concentration toxic to the cell. Extrapolated into the whole body clinical phenomena, the physiological Ca paradox has been expanded to include many pathological processes associated with aging; Ca deficiency leading to secondary hyperparathyroidism, Ca mobilization from bone, and its transfer to soft tissues with much less Ca content such as cartilage, vascular wall and other connective tissue, and intracellular compartment of variety of cells (Fujita and Palmieri, 2000). The list of the examples of the clinical Ca paradox is long, including hypertension, atherosclerosis, diabetes mellitus, obesity, immune dysfunction, degenerating diseases of the nervous system, and psychiatric disorders such as depression and panic syndrome (Fujita, 1986, 2002a, 2002b).

Frequent association of osteoporosis with calcified atherosclerosis is a typical example of whole body Ca paradox. Confronted by the impending risk of Ca deficiency and hypocalcemia which might cause serious disturbance of vital functions such as heart and brain activity, the bone storing more than 99% of Ca in the living organism has no choice but to release some of it to restore the serum Ca concentration. Because the difference in Ca concentration between bone and intracellular compartment may be as great as 10^8 fold, a small contribution of Ca from bone stores may overwhelm the ultramicro-intracellullar Ca concentration, that is, flooding of Ca in the intracellular compartment. By being repeatedly subjected to this process, bone may not only become osteoporotic, but soft tissue may also become calcified because of increased intracellular Ca concentrations. Cellular homeostasis and signal transduction may be disrupted, with eventual cellular dysfunction and even cell death. PTH, which inevitably mediates the Ca paradox by mobilizing Ca from bone, occupies an inevitable niche as a mediator of the Ca paradox for Ca mobilization from bone, and it occupies a key position in Ca paradox by stimulating Ca transfer from the extracellular bone fluid compartment to the major cytoplasmic compartment of cells (Bogin et al., 1981).

CA PARADOX AND PEROXIDE FREE RADICALS

The Ca paradox also generates oxidative stress because the Ca-loaded cells accumulate damaging free radicals of oxygen as a result of cytoplasmic and mitochondrial metabolic disturbance (Bracci, 1992). A marked decrease in plasma antioxidants has been reported in osteoporosis (Maggio et al., 2003). The final common path of the Ca paradox, an increase of intracellular free Ca ions, plays a crucial role in apoptosis induced by hydrogen peroxide. For example, incubation of ZC7901 cells with cadmium, that is, Cd^{2+}, which increases the generation of reactive oxygen species, raised cytosolic free Ca six-fold and induced apoptosis (Xiang and Shao, 2003). In addition, an increase of Ca influx into cytosol increases free radical production (Lipton and Nicotera, 1998). Thus, the two powerful candidates that may aggravate the aging process are potentially connected within the intracellular signal transduction system: oxygen stress creating peroxides and other free radicals and the Ca paradox resulting from an increase of cytosolic Ca. Each factor impinges on the other, which suggests that each may induce the other in an interactive manner, suggesting that these two processes are indeed inseparable deterrents of human health and longevity, but with two different faces.

DEGENERATIVE JOINT DISEASE AS CA PARADOX

Another group of diseases which may be explained by the Ca paradox are the degenerative joint diseases (Fujita, 1998).

Ca released from bone due to Ca deficiency and secondary hyperparathyroidism readily enters the adjacent cartilage which hardens, degenerates, and eventually is worn away, in response to excessive loading on the joints. An increase in direct contact between the two bones over the narrowed joint space generates osteophytes and hyperostotic zones especially in the vertebral and knee joints subjected to especially heavy stress load, which may lead to the development of osteoarthritis, typically characterized by severe pain on movement. Although primary cartilaginous degeneration may also contribute to the development of osteoarthritis, osteoporosis and osteoarthritis are one and inseparable because as bone loses Ca, cartilage gains it and degenerates. The best evidence supporting this hypothesis would be the dramatic analgesic effect of antiosteoporotic bisphosphonates, especially etidronate, on osteoarthritic pain (Fujita et al., 2001, 2009).

HOW TO OVERCOME THE CALCIUM PARADOX

CA SUPPLEMENTATION AND THE CA PARADOX

Because Ca paradox is caused by Ca deficiency, the best way to avoid it is to provide a sufficient Ca supply via a diet. The problem of Ca supplementation, however, is a rather low efficiency of intestinal absorption of Ca supplements compared with fat, water, and other electrolytes (Anderson, 1991; Toskes, 1996). The intestinal absorption of Ca from Ca supplements in common use was low, but a newly developed form raised anticipation that Ca efficiency could be significantly increased.

In 1988, oyster shell heated as high as 1000 became available for human testing. Following oral administration of this new Ca supplement in patients with hypocalcemia due to hypoparathyroidism and those with renal insufficiency, serum Ca concentration was effectively restored toward normal range. This finding went against the generally held concept of poor Ca absorption from other supplements. The new product was called active absorbable calcium (AACa) (Fujita et al., 1988). AACa also increased radial bone mineral density measured by single-photon absorptiometry after 12 and 24 months, but it decreased in subjects without Ca supplementation over the same period in Katsuragi Hospital, south of Osaka (Fujita et al., 1990). Addition of seaweed component heated at high temperature (heated algal ingredient) (Fujita et al., 2000) to AACa was then found to increase its absorbability (Uenishi et al., 2010), and this new preparation was called active absorbable algal calcium (AAACa) (Fujita et al., 2000).

KATSURAGI CALCIUM STUDY

A randomized, prospective, double-blind study comparing AAACa and Ca carbonate with placebo was then conducted on hospitalized women with a mean age of 80 years at Katsuragi

Hospital over a period of 2 years (Katsuragi Calcium Study) (Fujita et al., 1990) and reappraised (Fujita et al., 2004). AAACa increased spinal BMD, as measured by dual-energy X-ray absorptiometry (DXA), significantly over the level maintained by placebo, but the level achieved by Ca carbonate was not significantly different from the placebo level. Incident spinal fracture and degree of vertebral deformity evaluated by intraindividual variation of the combined mean BMD of L_1 to L_4 vertebrae, suggested as indicators of advanced osteoarthritis of the spine (Fujita et al., 2003), were also significantly less in the AAACa-supplemented group than in the placebo group. Serum intact and midportion PTH was significantly lower, and calcitonin higher, in AAACa, but not in either the Ca carbonate group or the placebo group at the 12th month of the study. When AAACa was given in all groups for additional 6 months following the completion of the study, serum PTH fell in the placebo group and was not different from the serum PTH of the AAA group any more.

Fat mass, measured by whole body DXA, significantly increased by approximately 23% in the placebo group but decreased by 5% in the AAACa-supplemented group, with a significant difference between the two, suggesting a possibility of decrease of the fat mass by Ca supplementation. No significant difference was noted between the Ca carbonate and placebo groups.

One review and one meta-analysis of the effect of Ca supplementation on BMD included results of the Katsuragi Calcium Study reporting the major effect of AAACa on bone mass (Tang et al., 2007; Nordin, 2009).

RED CELL CA CONTENT AND THE CA PARADOX

Finally, red cell Ca content rises in advancing age, and this phenomenon may be a possible manifestation of the Ca paradox. The red cell Ca falls to the typical level of younger subjects after effective Ca supplementation. AAACa caused a significantly greater decline in red cell Ca than either placebo or Ca carbonate supplementation did (Fujita et al., 2008). The red cell Ca increase is positively and significantly correlated with age, suggesting an increased Ca entry in the intracellular compartment with age. Supplementation with 900 mg Ca/day as AAACa significantly decreased red cell Ca content. The same amount of Ca as $CaCO_3$ slightly decreased the red cell Ca content, but the decrement was significantly less than that induced by AAACa. No significant fall of red blood cell Ca content was found in the placebo group, which received no Ca. The fall of red cell Ca content may be used as a test for the bioavailability of Ca in a supplement and hence the efficiency of Ca supplementation in inhibiting PTH secretion and preventing the Ca paradox.

SUMMARY

Japan is an Asian and Oceanic nation with the nutritional traditions of both, that is, characterized by low Ca intake. As a result of recent industrialization and lengthening of life span, the prevalence of osteoporosis and fractures has rapidly increased, with a peculiar pattern of a high rate of spinal compression fracture and a relatively low rate of hip fracture in Japan. The systemic Ca paradox consisting of low bone Ca content with paradoxically high Ca content of soft tissue and intracellular compartment characterizes Ca profile of Japanese elders with substantial calcified atherosclerosis, hypertension, degenerative diseases of the central nervous system, and degenerative joint diseases accompanying osteoporosis. Correction of Ca deficiency with highly absorbable Ca, such as AAACa, an ocean product consisting of shells and seaweed, may represent a significant advance to a victory over the Ca deficit. AAACa may be a merciful gift from the mother ocean surrounding Japan constantly watching it, the country which has suffered most from the Ca paradox. The high efficiency of Ca absorption of this supplement may well serve as the most powerful remedy for treating the Ca paradox all over the world.

REFERENCES

Anderson, J.J.B. 1991. Nutritional biochemistry of calcium and phosphorus. *J Nutr Biochem* 2:300–307.

Anderson, J.J.B. 2000. The important role of physical activity in skeletal development: How exercise may counter low calcium intake. *Am J Clin Nutr* 17:1384–1386.

Bogin, E., Massry, S.G., and Harary, I. 1981. Effect of parathyroid hormone on rat heart cells. *J Clin Invest* 67:1215–1227.

Bracci, R. 1992. Calcium involvement in free radical effects. *Calcif Tissue Int* 51:401–405.

Brown, E.M. 1991. Extracellular Ca^{2+} sensing, regulation of cell function, and role of Ca^{2+} and other ions as extracellular (first) messengers. *Physiol Rev* 71:371–411

Caniggia, A., Gennari, C., Bianchi, V., et al. 1963. Intestinal absorption of ^{45}Ca in senile osteoporosis. *Acta Med Scand* 173:613–617.

Chapuy, M.C., Durr, F., and Chapuy, P. 1983. Age-related changes in parathyroid hormone and 25-hydroxycholecalciferol levels. *J Gerontol* 38:19–22.

Conigrave, A.D., Quinin, S.J., and Brown, E.M. 2000. L-amino acid sensing by the extracellular Ca^{2+}-sensing receptor. *Proc. Natl. Acad Sci USA* 97:4814–4819.

Cummings, S.R., Cauley, J.A., Palermo, L., et al. 1994. Racial differences in hip axis length might explain racial differences in rates of hip fracture. Study of Osteoporotic Fractures Research Group. *Osteopor Int* 4:226–229.

Elkeles, A. 1957. A comparative radiological study of calcified atheroma in males and females over 50 years of age. *Lancet* 273:714–715.

Fujita, T. 1986. Aging and calcium. *Miner Electrolyte Metab* 12:149–156.

Fujita, T. 1998. Degenerative joint disease: An example of calcium paradox. *J Bone Miner Metab* 16:195–205.

Fujita, T. 2002a. Calcium and aging. In *Calcium in Internal Medicine*, Morii, H., Nishizawa, Y., and Massry, S.G., eds. Springer Verlag, London, pp. 399–415.

Fujita, T. 2002b. Calcium homeostasis and signaling in aging. In *Advances in Cell Aging and Gerontology 10*, Mattson, M.P., ed. Elsevier, Amsterdam, pp. 13–26.

Fujita, T., Fujii, Y., Goto, B., et al. 2000. Increase of intestinal calcium absorption and bone mineral density by heated algal ingredient (HAI) in rats. *J Bone Miner Metab* 18:165–169.

Fujita, T., Fujii, Y., Okada, S.F., et al. 2001. Analgesic effect of etidronate on degenerative joint disease. *J Bone Miner Metab* 19:251–256.

Fujita, T., Fukase, M., Miyamoto, H, et al. 1990. Increase of bone mineral density by calcium supplement with oyster shell electrolysate. *Bone Miner* 11:85–91.

Fujita, T., Fukase, M., Nakada, M., et al. 1988. Intestinal absorption of oyster shell electrolysate. *Bone Miner* 4:321–327.

Fujita, T., Ohgitani, S., Ohue, M., et al. 2008. Aging and calcium paradox: Increase of red cell calcium content with age and its reversal by calcium supplementation. In *Women and Aging: New Research*, Benninghouse, H. T., and Rosset, A.G., eds. Nova Science Publishers, New York, NY, pp. 529–538.

Fujita, T., Ohue, T., Fujii, Y., et al. 1990. Heated oyster shell-seaweed calcium (AAACa) on osteoporosis. *Calcif Tissue Int* 58:225–230.

Fujita, T., Ohue, M., Fujii, Y., et al. 2003. Intra-individual variation in lumbar bone mineral density as a measure of spondylotic deformity in the elderly. *J Bone Miner Metab* 21:98–102.

Fujita, T., Ohue, M., Fujii, Y., et al. 2004. Reappraisal of Katsuragi Calcium Study, a prospective, double-blind, placebo-controlled study of the effect of active absorbable algal calcium (AAACa) on vertebral deformity and fracture. *J Bone Miner Metab* 22:32–38.

Fujita, T., Ohue, M., Fujii, Y., et al. 2009. Comparison of the analgesic effect of bisphosphonates; alendronate and risedronate by electroalgometry utilizing the fall of skin impedance. *J Bone Miner Metab* 27:234–239.

Fujita, T., Okamoto, Y., Sakagami, Y., and Ota, K.M. 1984. Bone changes and aortic calcification in aging inhabitants of mountain versus seacoast communities in the Kii Peninsula. *J Am Geriat Soc* 32:124–128.

Fujita, T., Okamoto, Y., Tomita, T., et al. 1977. Calcium metabolism in aging inhabitants of mountain versus seacoast communities in the Kii Peninsula. *J Am Geriat Soc* 24:254–257.

Fujita, T., Orimo, H., Okano, K., et al. 1972. Radioimmunoassay of serum parathyroid hormone in postmenopausal osteoporosis. *Endocrinol Japon* 19:571–577

Fujita, T., and Palmieri, G.M.A. 2000. Calcium paradox disease: Calcium deficiency prompting secondary hyperparathyroidism and cellular calcium overload. *J Bone Miner Metab* 18:109–125.

Fujiwara, S., Ross, P.D. 1997. Epidemiological studies of osteoporosis in Japan. In *Osteoporosis in Asia*, Lau, E.M.C., Ho, S.C., Leung, S., et al., eds. World Scientific, Singapore, pp. 21–29.

Fujiwara, S., Sposto, R., Shiraki, M., et al. 1994. Levels of parathyroid hormone and calcitonin in serum among atomic bomb survivors. *Radiat Res* 137:96–103.

Goshima, K., Wakabayashi, S., and Masuda, A. 1980. Ionic mechanism of morphological changes in cultured myo-cardial cells on successive incubation in media without and with Ca2+. *J Mol Cell Cardiol* 12:1135–1157.

Hoogendijk, W.J., Lips, P., Dik, M.G., et al. 2008. Depression is associated with decreased 25-hydroxyvitamin D and increased parathyroid hormone levels in older adults. *Arch Gen Psychiatry* 65:508–512.

Insogna, K.L., Lewis, A.M., Lipinski, B.A., et al. 1981. Effect of age on serum immunoreactive parathyroid hormone and its biological effects. *J Clin Endocrinol Metab* 53:1072–1075.

Kerstetter, J.E., O'Brien, K.O., and Insogna, K.L. 2003. Low-protein intake: The impact on calcium and bone homeostasis in humans. *J Nutr* 133:855s–861s.

Lacey, J.M., Anderson, J.J.B., Fujita, T., et al. 1991. Correlates of cortical bone mass among premenopausal and postmenopausal Japanese women. *J Bone Miner Res* 6:651–659.

Lipton, S.A., and Nicotera, P. 1998. Calcium, free radicals and excitotoxins in neuronal apoptosis. *Cell Calcium* 23:165–171.

Maggio, D., Barabani, M., Pierandrei, M., et al. 2003. Marked decrease in plasma antioxidants in aged osteo-porotic women: Results of a cross-sectional study. *J Clin Endocrinol Metab* 88:1523–1527.

McKane, W.R., Khosla, S., Egan, K.S., et al. 1996. Role of calcium intake in modulating age-related increases in parathyroid function and bone resorption. *J Clin Endocrinol Metab* 81:1699–1703.

Ministry of Health, Welfare and Labor Committee for Dietary Reference Intakes for Japanese, 2009. *Dietary Reference Intakes for Japanese, 2010.* Daiichi Shuppan Publishing Co, LTD, Tokyo.

Nakamura, K., Hori, Y., Nashimoto, M., et al. 2003. Nutritional covariates of dietary calcium in elderly Japanese women: Results of a study using the duplicate portion sampling method. *Nutrition* 19:922–925.

Nakamura, K., Hori, Y., Nashimoto, M., et al. 2004. Dietary calcium, sodium, phosphorus, and protein and bone metabolism in elderly Japanese women: A pilot study using the duplicate portion sampling method. *Nutrition* 20:340–345.

Nakamura, K., Saito, T., Yoshihara, A., et al. 2009. Low calcium intake is associated with increased bone resorption in postmenopausal Japanese women. Yokogoshi Study. *Public Health Nutr* 12:1–5.

Nishimuta, M., Kodama, N., Morikuni, E., et al. 2004. Balances of calcium, magnesium and phosphorus in Japanese young adults. *J Nutr Soc Vitaminol* 50:19–25.

Nordin, B.E.C. 1966. International patterns of osteoporosis. *Clin Orthop Relat Res* 45:17–30.

Nordin, B.E.C. 1997. Calcium and osteoporosis. *Nutrition* 13:664–686.

Nordin, B.E.C. 2009. The effect of calcium supplementation on bone loss in 32 controlled trials in postmeno-pausal women. *Osteoporos Int* 20:2135–2143.

Orimo, H., Hashimoto, T., Yoshimura, N., et al. 1997. Nationwide incidence survey of femoral neck fracture in Japan, 1997. *J Bone Miner Metab* 15:100–106.

Roof, B.S., Piel, C.F., Hansen, J, et al. 1976. Serum parathyroid hormone levels and serum calcitonin levels from birth to senescence. *Mech Ageing Dev* 5:289–304.

Ross, P.D., Fujiwara, S., Huang, C., et al. 1995. Vertebral fracture prevalence in women in Hiroshima compared to Caucasians or Japanese in the US. *Int J Epidemiol* 24:1171–1177.

Tamaki, J., Iki, M., Hirano, Y., et al. 2009. Low bone mass is associated with carotid atherosclerosis in postmenopausal women: The Japanese Population-Based Osteoporosis (JPOS) Cohort Study. *Osteoporos Int* 20:53–60.

Tang, B.M.P., Eslick, G.D., Nowson, C., et al. 2007. Use of calcium or calcium in combination with vitamin D supplementation to prevent fractures and bone loss in people aged 50 years and older: A meta-analysis. *Lancet* 370:657–666.

Toskes, P.P. 1996. Malabsorption. In *Cecil Textbook of Medicine*, Bennett, J.C. and Plum, F., eds. WB Saunders, Philadelphia, PA, pp. 695–707.

Tsubaki T., and Yase, Y. 1988. *Amyotrophic Lateral Sclerosis. Recent Development in Research and Treatment.* Excerpta Medica, Amsterdam.

Uenishi, K., Fujita, T., Ishida, H. et al., 2010. Fractional absorption of activeabsorbavle calcium (AAACa) and calcium carbonate measured by a doublestable isotopoe method.

Uenishi, K., Ishida, H., Kamei, A., et al. 2001. Calcium requirement estimated by balance study in elderly Japanese people. *Osteopors Int* 12:858–863.

Ueno, K., Nakamura, K., Nishiwaki, T., et al. 2005. Intakes of calcium and other nutrients related to bone health in Japanese female college students: A study using the duplicate portion sampling method. *Tohoku J Exp Med* 206:319–326.

Wiske, P.S., Epstein, S., Bell, N.H., et al. 1979. Increase in immunoreactive parathyroid hormone with age. *New Engl J Med* 300:1419–1421.

Xiang, L.X., and Shao, J.Z. 2003. Role of intracellular Ca2+, reactive oxygen species, mitochondria transmem-brane potential, and antioxidant enzymes in heavy metal-induced apoptosis in fish cells. *Bull Environ Contam Toxicol* 71:114–122.

31 Diet and Bone Health of the Chinese Population

Suzanne C. Ho and Yu-ming Chen

CONTENTS

INTRODUCTION

Osteoporotic fracture is becoming a major public health problem in Asia. With the rapidly aging populations, it is projected that by year 2050, half of the world's hip fracture incidence will occur in Asia (Cooper et al., 1992). Hip and spine fractures are associated with substantial morbidity, mortality, and economic costs in China, but preventive efforts are still minimal (Dai et al., 2007). Low bone mineral density (BMD) or osteoporosis is the most important risk factor for osteoporotic factures. Established risk factor for osteoporosis are advanced age, genetic, menopause, low body weight, and lifestyle factor variables (NAMS, 2010).

Diet and nutrition are among the modifiable factors for the improvement of bone health. A balanced and bone-promoting diet forms the basis for pharmacologic approaches to the prevention or management of osteoporosis (Anon., 2010). Although many epidemiological studies have been conducted in the West, studies on osteoporosis and hip fractures among the Chinese population are relatively limited (Ho et al., 1993, 2008; Xu et al., 1996; Yan et al., 1999). However, dietary pattern and food culture among the Chinese, a population of over 1345 billion (China Popin, 2011), are quite different from that of the West. A plant-based diet with higher intakes of fruits and vegetables, fish, and soy food and lower intakes of calcium (Ca) and protein would mark some of the major differences (Zhai and Yang, 2006). This chapter focuses on the dietary intake of these components and bone health in the Chinese.

SOY AND BONE HEALTH

Soy has been suggested to have beneficial effects on a number of hormonally related diseases/conditions including dislipidemia, breast cancer, prostate cancer, menopausal symptoms, and osteoporosis. Soy is a traditional diet of the Chinese population. The soybean is the only commonly consumed food containing nutritionally relevant amounts of isoflavones, a class of phytoestrogens containing the three major constituents, genistein, daidzein, and glycitein. These diphenolic compounds are structurally similar to estrogen and possess mild estrogenic effects. Their preferential binding to estrogen receptor indicates that they act as selective estrogen receptor modulators (Setchell, 2001). The effects of soy and soy isoflavones on the related health conditions have received much research attention over the past two and a half decades. In vitro and animal studies have mainly indicated that soy or soy isoflavones may play a role in the reduction of bone loss (Arjmandi et al., 1998; Rickard et al., 2003; Setchell and Lydeking-Olsen, 2003). The bone-sparing effect of soy could be due to its estrogen-like effect of isoflavones in the inhibition of bone resorption or stimulation of bone formation or through its effect on estrogen receptors in bone cells (Fanti et al., 1998; Arjmandi et al., 2003). As reported by Arjmandi et al. (2003), soy could also have an anabolic effect on bone through the enhancement of insulin-like growth factor-I synthesis.

The beneficial effects observed in animal models, however, could not be confirmed by long-term randomized clinical trials (RCTs) of human subjects, and inconsistent findings have been reported (Potter et al., 1998; Alekel et al., 2000; Anderson et al., 2002; Chen et al., 2003; Uesugi et al., 2003; Gallagher et al., 2004; Harkness et al., 2004; Kreijkamp-Kaspers et al., 2004; Lydeking-Olsen et al., 2004; Arjmandi et al., 2005; Huang et al., 2006; Newton et al., 2006; Wu et al., 2006; Ye et al., 2006; Evans et al., 2007; Brink et al., 2008). Limited sample sizes and variations in intervention regimes and individual metabolic responses might partly explain the conflicting results. A meta-analysis of RCTs on isoflavone supplementation on BMD in women with a minimum treatment duration of 1 year showed no significant increase in BMD at the lumbar spine, total hip, or femoral neck (Liu et al., 2009). The meta-analysis suggested that ingesting a mean daily dose of 87-mg soy isoflavones for 1–2 years seemed unlikely to significantly improve BMD in women. Subanalyses showed a marginally significantly favorable effect on the spine BMD in the larger dose (≥80 mg/day, median 99 mg/day) of isoflavone group, but not in the lower dose group (<80/day, median 60 mg/day) (Liu et al., 2009). Confining the analyses to Asian women did not seem to alter the results (Liu et al., 2009). One recently published RCT investigating the 3-year effect of soy isoflavone tablets (80 and 120 mg) on BMD among Western postmenopausal women observed a modest protective effect of 120 mg of isoflavone intake at the femoral neck (only among the compliant subjects) (Alekel et al., 2010). Although most of the RCTs and epidemiological studies have BMD as the primary outcome, the few that have included bone mineral content (BMC) have reported beneficial changes in hip BMC and whole-body BMC (Chen et al., 2004). BMC has been proposed as a better indicator of nutrition-related changes in bone than BMD (Atkinson et al., 2008), which is derived from dividing BMC by the area of the region scanned.

Contradictory to the RCT findings, population-based epidemiological investigations among Chinese have generally shown a favorable association between higher soy/isoflavone intake and BMD and fracture rates. Three studies have found a positive relationship between soy or isoflavone intake and BMD or BMC at one or more bone sites. A cross-sectional study of 650 Chinese women showed that dietary isoflavone intake was associated with higher BMD at the spine, hip, and Ward's triangle (Mei et al., 2001) among postmenopausal women, although no association was found among premenopausal women. In another population-based study involving 454 Chinese postmenopausal women aged 48–62 years, BMD at the hip, spine, and total body was significantly higher in the fourth than in the first soy protein intake quartile, but protective effects were observed only among women who were 4 or more years beyond menopause (Ho et al., 2003).

Very few prospective studies on soy and bone changes have been published. One 38-month prospective study in women aged 30–40 years showed that the decrease (3.5%) in spinal BMD in the first isoflavone intake quartile was significantly greater than the loss (1.1%) in the fourth intake quartile (Ho et al., 2001). Another 30-month prospective study on the determinants of bone changes in perimenopausal women aged 45–55 years has revealed that higher soy intake quartiles (third and fourth) were associated with better whole-body BMC, even after adjustment for other potential confounders (Ho et al., 2008).

Although BMD measurement serves as an indicator of osteoporosis and an important predictor of fractures, it would be relevant to examine the relation of soy intake with the fracture end point. So far, only two published studies have examined habitual soy intake and hip fracture risk: one conducted among Chinese women in Shanghai (Zhang et al., 2005) and another in Singapore Chinese (Koh et al., 2009). Both studies reported a protective effect of higher soy intake in an equivalent to about ≥5 g soy protein consumed daily, which seemed to lower the fracture risk by about 30% when compared with the lower intake group. Thus, population-based epidemiological evidence in the Chinese population has so far provided a relatively consistent picture of a beneficial role of habitual soy intake on bone health.

In summary, the epidemiological literature suggests that soy intake is related to higher bone mass in Chinese. However, some caution is needed when drawing conclusions about the epidemiological studies because the data are limited and publication bias may exist. Additional RCTs and epidemiological investigations on the soy–bone linkage are clearly needed, especially prospective studies that include BMD, as well as BMC, and also fracture rates as outcomes.

CALCIUM AND BONE HEALTH

Adequate Ca intake is a major precondition of optimal bone health. The Chinese have habitually low Ca intake, with a range of mean intake around 350 to 550 mg/day for women (Ge et al., 1996; Ho et al., 2004) and around 300 to 400 mg/day for Mainland Chinese children in 2002 (Zhai and Yang, 2006). The dietary sources are also quite different from those of the Western populations, with 60% from plant sources and only about 25% from milk and dairy products (Ho et al., 1994; Ho, 1997). Ca intervention studies have mainly focused on Caucasian populations consuming an intake of over 700 mg Ca/day, and the effect of this amount of Ca on BMD seemed minimal (Winzenberg et al., 2006). Epidemiological and intervention studies in Chinese populations with habitual low Ca intake have generally shown that an adequate Ca intake (≥800 mg/day) improves bone mineral acquisition in children and adolescents (Lee et al., 1994b, 1995; Ho et al., 2005). Positive effects have been observed, whether the Ca was in the form of a supplement, fortified foods, or dairy products. Even a moderate supplement of 300 mg Ca/day over 18 months was observed to have enhanced bone acquisition in 7-year-old Chinese children with a usual low Ca intake of 280 mg/day (Lee et al., 1994). A 1-year Ca-fortified soy milk supplementation study was found to have a beneficial effect on hip BMD and BMC in adolescent girls aged 14 to 16 years (Ho et al., 2005). A higher Ca intake was also associated with 4%–7% higher BMD attained in young Chinese women aged 31–40 years (Ho et al., 1994).

Estrogen decline and greatly reduced ovarian production play a key role in early postmenopausal bone loss. An inconsistent relationship between dietary Ca intake and BMD in early postmenopausal women has been noted in Caucasian women (Dawson-Hughes et al., 1987; Shea et al., 2002). Few such studies are available in Chinese women with historically little use of hormonal therapy. A cross-sectional study found no correlation between Ca intake and bone mass (BMC) in Chinese (Chiu et al., 1997). Another cross-sectional study of women from five counties in China reported a positive association between dietary Ca intake and bone mass in middle-aged and elderly women, although the association was weakened after adjustment for other positive determinants (factors), such as age and body weight (Hu et al., 1994). A cross-sectional association between dietary Ca intake and bone mass was also noted in a study of Chinese perimenopausal women aged 45–55 years, but a follow-up over 30 months did not detect a significant long-term bone-preserving effect of Ca (Ho et al., 2008). It is likely that higher habitual Ca intake may not be effective in reducing bone loss in women transitioning through menopause or within the first few menopausal years (Ho et al., 2008). Another longitudinal study in a cohort of 454 slightly older postmenopausal Chinese women aged 48–62 years and within 12 years of menopause has shown that high habitual dietary Ca intake had a beneficial effect on bone loss at the whole body and some regions of the hip among those belonging to the highest intake quartile (but less than 600 mg/day) (Ho et al., 2004).

These cohorts of Chinese women were free from hormonal therapy (Ho et al., 2004, 2008). The results correlate with those of a study conducted among Canadian postmenopausal women, not taking estrogen, whose total Ca intake had a positive effect on BMD at cortical bone sites, such as hip, femoral neck, and total body, although a more significant proportion of variance of BMD was accounted for by years since menopause and body weight (Suzuki et al., 2003).

An intake of Ca exceeding 900 mg/day seemed to be helpful in the prevention of cortical bone loss in postmenopausal Chinese women (Ho et al., 2004). A 2-year intervention study with 50-g high-Ca milk powder supplementation providing an additional Ca of 550 to 650 mg/day to postmenopausal Chinese women aged 55–59 years demonstrated a mild retardation of bone loss, and the effect was more significant at the femoral neck than at the spine (Lau et al., 2001). Although prospective studies on dietary Ca intake and fractures in Chinese subjects are lacking, case–control studies have shown increased risks of vertebral fracture and hip fracture in older Chinese women with low Ca intakes (Chan et al., 1996; Lau et al., 2001).

Ca absorption, it has been proposed, may be more efficient in populations with low Ca intake. The limited Ca absorption studies in Chinese populations have shown a high absorption efficiency in children (Lee et al., 1994, 2005) as well as in postmenopausal women (Kung et al., 1998; Chen et al., 2007). A small study in 12 children with usual intake of 300 mg Ca/day had a mean fractional true Ca absorption (TFCA) of 63 ± 11%, whereas in another study, Chinese girls aged 9–17 years had a TFCA of 60% ± 14% (Lee et al., 2002). A Ca absorption study conducted in healthy postmenopausal Chinese women aged 49–64 years with a similar level of Ca intake found that a TFCA of 57% ± 12% and a mean Ca intake of about 1300 mg/day were required to reach the plateau Ca retention. This amount of Ca seemed to concur with a similar proposed level of 1300 mg/day of intake to allow maximal Ca retention for adolescence, although the study was conducted in Caucasian adolescents (Weaver et al., 2006).

Thus, with such relatively low Ca intakes in the Chinese population, an increase in dietary intake of this mineral through both traditional food items, such as tofu, green leafy vegetables, small fish with bone, some seeds and nuts (e.g., sesame), as well as some Ca-fortified foods like soymilk, and also dairy products would be useful to increase the overall dietary Ca intake. Ca supplements could achieve the same high amounts of Ca needed for bone development and maintenance, but they are not as healthful as foods that contain many nutrients.

FRUITS, VEGETABLES, AND BONE HEALTH

Nutrients, such as vitamin K, vitamin C, and alkaline ions, found abundantly in fruits and vegetables, have been reported to be associated with better human bone indices by Tucker et al. (1999). These findings have led to the examination of linkages between fruit and vegetable consumption and bone health. New et al. (1997) reported the association of fruit and vegetable with bone health in a cross-sectional study. They found that BMD at the lumbar spine, femoral neck, greater trochanter, and Ward's triangle was significantly lower by 3.4%–4.8% in middle-aged (44–50 years) women who reported a low intake of fruit in early adulthood than that in those who reported a medium or high intake. A few other studies have also reported the beneficial associations between fruit and vegetable consumption and BMD and/or bone size among children and adults (New et al., 1997; Tucker et al., 1999; New et al., 2000; Tucker et al., 2001, 2002; New and Millward 2003; Macdonald et al., 2004; McGartland et al., 2004; Tylavsky et al., 2004). Similar positive associations between fruit and vegetable intake and BMD, BMC, or lower fracture rates were also observed in most (Tucker et al., 1999; Tylavsky et al., 2004; Vatanparast et al., 2005; Prynne et al., 2006), but not all (Whiting et al., 2002; Kaptoge et al., 2003; Thorpe et al., 2008), Western studies. The findings in Chinese populations are consistent with the results from Western populations.

The Chinese population has traditionally consumed a plant-based diet. A typical Chinese diet is composed of higher components of vegetables and fruits and lower intake of protein than that of their Western counterparts (Leung et al., 1997; Zhai and Yang, 2006). A Chinese national survey found a higher intake of fruits and vegetables (320 g/day) among the Chinese (Zhai and Yang, 2006) compared with 3.5 ± 1.8 servings (~280 g/day) among American women at 52 years of age (Djousse et al., 2004).

Five studies reported positive associations of intake of vegetables and fruits with BMD and BMC in Chinese adults (Dawson-Hughes 1998; Li et al., 2001; Chen et al., 2006; Zalloua et al., 2007; Ho et al., 2008). The largest study by Zalloua et al. (2007) was conducted among 5848 men and 6207 women aged 25–64 years in rural Anhui, China. Greater fruit intake was significantly associated with higher total body BMD in men ($p > .05$) and in women ($p < .05$), and at the hip, in men (≤45 years) ($p < .05$). The risks for low BMD (quartile one) were 11% to 27% lower among subjects with high fruit intake (>250 vs. ≤250 g/week). Similar results were observed by Li et al. (2001) in a nationwide study of 1299 men and 1391 women (50–97 years) in Mainland China. They found significant positive associations between vegetable intake and hip BMD in urban men and between combined vegetable and fruit intake and hip BMD in urban women, but no significant association was observed in rural men and women (Li et al., 2001). Two cross-sectional studies conducted in Hong Kong also found that greater fruit and vegetable intake was associated with greater bone mass in both perimenopausal (Ho et al., 2008) and postmenopausal midlife women (Chen et al., 2006). However, combined fruit and vegetable intake was not observed to have a protective effect for women transitioning through menopause (Ho et al., 2008) (Table 31.1).

The 2000–2001 Nutrition and Health Survey in Taiwan Elementary School Children found that frequency of vegetable or fruit consumption was positively and significantly related to the broadband ultrasound attenuation (in dB/MHz) in both boys and girls (Lin et al., 2007). A similar result was observed in a small study in Guangzhou children aged 8–12 years (Yu et al., 1998). However, inconsistent results were observed in a school-based cohort study in Beijing of 757 children aged 10 years (Zhang et al., 2010). Zhang et al. (2010) found that greater fruit consumption was associated with lower 5-year bone mass (BMC) accrual at the distal forearm but a higher increase in BMD at the proximal forearm. Higher vegetable intake was noted to be associated with a lower increase in total body BMD but a higher BMD increase at the distal forearm in the multivariate regression model (Table 31.1).

Two case–control studies examined the association between consumption of vegetables and fruits and bone fractures in Chinese. Xu et al. (2009) assessed the relationship between fruits and vegetables and the risk of forearm fracture in Chinese postmenopausal women aged 50–70 years. A total of 209 individuals with new forearm fractures and 209 age- and district-matched community controls were selected in Chengdu, China. The estimated odds ratio (95% confidence interval) [ORs (95%CI)] for forearm fracture was 0.53 (0.42–0.67) for each quintile increase in vegetable intake after adjustment for potential confounders. Another hospital-based study determined the effect of fruit and vegetable intake on the risk of hip fractures in middle-aged and elderly adults (55–80 years) in Guangzhou (Ouyan et al., 2008). This fracture study enrolled 279 incident cases and 279 age-, gender-, and district-matched hospital or community-based controls. As compared with those of the lowest quartile group of fruit and vegetable intake (158 g/day), the ORs (95%CI) for hip fractures were 0.64 (0.39, 1.03), 0.53 (0.30, 0.85), and 0.51 (0.27, 0.80) in Quartiles II (274 g/day), III (421 g/day), and IV (620 g/day), respectively. The results of these two studies (Ouyan et al., 2008; Xu et al., 2009) suggested that greater consumption of vegetables and fruits might be beneficial for the prevention of osteoporotic bone fractures in Chinese populations (Table 31.1).

Several mechanisms might explain the potential beneficial effects of fruits and vegetables on bone health. Among them, the acid–base homeostatic theory has been addressed extensively in previous reviews in explaining the potential favorable effects of fruits and vegetables on bone health (Bushinsky and Frick, 2000; Lemann et al., 2003; New, 2003; Krieger et al., 2004). Alkaline bone mineral may play a role in the defense against modest metabolic acidosis. The abundant base cations (potassium, Ca, and magnesium) in fruits and vegetables act as buffers for organic acids and, thus, prevent acidosis-induced bone loss. Many human studies found an association between greater intakes of potassium (Jones et al., 2001; Jehle et al., 2006) and magnesium (Dimai et al.,

TABLE 31.1

A Summary of the Results of Studies on Fruit and Vegetables on Bone Health in Chinese

Study	Study Design	Study Size	Age, Mean (SD) or Range	Dietary Marker	Outcome	Association
Xu et al., 2009	CC	F: 209/F: 209	50–70	Veg	Forearm fracture	Positive
Ouyan et al., 2008	CC	279/279 M: 38%	68.7 (6.7)	F&V	Hip fracture	Positive
Yan et al., 2005	CC	348 (M: 107)/210 (M: 57)	62.1	Green veg	Osteoporosis	Positive
Ho et al., 2008	CS, cohort	F: 438	45–55	F&V	BMD BMC	Positive (TH BMC, TB BMC) in cross-sectional data; NS with 30-m bone changes
Chen et al., 2006	CS	F: 670	48–63	F&V	BMD	Positive (BMD at the TB, LS, TH)
Zalloua et al., 2007	CS	M: 5848 F: 6207	24–67	F&V	BMD	Fru: positive (TB BMD) in women but not in men Veg: NS with the TB and TH BMD
Hu et al., 1998	CS	F: 434	46 (20–65)	Green veg.	Radius BMD	Positive
Li et al., 2001	CS	M: 1299 F: 1391	M: 63.9 (50–92) F: 62.9 (50–97)	F&V	Hip BMD	Positive in urban men (veg only) and women (F&V) NS in rural men and women
Lin et al., 2007	CS	M: 1154 F: 1006	9.5 (0.1)	F&V	BUA	Positive in girls but not in boys
Zhang et al., 2009	Cohort	F: 757	10.1 (0.4)	F&V (in protein)	5-year changes in BMD BMC	Positive: fru and proximal forearm BMD Negative: fru & distal forearm BMC, veg & TB BMD

Notes: Abbreviations: SD: study design; CC: case–control; CS: cross-sectional. Dietary marker, results: fru: fruit; F&V: fruit and vegetable; veg: vegetable. Dietary measurement: Outcome, associations: BMC: bone mineral content; BMD: bone mineral density; BUA: broadband ultrasound attenuation; LS: lumbar spine; NS: no significant association; negative: adverse association with statistically significance; positive: favorable association with statistically significance; TB: total body; TH: total hip. M: male; F: female.

1998; Carpenter et al., 2006) and lower dietary endogenous acid load (New et al., 2004; Alexy et al., 2005; Welch et al., 2007; Chan et al., 2008) with better bone indices. In addition, thousands of biologically protective phytochemicals have been identified in fruits and vegetables. Plants are rich in Ca, magnesium, vitamin K, numerous antioxidant compounds, and phytochemicals, such as polyphenols, carotenoids, tocopherols, tocotrienols, glutathione, and ascorbic acid (Benzie, 2003). The favorable effects of Ca and vitamin K on bone have long been established (Cockayne et al., 2006; Tang et al., 2007). Several recent studies have suggested that oxidative stress might play a role in the progress of osteoporosis, and dietary antioxidants from fruits and vegetables might reduce oxidative stress and prevent osteoporosis (Key et al., 1990; Yang et al., 2001; Bai et al., 2004; Altindag et al., 2008). A few biologically active phytochemicals, such as quercetin, rutin, and hesperidin, have been identified from fruits and vegetables and found to have a beneficial effect on bone health in animal and in vitro studies (Muhlbauer and Li, 1999; Muhlbauer, 2001; Chiba et al., 2003; Wong and Rabie, 2008). Further high-quality RCTs as well as human studies are needed to demonstrate the acid–base hypothesis and examine the effects of phytochemicals contained in fruits and vegetables on bone indices. These results would be of particular relevance to populations with plant-based diets.

FISH AND BONE HEALTH

A few studies have examined the association between fish or seafood consumption and bone health in other populations. In the Nurses' Health Study, a dose–response relationship was found between a greater intake of dark fish and a lower risk of hip fractures among 72,337 postmenopausal women during 18 years of follow-up (Feskanich et al., 2003). Suzuki et al. (1997) found a 42% (9%–64%) lower risk for hip fractures in subjects with fish consumption 3–4 times per week compared with <2 times per week in a case–control study involving 249 cases and 498 controls of elderly Japanese men and women. A similar association between fish or seafood intake and bone health was found in another study (Terano, 2001). In contrast, two other studies reported no significant association between any fish consumption and the risk of bone fractures: the 5.2-year follow-up of the EPIC-Oxford study including 7947 men and 26,749 women aged 20–80 years (Appleby et al., 2007) and the 12-year follow-up study of a Japanese cohort of 4573 people (mean age 58.5 years) (Fujiwara et al., 1997).

Nine studies (Yu et al., 1998; Huo and Li 2000; Liu et al., 2001, 2002; Yan et al., 2005; Xu et al., 2006; Zalloua et al., 2007; Ouyan et al., 2008; Chen et al., 2010) have examined the association between fish or seafood and bone health among Chinese subjects. The large population-based study by Zalloua et al. (2007) showed that increased seafood consumption was significantly associated with greater BMD in women, and the association was most noticeable in the premenopausal group. A 34% lower risk for low BMD (quartile one) was noted in premenopausal women with high seafood intake (>250 vs. ≤250 g/week) (Zalloua et al., 2007). A study in postmenopausal Chinese women in Hong Kong showed that greater marine fish consumption was dose-dependently associated with a decreased risk for osteoporosis (Chen et al., 2010). The ORs (95%CI) for osteoporosis (T score <−2.5) in the top quintile group (vs. the bottom group) were 0.23 (0.08–0.66), 0.12 (0.03–0.59), and 0.06 (0.01–0.44) at the whole body, total hip, and femur neck, respectively (Chen et al., 2010). However, no independent association between the consumption of freshwater fish or shellfish and bone mass was observed (Chen et al., 2010). A similar beneficial effect of fish intake was noted in two other studies (Liu et al., 2001; Yan et al., 2005) in adult or older populations, but not in children (Yu et al., 1998) (Table 31.2).

Four studies found an inverse association between the consumption of fish and/or seafood with the risk of fracture at the forearm (Xu et al., 2006), hip (Huo and Li, 2000; Ouyan et al., 2008), or lumbar spine (Li et al., 2002). In a population-based cross-sectional study including 2380 men and 2723 women aged 50–97 years in five provinces of China, Li et al. (2002) found that frequent consumption of fish (vs. seldom) was associated with a 31% ($p < .01$) lower risk of vertebral fractures in men but had no significant effect in women after adjusting for potential covariates. Xu et al. (2006) and Huo and Li (2000) also found a favorable effect of fish consumption on hip fracture (Huo and

TABLE 31.2
A Summary of the Results of Studies on Fish Consumption and Bone Health in Chinese

Study	Study Design	Study Size	Age, Mean (SD) or Rang	Dietary Marker	Outcome	Association
Xu et al., 2006	CC	F: 209/209	50–70	Fish	Forearm fractures	Positive
Ouyan et al., 2008	CC	279/279 M: 38%	68.7 ± 6.7	Fish	Hip fractures	NS
Chen et al., 2009	CS	F: 685	48–63	Fish	BMD, Osteoporosis	Positive: sea fish NS: freshwater fish
Zalloua et al., 2007	CS	M: 5848 F: 6207	24–67	Seafood	BMD	TB BMD: positive in women, NS in men
Yan et al., 2005	CC	348 (M: 107)/210 (M: 57)	Mean 62.1	Fish	Osteoporosis BMD <–2SD	Positive
Huo and Li, 2000	CC	201/402 M 41.3%	50–91	Fish	Hip fracture	NS

Note: Abbreviations: see Table 31.1.

Li, 2000) or forearm fracture (Xu et al., 2006) in case–control studies. However, no significant association between total fish or marine fish and hip fracture was noted in a hospital-based case–control study involving 279 cases and 279 matched controls of men and women aged 55–80 years (Ouyan et al., 2008). Besides differences in methodology, target populations and outcome measures, dietary variations, and accuracy and precision of dietary assessment methods might attenuate the association and contribute to the inconsistency of the observed results (Willett, 1998) (Table 31.2).

Plausible mechanisms that may explain the potential favorable association between fish and bone health have been suggested. Fish, particularly sea fish, are the major source of long-chain n-3 fatty acids of eicosapentaenoic acid and docosahexaenoic acid. Many studies have shown the beneficial effects of n-3 fatty acids on bone health in both humans and animals (Sun et al., 2003; Watkins et al., 2006; Shen et al., 2007; Salari et al., 2008). A higher ratio of n-3 to n-6 fatty acids has been observed to be associated with higher BMD at the hip in community-dwelling men and women aged 45–90 years (Weiss et al., 2005). The beneficial effects of dietary n-3 fatty acids on bone may be mediated through increases in intestinal Ca absorption and in the synthesis of bone collagen and decreases in urinary Ca loss (Claassen et al., 1995a, 1995b; Kruger and Horrobin, 1997), in prostaglandin synthesis (Liu et al., 2004), and in inflammatory cytokines, for example, interleukin-1, interleukin-6, and tumor necrosis factor (Caughey et al., 1996; Sun et al., 2003). Other nutrients, such as high-quality protein, Ca, and vitamin D, contained in fish may also contribute to the potential beneficial effects on bone.

Until now, all the studies on fish intake and bone health were observational, cross-sectional, or case–control so that a temporal relationship cannot be established. About half of the studies assessed dietary intake by using only one or a few simple questions. The accuracy and precision of dietary assessment might be poorer than those using a validated food frequency questionnaire. Therefore, the potential beneficial effect of fish or seafood consumption on bone health among Chinese needs to be confirmed by well-conducted cohort studies or RCTs.

CONCLUSION

In conclusion, the Chinese diet is typically rich in fruits, vegetables, soy foods, and fish and other seafood. All these foods may have favorable effects on bone health, but more evidence is required to demonstrate these hypotheses and to test the potential mechanisms of action of specific food components. The low Ca intake of a typical Chinese diet deserves attention, and more effort is required to increase Ca intake through the careful selection of food choices.

Besides dietary intake, bone health is affected by many factors, including genetics, age, hormones, overall dietary pattern and supplemental factors, level and type of physical activity, and lifestyle, including smoking, drinking of alcohol, caffeine intake, and psychological factors (Marcus et al., 2008). The role of vitamin D exposure also needs to be explored. Also, because the dietary and lifestyle patterns are rapidly changing, it is paramount to explore ways to promote and retain the healthy bone-promoting lifestyle conditions.

REFERENCES

Alekel, D.L., Germain, A.S., Peterson, C.T., et al. 2000. Isoflavone-rich soy protein isolate attenuates bone loss in the lumbar spine of perimenopausal women. *Am J Clin Nutr* 72:844–852.

Alekel, D.L., Van Loan, M.D., Koehler, K.J., et al. 2010. The soy isoflavones for reducing bone loss (SIRBL) study: A 3-y randomized controlled trial in postmenopausal women. *Am J Clin Nutr* 91:218–230.

Alexy, U., Remer, T., Manz, F., et al. 2005. Long-term protein intake and dietary potential renal acid load are associated with bone modeling and remodeling at the proximal radius in healthy children. *Am J Clin Nutr* 82:1107–1114.

Altindag, O., Erel, O., Soran, N., et al. 2008. Total oxidative/anti-oxidative status and relation to bone mineral density in osteoporosis. *Rheumatol Int* 28:317–321.

Anderson, J.J., Chen, X., Boass, A., et al. 2002. Soy isoflavones: No effects on bone mineral content and bone mineral density in healthy, menstruating young adult women after one year. *J Am Coll Nutr* 21:388–393.

Appleby, P., Roddam, A., Allen, N., et al. 2007. Comparative fracture risk in vegetarians and nonvegetarians in EPIC-Oxford. *Eur J Clin Nutr* 61:1400–1406.

Arjmandi, B.H., Getlinger, M.J., Goyal, N.V., et al. 1998. Role of soy protein with normal or reduced isoflavone content in reversing bone loss induced by ovarian hormone deficiency in rats. *Am J Clin Nutr* 68(6 supp):1358S–1363S.

Arjmandi, B.H., Khalil, D.A., Smith, B.J., et al. 2003. Soy protein has a greater effect on bone in postmenopausal women not on hormone replacement therapy, as evidenced by reducing bone resorption and urinary calcium excretion. *J Clin Endocrinol Metab* 88:1048–1054.

Arjmandi, B.H., Lucas, E.A., Khalil, D.A., et al. 2005. One year soy protein supplementation has positive effects on bone formation markers but not bone density in postmenopausal women. *Nutr J* 4:1–9.

Atkinson, S.A., McCabe, G.P., Weaver, C.M., et al. 2008. Are current calcium recommendations for adolescents higher than needed to achieve optimal peak bone mass? The controversy. *J Nutr* 138:1182–1186.

Bai, X.C., Lu, D., Bai, J., et al. 2004. Oxidative stress inhibits osteoblastic differentiation of bone cells by ERK and NF-kappaB. *Biochem Biophys Res Commun* 314:197–207.

Benzie, I.F. 2003. Evolution of dietary antioxidants. *Comp Biochem Physiol A Mol Integr Physiol* 136:113–126.

The Board of Trustees of The North American Menopause Society, 2010. Management of osteoporosis in postmenopausal women: 2010 position statement of the North American Menopause Society. *Menopause* 17:25–54; quiz 55–56.

Brink, E., Coxam, V., Robins, S., et al. 2008. Long-term consumption of isoflavone-enriched foods does not affect bone mineral density, bone metabolism, or hormonal status in early postmenopausal women: A randomized, double-blind, placebo controlled study. *Am J Clin Nutr* 87:761–770.

Bushinsky, D.A., and Frick, K.K. 2000. The effects of acid on bone. *Curr Opin Nephrol Hypertension* 9:369–379.

Carpenter, T.O., DeLucia, M.C., Zhang, J.H., et al. 2006. A randomized controlled study of effects of dietary magnesium oxide supplementation on bone mineral content in healthy girls. *J Clin Endocrinol Metab* 91:4866–4872.

Caughey, G.E., Mantzioris, E., Gibson, R.A., et al. 1996. The effect on human tumor necrosis factor alpha and interleukin 1 beta production of diets enriched in n-3 fatty acids from vegetable oil or fish oil. *Am J Clin Nutr* 63:116–122.

Chan, H.H., Lau, E.M., Woo, J., et al. 1996. Dietary calcium intake, physical activity and the risk of vertebral fracture in Chinese. *Osteoporos Int* 6:228–232.

Chan, R.S., Woo, J., Chan, D.C., et al. 2008. Bone mineral status and its relation with dietary estimates of net endogenous acid production in Hong Kong Chinese adolescents. *Br J Nutr* 100:1283–1290.

Chen, Y.M., Ho, S.C., Lam, S.S., et al. 2003. Soy isoflavones have a favorable effect on bone loss in Chinese postmenopausal women with lower bone mass: A double-blind, randomized, controlled trial. *J Clin Endocrinol Metab* 88:4740–4747.

Chen, Y.M., Ho, S.C., Lam, S.S., et al. 2004. Beneficial effect of soy isoflavones on bone mineral density was modified by years since menopause, body weight, and calcium intake: A double-blind randomized-controlled trial. *Menopause* 11:246–254.

Chen, Y.M., Ho, S.C., and Lam, S.S. 2010. Higher sea fish intake is associated with greater bone mass and lower osteoporosis risk in postmenopausal Chinese women. *Osteoporos Int* 21:939–946.

Chen, Y.M., Ho, S.C., and Woo, J.L. 2006. Greater fruit and vegetable intake is associated with increased bone mass among postmenopausal Chinese women. *Br J Nutr* 96:745–751.

Chen, Y.M., Teucher, B., Tang, X.Y., et al. 2007. Calcium absorption in postmenopausal Chinese women: A randomized crossover intervention study. *Br J Nutr* 97:160–166.

Chiba, H., Uehara, M., Wu, J., et al. 2003. Hesperidin, a citrus flavonoid, inhibits bone loss and decreases serum and hepatic lipids in ovariectomized mice. *J Nutr* 133:1892–1897.

China Popin. 2011. The China Population and Development Research Centre. Retrieved from http://www.cpdrc.org.cn/en/eindex.htm on 7 June 2011.

Chiu, J.F., Lan, S.J., Yang, C.Y., et al. 1997. Long-term vegetarian diet and bone mineral density in postmenopausal Taiwanese women. *Calcif Tissue Int* 60:245–249.

Claassen, N., Coetzer, H., Steinmann, C.M., et al. 1995a. The effect of different n-6/n-3 essential fatty acid ratios on calcium balance and bone in rats. *Prostaglandins Leukot Essent Fatty Acids* 53:13–19.

Claassen, N., Potgieter, H.C., Seppa, M., et al. 1995b. Supplemented gamma-linolenic acid and eicosapentaenoic acid influence bone status in young male rats: Effects on free urinary collagen crosslinks, total urinary hydroxyproline, and bone calcium content. *Bone* 16:385S–392S.

Cockayne, S., Adamson, J., Lanham-New, S., et al. 2006. Vitamin K and the prevention of fractures: Systematic review and meta-analysis of randomized controlled trials. *Arch Intern Med* 166:1256–1261.

Cooper, C., Campion, G., and Melton, L.J., III. 1992. Hip fractures in the elderly: A world-wide projection. *Osteoporos Int* 2:285–289.

Dai, K., Zhang, Q., Fan, T., et al. 2007. Osteoporotic Hip Fracture in China Study Team. Estimation of resource utilization associated with osteoporotic hip fracture and level of post-acute care in China. *Curr Med Res Opin* 23:2937–2943.

Dawson-Hughes, B. 1998. Vitamin D and calcium: Recommended intake for bone health. *Osteoporos Int* 8: S30–S34.

Dawson-Hughes, B., Jacques, P., and Shipp, C. 1987. Dietary calcium intake and bone loss from the spine in healthy postmenopausal women. *Am J Clin Nutr* 46:685–687.

Dimai, H.P., Porta, S., Wirnsberger, G., et al. 1998. Daily oral magnesium supplementation suppresses bone turnover in young adult males. *J Clin Endocrinol Metab* 83:2742–2748.

Djousse, L., Arnett, D.K., Coon, H., et al. 2004. Fruit and vegetable consumption and LDL cholesterol: The National Heart, Lung, and Blood Institute Family Heart Study. *Am J Clin Nutr* 79:213–217.

Evans, E.M., Racette, S.B., Van Pelt, R.E., et al. 2007. Effects of soy protein isolate and moderate exercise on bone turnover and bone mineral density in postmenopausal women. *Menopause* 14:481–488.

Fanti, P., Monier-Faugere, M.C., Geng, Z., et al. 1998. The phytoestrogen genistein reduces bone loss in short-term ovariectomized rats. *Osteoporos Int* 8:274–281.

Fujiwara, S., Kasagi, F., Yamada, M., et al. 1997. Risk factors for hip fracture in a Japanese cohort. *J Bone Miner Res* 12:998–1004.

Huo, D., and Li, L. 2000. A case–control study on risk factors for hip fracture in the middle-aged and elderly in Beijing. *Chin J Epidemiol* 21:37–40.

Feskanich, D., Willett, W.C., and Colditz, G.A. 2003. Calcium, vitamin D, milk consumption, and hip fractures: A prospective study among postmenopausal women. *Am J Clin Nutr* 77:504–511.

Gallagher, J.C., Satpathy, R., Rafferty, K., et al. 2004. The effect of soy protein isolate on bone metabolism. *Menopause* 11:290–298.

Ge, K.Y., Zhai, F.Y., and Yan, H.C. 1996. *Dietary and Nutritional Status of the Chinese Population*. Beijing: People's Medical Publishing House (in Chinese).

Harkness, L.S., Fiedler, K., Sehgal, A.R., et al. 2004. Decreased bone resorption with soy isoflavone supplementation in postmenopausal women. *J Women's Health* 13:1000–1007.

Ho, S.C. 1997. Attainment of peak bone mass and dietary factors in Chinese women. In Lau, M.C., Ho, S.C., Leung, S., and Woo, J., eds. *Osteoporosis in Asia: Crossing the Frontiers*. Singapore: World Scientific Publishing Co PTE Ltd.

Ho, S.C., Bacon, E., Harris, T., et al. 1993. Hip fracture rates in Hong Kong and the United States, 1988 through 1989. *Am J Public Health* 83:694–697.

Ho, S.C., Chan, S.G., Yi, Q., et al. 2001. Soy intake and the maintenance of peak bone mass in Hong Kong Chinese women. *J Bone Miner Res* 16:1363–1369.

Ho, S.C., Chan, S.G., Yip, Y.B., et al. 2008. Change in bone mineral density and its determinants in pre- and per-imenopausal Chinese women: The Hong Kong perimenopausal women osteoporosis study. *Osteoporos Int* 19:1785–1796.

Ho, S.C., Chen, Y.M., Woo, J.L.F., et al. 2004. High habitual calcium intake attenuates bone loss in early postmenopausal Chinese women: An 18 month followup study. *J Clin Endocrinol Metab* 89:2166–2170.

Ho, S.C., Guldan, G.S., Woo, J., et al. 2005. A prospective study of the effects of 1-year calcium-fortified soy milk supplementation on dietary calcium intake and bone health in Chinese adolescent girls aged 14–16. *Osteoporos Int* 16:1907–1916.

Ho, S.C., Leung, P.C., Swaminathan, R., et al. 1994. Determinants of bone mass in Chinese women aged 21–40. II. Pattern of dietary calcium intake and association with bone mineral density. *Osteoporosis Int* 4:167–175.

Ho, S.C., Woo, J., Lam, S., et al. 2003. Soy protein consumption and bone mass in early postmenopausal Chinese women. *Osteoporos Int* 14:835–842.

Hu, Y.F., Zhao, X. H., Bai, J., Ling, Y. 1998. Relationship between dietary habits and bone density of women in Beijing. *Chin J Osteoporos* 4:27–30.

Hu, J.F., Zhaom, X.H., Chen, J.S., et al. 1994. Bone density and lifestyle characteristics in premenopausal and postmenopausal Chinese women. *Osteoporosis Int* 4:288–297.

Huang, H.Y., Yang, H.P., Yang, H.T., et al. 2006. One-year soy isoflavone supplementation prevents early postmenopausal bone loss but without a dose dependent effect. *J Nutr Biochem* 17:509–517.

Jehle, S., Zanetti, A., Muser, J., et al. 2006. Partial neutralization of the acidogenic Western diet with potassium citrate increases bone mass in postmenopausal women with osteopenia. *J Am Soc Nephrol* 17:3213–3222.

Jones, G., Riley, M.D., and Whiting, S. 2001. Association between urinary potassium, urinary sodium, current diet, and bone density in prepubertal children. *Am J Clin Nutr* 73:839–844.

Kaptoge, S., Welch, A., McTaggart, A., et al. 2003. Effects of dietary nutrients and food groups on bone loss from the proximal femur in men and women in the 7th and 8th decades of age. *Osteoporos Int* 14:418–428.

Key, L.L., Jr., Ries, W.L., Taylor, R.G.., et al. 1990. Oxygen derived free radicals in osteoclasts: The specificity and location of the nitroblue tetrazolium reaction. *Bone* 11:115–119.

Koh, W.P., Wu, A.H., Wang, R., et al. 2009. Gender-specific associations between soy and risk of hip fracture in the Singapore Chinese health study. *Am J Epidemiol* 170:901–909.

Kreijkamp-Kaspers, S., Kok, L., Grobbee, D.E., et al. 2004. Effect of soy protein containing isoflavones on cognitive function, bone mineral density, and plasma lipids in postmenopausal women: A randomized controlled trial. *JAMA* 292:65–74.

Krieger, N.S., Frick, K.K., and Bushinsky, D.A. 2004. Mechanism of acid-induced bone resorption. *Curr Opin Nephrol Hypertension* 13:423–436.

Kruger, M.C., and Horrobin, D.F. 1997. Calcium metabolism, osteoporosis and essential fatty acids: A review. *Prog Lipid Res* 36:131–151.

Kung, A.W., Luk, K.D., Chu, L.W., et al. 1998. Age-related osteoporosis in Chinese: An evaluation of the response of intestinal calcium absorption and calcitropic hormones to dietary calcium deprivation. *Am J Clin Nutr* 68:1291–1297.

Lau, E.M., Woo, J., Lam, V., et al. 2001. Milk supplementation of the diet of postmenopausal Chinese women on a low calcium intake retards bone loss. *J Bone Miner Res* 16:1704–1709.

Lee, W.T.K., Cheung, C.S.K., Tse, Y.K., et al. 2005. Generalized low bone mass of girls with adolescent idiopathic scoliosis is related to inadequate calcium intake and weight bearing physical activity during peripubertal period. *Osteoporos Int* 16:1024–1035.

Lee, W.T., Jiang, J., Hu, P., Hu, X., Roberts, D.C., Cheng, J.C. 2002. Use of stable calcium isotopes (42Ca & 44Ca) in evaluation of calcium absorption in Beijing adolescents with low vitamin D status. *Food Nutr Bull* 23:42–47.

Lee, W.T., Leung, S.S., Fairweather-Tait, S.J., et al. 1994a. True fractional calcium absorption in Chinese children measured with stable isotopes (42Ca and 44Ca). *Br J Nutr* 72:883–897.

Lee, W.T.K., Leung, S.S.F., Leung, D.M.Y., et al. 1995. A randomized double-blind controlled calcium supplementation trial, and bone and height acquisition in children. *Br J Nutr* 74:125–139.

Lee, W.T.K., Leung, S.S.F., Wang, S.H., et al. 1994b. Double-blind controlled calcium supplementation and bone mineral accretion in children accustomed to low calcium diet. *Am J Clin Nutr* 60:744–752.

Lemann, J, Jr., Bushinsky, D.A., and Hamm, L.L. 2003. Bone buffering of acid and base in humans. *Am J Physiol Renal Physiol* 285:F811–F832.

Leung, S.S., Ho, S.C., Woo, J., et al. 1997. *Hong Kong Adult Dietary Survey.* Hong Kong: The Chinese University of Hong Kong.

Li, N., Ou, P., Yang, D., et al. 2001. Correlation analysis of bone mineral density and diet-customs in the middle-aged and elderly population in parts of China. *Mod Rehabil* 5:100–101.

Li, N., Ou, P., Zhu, H., et al. 2002. Comparison study on risk factors of vertebral fracture between men and women in middle-aged and elderly population in parts area of China. *China Public Health* 18:782–784.

Lin, Y., Tu, S., and Pan, W. 2007. Bone mass status of school-aged children in Taiwan assessed by quantitative ultrasound: The Nutrition and Health Survey in Taiwan Elementary School Children (NAHSIT Children 2001–2002). *Asia Pac J Clin Nutr* 16 585–592.

Liu, J., Ho, S.C., Su, Y.X., et al. 2009. Effect of long-term intervention of soy isoflavones on bone mineral density in women: A meta-analysis of randomized controlled trials. *Bone* 44:948–953.

Liu, H., Hong, X., Liu, X., et al. 2001. Analysis of factors affecting bone mass density of menopausal women in village. *China Public Health* 17:787–789.

Liu, D., Veit, H.P., and Denbow, D.M. 2004. Effects of long-term dietary lipids on mature bone mineral content, collagen, crosslinks, and prostaglandin E2 production in Japanese quail. *Poult Sci* 83:1876–1883.

Lydeking-Olsen, E., Beck-Jensen, J.E., Setchell, K.D., et al. 2004. Soymilk or progesterone for prevention of bone loss: A 2 year randomized, placebo-controlled trial. *Eur J Nutr* 43:246–257.

Macdonald, H.M., New, S.A., Golden, M.H.N., et al. 2004. Nutritional associations with bone loss during the menopausal transition: Evidence of a beneficial effect of calcium, alcohol, and fruit and vegetable nutrients and of a detrimental effect of fatty acids. *Am J Clin Nutr* 79:155–165.

McGartland, C.P., Robson, P.J., Murray, L.J., et al. 2004. Fruit and vegetable consumption and bone mineral density: The Northern Ireland Young Hearts Project. *Am J Clin Nutr* 80:1019–1023.

Marcus, R., Feldman, D., Nelson, D.A., Rosen, C. J. 2008. *Osteoporosis* (volume 1). 3rd ed., Elsevier Academic Press, San Diego.

Mei, J., Yeung, S.S., and Kung, A.W. 2001. High dietary phytoestrogen intake is associated with higher bone mineral density in postmenopausal but not premenopausal women. *J Clin Endocrinol Metab* 86:5217–5221.

Muhlbauer, R.C. 2001. Rutin cannot explain the effect of vegetables on bone metabolism. *J Bone Miner Res* 16:970–971.

Muhlbauer, R.C., and Li, F. 1999. Effect of vegetables on bone metabolism. *Nature* 401:343–344.

New, S.A. 2003. Intake of fruit and vegetables: Implications for bone health. *Proc Nutr Soc* 62:889–899.

New, S.A., Bolton-Smith, C., Grubb, D.A., et al. 1997. Nutritional influences on bone mineral density: A cross-sectional study in premenopausal women. *Am J Clin Nutr* 65:1831–1839.

New, S.A., MacDonald, H.M., Campbell, M.K., et al. 2004. Lower estimates of net endogenous non-carbonic acid production are positively associated with indexes of bone health in premenopausal and perimenopausal women. *Am J Clin Nutr* 79:131–138.

New, S.A., and Millward, D.J. 2003. Calcium, protein, and fruit and vegetables as dietary determinants of bone health. *Am J Clin Nutr* 77:1340–1341.

New, S.A., Robins, S.P., Campbell, M.K., et al. 2000. Dietary influences on bone mass and bone metabolism: Further evidence of a positive link between fruit and vegetable consumption and bone health? *Am J Clin Nutr* 71:142–151.

Newton, K.M., LaCroix, A.Z., Levy, L., et al. 2006. Soy protein and bone mineral density in older men and women: A randomized trial. *Maturitas* 55:270–277.

Ouyan, W., Wu, B., Tu, S., et al. 2008. Consumption of various food and hip fractures in middle-aged and elderly Chinese: A case–control study. Guangzhou: Sun Yat-sen University.

Potter, S.M., Baum, J.A., Teng, H., et al. 1998. Soy protein and isoflavones: Their effects on blood lipids and bone density in postmenopausal women. *Am J Clin Nutr* 68:1375S–1379S.

Prynne, C.J., Mishra, G.D., O'Connell, M.A., et al. 2006. Fruit and vegetable intakes and bone mineral status: A cross sectional study in 5 age and sex cohorts. *Am J Clin Nutr* 83:1420–1428.

Rickard, D.J., Monroe, D.G., Ruesink, T.J., et al. 2003. Phytoestrogen genistein acts as an estrogen agonist on human osteoblastic cells through estrogen receptors α and β. *J Cell Biochem* 89:633–646

Salari, P., Rezaie, A., Larijani, B., et al. 2008. A systematic review of the impact of n-3 fatty acids in bone health and osteoporosis. *Med Sci Monit* 14:RA37–RA44.

Setchell, K.D. 2001. Soy isoflavones: Benefits and risks from nature's selective estrogen receptor modulators (SERMs). *J Am Coll Nutr* 20:354S–362S; discussion 81S–83S.

Setchell, K.D., and Lydeking-Olsen, E. 2003. Dietary phytoestrogens and their effect on bone evidence from in vitro and in vivo, human observational, and dietary intervention studies. *Am J Clin Nutr* 73(suppl):593S–609S.

Shea, B., Wells, G., Cranney, A., et al. 2002. Meta-analyses of therapies for postmenopausal osteoporosis. VII. Meta-analysis of calcium supplementation for the prevention of postmenopausal osteoporosis. *Endocr Rev* 23:552–559.

Shen, C.L., Yeh, J.K., Rasty, J., et al. 2007. Improvement of bone quality in gonad-intact middle-aged male rats by long-chain n-3 polyunsaturated fatty acid. *Calcif Tiss Int* 80:286–293.

Sun, D., Krishnan, A., Zaman, K., et al. 2003. Dietary n-3 fatty acids decrease osteoclastogenesis and loss of bone mass in ovariectomized mice. *J Bone Miner Res* 18:1206–1216.

Suzuki, T., Yoshida, H., Hashimoto, T., et al. 1997. Case–control study of risk factors for hip fractures in the Japanese elderly by a Mediterranean Osteoporosis Study (MEDOS) questionnaire. *Bone* 21:461–467.

Suzuki, Y., Whiting, S.J., Davison, K.S., et al. 2003. Total calcium intake is associated with cortical bone mineral density in a cohort of postmenopausal women not taking estrogen. *J Nutr Health Aging* 7:296–299.

Tang, B.M., Eslick, G.D., Nowson, C., et al. 2007. Use of calcium or calcium in combination with vitamin D supplementation to prevent fractures and bone loss in people aged 50 years and older: A meta-analysis. *Lancet* 370:657–666.

Terano, T. 2001. Effect of omega 3 polyunsaturated fatty acid ingestion on bone metabolism and osteoporosis. *World Rev Nutr Diet* 88:141–147.

Thorpe, D.L., Knutsen, S.F., Beeson, W.L., et al. 2008. Effects of meat consumption and vegetarian diet on risk of wrist fracture over 25 years in a cohort of peri- and postmenopausal women. *Public Health Nutr* 11:564–572.

Tucker, K.L., Chen, H., Hannan, M.T., et al. 2002. Bone mineral density and dietary patterns in older adults: The Framingham Osteoporosis Study. *Am J Clin Nutr* 76:245–252.

Tucker, K.L., Hannan, M.T., Chen, H., et al. 1999. Potassium, magnesium, and fruit and vegetable intakes are associated with greater bone mineral density in elderly men and women. *Am J Clin Nutr* 69:727–736.

Tucker, K.L., Hannan, M.T., and Kiel, D.P. 2001. The acid–base hypothesis: Diet and bone in the Framingham Osteoporosis Study. *Eur J Nutr* 40:231–237.

Tylavsky, F.A., Holliday, K., Danish, R., et al. 2004. Fruit and vegetable intakes are an independent predictor of bone size in early pubertal children. *Am J Clin Nutr* 79:311–317.

Uesugi, T., Toda, T., Okuhira, T., et al. 2003. Evidence of estrogenic effect by the three-month intervention of isoflavone on vaginal maturation and bone metabolism in early postmenopausal women. *Endocrinol J* 50:613–619.

Vatanparast, H., Baxter-Jones, A., Faulkner, R.A., et al. 2005. Positive effects of vegetable and fruit consumption and calcium intake on bone mineral accrual in boys during growth from childhood to adolescence: The University of Saskatchewan Pediatric Bone Mineral Accrual Study. *Am J Clin Nutr* 82:700–706.

Watkins, B.A., Li, Y., and Seifert, M.F. 2006. Dietary ratio of n-6/n-3 PUFAs and docosahexaenoic acid: Actions on bone mineral and serum biomarkers in ovariectomized rats. *J Nutr Biochem* 17:282–289.

Weaver, C.M. 2006. Pre-puberty and adolescence. In *Calcium in Human Health*, Weaver, C.M., and Heaney, R.P., eds. Totowa, NJ: Humana Press, pp. 281–296.

Weiss, L.A., Barrett-Connor, E., and von Muhlen, D. 2005. Ratio of n-6 to n-3 fatty acids and bone neral density in older adults: The Rancho Bernardo Study. *Am J Clin Nutr* 81:934–938.

Welch, A.A., Bingham, S.A., Reeve, J., et al. 2007. More acidic dietary acid–base load is associated with reduced calcaneal broadband ultrasound attenuation in women but not in men: Results from the EPIC-Norfolk cohort study. *Am J Clin Nutr* 85:1134-41.

Whiting, S.J., Boyle, J.L., Thompson, A., et al. 2002. Dietary protein, phosphorus and potassium are beneficial to bone mineral density in adult men consuming adequate dietary calcium. *J Am Coll Nutr* 21:402–409.

Willett, W. 1998. *Nutritional Epidemiology*. 2nd ed. New York, NY: Oxford University Press, Inc.

Winzenberg, T., Shaw, K., Fryer, J., et al.. 2006. Effect of calcium supplementation on bone density in health children: Meta-analysis of randomized controlled trials. *BMJ* 333:775–781.

Wong, R.W., and Rabie, A.B. 2008. Effect of quercetin on bone formation. *J Orthop Res* 26:1061–1066.

Wu, J., Oka, J., Tabata, I., et al. 2006. Effects of isoflavone and exercise on BMD and fat mass in postmenopausal Japanese women: A 1-year randomized placebo-controlled trial. *J Bone Miner Res* 21:780–789.

Xu, L., Dibley, M., D'Este, C., et al. 2009. Food groups and risk of forearm fractures in postmenopausal women in Chengdu, China. *Climacteric* 12:222–229.

Xu, L., Lu, A., Zhaom, X., et al. 1996. Very low rates of hip fracture in Beijing, People's Republic of China: The Beijing osteoporosis project. *Am J Epidemiol* 144:901–907.

Xu, L., Phillips, M., D'Este, C., et al. 2006. Diet, activity, and other lifestyle risk factors for forearm fracture in postmenopausal women in China: A case–control study. *Menopause* 13:102–110.

Yan, X., Yang, Y., Wang, X., et al. 2005. Association between dietary factors and osteoporosis. *Chin Prev Med* 6:340–342.

Yan, L., Zhou, B., Prentice, A., et al. 1999. Epidemiological study of hip fracture in Shenyang, People's Republic of China. *Bone* 24:151–155.

Yang, S., Madyastha, P., Bingel, S., et al. 2001. A new superoxide-generating oxidase in murine osteoclasts. *J Biol Chem* 276:5452–5458.

Ye, Y.B., Tang, X.Y., Verbruggen, M.A., et al. 2006. Soy isoflavones attenuate bone loss in early postmenopausal Chinese women: A single-blind randomized, placebo-controlled trial. *Eur J Nutr* 45:327–334.

Yu, W., Pan, M., Zhang, Y., et al. 1998. Association of food frequency and bone density in school children in Guangdong, China. *Chinese General Practice* 1:38–40.

Zalloua, P.A., Hsu, Y.H., Terwedow, H., et al. 2007. Impact of seafood and fruit consumption on bone mineral density. *Maturitas* 56:1–11.

Zhai, F., and Yang, X. 2006. 2002. *National Nutrition and Health Survey in Chinese Residents: Part II*. Beijing: People's Medical Publishing House.

Zhang, Q., Ma, G., Greenfield, H., et al. 2010. The association between dietary protein intake and bone mass accretion in pubertal girls with low calcium intakes. *Br J Nutr* 103:714–723.

Zhang, X., Shu, X.O., Li, H., et al. 2005. Prospective cohort study of soy food consumption and risk of bone fracture among postmenopausal women. *Arch Intern Med* 165:1890–1895.

Part V

Osteopenia and Osteoporosis

32 Prevention of Bone Loss with Exercise

Anna Nordström and Peter Nordström

CONTENTS

INTRODUCTION

Osteoporosis is a global health care problem, increasing largely due to improved health care, preventive health measures, and subsequent delay in mortality (Anon., 1993). It is characterized by reduced bone mass, microstructural deterioration with advancing age, and an increase in fracture rate. Knowledge concerning factors affecting the incidence of osteoporosis is critical for the possibility to successfully minimize the impact of the fractures, as a result of a weak and osteoporotic bone, that are an increasing cause of mortality and painful physical impairment of the elderly, particularly in the Western world (Browner et al., 1996; Cooper et al., 1993; Nevitt et al., 1998). Osteoporosis is a multifactorial disease, and it depends on both environmental and genetic factors. Some factors cannot be influenced such as genetic factors that have been estimated to be responsible for about 50%–70% of the variance in bone mass (Eisman, 1999; Jouanny et al., 1995; Seeman et al., 1989; Slemenda et al., 1991), but other lifestyle factors, known to influence bone mass, a such as nutritional intake, smoking, and exercise, can be influenced (Cummings et al., 1995). Exercise has been recommended for prevention and even treatment of osteoporosis because it potentially can increase bone mass and strength in the early years of life and reduce the risk of falling in older populations. This chapter focuses on describing the effects of exercise on bone tissue, the development of bone mass, peak bone mass, osteoporosis fracture prevention.

BONE RESPONSE TO LOAD

In 1892, the German anatomist Julius Wolff stated that bone tissue adapts to the loads it is subjected to. Wolff's law states that if a bone is subjected to heavy loading, it will remodel itself to become stronger; conversely, the bone will lose strength if loading is decreased (Wolff, 1892). He specifically proposed that bone trabeculi become aligned with the predominant loads, a principle that has since been confirmed in animal experiments (Pontzer et al., 2006; Teng et al., 1997). More recently, Frost presented a very comprehensive mechanostat theory on how bone modeling and remodeling allow bones to adapt to changing loads (Frost, 1987, 2003). In both animal and human studies, researchers have found ample support for the principles originally outlined by Wolf.

Bone adapts to its mechanical load, but the mechanism by which it occurs is poorly understood. Bone changes structure and mass in response to dynamic and static loads. Bending loads causes deformations in the bone matrix that generates fluid pressure differences through the extracellular spaces in canaliculi and lacunae from the compression to the tension side. The resulting fluid shear stress has been suggested to be one way by which the bone cell network senses mechanical loading. The fluid flow that is generated causes shearing stresses on the cell membranes in both osteoblastic and osteocytic cell lines, disrupts junctional communication, rearranges junctional proteins, and determines de novo synthesis of specific connexins to an extent that depends on the magnitude of the shear stress. The disconnection as a result of the fluid shear stress on the bone cell network may be part of the signal whereby the disconnected cells or the remaining network initiates focal bone remodeling (Thi et al., 2003). Rat studies have suggested that there is both an immediate and a delayed response in bone formation produced by mechanical stimulation (Chow et al., 1998; Turner et al., 1998). The immediate response is mediated through an activation of bone lining cells into osteoblasts (Chow et al., 1998), and the delayed response is the result of preosteoblast proliferation and differentiation into osteoblasts (Turner et al., 1998). The general belief is that bone tissue adapts to the stress acting on it, forming an equilibrium that covers normal daily strains. According to Frost, a threshold, "the minimum effective strain," exists; when the mechanical stimulus is too low, remodeling removes bone, and when it is too high creating an overload, remodeling adds bone (Frost, 1988). A schematic picture of the relationship between daily stress stimulus and bone remodeling is presented in Figure 32.1.

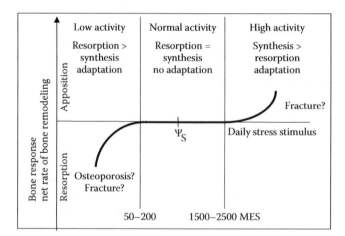

FIGURE 32.1 A hypothetical presentation of the impact on bone remodeling from reduced or increased physical activity. Daily stress stimulus is presented on the *x* axis, and the response of the bone to stimuli is presented on the *y* axis. The mechanobiologic response drives the bone toward equilibrium where no adaptation occurs where the resorption equals synthesis, the so called stress stimulus set point (Ψ_S). There will be a net resorption when the mechanical daily stress stimulus is less than the stress stimulus set point and a net apposition when the mechanical daily stress is higher. (Adapted from Turner, C.H., *Bone*, 12, 203–17, 1991; Carter, D.R., *Crit Rev Biomed Eng*, 8, 1–28, 1982.)

EXPERIMENTAL STUDIES OF SKELETAL LOADING

Studies in animals have revealed that the best osteogenic response is achieved by intense and regular dynamic skeletal loading; only a low number of loading cycles per day is necessary, and increasing the number of loading cycles does not confer additional benefits (Raab-Cullen et al., 1994; Robling et al., 2002; Rubin & Lanyon, 1987; Umemura et al., 1997). In response to loading, trabecular orientation is altered, new bone is formed, and increases in bone weight, cortical area, and breaking strength have been observed (Lanyon et al., 1982; Pontzer et al., 2006; Umemura et al., 1997). Thus, it seems that exercise should be weight bearing and dynamic, with high magnitude strains applied at a high rate with relatively few repetitions (O'Connor et al., 1982; Raab-Cullen et al., 1994; Rubin & Lanyon, 1984, 1985), and probably from different angles (Lanyon et al., 1986, 1992) to optimize the osteogenic effect.

IMMOBILIZATION, INACTIVITY, AND MICROGRAVITY

The importance of weight-bearing loading to uphold bone density becomes apparent in studies investigating what happens to the skeleton when it is unloaded. A model that has been used to study disuse osteoporosis is microgravity-induced bone loss. Holick estimated a 1%–2% loss each month of bone mineral density (BMD) at different skeletal sites when the skeleton is exposed to microgravity (Holick, 1998). Several studies, although with small cohorts, have shown a loss of BMD (g/cm^2) at predominantly weight-bearing sites, such as the calcaneus and tibia, whereas there have been no loss of bone in nonweight-bearing sites, such as the radius (Rambaut & Johnston, 1979; Rambaut et al., 1975; Vico et al., 2000).

Another model to study disuse osteoporosis is bed rest. LeBlanc et al. studied six patients that were confined to bed rest for 17 weeks (Leblanc et al., 1990). The patients exhibited BMD loss in the leg that was estimated to be 0.4% per month. Another study showed BMD decreases of 0.95% per month in the greater trochanter, but no decreases was detected at the radius after 12 weeks of bed rest (Zerwekh et al., 1998). Several other studies come to the same conclusion that during periods of bed rest, the most prominent loss of BMD occurs in weight-bearing skeletal sites (Watanabe et al., 2004; Zerwekh et al., 1998).

Bone loss following unloading has also been observed in clinical settings. Limb disuse or immobilization resulting from painful joint disease, trauma, or surgery results in bone loss predominantly in the affected limb (Houde et al., 1995; Kannus et al., 1995; Leppala et al., 1998; Sambrook et al., 1990). In patients with hemiparesis due to stroke, there is rapid bone loss on the affected side that is subjected to less loading; in contrast, there is increased bone density on the nonaffected side, possibly due to increased loading on the healthy side (Ramnemark et al., 1999a, 1999b), but it has also been proposed that bone minerals are relocated to the healthy side. This phenomenon has also been observed in patients with spinal cord injuries in which rapid bone loss occurred in paralyzed areas: Although quadriplegics suffer bone loss in both arms and legs, paraplegics lose bone primarily in the lower limbs while maintaining BMD better in the arms (Demirel et al., 1998; Frey-Rindova et al., 2000; Garland et al., 1992).

EXERCISE AND INFANTS

Even in such young ages as infancy, there seems to be a positive effect of exercise on bone accretion (Litmanovitz et al., 2003; Moyer-Mileur et al., 2000; Nemet et al., 2002). The intervention studies have been performed on premature infants that are at risk of osteopenia due to early birth and the following hospitalization in neonatal intensive care units without sensory and physical stimulation. Moyer-Mileur and colleagues designed a passive motion exercise program with gentle compression of the upper and lower extremities that was performed daily. The result showed greater gains in bone mineral content (BMC, g) and bone area (BA) and body weight in the active group compared with controls (Moyer-Mileur et al., 2000).

EXERCISE AND CHILDREN

It is of major importance to study the impact of exercise on the growing skeleton during the prepubertal and peripubertal period because about 40% of the total amount of bone mineral is accumulated during this time (Bonjour et al., 1991). Weight-bearing exercise may reduce fracture risk by increasing the amount of bone accrual during growth. The effect of weight-bearing exercise on the skeleton is especially difficult to study in the growing skeleton because dual-energy x-ray absorptiometry (DXA) measures BMC unadjusted for bone size. As BMC is size dependent, a higher BMC could be due to increased size rather than an increase in true bone density. In addition, skeletal maturation differs between regions in adolescence due to different pubertal maturation (MacKelvie et al., 2002; Tanner, 1962).

Randomized controlled intervention studies have shown that weight-bearing exercise may increase both bone size and BMD at weight-bearing sites in 6- to 12-year-old boys and girls (Bradney et al., 1998; Fuchs et al., 2001; MacKelvie et al., 2001, 2003; McKay et al., 2000; Morris et al., 1997) (Table 32.1). Thus, exercise in children may increase bone density not only by remodeling but also by apposition of new bone on the endocortical and periosteal surfaces of the bone, a process called bone modeling. It has also been observed that the effects of weight-bearing activity are site and region specific because jumping sports primarily improve BMD in the lower limbs whereas racket sports lead to bone mass improvements in the playing arm. The intervention programs in these studies were conducted in school settings and ranged in duration from 10 to 30 min and in frequency from three to five times a week, emphasizing that only a limited amount of physical activity is needed to achieve significant effects on bone mass accrual during childhood. In summary, physical activity seems to have beneficial effects on both the bone mineral accrual and structural geometry in the growing skeleton of both boys and girls.

The transition period between childhood and adolescence represents a time when biological factors associated with bone growth and development differ noticeably depending on a child's level of maturity. This is further complicated by rapid biological changes observed during growth within a relatively short time frame. However, this is also a time that has been suggested to be an opportune time to intervene with exercise, that is, in Tanner stage 2–4 when the insulin growth factor 1 (IGF1) levels peak due to the notion that IGF1 could be a mediator or promoter of the effect of exercise (Libanati et al., 1999; Mora et al., 1999).

EXERCISE AND ADOLESCENTS

The literature to date is very limited concerning exercise and effects in adolescence. There are several limitations of the studies, notably small sample sizes and estimations of putative interactions with gender and puberty.

Retrospective and observational longitudinal studies suggest that exercise positively influences bone accrual in both boys and girls (Bailey et al., 1996; Lehtonen-Veromaa et al., 2000; Slemenda et al., 1994; Welten et al., 1994) (Table 32.2).

The number of controlled intervention studies that exists has failed to show consistent data of any effect of exercise on BMD accrual in adolescence girls (Blimkie et al., 1996; Snow-Harter et al., 1992; Witzke & Snow, 2000) (Table 32.2). This could be due to that one of the studies had used resistance training as intervention and all studies had shorter intervention times than 1 year. No such studies have been performed in boys.

In summary, exercise may positively affect BMD, but not BA, in both boys and girls during adolescence, although this is based on data from predominantly observational studies. Thus, the

TABLE 32.1

Bone Mass Response to Exercise Observed in Nonrandomized Controlled Intervention Study and Randomized Controlled Interventional Studies of Children

Reference	Participants	Study Period	Intervention/ Exercise	Measurements	Results
Nonrandomized interventional study					
Morris et al., 1997	71 girls 9–10 years	10 months	High impact 3 times a week, school intervention	BMC, BMD, BA of PF, FN, LS, TB	All BMD, BMC sites and FN BA increased significantly in IG than CG.
Randomized interventional studies					
McKay et al., 2000	144 children 6–10 years	8 months	High impact 3 times a week, school intervention	BMD, BMC, BA of TB, LS, PF	TR BMD increased significantly more in the IG than CG.
Fuchs et al., 2001	51 boys, 38 girls 5.9–9.8 years	7 months	High impact 3 times a week, school intervention	BMD, BMC, BA of LS, FN	FN, LS BMC, LS BMD and FN BA increased significantly.
Macdonald et al., 2007	281 boys and girls, 129 controls 10.2 ± 0.6 at baseline	High impact 5 times a week	16 months	BSI of the DT and SSIp of the TMS as assessed by pQCT	BSI increased significantly more in prepubertal boys than postpubertal boys and girls.
MacKelvie et al., 2004	64 boys 8.8–12.1 years	20 months	High impact 3 times a week, school intervention	BMC, BA of TB, PF, LS	FN BMC increased significantly in IG than CG.
MacKelvie et al., 2003	75 girls age 8.8–11.7 years	20 months	High impact, 3 times a week, school intervention	BMC of TB, PF, LS	FN, LS BMC increased significantly in IG than CG.
Bradney et al., 1998	40 boys 8.4–11.8 years	8 months	Weight bearing 3 times a week, school intervention	BMD, BMC of TB, LS	TB, LS, legs BMD increased significantly in IG than CG.
Alwis et al., 2008	80 boys 7–9 years	2 years	General physical activity school-based intervention, 40 min, 3 times a week	BMC of TB, LS, FN	LS BMD increased significantly more in IG than CG.

Notes: BMD = bone mineral density, BMC = bone mineral content, BA = bone area, TB = total body, LS = lumbar spine, FN = femoral neck, PF = proximal femur, TR = femur trochanter, IG = intervention group, CG = control group, DT = distal tibia, TMS = tibial midshaft, BSI = bone strength index, SSIp = polar strength strain index, pQCT = peripheral dual-energy x-ray absorptiometry.

effect of exercise on bone accrual might be bone remodeling rather than modeling in this age group. On the other hand, to our knowledge, no study has used computed tomography to investigate any possible effects on endocortical bone apposition in this age group. Further research is needed to investigate the effect of exercise on bone accrual during different maturational stages especially regarding boys.

TABLE 32.2
Effects on Exercise in Intervention Studies in Adolescents

Reference	Design	Participants	Study Period	Intervention/ Exercise	Measurements	Results
Cross-sectional studies						
Nordström & Lorentz on, 1996		44 boys age 16.8 years		Ice hockey players and CG	BMD of TB, head, pelvis, ala ossis ilii, FN, TR, femur diaphysis, tibia diaphysis	TB, FN, TR, pelvis BMD higher in ice hockey players vs. CG
Retrospective studies						
Welten et al., 1994		84 boys, 98 girls age 27 years		Interview evaluating exercise levels	BMD of LS	LS association significant
Observational longitudinal studies						
Bailey et al., 1996		60 boys, 53 girls age 8–14 years	6 years	Divided into inactive, average active, and active	BMC of TB, LS, PF	TB, FN, BMC increased significantly in active vs. inactive
Lehtonen-Veromaa et al., 2000		155 girls age 9–15 years Tanner stage Registered	1 year	Gymnasts, runners, CG	BMD, BA of PF, LS	FN, TR BMD increased significantly in gymnasts than CG and runners
Slemenda et al., 1994		90 twins 6–14 years Tanner stage registered	3 years	Correlation analysis	BMD of R, PF, LS	R, PF, LS BMD significantly correlated to physical activity
Gustavsson et al., 2003		56 boys age 16 years	3 years	Athletes, CG	BMD of TB, FN, H, LS vBMD of FN	Athletes gained significantly more in nondominant H, FN BMD than CG
Nordström et al., 2008		46 boys, age 17 years	4 years	Ice hockey players, badminton players, CG	BMD of FN, H, PF, LS BMC of FN, H, PF, LS	FN BMD, BMC, and hip BMC significantly higher gain in badminton players than in CG Greater gain in hip BMC and BA in ice hockey players
Intervention studies						
Blimkie et al., 1996	RCT	36 girls 14–18 years	26 weeks	Resistance training 3 times a week	BMD, BMC of TB, LS	NS
Witzke & Snow, 2000	CT	53 girls age 13–15 years	9 months	High impact 3 times a week school intervention	BMC of TB, LS, PF	NS
Snow-Harter et al., 1992	RCT	52 women 19.9 ± 0.7 years	8 months	Weight lifting or running 3 times a week + controls	BMD, BMC of LS, FN	LS BMD increased significantly in IG vs. CG

TABLE 32.2 (Continued)
Effects on Exercise in Intervention Studies in Adolescents

Reference	Design	Participants	Study Period	Intervention/ Exercise	Measurements	Results
Weeks et al., 2008	RCT	46 boys, 53 girls 13.8 years	8 months	High impact 2 times a week	Calcaneal BUA, BMC, BMD, and BA of the FN, TR, LS, and TB	Calcaneal BUA as well as FN, TB, and LS BMC increased significantly more in the IG than in the CG
Kato et al., 2006	RCT	36 young women age 20 years	6 months	10 maximal jumps/ day 3 times a week	BMD of the LS, FN, Ward's, and TR	FN and LS BMD increased significantly more in the IG than in the CG
Heinonen, et al., 2000	CT	139 girls age 10–15 years	9 months	Step aerobics + extra jumping 2 times a week	BMC of the LS and PF	LS and PF BMD increased significantly more at post than pre and than CG

Notes: BMD = bone mineral density, BMC = bone mineral content, BA = bone area, H = humerus LS = lumbar spine, R = radius, FN = femoral neck, TB = total body, PF = proximal femur, TR = trochanter, CG = control group, IG = intervention group, NS = nonsignificant, BUA = broadband ultrasound attenuation, Pre = premenarcheal group, Post = postmenarcheal group, vBMD = volumetric BMD, RCT = Randomized controlled trial, CT = Clinical trial.

SUMMARY AND TRAINING ADVICE FOR PROMOTING BONE ACCRUAL IN YOUNG INDIVIDUALS

The young skeleton seems to adapt better and quicker to altered external stimuli than does the older skeleton. To achieve a high osteogenic stimuli, the activity should be weight bearing and gives rise to dynamic deformations of the skeleton in different loading directions. Thus, different ball sports such as badminton and tennis have been associated with higher bone mass than does swimming.

- Weight-bearing activity that includes jumping and fast directional changes, for example, gymnastics, track and field, and different ball sports.
- Training should be varied and at least three times a week and 45 min in length to achieve a good effect.

EXERCISE AND MEN

Data from retrospective studies imply that weight-bearing exercise seems to be associated with higher BMD at weight-bearing sites (Delvaux et al., 2001; Neville et al., 2002; Nguyen et al., 2000) (Table 32.3). To date, the strongest evidence of an exercise effect on men after puberty is observational studies of athletes (Gustavsson et al., 2003; Nordström and Lorentzon, 1996; Nordström et al., 2008). In summary, these studies suggest that physical activity in young adult males results in high and important gains in BMD, especially at the clinically important proximal femur. These gains seem to be site specific and related to the strains created locally in the bone.

One randomized controlled study has been performed with men using weight lifting as intervention (Fujimura et al., 1997) (Table 32.3). The study period was 4 months and included 17 subjects. The study failed to find an effect of exercise on BMD. The reason for these results might be the

TABLE 32.3
Effects of Exercise Intervention Studies in Men

Reference	Participants	Study Period	Intervention/ Exercise	Measurements	Results
Cross-sectional studies					
Neville et al., 2002	250 men age 20–25 years		Questionnaire evaluating exercise levels	BMD, BMC of LS, FN	LS, FN BMD and BMC association significant in exercisers
Retrospective studies					
Nguyen et al., 2000	690 men age 60 years and above		Interview evaluating exercise levels	BMD of LS, FN	FN BMD and exercise association significant but not after adjusted for age and BMI
Lynch et al., 2007	16 former professional football players, controls 66 ± 6 years		Self-reported questionnaire evaluating exercise levels	BMC and BMD of TB, LS, and PF	TB BMC and BMD, as well as LS and FN BMD were significantly increased in FP
Longitudinal observational studies					
Delvaux et al., 2001	126 men age 40 years		Questionnaire evaluating exercise levels	BMD, BMC of TB, LS	TB, LS BMD and BMC association significant in exercisers
Randomized Interventional studies					
Fujimura et al., 1997	17 males 23–31 years	4 months	Weight training 3 times a week	BMD of TB, LS, FN, R	NS

Notes: BMD = bone mineral density, BMC = bone mineral content, LS = lumbar spine, PF = proximal femur, FN = femoral neck, TB = total body, R = radius, BMI = body mass index, FP = football players, NS = nonsignificant.

nondynamic type of activity in which study participants participated or the duration the follow-up of 4 months, which is too short of a period of time to detect any changes in BMD by DXA.

EXERCISE AND PREMENOPAUSAL WOMEN

Intervention studies performed in premenopausal women have shown a positive osteogenic effect of high-impact exercise that seems to be site specific (Bassey et al., 1998; Heinonen et al., 1996, 1999; Winters & Snow, 2000) (Table 32.4). Studies that have used resistance or weight training as an intervention have shown inconsistent findings (Gleeson et al., 1990; Lohman et al., 1995; Sinaki et al., 1996) (Table 32.4). Possibly, some of the training programs have not imposed enough deformation of the skeleton to increase BMD. The cohorts of these intervention studies are rather small and with high dropout rates of up to 30%.

NEGATIVE EFFECTS OF EXERCISE ON BONE

Exercise can however have a negative impact on BMD in certain situations. In long-distance runners on competitive level that train tremendously (average of >70 km/week), BMD has even been lower than that in controls (Hetland et al., 1993a, 1993b; Louis et al., 1991; Robinson et al., 1995). In women, training intensity has been related to changes in sex hormones, and it has

TABLE 32.4
Effects of Exercise Intervention Studies in Premenopausal Women

Reference	Design	Participants	Study Period	Intervention/ Exercise	Measurements	Results
Heinonen et al., 1996	RCT	98 women 35–45 years	18 months	High impact 3 times a week	BMD of R, FN, LS	FN, LS BMD increased significantly in IG vs. CG
Heinonen et al., 1999	Follow-up study	49 women 35–45 years	8 months	High impact 3 times a week continued training	BMD of R, LS, PF	FN BMD increased significantly in IG vs. CG
Lohman et al., 1995	RCT	56 women 28–39 years	18 months	Resistance Calcium supplement	BMD of TB, LS, PF	TR, LS BMD increased significantly in IG vs. CG
Gleeson et al., 1990	CT	68 women	12 months	Weight lifting Calcium supplement	BMD of LS	NS
Bassey et al., 1998	RCT	55 women mean age 37.5 years	5 months	High impact 3 times a week	BMD of PF, LS	TR BMD increased significantly in IG vs. CG
Sinaki et al., 2004	RCT	96 women 30–40 years	3 years	Weight lifting Calcium supplement	BMD of LS, PF, R	NS
Winters & Snow, 2000	CT	65 women 30–45 years	12 months	High impact	BMD of TB, TR, FN, LS	TR BMD increased significantly in IG vs. CG
Vainionpaa et al., 2005	RCT	120 women 35–40 years	12 months	High impact 3 times a week and daily home exercise program	BMD of FN, TR, ITR, W, F, L1–L4, LT, uR, R, U	FN, TR, ITR, F, L1 increased significantly in IG vs. CG

Notes: BMD = bone mineral density, LS = lumbar spine, FN = femoral neck, TB = total body, PF = proximal femur, TR = trochanter, R = radius, L1 = first lumbar vertebrae, L4 = fourth lumbar vertebrae, IG = intervention group, CG = control group, NS = nonsignificant, ITR = intertrochanter region, RCT = Randomized controlled trial, CT = clinical trial, W = Ward's triangle, F = femur, LT = lumbar total, uR = ultradistal radius, U = ulna.

been speculated that the decreased bone mass in female long-distance running can be related to changes in hormone levels and menstruation disturbances (lowered estrogen levels and elevated cortisol levels) (Hetland et al., 1993). Amenorrhea in athletes due to intensive endurance exercise has a negative impact on bone mass, especially on trabecular bone (Drinkwater et al., 1986; Micklesfield et al., 1995; Seeman et al., 1982, 1992). Not only women are affected, but very tough endurance training can also reduce gonad hormone levels in male athletes with negative effects on bone mass (Drinkwater et al., 1986; Micklesfield et al., 1995; Seeman et al., 1982, 1992; Wheeler et al., 1984).

EXERCISE AND POSTMENOPAUSAL WOMEN

Kemmler and coworkers designed an exercise program for prevention of osteoporosis in early post-menopausal women. The exercise program consisting of four sessions of 60–70 min of endurance, jumping, strength, and flexibility was prescribed together with daily intake of 1.5 g of calcium and 500 IU of cholecalciferol for 26 months (Kemmler et al., 2004). In this nonrandomized study, there was a prevention of bone mass loss in the lumbar spine and hip (DXA measurement) in the exercise group. In the spine, even an increase in BMD could be achieved in the exercise group, whereas women in the control group significantly lost bone mass in the hip and lumbar spine. In the control group, the decrease in BMD was much higher in the metabolically more active trabecular bone than in the cortical compartments (quantitative computed tomography measurement). When examining the evidence in the form of randomized controlled studies, there seems to be a weak positive effect of exercise in postmenopausal women on BMD at sites that are exposed to mechanical strains when examining randomized controlled intervention studies (Table 32.5). The studies performed are mostly limited in time to 1 year, have a low number of participants, and have investigated different forms of exercise. Furthermore, ethnicity, hormone replacement therapy (HRT) treatment, calcium substitution, and smoking are not always accounted for (Holm et al., 2008; Prince et al., 1995).

TABLE 32.5
Effects of Randomized Controlled Exercise Interventions Studies in Postmenopausal Women

Reference	Participants	Study period	Intervention/ Exercise	Measurements	Results
Kerr et al., 1996	56 women 40–70 years	1 year	Endurance resistance or high load resistance, one side used as CG	BMD of R, PF	PF, R BMD increased significantly in high load vs. CG and R BMD in endurance resistance
Sandler et al., 1987	255 women 49–65 years	3 years	Walking	BMD of R measured with CT	NS
Prince et al., 1995	168 women 50–70 years	2 years	Weight lifting and/or calcium supplement	BMD of LS, PF	PF BMD exercise + calcium increased significantly vs. calcium
Nelson et al., 1994	40 women 50–70 years	1 year	Weight lifting 2 times a week	BMD, BMC of TB, FN, LS	FN, LS BMD increased significantly in IG vs. CG
Grove and Londeree, 1992	15 women 49–64 years	1 year	High impact, low impact, CG	BMD of LS	LS BMD in CG decreased significantly, maintenance in IG
Brooke-Wavell et al., 1997	84 women 60–70 years	1 year	Walking or CG	BMD of LS, FN, C	BMD C increased significantly in IG vs. CG
Bassey et al., 1998	44 women 50–60 years	1 year	Weight bearing or CG	BMD of PF, LS, R	NS
Karinkanta et al., 2007	149 women 70–78 years	1 year	Resistance, balance jumping, or combination, control	BMD, BMC, and pQCT of the FN, DT, TS, Rs, DR	TS bone strength index decreased significantly less in combination than in control
Chan et al., 2004	132 postmenopausal women 54 ± 3.5 years	1 year	TCC 45 min, 5 times a week, CG	BMD of LS, PF, and pQCT of distal tibia	No significant loss of BMD at FN in TCC compared with significant losses in CG; pQCT tBMD, iBMD, cBMD loss were significantly slower in TCC vs. CG

Notes: BMD = bone mineral density, BMC = bone mineral content, LS = lumbar spine, FN = femoral neck, PF = proximal femur, R = radius, TB = total body, CT = computerized tomography, IG = intervention group, CG = control group, NS = nonsignificant. pQCT = peripheral quantitative computerized tomography, DT = distal tibia, DR = distal radius, tBMD = trabecular BMD, iBMD = integral BMD, cBMD = cortical tissue density, R = radius, TS = tibial shaft, and C = calcaneus Tai Chi Chun (TCC) exercise.

Thus, there seems to be a positive effect of exercise in postmenopausal women; however, when prescribing exercise to this subpopulation, the risk and significance of sport accidents and injuries should not be neglected.

EXERCISE AND FRACTURES

Although most studies suggest that a history of high levels of exercise is associated with lower hip fracture incidence, there are no prospective studies evaluating whether lifelong exercise protects against fragility fractures in old age (Gregg et al., 1998; Wickham et al., 1989). Observational studies indicate that exercise is associated with a reduction in fractures (Cummings et al., 1995; Farmer et al., 1989, Kujala et al., 2000, Paganini-Hill et al., 1991) (Table 32.6). Several studies have also reported a dose–response relationship when comparing the most active with the least active individuals, which supports the theory that activity reduces the hip fracture risk (Coupland et al., 1993; Gregg et al., 2000; Paganini-Hill et al., 1991). Thus, there seems to be a protective effect of current exercise against hip fractures in both men and women. However, it could also be that the studies reflect the overall health of the participants, that is, participants with worse health tend to exercise less and are more prone to fall and therefore susceptible to fractures (Gregg et al., 1998).

SUMMARY AND TRAINING ADVICE FOR PROMOTING BONE ACCRUAL IN MIDDLE-AGED INDIVIDUALS

Peak bone mass is archived in the second decade of life, and during middle age, bone loss becomes apparent. The skeleton is no longer so adaptive to mechanical stimuli, and meanwhile, muscle, tendons, and ligaments begin to lose strength. Thus, training advice is built on maintaining bone strength. Not only the maintenance of bone strength but also the preservation of balance, coordination, and muscle strength is in focus. Elderly should avoid intensive training in certain sports that leads to high strains on the skeleton and connective tissue, which increases risk for injuries.

- Weight-bearing activity that is not as strenuous on the skeleton, tendons, and muscles as the exercises prescribed in younger ages is recommended. These include jogging, cross-country skiing, pull walking, dance, walking, and resistance training. Specific balance training such as Tai Chi has been shown to decrease the risk of falling.
- The activity should be varied, three times per week on an average of 45 min each time.

TABLE 32.6
Observational Studies of Physical Activity and Fracture Incidence

Reference	Participants	Study Period	Intervention/Exercise	Results
Cummings et al., 1995	9516 women 65 years or older	4.1 years	Questionnaire + interview to assess exercise levels	Significant fracture reduction associated with physical activity
Gregg et al., 1998	9704 women 65 years or older	7.6 years	Questionnaire to assess exercise levels	Significant fracture reduction associated with physical activity
Farmer et al., 1989	3595 women 40–77 years	10 years	Questionnaire to assess exercise levels	Significant fracture reduction associated with physical activity
Kujala et al., 2000	3262 men 44 years or older	21 years	Questionnaire to assess exercise levels	Significant fracture reduction associated with physical activity
Paganini-Hill et al., 1991	5049 men age 73 years	7 years	Questionnaire to assess exercise levels	Significant fracture reduction associated with physical activity

REFERENCES

Alwis, G., Linden, C., Ahlborg, H.G., et al. 2008. A 2-year school-based exercise programme in pre-pubertal boys induces skeletal benefits in lumbar spine. *Acta Paediatr* 97:1564–1571.

Anon. 1993. Consensus development conference: Diagnosis, prophylaxis, and treatment of osteoporosis. *Am J Med* 94:646–650.

Bailey, D.A., Faulkner, R.A., McKay, H.A.1996. Growth, physical activity, and bone mineral acquisition. *Exerc Sport Sci Rev* 24:233–266.

Bassey, E.J., Rothwell, M.C., Littlewood, J.J., et al. 1998. Pre- and postmenopausal women have different bone mineral density responses to the same high-impact exercise. *J Bone Miner Res* 13:1805–1813.

Blimkie, C.J., Rice, S., Webber, C.E., et al. 1996. Effects of resistance training on bone mineral content and density in adolescent females. *Can J Physiol Pharmacol* 74:1025–1033.

Bonjour, J.P., Theintz, G., Buchs, B., et al. 1991. Critical years and stages of puberty for spinal and femoral bone mass accumulation during adolescence. *J Clin Endocrinol Metab* 73:555–563.

Bradney, M., Pearce, G., Naughton, G., et al. 1998. Moderate exercise during growth in prepubertal boys: Changes in bone mass, size, volumetric density, and bone strength: A controlled prospective study. *J Bone Miner Res* 13:1814–1821.

Brooke-Wavell, K., Jones, P.R., Hardman, A.E.1997. Brisk walking reduces calcaneal bone loss in post-menopausal women. *Clin Sci (Lond)* 92:75–80.

Browner, W.S., Pressman, A.R., Nevitt, M.C., et al. 1996. Mortality following fractures in older women. The study of osteoporotic fractures. *Arch Intern Med* 156:1521–1525.

Carter, D.R. 1982. The relationship between in vivo strains and cortical bone remodeling. *Crit Rev Biomed Eng* 8:1–28.

Chan, K., Qin, L., Lau, M., et al. 2004. A randomized, prospective study of the effects of Tai Chi Chun exercise on bone mineral density in postmenopausal women. *Arch Phys Med Rehabil* 85:717–722.

Chow, J.W., Wilson, A.J., Chambers, T.J., et al. 1998. Mechanical loading stimulates bone formation by reactivation of bone lining cells in 13-week-old rats. *J Bone Miner Res* 13:1760–1767.

Cooper, C., Atkinson, E.J., Jacobsen, S.J., et al. 1993. Population-based study of survival after osteoporotic fractures. *Am J Epidemiol* 137:1001–1005.

Coupland, C., Wood, D., Cooper, C. 1993. Physical inactivity is an independent risk factor for hip fracture in the elderly. *J Epidemiol Community Health* 47:441–443.

Cummings, S.R., Nevitt, M.C., Browner, W.S., et al. 1995. Risk factors for hip fracture in white women. Study of Osteoporotic Fractures Research Group [see comments]. *N Engl J Med* 332:767–773.

Delvaux, K., Lefevre, J., Philippaerts, R., et al. 2001. Bone mass and lifetime physical activity in Flemish males: A 27-year follow-up study. *Med Sci Sports Exerc* 33:1868–1875.

Demirel, G., Yilmaz, H., Paker, N., et al. 1998. Osteoporosis after spinal cord injury. *Spinal Cord* 36:822–825.

Drinkwater, B.L., Nilson, K., Ott, S., et al. 1986. Bone mineral density after resumption of menses in amenorrheic athletes. *JAMA* 256:380–382.

Eisman, J.A. 1999. Genetics of osteoporosis. *Endocrinol Rev* 20:788–804.

Farmer, M.E., Harris, T., Madans, J.H., et al. 1989. Anthropometric indicators and hip fracture. The NHANES I Epidemiologic Follow-up Study. *J Am Geriatr Soc* 37:9–16.

Frey-Rindova, P., de Bruin, E.D., Stussi, E., et al. 2000. Bone mineral density in upper and lower extremities during 12 months after spinal cord injury measured by peripheral quantitative computed tomography. *Spinal Cord* 38:26–32.

Frost, H.M. 1987. Bone "mass" and the "mechanostat": A proposal. *Anat Rec* 219:1–9.

Frost, H.M. 1988. Vital biomechanics: Proposed general concepts for skeletal adaptations to mechanical usage. *Calcif Tissue Int* 42:145–156.

Frost, H.M. 2003. Bone's mechanostat: A 2003 update. *Anat Rec* 275A:1081–1101.

Fuchs, R.K., Bauer, J.J., Snow, C.M.2001. Jumping improves hip and lumbar spine bone mass in prepubescent children: A randomized controlled trial. *J Bone Miner Res* 16:148–156.

Fujimura, R., Ashizawa, N., Watanabe, M., et al. 1997. Effect of resistance exercise training on bone formation and resorption in young male subjects assessed by biomarkers of bone metabolism. *J Bone Miner Res* 12:656–662.

Garland, D.E., Stewart, C.A., Adkins, R.H., et al. 1992. Osteoporosis after spinal cord injury. *J Orthop Res* 10:371–378.

Gleeson, P.B., Protas, E.J., LeBlanc, A.D., et al. 1990. Effects of weight lifting on bone mineral density in premenopausal women. *J Bone Miner Res* 5:153–158.

Gregg, E.W., Cauley, J.A., Seeley, D.G., et al. 1998. Physical activity and osteoporotic fracture risk in older women. Study of Osteoporotic Fractures Research Group. *Ann Inten Med* 129:81–88.

Gregg, E.W., Pereira, M.A., Caspersen, C.J. 2000. Physical activity, falls, and fractures among older adults: A review of the epidemiologic evidence. *J Am Geriatr Soc* 48:883–893.

Grove, K.A., Londeree, B.R. 1992. Bone density in postmenopausal women: High impact vs. low impact exercise. *Med Sci Sports Exerc* 24:1190–1194.

Gustavsson, A., Thorsen, K., Nordström, P. 2003. A 3-year longitudinal study of the effect of physical activity on the accrual of bone mineral density in healthy adolescent males. *Calcif Tissue Int* 73:108–114.

Heinonen, A., Kannus, P., Sievanen, H., et al. 1996. Randomised controlled trial of effect of high-impact exercise on selected risk factors for osteoporotic fractures. *Lancet* 348:1343–1347.

Heinonen, A., Kannus, P., Sievanen, H., et al. 1999. Good maintenance of high-impact activity-induced bone gain by voluntary, unsupervised exercises: An 8-month follow-up of a randomized controlled trial. *J Bone Miner Res* 14:125–128.

Heinonen, A., Sievanen, H., Kannus, P., et al. 2000. High-impact exercise and bones of growing girls: A 9-month controlled trial. *Osteoporos Int* 11:1010–1017.

Hetland, M.L., Haarbo, J., Christiansen, C. 1993a. Low bone mass and high bone turnover in male long distance runners. *J Clin Endocrinol Metab* 77:770–775.

Hetland, M.L., Haarbo, J., Christiansen, C., et al. 1993b. Running induces menstrual disturbances but bone mass is unaffected, except in amenorrheic women. *Am J Med* 95: 53–60.

Holick, M.F. 1998. Perspective on the impact of weightlessness on calcium and bone metabolism. *Bone* 22:105S–111S.

Holm, L., Olesen, J.L., Matsumoto, K., et al. 2008. Protein-containing nutrient supplementation following strength training enhances the effect on muscle mass, strength, and bone formation in postmenopausal women. *J Appl Physiol* 105:274–281.

Houde, J.P., Schulz, L.A., Morgan, W.J., et al. 1995. Bone mineral density changes in the forearm after immobilization. *Clin Orthop* 317:199–205.

Jouanny, P., Guillemin, F., Kuntz, C., et al. 1995. Environmental and genetic factors affecting bone mass. Similarity of bone density among members of healthy families. *Arthritis Rheum* 38:61–67.

Kannus, P., Leppala, J., Lehto, M., et al. 1995. A rotator cuff rupture produces permanent osteoporosis in the affected extremity, but not in those with whom shoulder function has returned to normal. *J Bone Miner Res* 10:1263–1271.

Karinkanta, S., Heinonen, A., Sievanen, H., et al. 2007. A multi-component exercise regimen to prevent functional decline and bone fragility in home-dwelling elderly women: Randomized, controlled trial. *Osteoporos Int* 18:453–462.

Kato, T., Terashima, T., Yamashita, T., et al. 2006. Effect of low-repetition jump training on bone mineral density in young women. *J Appl Physiol* 100:839–843.

Kemmler, W., Lauber, D., Weineck, J., et al. 2004. Benefits of 2 years of intense exercise on bone density, physical fitness, and blood lipids in early postmenopausal osteopenic women: Results of the Erlangen Fitness Osteoporosis Prevention Study (EFOPS). *Arch Intern Med* 164:1084–1091.

Kerr, D., Morton, A., Dick, I., et al. 1996. Exercise effects on bone mass in postmenopausal women are site-specific and load-dependent. *J Bone Miner Res* 11:218–225.

Kujala, U.M., Kaprio, J., Kannus, P., et al. 2000. Physical activity and osteoporotic hip fracture risk in men. *Arch Intern Med* 160:705–708.

Lanyon, L.E. 1992. Control of bone architecture by functional load bearing. *J Bone Miner Res* 7 (Suppl 2):S369–S375.

Lanyon, L.E., Goodship, A.E., Pye, C.J., et al. 1982. Mechanically adaptive bone remodelling. *J Biomech* 15:141–154.

Lanyon, L.E., Rubin, C.T., Baust, G. 1986. Modulation of bone loss during calcium insufficiency by controlled dynamic loading. *Calcif Tissue Int* 38:209–216.

Leblanc, A.D., Schneider, V.S., Evans, H.J., et al. 1990. Bone mineral loss and recovery after 17 weeks of bed rest. *J Bone Miner Res* 5:843–850.

Lehtonen-Veromaa, M., Mottonen, T., Irjala, K., et al. 2000. A 1-year prospective study on the relationship between physical activity, markers of bone metabolism, and bone acquisition in peripubertal girls. *J Clin Endocrinol Metab* 85:3726–3732.

Leppala, J., Kannus, P., Natri, A., et al. 1998. Bone mineral density in the chronic patellofemoral pain syndrome. *Calcif Ttissue Int* 62:548–553.

Libanati, C., Baylink, D.J., Lois-Wenzel, E., et al. 1999. Studies on the potential mediators of skeletal changes occurring during puberty in girls. *J Clin Endocrinol Metab* 84:2807–2814.

Litmanovitz, I., Dolfin, T., Friedland, O., et al. 2003. Early physical activity intervention prevents decrease of bone strength in very low birth weight infants. *Pediatrics* 112:15–19.

Lohman, T., Going, S., Pamenter, R., et al. 1995. Effects of resistance training on regional and total bone mineral density in premenopausal women: A randomized prospective study. *J Bone Miner Res* 10:1015–1024.

Louis, O., Demeirleir, K., Kalender, W., et al. 1991. Low vertebral bone density values in young non-elite female runners. *Int J Sports Med* 12:214–217.

Lynch, N.A., Ryan, A.S., Evans, J., et al. 2007. Older elite football players have reduced cardiac and osteoporosis risk factors. *Med Sci Sports Exerc* 39:1124–1130.

Macdonald, H.M., Kontulainen, S.A., Khan, K.M., et al. 2007. Is a school-based physical activity intervention effective for increasing tibial bone strength in boys and girls? *J Bone Miner Res* 22:434–446.

MacKelvie, K.J., Khan, K.M., McKay, H.A. 2002. Is there a critical period for bone response to weight-bearing exercise in children and adolescents? A systematic review. *Br J Sports Med* 36:250–257; discussion 257.

MacKelvie, K.J., Khan, K.M., Petit, M.A., et al. 2003. A school-based exercise intervention elicits substantial bone health benefits: A 2-year randomized controlled trial in girls. *Pediatrics* 112:e447.

MacKelvie, K.J., McKay, H.A., Khan, K.M., et al. 2001. A school-based exercise intervention augments bone mineral accrual in early pubertal girls. *J Pediatr* 139:501–507.

MacKelvie, K.J., Petit, M.A., Khan, K.M., et al. 2004. Bone mass and structure are enhanced following a 2-year randomized controlled trial of exercise in prepubertal boys. *Bone* 34:755–764.

McKay, H.A., Petit, M.A., Schutz, R.W., et al. 2000. Augmented trochanteric bone mineral density after modified physical education classes: A randomized school-based exercise intervention study in prepubescent and early pubescent children. *J Pediatr* 136:156–162.

Micklesfield, L.K., Lambert, E.V., Fataar, A.B., et al. 1995. Bone mineral density in mature, premenopausal ultramarathon runners. *Med Sci Sports Exerc* 27:688–696.

Mora, S., Pitukcheewanont, P., Nelson, J.C., et al. 1999. Serum levels of insulin-like growth factor I and the density, volume, and cross-sectional area of cortical bone in children. *J Clin Endocrinol Metab* 84:2780–2783.

Morris, F.L., Naughton, G.A., Gibbs, J.L., et al. 1997. Prospective ten-month exercise intervention in premenarcheal girls: Positive effects on bone and lean mass. *J Bone Miner Res* 12:1453–1462.

Moyer-Mileur, L.J., Brunstetter, V., McNaught, T.P., et al. 2000. Daily physical activity program increases bone mineralization and growth in preterm very low birth weight infants. *Pediatrics* 106:1088–1092.

Nelson, M.E., Fiatarone, M.A., Morganti, C.M., et al. 1994. Effects of high-intensity strength training on multiple risk factors for osteoporotic fractures. A randomized controlled trial. *JAMA* 272:1909–1914.

Nemet, D., Dolfin, T., Litmanowitz, I., et al. 2002. Evidence for exercise-induced bone formation in premature infants. *Int J Sports Med* 23:82–85.

Neville, C.E., Murray, L.J., Boreham, C.A., et al. 2002. Relationship between physical activity and bone mineral status in young adults: The Northern Ireland young hearts project. *Bone* 30:792–798.

Nevitt, M.C., Ettinger, B., Black, D.M., et al. 1998. The association of radiographically detected vertebral fractures with back pain and function: A prospective study. *Ann Intern Med* 128:793–800.

Nguyen, T.V., Center, J.R., Eisman, J.A. 2000. Osteoporosis in elderly men and women: Effects of dietary calcium, physical activity, and body mass index. *J Bone Miner Res* 15:322–331.

Nordström, A., Hogstrom, M., Nordström, P. 2008. Effects of different types of weight-bearing loading on bone mass and size in young males: A longitudinal study. *Bone* 42:565–571.

Nordström, P., Lorentzon, R. 1996. Site-specific bone mass differences of the lower extremities in 17-year-old ice hockey players. *Calcif Tissue Int* 59:443–448.

O'Connor, J.A., Lanyon, L.E., MacFie, H.1982. The influence of strain rate on adaptive bone remodelling. *Journal of Biomechanics* 15:767–781.

Paganini-Hill, A., Chao, A., Ross, R.K., et al. 1991. Exercise and other factors in the prevention of hip fracture: The Leisure World study. *Epidemiology* 2:16–25.

Pontzer, H., Lieberman, D.E., Momin, E., et al. 2006. Trabecular bone in the bird knee responds with high sensitivity to changes in load orientation. *J Exp Biol* 209:57–65.

Prince, R., Devine, A., Dick, I., et al. 1995. The effects of calcium supplementation (milk powder or tablets) and exercise on bone density in postmenopausal women. *J Bone Miner Res* 10:1068–1075.

Raab-Cullen, D.M., Akhter, M.P., Kimmel, D.B., et al. 1994. Bone response to alternate-day mechanical loading of the rat tibia. *J Bone Miner Res* 9:203–211.

Rambaut, P.C., Johnston, R.S. 1979. Prolonged weightlessness and calcium loss in man. *Acta Astronaut* 6:1113–1122.

Rambaut, P.C., Leach, C.S., Johnson, P.C. 1975. Calcium and phosphorus change of the Apollo 17 crew members. *Nutr Metab* 18:62–69.

Ramnemark, A., Nyberg, L., Lorentzon, R., et al. 1999a. Progressive hemiosteoporosis on the paretic side and increased bone mineral density in the nonparetic arm the first year after severe stroke. *Osteoporos Int* 9:269–275.

Ramnemark, A., Nyberg, L., Lorentzon, R., et al. 1999b. Hemiosteoporosis after severe stroke, independent of changes in body composition and weight. *Stroke; J Cerebral Circul* 30:755–760.

Robinson, T.L., Snow-Harter, C., Taaffe, D.R., et al. 1995. Gymnasts exhibit higher bone mass than runners despite similar prevalence of amenorrhea and oligomenorrhea. *J Bone Miner Res* 10:26–35.

Robling, A.G., Hinant, F.M., Burr, D.B., et al. 2002. Improved bone structure and strength after long-term mechanical loading is greatest if loading is separated into short bouts. *J Bone Miner Res* 17:1545–1554.

Rubin, C.T., Lanyon, L.E.1984. Regulation of bone formation by applied dynamic loads. *J Bone Joint Surg Am* 66:397–402.

Rubin, C.T., Lanyon, L.E.1985. Regulation of bone mass by mechanical strain magnitude. *Calcif Tissue Int* 37:411–417.

Rubin, C.T., Lanyon, L.E. 1987. Kappa Delta Award paper. Osteoregulatory nature of mechanical stimuli: Function as a determinant for adaptive remodeling in bone. *J Orthop Res* 5:300–310.

Sambrook, P.N., Shawe, D., Hesp, R., et al. 1990. Rapid periarticular bone loss in rheumatoid arthritis. Possible promotion by normal circulating concentrations of parathyroid hormone or calcitriol (1,25-dihydroxyvitamin D3). *Arthritis Rheum* 33:615–622.

Sandler, R.B., Cauley, J.A., Hom, D.L., et al. 1987. The effects of walking on the cross-sectional dimensions of the radius in postmenopausal women. *Calcif Tissue Int* 41:65–69.

Seeman, E., Hopper, J.L., Bach, L.A., et al. 1989. Reduced bone mass in daughters of women with osteoporosis. *N Engl J Med* 320:554–558.

Seeman, E., Szmukler, G.I., Formica, C., et al. 1992. Osteoporosis in anorexia nervosa: The influence of peak bone density, bone loss, oral contraceptive use, and exercise. *J Bone Miner Res* 7:1467–1474.

Seeman, E., Wahner, H.W., Offord, K.P., et al. 1982. Differential effects of endocrine dysfunction on the axial and the appendicular skeleton. *J Clin Invest* 69:1302–1309.

Sinaki, M., Canvin, J.C., Phillips, B.E., et al. 2004. Site specificity of regular health club exercise on muscle strength, fitness, and bone density in women aged 29 to 45 years. *Mayo Clin Proc* 79:639–644.

Sinaki, M., Wahner, H.W., Bergstralh, E.J., et al. 1996. Three-year controlled, randomized trial of the effect of dose-specified loading and strengthening exercises on bone mineral density of spine and femur in nonathletic, physically active women. *Bone* 19:233–244.

Slemenda, C.W., Christian, J.C., Williams, C.J., et al. 1991. Genetic determinants of bone mass in adult women: A reevaluation of the twin model and the potential importance of gene interaction on heritability estimates. *J Bone Miner Res* 6:561–567.

Slemenda, C.W., Reister, T.K., Hui, S.L., et al. 1994. Influences on skeletal mineralization in children and adolescents: Evidence for varying effects of sexual maturation and physical activity. *J Pediatr* 125:201–207.

Snow-Harter, C., Bouxsein, M.L., Lewis, B.T., et al. 1992. Effects of resistance and endurance exercise on bone mineral status of young women: A randomized exercise intervention trial. *J Bone Miner Res* 7:761–769.

Tanner, J.M. 1962. *Growth at Adolescence*. Blackwell Scientific Publications, Philadelphia.

Teng, S., Choi, I.W., Herring, S.W., et al. 1997. Stereological analysis of bone architecture in the pig zygomatic arch. *Anat Rec* 248:205–213.

Thi, M.M., Kojima, T., Cowin, S.C., et al. 2003. Fluid shear stress remodels expression and function of junctional proteins in cultured bone cells. *Am J Physiol Cell Physiol* 284:C389–C403.

Turner, C.H. 1991. Homeostatic control of bone structure: An application of feedback theory. *Bone* 12:203–217.

Turner, C.H., Owan, I., Alvey, T., et al. 1998. Recruitment and proliferative responses of osteoblasts after mechanical loading in vivo determined using sustained-release bromodeoxyuridine. *Bone* 22:463–469.

Umemura, Y., Ishiko, T., Yamauchi, T., et al. 1997. Five jumps per day increase bone mass and breaking force in rats. *J Bone Miner Res* 12:1480–1485.

Vainionpaa, A., Korpelainen, R., Leppaluoto, J., et al. 2005. Effects of high-impact exercise on bone mineral density: A randomized controlled trial in premenopausal women. *Osteoporos Int* 16:191–197.

Vico, L., Collet, P., Guignandon, A., et al. 2000. Effects of long-term microgravity exposure on cancellous and cortical weight-bearing bones of cosmonauts. *Lancet* 355:1607–1611.

Watanabe, Y., Ohshima, H., Mizuno, K., et al. 2004. Intravenous pamidronate prevents femoral bone loss and renal stone formation during 90-day bed rest. *J Bone Miner Res* 19:1771–1778.

Weeks, B.K., Young, C.M., Beck, B.R. 2008. Eight months of regular in-school jumping improves indices of bone strength in adolescent boys and Girls: The POWER PE study. *J Bone Miner Res* 23:1002–1011.

Welten, D.C., Kemper, H.C., Post, G.B., et al. 1994. Weight-bearing activity during youth is a more important factor for peak bone mass than calcium intake. *J Bone Miner Res* 9:1089–1096.

Wheeler, G.D., Wall, S.R., Belcastro, A.N., et al. 1984. Reduced serum testosterone and prolactin levels in male distance runners. *JAMA* 252:514–516.

Wickham, C.A., Walsh, K., Cooper, C., et al. 1989. Dietary calcium, physical activity, and risk of hip fracture: A prospective study. *BMJ* 299:889–892.

Winters, K.M., Snow, C.M. 2000. Detraining reverses positive effects of exercise on the musculoskeletal system in premenopausal women. *J Bone Miner Res* 15:2495–2503.

Witzke, K.A., Snow, C.M. 2000. Effects of plyometric jump training on bone mass in adolescent girls. *Med Sci Sports Exerc* 32:1051–1057.

Wolff, J. 1892. *Das Gesetz der Transformation der Knochen.* Bei Hirschwald, Leipzig.

Zerwekh, J.E., Ruml, L.A., Gottschalk, F., et al. 1998. The effects of twelve weeks of bed rest on bone histology, biochemical markers of bone turnover, and calcium homeostasis in eleven normal subjects. *J Bone Miner Res* 13:1594–1601.

33 The Bone–Vascular Axis in Chronic Kidney Disease

Philip J. Klemmer and John J.B. Anderson

CONTENTS

INTRODUCTION

Chronic kidney disease (CKD) results from functional abnormalities of any one of the three anatomical substructures in the kidney: the glomeruli, the tubules, or the interstitium. An estimation of overall kidney function is made by measurement of serum creatinine concentration, which can be used to estimate the glomerular filtration rate. Kidney function may decline as a result of congenital or acquired disease or as a result of functional decline related to aging. This chapter examines the interrelationships among abnormal mineral metabolism, bone disease, and vascular calcification in patients with CKD. Discussion of pharmacologic options in the treatment of patients with CKD is also offered.

THE BONE–VASCULAR AXIS IN CKD

CKD is a growing public health epidemic that effects 13% of the U.S. population—approximately 26 million adults in the United States (Coresh et al., 2007). Once established, CKD tends to progress inexorably toward end-stage renal disease (ESRD), which necessitates renal replacement therapy, either dialysis or renal transplantation, to support life. More than 519,000 Americans currently rely on dialysis, and 16,000 individuals each year receive renal transplantation. The number of Americans on dialysis continues to grow, largely reflecting the aging of our population and the increasing prevalence of obesity-associated metabolic syndrome, which has adverse effects on kidney function (National Institutes of Health, 2009). Indeed, diabetes and hypertension, two components of the metabolic syndrome that have strong links to nutrition, are responsible for over half of advanced CKD requiring dialysis or kidney transplantation.

Cardiovascular disease (CVD) and CKD are interrelated and, in a sense, may be viewed as "different sides of the same coin." Indeed, CKD is an independent risk factor for the development of CVD (Foley et al., 1998). Patients on dialysis suffer an extraordinarily high annual death rate, exceeding 22% (Block et al., 2004; Go et al., 2004). More than half of these deaths are the consequence of CVD (Foley et al., 1998). The majority of patients with lesser degrees of CKD die from CVD before ever reaching dialysis or renal transplantation.

The reason for this high rate of CVD-related morbidity and mortality in CKD patients is not fully understood. Certainly, the high prevalence of traditional cardiovascular risk factors—hypertension, diabetes mellitus, dyslipidemia, and tobacco use—among CKD patients may account for some, but not all, of this excess morbidity and mortality. The presence of any degree of CKD accelerates the development of CVD independently of the traditional Framingham CVD risk factors. Disturbances in mineral metabolism and renal osteodystrophy (ROD) are common in CKD patients and tend to worsen as ESRD is approached.

In recent years, links between dysregulated mineral and bone metabolism, on one hand, and between disordered mineral metabolism and vascular calcification, on the other, have been established in in vitro and in vivo investigations, as well as in epidemiologic studies (Block et al., 1998; Giachelli et al., 2001; Jono et al., 2000; Reynolds et al., 2004; Schoppet et al., 2008). Vascular calcification and bone disease are linked by common physiological control mechanisms. The term *calcification paradox* is derived from the observation that CKD patients frequently develop extensive vascular calcification at the same time that they paradoxically lose bone mineral density (BMD) because of disturbances in bone turnover resulting predominantly from secondary hyperparathyroidism, that is, high bone turnover. Under some conditions, adynamic bone disease resulting from low bone turnover may occur (Persy and D'Haese, 2009).

Each of these two bone diseases is associated with kidney dysfunction. ROD may be linked with growth abnormalities in children and with bone fractures in adults as well as in children. Vascular calcification in CKD patients, even very young patients (Goodman et al., 2000), occurs in two locations: the vascular media of large conduit arteries, where it is called Mönckeberg sclerosis, and the intimal region of smaller arteries, where it is associated with atherosclerotic plaques. Vascular calcifications in both locations are associated with high rates of cardiovascular morbidity and mortality in CKD patients (Blacher et al., 2001; Raggi et al., 2002). The molecular mechanisms that normally regulate bone formation and remodeling is thought to be activated at these ectopic vascular sites, which promotes or accelerates vascular calcification. Disturbances in these same control mechanisms at these inappropriate sites of bone formation account for the high prevalence of ROD in CKD patients (London et al., 2004).

Of interest, the same reciprocal relationship between low bone density (osteoporosis) and vascular calcification has been noted in older adults in the absence of CKD (Demer and Tintut, 2009). In addition, high degrees of cardiovascular calcification (CVC) have been shown to be directly associated with adverse cardiovascular outcomes in diverse populations with normal kidney function (Detrano et al., 2008). To reduce the burdens of CVD and ROD in CKD patients, efforts have been made to understand the dysregulated signaling, which leads to the calcification paradox.

RENAL OSTEODYSTROPHY

ROD is a heterogeneous disorder of bone remodeling that eventually affects most patients with moderate to severe degrees of CKD. Multiple metabolic disorders lead to ROD. Although largely asymptomatic in its earliest stages, ROD leads to growth retardation in children and adolescents and loss of bone strength in all age groups. The interactions among ROD, vascular calcification, and disordered mineral metabolism must be considered when treating these disorders. Observational studies suggest that abnormalities of these complex interactions affect cardiovascular morbidity and mortality in patients with CKD. ROD typically begins after 50% of renal function has been lost (Adragao et al., 2009).

The principal histological changes in ROD encompass changes in bone turnover, mineralization, and bone volume. Typically, CKD patients have one of three patterns of histological change on bone biopsy: (1) high turnover, termed secondary hyperparathyroidism or osteitis fibrosa cystica, in its most advanced form; (2) adynamic bone disease that usually reflects relative hypoparathyroidism;

and (3) vitamin-D-deficiency–related osteomalacia, which is also a low bone turnover disease. All forms of ROD usually decrease BMD and lead to osteopenic changes in bone ultrastructure. ROD is associated with progressive vascular calcification in patients with CKD. Treatment of ROD may have indirect effects (beneficial or detrimental) on patient survival because of the pathophysiological linkage between ROD and CVC.

Because most CKD patients do not undergo bone biopsy, the clinician must utilize clinical, biochemical, and radiographic data to categorize and treat CKD patients with ROD. Most patients with advanced CKD have histological changes characteristic of secondary hyperparathyroidism on bone biopsy. This high bone turnover state is characterized by both increased activity of osteoblasts and osteoclasts and low bone volume, but no defect in bone mineralization exists.

The traditional pathophysiological explanation for this histological pattern is centered on the parathyroid gland. According to this view, patients with progressive loss of renal function develop elevated levels of parathyroid hormone (PTH) that result in skeletal abnormalities associated with hyperparathyroidism. Elevation in serum PTH concentrations in CKD has been thought to be the consequence of reduction in normal inhibitory factors on PTH secretion and parathyroid cell growth. Loss of negative inhibition on the parathyroid occurs as the result of lower serum concentrations of 1,25-dihydroxy vitamin D as well as reduced number of vitamin D and calcium-sensing receptors on the parathyroid cell membrane. In addition, hyperphosphatemia and intermittent postprandial hypocalcemia directly stimulate parathyroid growth and PTH secretion. As a consequence of these combined stimuli, parathyroid hyperplasia develops, which results in further increases of PTH secretion and the stimulation of bone remodeling.

Recently, Hruska et al. (2007) have challenged this mechanistic view of hyperparathyroid-induced bone disease in CKD. According to this alternative view, the primary abnormality in CKD resides at the level of skeleton rather than at the parathyroid gland. Early in the course of CKD, a defect in normal skeletal anabolism occurs due to resistance to the action of PTH on osteoblasts. The mechanism of this skeletal resistance to the anabolic effects of PTH is unknown but may involve suppression of 1,25-vitamin D synthesis because of elevated serum concentration of FGF-23 in the early stages of CKD. The skeletal resistance to PTH causes compensatory PTH hypersecretion in an attempt to maintain normal bone remodeling. This theory explains why many CKD patients have elevated levels of PTH in the absence of major abnormalities in serum concentrations of inorganic phosphate or calcium ions. This theory also helps explain why these CKD patients rarely have hypercalcemia despite of a significant chronic elevation of serum PTH concentrations.

The initial resistance in the skeleton to the anabolic effects of PTH eventually leads to further parathyroid hyperplasia and superphysiological concentrations of PTH in the serum. Eventually, a predominant skeletal catabolic action of PTH occurs, which increases the high bone turnover by stimulating high osteoblastic and even higher osteoclastic activity. This alternative view of Hruska et al. also helps explain the development of adynamic bone disease, which frequently results from excessive inhibition of PTH secretion following the administration of calcium (as part of calcium-containing phosphate binders), that is, the use of dialysate containing supraphysiological concentrations of calcium, excessive active vitamin D therapy, or complete surgical parathyroidectomy. PTH concentrations below 150 pg/mL have been associated with adynamic bone disease in dialysis patients (Kalantar-Zadeh et al., 2006).

Both high and low bone turnover states may contribute to CVC in CKD patients, albeit by different mechanisms. High bone turnover states are characterized by an efflux of calcium and phosphate from bone. Talmage (1996) has postulated that the bone space (or bone envelope) provides a vast store of calcium available for immediate exchange with the extracellular fluids (see Chapter 7). This efflux from the bone membrane exceeds that from structural bone by at least 15-fold. The effect of PTH on the regulation of ionic calcium flux across the bone envelope is the major mechanism by which normocalcemia is maintained. Patients with secondary hyperparathyroidism may have even greater levels of calcium fluxes from structural bone than do normal individuals because of excessive osteoclastic bone resorption. CKD patients with severe secondary hyperparathyroidism frequently develop severe hyperphosphatemia as a result of high phosphate efflux from the skeleton. Dietary phosphate restriction and use of phosphate binders frequently fail to control hyperphosphatemia in these patients because much of the phosphate in the serum is derived from phosphate ions released into the blood as a result of skeletal resorption, that is, it is unaffected by binders within the gut.

Effective treatment in these patients has been achieved by lowering PTH hypersecretion with the use of calcimimetic drugs or, alternatively, with subtotal surgical parathyroidectomy. Because hyperphosphatemia promotes CVC, the hyperparathyroid form of ROD is intimately linked to cardiovascular morbidity and mortality in CKD patients (Block et al., 2004). Adynamic bone disease may promote CVC through a different mechanism. Osteoblast-like cells on the bone envelope normally mediate the efflux and influx of 6000 mg/day of calcium (Talmage, 1996). During brief periods of positive calcium balance in normal adults, the bone envelope buffers these excess ions for a brief period of time prior to renal excretion. This action helps maintain minute-to-minute normocalcemia. The CKD patients with adynamic bone disease and functional hypoparathyroidism lose calcium and phosphate-buffering capacity in the bone envelope. Because positive calcium balance cannot be buffered, excess calcium load deposits in soft tissue, including in diverse vascular locations. Calcium deposition at two sites, the intimal spaces associated with atherosclerotic plaque and the medial layers of arteries and arterioles, may accelerate preexistent CVC. High morbidity and mortality rates in CKD5 patients are directly associated with the degree of CVC. Supporting this view, Malluche has shown, in CKD5 patients, a direct association between histological changes of adynamic bone disease and advanced CVC (Adragao et al., 2004).

Patients with adynamic bone disease require an upward adjustment of PTH serum concentrations to restore normal bone remodeling and normal calcium buffer capacity of the bone envelope to avoid calcium loading in soft tissues and vascular sites. Therapeutic maneuvers that may allow PTH to increase to a more appropriate level include decreasing or eliminating calcium from calcium-based phosphate binders, decreasing usage of active vitamin D, or lowering dialysate calcium concentrations to physiological levels. All of these maneuvers decrease the inhibition of PTH secretion, thereby helping to restore normal bone remodeling. Achieving an optimal level of PTH in CKD is difficult without the aid of bone histological sections. Without information on bone histomorphology, a clinician is typically left only with biochemical parameters and radiographs to help make judgments with regard to speculated bone histological changes. A CKD3 patient is typically first treated with ergocalciferol or cholecalciferol and a low-phosphate diet if PTH levels are elevated, serum phosphorus and calcium concentrations are within physiological range, and serum 25-hydroxyvitamin D concentrations are below 30 µg/mL. As the CKD progresses toward CKD5, hyperphosphatemia usually develops and requires initiation of phosphate binders to be taken orally along with meals.

Until recently, clinical guidelines recommended a serum phosphate concentration equal to or less than 5.5, PTH level of 150–300, and serum calcium of 9.2–10.2 as therapeutic goals for the clinician (Craver et al., 2007). More recently, the upper limit of PTH recommended in CKD5 has been increased to approximately 600 (Eckardt et al., 2009). These guidelines changes have been directed at avoiding oversuppression of PTH and resultant adynamic bone disease that is strongly considered to advance progressive CVC. An observational study has shown that PTH is only weakly associated with all-cause mortality in dialysis patients, whereas elevated serum phosphate is much more strongly linked with these events (Block et al., 2004). Although protein is a rich source of phosphate, CKD patients are not advised to limit intake of dietary protein from meats, fish, poultry, or eggs because protein malnutrition and hypoalbuminemia have profound adverse effects on patient survival.

The judicious use of phosphate binders with meals helps reduce the phosphate absorption from these dietary sources. Yet, no large prospective studies have been reported that demonstrate improved morbidity and mortality in CKD5 patients treated with various phosphate binders, active vitamin

D, or active vitamin D analogs or calcimimetics. Beyond these therapeutic interventions, other strategies to improve ROD and CVD outcomes are currently being explored, including increasing dialysis time by means of slow nightly dialysis. Longer dialysis time is known to remove excess phosphate, and it lessens the need for expensive phosphate-binding medications that may be unpalatable. Finally, renal transplantation mitigates many of the skeletal effects of hyperphosphatemia and low serum concentrations of 1,25-dihydroxy cholecalciferol.

VASCULAR CALCIFICATION

Vascular calcification has been known to be associated with CVD for over 100 years (Virchow, 1855). CKD patients, particularly diabetics and those who have been treated with dialysis over many years, demonstrate high degrees of vascular calcification (Schoppet et al., 2008). Rapid sequence tomography (a research tool) has provided a means of measuring the degree of vascular calcification in coronary arteries, thus providing a coronary artery calcium score (CACS). A high CACS, particularly those above 400, is associated with a higher rate of cardiovascular morbidity and mortality inpatients with and without CKD (Moe and Chertow, 2006). Traditional cardiovascular risk factors—hypertension, diabetes, hyperlipidemia, and smoking—all promote vascular calcification in CKD patients. Beyond these traditional risk factors, CKD patients have a particularly high burden of vascular calcification that appears to be at least partially related to disordered mineral and bone metabolism. In addition, concern has been raised whether some of current treatment strategies of these disorders may actually hasten the progression of vascular calcification in CKD patients (Moe and Chertow, 2006).

Vascular calcification occurs in two locations: in the media of the aorta, where it causes vascular stiffening, and in the intimal space of medium and small muscular arteries (including coronary arteries), where it is located within atherosclerotic plaques. Aortic calcification leads to cardiovascular events by causing isolated systolic hypertension, reduced coronary artery filling in diastole, and left ventricular hypertrophy. These abnormalities promote the development of congestive heart failure, a major cause of death in CKD. Intimal calcification occurs in the majority of atherosclerotic plaques. This fixed association has made the CACS a quantitative measure of total atherosclerotic burden, thus providing a strong predictor of cardiovascular events (Braun et al., 1996). Calcium in atherosclerotic plaques leads to vascular narrowing, reduction in blood flow, and in some cases, plaque instability and acute ischemic events, including stroke and myocardial infarction. Over half of the annual mortality among dialysis patients has been attributed to CVD. This very high incidence of events cannot be fully attributed to traditional cardiovascular risk factors. Disordered mineral metabolism and bone disease may possibly accelerate vascular damage in CKD patients by promoting vascular calcification.

Figure 33.1 provides a schematic illustration of vascular calcification, including multiple potential mechanisms.

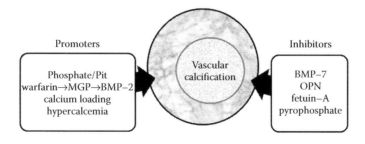

FIGURE 33.1 Schematic drawing of vascular calcification. Inhibitors (right) and promoters (left) of vascular calcification.

HYPERPHOSPHATEMIA

The serum biochemical environment in the CKD patient promotes vascular calcification. Multiple factors involved in this "perfect storm" include hyperphosphatemia, calcium loading, oxidative stress, active vitamin D deficiency, and decreases in serum inhibitors of vascular calcification, including alpha fetuin, pyrophosphate, and vitamin-K-dependent GLA protein. Evidence supporting the role of hyperphosphatemia in the promotion of vascular calcification comes from in vitro studies in which vascular smooth muscle cells (VSMCs) were incubated in graduated concentrations of phosphate. In this system, the hyperphosphatemic environment causes a phenotype change of a VSMC into an osteoblastic cell lineage.

Osteoid formation produced by these osteoblasts leads to the formation of extracellular calcium apatite (Giachelli et al., 2001; Jono et al., 2000; Proudfoot and Shanahan, 2001). These studies support the possibility that vascular calcification is an actively regulated process rather than a passive response to primary vascular injury. The importance of targeting phosphate as a means of controlling vascular calcification is underscored by the fact that half of dialysis patients have serum phosphate concentrations greater than 5.5 mg/dL and are thereby exposed to the heterotopic mineralization effects of hyperphosphatemia. Retrospective analyses of large databases have shown that most dialysis patients today have an elevated serum phosphate concentration, which, after correction for a number of relevant confounders, remains strongly associated with morbidity and mortality. Control of hyperphosphatemia requires reduction of dietary phosphate from nonprotein sources (primarily dairy and processed foods) and the use of phosphate-binding medications taken with meals. Adequate duration of dialysis is also critical. Controlling phosphate ion efflux from resorbing bone stores in patients with severe hyperparathyroidism may require calcimimetic therapy or subtotal parathyroidectomy.

Multiple clinical practice recommendations have published target values for serum phosphate as well as other biochemical parameters in CKD based on observational data describing risk relationships between abnormal serum values and clinically important outcomes. However, to date, no large long-term randomized clinical trials reporting patient morbidity and mortality have been completed supporting these recommendations. The upper limit of ideal serum phosphate concentration in CKD has not been established. Until recently, serum concentrations above 5.5 mg/dL have been considered elevated. More recently, practice guidelines have encouraged clinicians to consider time-average trends on monthly biochemistries rather than single threshold biochemical values. Most would agree that lowering serum phosphate concentrations to within the normal range is fundamental for reducing the risk of ROD as well as of vascular calcification.

Clinical reality shows that serum phosphate, calcium, and PTH concentrations are interrelated. Therapeutic efforts to lower one biochemical risk may result in the elevation of another biochemical risk factor. For example, use of excessive calcium-based phosphate binders may control hyperphosphatemia and the price of hypercalcemia and calcium loading. Likewise, excessive use of active vitamin D or vitamin D analogues my promote calcium loading, hypercalcemia, and adynamic bone disease.

HYPERCALCEMIA AND CALCIUM LOADING

The possible role of hypercalcemia and/or positive calcium balance (called calcium loading) in promoting vascular calcification in CKD is less clear than that of hyperphosphatemia. In vitro studies have suggested that hypercalcemia acts synergistically with hyperphosphatemia to promote extracellular mineralization by VSMC (Proudfoot and Shanahan, 2001).

Two clinical studies (Block et al., 2007; Chertow et al., 2002) have shown differences in rates of progression of vascular calcification in dialysis patients treated with calcium acetate or calcium carbonate, both calcium-based phosphate binders compared with sevelamer, a non-calcium-containing phosphate binder. Over a 2-year course of therapy, patients treated with sevelamer showed insignificant degrees of progression of CACS. Over the same period, the patients treated with calcium-based phosphate binders showed significant progression of CACS. In one of these studies (Block et al., 2007), the patients treated with sevelamer had a significant reduction in mortality as well. One study comparing sevelamer hydrochloride with calcium-containing phosphate binders found no differences in all-cause or cause-specific mortality rates (Suki et al., 2007). One study in children and young adults on dialysis showed an association between total calcium intake from phosphate binders and the degree of coronary artery calcification (Goodman et al., 2000).

Unlike sevelamer and lanthanum carbonate, patients treated with calcium acetate absorb significant amounts of calcium cations, and this may contribute to calcium loading events in the absence of hypercalcemia (Sheikh et al., 1989). Active vitamin therapy used to suppress hypersecretion of PTH may further enhance calcium loading by increasing the efficiency intestinal calcium absorption. Because dialysis patients have virtually no urinary calcium excretion and those with adynamic bone disease may lack normal calcium buffering capacity in the bone envelope, these patients may deposit excess calcium in soft tissues, including vascular locations. New analogues of 1,25-dihydroxycholecalciferol have been shown to have less calcimimetic effect than does the natural active vitamin D in patients with CKD. It is unknown whether these analogues are less likely to promote calcium loading with 1,25-dihydroxycholecalciferol. Calcimimetics are less likely to cause calcium loading than active vitamin D or vitamin D analogues are because they act at the level of bone and they do not enhance the intestinal absorption of calcium. Unlike calcium-based phosphate binders which decrease serum phosphate concentrations at the expense of increasing serum calcium concentrations, calcimimetics decrease serum concentrations of PTH, calcium, and phosphate. A study is currently in progress examining whether all-cause mortality in dialysis patients is reduced by calcimimetic therapy (Chertow et al., 2007).

SUMMARY

Patients with CKD suffer from increased morbidity and mortality as the result of abnormal mineral metabolism and its effect on the bone–vascular interface. Hyperphosphatemia appears to be the most important mutable biochemical perturbation accelerating vascular calcification and promoting ROD. Several barriers prevent adequate control of elevated serum phosphate in CKD patients including high dietary phosphate intakes resulting from the ubiquitous use of phosphate-rich processed foods and the pill burden of phosphate binders. The high cost of non-calcium-based phosphate binders and calcimimetic therapy also account for suboptimal therapy. In the future, it is hoped that improved therapies can be developed which can control hyperphosphatemia at lower cost while not exposing the CKD patient to the risks of calcium loading. Most importantly, randomized control trials using currently available therapies need to examine not only biochemical surrogate outcomes but morbidity and mortality in CKD populations.

REFERENCES

Adragao, T., Herberth, J., Monier-Faugere, M.C., et al. 2009. Low bone volume—A risk factor for coronary calcifications in hemodialysis patients. *Clin J Am Soc Nephrol* 4: 450–455.

Adragao, T., Pires, A., Lucas, C., et al. 2004. A simple vascular calcification score predicts cardiovascular risk in haemodialysis patients. *Nephrol Dial. Transplant* 19: 1480–1488.

Blacher, J., Guerin, A.P., Pannier, B., et al. 2001. Arterial calcifications, arterial stiffness, and cardiovascular risk in end-stage renal disease. *Hypertension* 38: 938–942.

Block, G.A., Hulbert-Shearon, T.E., Levin, N.W., et al. 1998. Association of serum phosphorus and calcium × phosphate product with mortality risk in chronic hemodialysis patients: A national study. *Am J Kidney Dis* 31: 607–617.

Block, G.A., Klassen, P.S., Lazarus, J.M., et al. 2004. Mineral metabolism, mortality, and morbidity in maintenance hemodialysis. *J Am Soc Nephrol* 15: 2208–2218.

Block, G.A., Raggi, P., Bellasi, A., et al. 2007. Mortality effect of coronary calcification and phosphate binder choice in incident hemodialysis patients. *Kidney Int* 71: 438–441.

Braun, J., Oldendorf, M., Moshage, W., et al. 1996. Electron beam computed tomography in the evaluation of cardiac calcification in chronic dialysis patients. *Am J Kidney Dis* 27: 394–401.

Chertow, G.M., Burke, S.K., and Raggi, P. 2002. Sevelamer attenuates the progression of coronary and aortic calcification in hemodialysis patients. *Kidney Int* 62: 245–252.

Chertow, G.M., Pupim, L.B., Block, G.A., et al. 2007. Evaluation of cinacalcet therapy to lower cardiovascular events (EVOLVE): Rationale and design overview. *Clin J Am Soc Nephrol* 2: 898–905.

Coresh, J., Selvin, E., Stevens, L.A., et al. 2007. Prevalence of chronic kidney disease in the United States. *JAMA* 298: 2038–2047.

Craver, L., Marco, M.P., Martinez, I., et al. 2007. Mineral metabolism parameters throughout chronic kidney disease stages 1–5—achievement of K/DOQI target ranges. *Nephrol Dial Transplant* 22: 1171–1176.

Demer, L.L., and Tintut, Y. 2009. Mechanisms linking osteoporosis with cardiovascular calcification. *Curr Osteoporos Rep* 7: 42–46.

Detrano, R., Guerci, A.D., Carr, J.J., et al. 2008. Coronary calcium as a predictor of coronary events in four racial or ethnic groups. *New Engl J Med* 358: 1336–1345.

Eckardt, K.U., Kasiske, B.L., and KDIGO Work Group. 2009. KDIGO clinical practice guideline for the diagnosis, evaluation, prevention, and treatment of chronic kidney disease–mineral and bone disorder (CKD–MBD). *Kidney Int* 76: S1–s130.

Foley, R.N., Parfrey, P.S., and Sarnak, M.J. 1998. Epidemiology of cardiovascular disease in chronic renal disease. *J Am Soc Nephrol* 9: S16–S23.

Giachelli, C.M., Jono, S., Shioi, A., et al. 2001. Vascular calcification and inorganic phosphate. *Am J Kidney Dis* 38: S34–S37.

Go, A.S., Chertow, G.M., Fan, D., et al. 2004. Chronic kidney disease and the risks of death, cardiovascular events, and hospitalization. *New Engl. J Med* 351: 1296–1305.

Goodman, W.G., Goldin, J., Kuizon, B.D., et al. 2000. Coronary-artery calcification in young adults with end-stage renal disease who are undergoing dialysis. *New Engl J Med* 342: 1478–1483.

Hruska, K.A., Saab, G., Mathew, S., et al. 2007. Renal osteodystrophy, phosphate homeostasis, and vascular calcification. *Semin Dial* 20: 309–315.

Jono, S., McKee, M.D., Murry, C.E., et al. 2000. Phosphate regulation of vascular smooth muscle cell calcification. *Circ Res* 87: E10–E17.

Kalantar-Zadeh, K., Kuwae, N., Regidor, D.L., et al. 2006. Survival predictability of time-varying indicators of bone disease in maintenance hemodialysis patients. *Kidney Int* 70: 771–780.

London, G.M., Marty, C., Marchais, S.J., et al. 2004. Arterial calcifications and bone histomorphometry in end-stage renal disease. *J Am Soc Nephrol* 15: 1943–1951.

Moe, S.M., and Chertow, G.M. 2006. The case against calcium-based phosphate binders. *Clin J Am Soc Nephrol* 1: 697–703.

National Institutes of Health, 2009. U.S. *Renal Data System, USRDS 2009 Annual Data Report: Atlas of Chronic Kidney Disease and End-Stage Renal Disease in the United States*. NIH, Bethesda, MD.

Persy, V., and D'Haese, P. 2009. Vascular calcification and bone disease: The calcification paradox. *Trends Mol Med* 15: 405–416.

Proudfoot, D., and Shanahan, C.M. 2001. Biology of calcification in vascular cells: Intima versus media. *Herz* 26: 245–251.

Raggi, P., Boulay, A., Chasan-Taber, S., et al. 2002. Cardiac calcification in adult hemodialysis patients. A link between end-stage renal disease and cardiovascular disease? *J Am Coll Cardiol* 39: 695–701.

Reynolds, J.L., Joannides, A.J., Skepper, J.N., et al. 2004. Human vascular smooth muscle cells undergo vesicle-mediated calcification in response to changes in extracellular calcium and phosphate concentrations: A potential mechanism for accelerated vascular calcification in ESRD. *J Am Soc Nephrol* 15: 2857–2867.

Schoppet, M., Shroff, R.C., Hofbauer, L.C., et al. 2008. Exploring the biology of vascular calcification in chronic kidney disease: What's circulating? *Kidney Int* 73: 384–390.

Sheikh, M.S., Maguire, J.A., Emmett, M., et al. 1989. Reduction of dietary phosphorus absorption by phosphorus binders. A theoretical, in vitro, and in vivo study. *J Clin Invest* 83: 66–73.

Suki, W.N., Zabaneh, R., Cangiano, J.L., et al. 2007. Effects of sevelamer and calcium-based phosphate binders on mortality in hemodialysis patients. *Kidney Int* 72: 1130–1137.

Talmage, R.V., 1996. Foreword. In *Calcium and Phosphorus in Health and Disease*, Anderson, J.J.B., and Garner, S.C., eds. CRC Press, Boca Raton, FL.

Virchow, R. 1855. Kalk-Metastasen. *Virchows Arch* 8: 103–113.

34 Contribution of Clinical Risk Factors to the Assessment of Hip Fracture Risk and Treatment Decision Making

Guizhou Hu, Martin M. Root, and John J.B. Anderson

CONTENTS

INTRODUCTION

Osteoporosis is a seriously debilitating disease, particularly among postmenopausal white women in Western countries. Among women over 50 years in the United States, about one in six can anticipate a hip, vertebral, or forearm fracture sometime in their life. Among men, the risk is about 1 in 20 (Cummings and Melton, 2002). About 54% of women in this age group are osteopenic, and 30% are osteoporotic. By the age of 80 years, almost 70% of women become osteoporotic (Melton, 1995). In addition, the mortality risk approximately doubles in the first year after an osteoporotic fracture after the age of 60 years (Center et al., 1999). By 2025, annual costs of osteoporotic fractures are projected to increase by 50% to about $25 billion (Burge et al., 2007). These statistics are similar in Canada where osteoporosis affects one in four women and more than one in eight men over the age of 50 years (Goeree et al., 1996).

The diagnosis of osteoporosis has typically been based on the measurement of bone mineral density (BMD) (Hui et al., 1988, 1989). The objective of osteoporosis treatment is to prevent fractures. However, research has shown that the risk of fracture is dependent not only on BMD but also on a number of clinical risk factors. Therefore, potential misclassification could result if the treatment decision for osteoporosis is solely based on BMD. In this chapter, the magnitude of this misclassification problem and the clinical consequences of it are reviewed.

In clinical practice, clinical risk factors are often considered only in the initial step of finding patients for BMD measurement. For example, clinicians may consider family history of fragility fracture, previous fragility fracture, low body mass index (BMI), and the long-term use of corticosteroids as a way to identify patients to be referred for BMD measurement. The presence of clinical risk factors, however, is often not considered in the later treatment decision-making process. A growing view in the literature suggests that the assessment of fracture risk is enhanced by integrating many clinical risk factors with BMD (Kanis and Glüer, 2000; Kanis et al., 2002). A similar integrated strategy has been used successfully for years in the heart disease prevention and treatment guidelines (Expert Panel on Detection Evaluation and Treatment of High Blood Cholesterol in Adults, 2001). Numerous risk factors are combined to assess risk level, and then treatment goals are set by risk level. To implement such a strategy in hip fracture prevention, a comprehensive risk assessment model would be required that integrates clinically relevant risk factors with BMD.

Studies, including comprehensive meta-analyses, have shown that many clinical risk factors are associated with fracture risk, and these are independent of age and BMD (Kanis et al., 2005a). Published reports on the integration of multiple clinical risk factors, which assess the combination of risk factors to overall fracture risk, are limited. Multivariate hip fracture risk prediction models were developed using data from the Study of Osteoporotic Fractures (SOF) (Black et al., 2001; Cummings et al., 1995). These models were limited to the risk factors that were available and also were statistically significant in that study sample data. These models did not always include other important risk factors, such as smoking, low BMI, alcohol abuse, systemic corticosteroids medication, and diagnosis of rheumatoid arthritis, which have been reported as independently associated with fracture risk in recent meta-analyses (Kanis et al., 2004b, 2005a). Leslie and others reported a fracture model that was based not only on the findings of SOF but also on the results from other studies in the literature (Leslie et al., 2002, 2003). However, the way the model was assembled assumed independence among the risk factors considered. In other words, the univariate (or age and BMD adjusted) associations were assumed to be the same as the multivariate associations. This assumption would, to a certain extent, overestimate the contribution of each risk factor.

In the present study, a multivariate hip fracture risk assessment model was developed. This model includes age and BMD as well as clinical risk factors that were reported in a recent series of meta-analyses. A statistical approach that we previously described was used to adjust the correlations among the risk factors (Hu and Root, 2005; Samsa et al., 2005). This model was then used to consider the effect of adding clinical risk factors to the treatment decision for osteoporosis.

METHODS

POPULATION

The study population was selected from the Third National Health and Nutritional Examination Survey (NHANES III) and included subjects over 45 years old with no missing BMD values assessed at the femoral neck by dual-energy x-ray absorptiometry (DXA). A detailed description of the data was reported elsewhere (National Center for Health Statistics, 1994). Table 34.1 shows the general characteristics of the study sample.

BASELINE MODEL: BMD AND AGE-ONLY MODEL

A baseline regression model that describes the relationship of the 10-year probability of hip fracture risk with age and BMD assessed at the femoral neck by DXA was derived from a fitted regression model using the data reported by Kanis et al. (2001). The original data came from a population survey from Malmo, Sweden. Natural log transformation was applied to the probability to make most of the association linear, as shown in Figure 34.1.

TABLE 34.1

**General Characteristics of the NHANES III Subsample
(Aged >45 Years, with BMD result, *n* = 6692)**

Age	64 ± 12
BMI	27 ± 5
T score (femoral neck)	−1.1 ± 1.2
Female	50.9%
White	74.9%
Parental history of hip fracture	9.1%
Prior fracture after the age of 50 years	0.45%
Current smoking	20.7%
Alcohol intake >2 drinks daily	2.2%
Ever use of systemic corticosteroids	1.7%
Rheumatoid arthritis	6.5%
Low BMI (<20 kg/m²)	4.8%

Notes: NHANES III = Third National Health and Nutritional Examination
Survey; BMD = bone mineral density; SD = standard deviation;
BMI = body mass index.

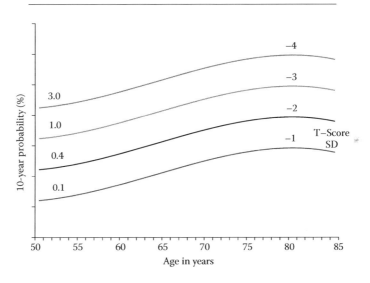

FIGURE 34.1 Ten-year probability of hip fracture according to age and *T* score assessed at the femoral neck by DXA. A fitted regression line is based on the model reported by Leslie, Metge, and Salamon (2002). (From data reported by Leslie, W.D., Metge, C., Salamon, E.A., et al., *J Clin Densitom*, 5, 117–30, 2002. With permission.)

Full Model: Baseline Model Plus Major Clinical Risk Factors

Clinical risk factors integrated into the baseline model included (1) prior fracture after the age of 50 years, (2) parental history of hip fracture or diagnosis of osteoporosis, (3) current smoking, (4) alcohol drinking more than two drinks per day, (5) BMI less than 20 kg/m², (6) ever use of systemic corticosteroids, and (7) a diagnosis of rheumatoid arthritis. A statistical method called synthesis analysis, which we previously described, was used to integrate these risk factors into the baseline model (Hu and Root, 2005; Samsa et al., 2005). The objective was to build a multivariate regression model from the univariate regression coefficients and the correlation coefficients among the risk factors. Univariate regression coefficients could come from the published literature. The correlation

TABLE 34.2
**Reported RR for Hip Fracture Associated with
Clinical Risk Factors Adjusted for Age and BMD in
Meta-analyses**

Clinical Risk Factors (with References)	RR
Parental history of hip fracture (Kanis et al., 2004a)	2.28
Prior fracture after the age of 50 years (Kanis et al., 2004a)	1.62
Current smoking (Kanis et al., 2005c)	1.60
Alcohol intake >2 drinks daily (Kanis et al., 2005b)	1.70
Ever use of systemic corticosteroids (Kanis et al., 2004b)	2.25
Rheumatoid arthritis (Kanis et al., 2005a)	1.73
Lower BMI (<20 kg/m^2) (De Laet et al., 2005)	1.42

Notes: Data from several reports. RR = relative risk; BMD = bone mineral density; BMI = body mass index.

coefficients among risk factors could come from a cross-sectional data set such as NHANES III.
The univariate regression coefficients (or relative risks), in this case, were age- and BMD-adjusted
relative risks, as shown in Table 34.2, and were derived from a series of recently published meta-
analyses by Kanis et al. (2004a, 2005a).

The adjustment on the correlations among the considered risk factors was accomplished from
the following four-step iterative process. In Step 1, the baseline model plus the first clinical risk
factor with its age and BMD-adjusted regression coefficient were first applied to a cross-sectional
population data set (NHANES III), which contained all the clinical risk factor measurements. Each
individual in the data set had a predicted risk based on age, BMD, and the first risk factor. In Step 2,
regression is used to assess the relationship between the predicted risk from Step 1 and the second
clinical risk factor in the data. This approach generates a regression coefficient that represents the
relation between Risk Factor 2 and hip fracture risk that has already been captured by age, BMD,
and Risk Factor 1. In Step 3, comparison of the regression coefficient derived from Step 2 is made
with the age- and BMD-adjusted regression coefficient from the published meta-analysis, as shown
in Table 34.2. The risk factor was then included into the model after the component of the regression coefficient from Step 2 was removed from the age- and BMD-adjusted regression coefficient.
In Step 4, Steps 1–3 are repeated until all risk factors are included.

Two Model Comparisons

The impact of the clinical risk factors on the fracture risk assessment and, in turn, on the osteoporosis treatment decision can be evaluated through a comparison of the full multivariate model and
the baseline BMD and age-only model. Both models were applied to the NHANES III population,
and the difference in risk predictions was calculated. The prediction outcome is expressed as log-
transformed 10-year probability. Clinicians tend to have more familiarity with the clinical significance of BMD *T* scores rather than a 10-year probability, let alone a log-transformed probability.
Therefore, the 10-year probability difference was converted to an equivalent change in *T* score of
BMD using the age–*T* score–risk equation. For example, if the reported difference between models
is equal to 1 unit, then the difference of predicted risk between the two models is equivalent to a
1-unit change of *T* score, which, by definition, is 1 standard deviation of BMD.

Potential Misclassification of Using −2.5 *T* Score as Treatment Cutoff Point

The impact of the clinical risk factors on osteoporosis treatment decision making was examined
through evaluation of potential misclassification of using a BMD −2.5 *T* score, which is the World

---

TABLE 34.3
10-Year Hip Fracture Probability
According to Age at Which
Intervention Is Cost-Effective

Age (Years)	Probability (%)
50	1.10
55	1.81
60	2.64
65	3.70
70	5.24
75	6.87
80	8.52
85	8.99
90	7.12

Source: Reprinted from *The Lancet*, 359, Kanis, J.A., Diagnosis of osteoporosis and assessment of fracture risk, 1929–36, Copyright 2002, with permission from Elsevier.

Health Organization criterion for osteoporosis diagnosis, as the treatment decision cutoff point (Royal College of Physicians, 1999). We assumed the decision for osteoporosis treatment should be made strictly according to the probability of fracture risk from the full model. Misclassification would then occur if only BMD is considered as the treatment threshold. A false negative misclassification is a situation of missing treatment to patients who should receive it. In other words, the patient's BMD is not below −2.5, but the patient has a high fracture risk and should receive treatment. In a false positive misclassification, the patient is receiving treatment but is not at high risk of fracture. The magnitude of the potential misclassification is dependent on the assumed treatment threshold, which is the probability risk level above which treatment is believed to be cost-effective. The above-mentioned potential misclassifications were evaluated under the following two treatment threshold assumptions:

1. For a given age, set the fracture risk probability associated with a −2.5 T score in the absence of any clinical risk factors as the treatment threshold. Under this assumption, only false negative misclassifications of using the −2.5 T score would occur.
2. For a given age, set the fracture risk probability, which is derived from a cost-effective study in the literature, as a treatment threshold (Kanis, 2002). The probabilities are listed in Table 34.3 and plotted in Figure 34.3. In this case, both the false positive rate and the false negative rate of using the −2.5 T score would occur.

Other commonly used terms of misclassification are sensitivity and specificity. *Sensitivity*, in this case, is defined as the proportion of subjects who have a T score less than or equal to −2.5 among those who have a risk above the treatment threshold. One minus sensitivity is the false negative or missing treatment rate. *Specificity*, in this case, is defined as the proportion of subjects who have a T score above −2.5 among those who have a risk below the treatment threshold.

RESULTS

The BMD and age-only model is presented in Figure 34.1. The two predictors in this model are BMD T score and age in years. The outcome is log-transformed 10-year probability of hip fracture.

After log transformation, the 10-year risk and *T* score are linearly associated. The transformed risk is also most linearly associated with age in the range of 55–70 years, with curvature below age 55 and above 75 years. Because the clinical risk factors are not considered in this model, the graph represents the situation where each clinical risk factor is at the population-average level. When individuals' specific levels of clinical risk factors are taken into account, the full model generates different predicted risks from the BMD and age-only model. The distribution of such differences in terms of *T* score equivalents between the two models in the population is shown in Table 34.4. The *T* score equivalents were calculated such that each unit of *T* score change was associated with a change of 1.01 in the log-transformed 10-year probability in the baseline model (Figure 34.1). About 62% of the people who had none of the clinical risk factors had a difference value between −0.28 and −0.22, with an approximate average of −0.25. This average indicates that the BMD and age-only model would overestimate their risk by about 0.25 *T* score equivalent units compared with the full model.

As shown in Figure 34.2, among the individuals without major clinical risk factors, the probability curves of the full model shifted downward by about 0.25 *T* score equivalents over the BMD

TABLE 34.4
Distribution of Difference of Hip Fracture Risk Predictions between Baseline Model and Full Model in NHANES III Subsample (Aged >45 Years, with BMD result, *n* = 6692)

Percentile (%)	Difference in Log of 10-Year Probability	*T* Score Equivalents[a]
0–62	−0.29 to −0.23	−0.28 to −0.22
63–99	−0.01 to 0.97	−0.01 to 0.96
>99	>1.01	>1.00

Notes: NHANES III = Third National Health and Nutritional Examination Survey; BMD = bone mineral density; DXA = dual-energy x-ray absorptiometry.

[a] *T* score equivalent is defined as the amount of hip fracture risk change that can be produced by the amount of changes of *T* score assessed at the femoral neck by DXA.

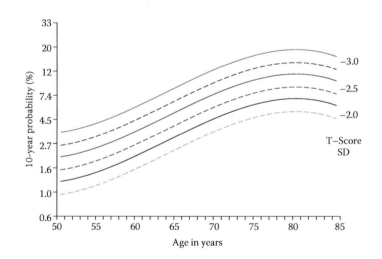

FIGURE 34.2 Ten-year probability of hip fracture according to age and *T* score assessed at the femoral neck by DXA. Comparison of full model (dotted lines) and baseline model (solid lines) among 62% of NHANES III subsample (aged >45 years who do not have any identifiable clinical risk factors).

TABLE 34.5
Examples on 10-Year Hip Fracture Risk Prediction Difference between Full Model and Baseline (BMD and Age Only)

Patient	10-Year Probability of Hip Fracture	
	BMD and Age-Only Model	Full Model
Patient 1: female, aged 65 years, BMD *T* score of –2.5 had family history of osteoporosis, had a fall at age 60 years, current smoking, not drinking alcohol, never use corticosteroids, had rheumatoid arthritis, BMI = 26	5.4	29.1
Patient 2: female, aged 65 years, BMD *T* score of –2.5, no family history of osteoporosis, no fall history, never smoke, not drinking alcohol, never use corticosteroids, no rheumatoid arthritis, BMI = 26	5.4	4.1

Notes: BMD = bone mineral density; BMI = bone mass index.

and age-only model (dotted lines vs. the solid lines). For the next approximately 37% of the population which had little clinical risk, the predicted risk from the full model differed with the BMD and age-only model by −0.01 to 0.96 *T* score equivalents. The remaining 1% of the population had many clinical risk factors; their predicted fracture risk from the full model was more than 1 unit higher than that of the BMD and age-only model. In other word, when not considering clinical risk factors for those patients, their estimated fracture risk was underestimated by an amount which was equivalent to more than 1 unit of *T* score change, a very significant clinical difference. Examples of the model difference are shown in Table 34.5.

If the treatment threshold was set at the probability level corresponding to a *T* score of −2.5 without any clinical risk factors, which is the middle dotted line in Figure 34.2, then 1299 patients out of the 6629 total population had a predicted risk higher than the threshold. Among them, 882 patients had BMD *T* scores below −2.5, which generates a sensitivity of 882/1299 or 67% (Table 34.6, top panel). The false negative rate would then be 100% minus 67% or 33%.

If the treatment threshold was set at the probability level according to Table 34.3 and Figure 34.3, then 1478 patients had a predicted risk higher than the threshold. The sensitivity and specificity were 849/1478 (57%) and 5172/5205 (99%). (Table 34.5, bottom panel) The false negative rate was 43%. Also, among the 882 patients with a BMD *T* score below −2.5, 33 (4%) of patients had a fracture risk that was below the treatment threshold, which is a false positive, or no need to be treated.

DISCUSSION

The present study has identified about 1% of the general population who have many clinical risk factors, and the clinical risk factors could contribute to an increased fracture risk by the equivalent of a decrease of more than 1 *T* score unit of BMD. For example, a given 65-year-old female patient has a BMD *T* score of −2.0. A 1% chance exists that this patient could have many clinical risk factors that could put her at the same risk of another 65-year-old woman who has a *T* score below −3.0 with the absence of major clinical risk factors.

Simply using a *T* score of −2.5 as the treatment cutoff point without considering clinical risk factors would have a sensitivity in the range of 57% to 67%, depending on the treatment threshold assumptions as a case-finding strategy. The clinical significance is that 33% to 43% of cases would

TABLE 34.6
Potential Misclassification of Using –2.5 *T* Score Assessed at Femoral Neck by DXA as Treatment Cutoff Point with Two Treatment Thresholds Assumption in NHANES III Subsample (Aged >45 Years, with BMD result, *n* = 6692)

Treatment Threshold: Risk Corresponding to *T* Score of –2.5 without Clinical Risk Factors (Middle Dotted Line in Figure 34.2)

	Risk ≥ Threshold	Risk < threshold	Total
T score ≤–2.5	882	0	882
T score >–2.5	417	5393	5810
Total	1299	5393	6692

Treatment Threshold: Risk Value Derived from Cost-Effective Study (Triangles in Figure 34.3)

	Risk ≥ Threshold	Risk < Threshold	Total
T score ≤–2.5	849	33	882
T score >–2.5	638	5172	5810
Total	1487	5205	6692

Notes: NHANES III = Third National Health and Nutritional Examination Survey; BMD = bone mineral density; DXA = dual-energy x-ray absorptiometry.

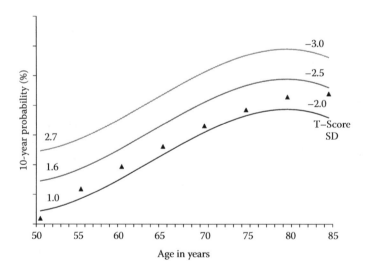

FIGURE 34.3 Ten-year probability of hip fracture according to age and *T* score assessed at the femoral neck by DXA. The triangles denote the probabilities above which interventions are cost-effective, as reported by Kanis (2002). (Reprinted from *The Lancet*, 359, 1929–36, Kanis, J.A., Diagnosis of osteoporosis and assessment of fracture risk, 2002, with permission from Elsevier.)

be false negatives and therefore miss the opportunity to be treated although they have a fracture probability higher than the treatment threshold based on known clinical risk factors. Also, up to an estimated 4% of patients who would receive the treatment actually would not need it.

A T score of less than or equal to −2.5 may seem to be too strict a criterion, as only 882 out of 6692, or 13% of the population, qualified for treatment (Table 34.6). However, 19% to 22% of the population had a risk above the treatment threshold in terms of fracture probability based on the full model (Table 34.6). Relaxing the T score cutoff point, say to −2.0, would increase the sensitivity even without considering clinical risk factors, but the specificity would inevitably decrease with an increase of the percentage of false positives at the same time.

The cost-effectiveness study indicated that the osteoporosis intervention threshold should be set according to the probability of fracture risk (Kanis and Glüer, 2000; Kanis et al., 2002). For example, absolute estimates of cardiovascular disease risk have been used to develop cholesterol treatment guidelines (Expert Panel on Detection Evaluation and Treatment of High Blood Cholesterol in Adults, 2001). Treatment guidelines for osteoporosis, however, are primarily based on BMD alone, although evidence clearly shows that many clinical risk factors have an independent contribution to hip fracture risk. Understanding the magnitude of the effect of these clinical risk factors on the overall hip fracture risk assessment and how these factors influence the treatment decision are very important.

The present study includes both males and females based on the assumptions that, at a given BMD level, the risk of having a hip fracture is the same and also that the effects of clinical risk factors on the hip fracture risk are the same regardless of gender (Kanis et al., 2001). These assumptions are made although, in general, women after menopause have significantly lower BMD than do men.

The full model in this study includes seven major clinical risk factors that were reported in a series of meta-analyses. A few other clinical factors were reported to be predictive of hip fracture risk but were not included in this study, either because they would be difficult to measure, such as distance depth perception or contrast sensitivity, or because they are not likely to be independent of BMD, such as dietary calcium intake, exercise level, or diabetes (Janghorbani et al., 2007; Kanis et al., 2005a). Should the full model include additional independent clinical risk factors, the magnitude of the impact on the risk assessment and osteoporosis treatment decision would be even more significant.

As shown on the Figure 34.1, hip fracture risk increases with age at any given BMD T score level. An economic study on the cost-effectiveness of osteoporosis treatment showed that the hip fracture risk treatment threshold above which the treatment is cost-effective also increases with age, as indicated in Table 34.3 and Figure 34.3. The slopes of the above two age-related increases appear to be parallel (Figure 34.3). Therefore, if we put clinical risk factors aside, age does not need to be considered in treatment decisions. In other word, the same BMD T score cutoff point can be used for the treatment decision regardless of age. For this reason, age should not be treated as another "clinical" risk factor. The comparisons made in the present study are between the full model and BMD and age-only model, not between the full model and BMD-only model, as suggested in another reported study (Leslie et al., 2003).

Limitations of the present study include that it only examined a U.S. population and the considered clinical risk factors were limited to those that were available in the NHANES III data set. In addition, only hip fracture risk, which is only part of the risk of osteoporosis, was investigated. Further study on the contribution of clinical risk factors to fracture risk assessment of other skeletal sites remains.

SUMMARY

Several major clinical risk factors have been shown to have significant impacts on osteoporosis risk assessment and the treatment decision making. Integration of such clinical risk factors with bone density and age in the clinical decision making process is, thus, very important. The relatively simple mathematical model used in this study could be used by clinicians to improve greatly the sensitivity and specificity in case-finding strategies.

ACKNOWLEDGMENT

This project was entirely funded by BioSignia, Inc.

REFERENCES

Black, D.M., Steinbuch, M., Palermo, L., et al. 2001. An assessment tool for predicting fracture risk in post-menopausal women. *Osteoporos Int* 12:519–528.

Burge, R., Dawson-Hughes, B., and Solomon, D.H. 2007. Incidence and economic burden of osteoporosis-related fractures in the United States, 2005–2025. *J Bone Miner Res* 22.

Center, J.R., Nguyen, T.V., Schneider, D., et al. 1999. Mortality after all major types of osteoporotic fracture in men and women: An observational study. *Lancet* 353:878–882.

Cummings, S., and Melton, L.J. 2002. Epidemiology and outcomes of osteoporotic fractures. *Lancet* 359:1761–1767.

Cummings, S.R., Nevitt, M.C., Browner, W.S., et al. 1995. Risk factors for hip fracture in white women. Study of Osteoporotic Fractures Research Group. *N Engl J Med* 332:767–773.

De Laet, C., Kanis, J.A., Odén, A., et al. 2005. Body mass index as a predictor of fracture risk: A meta-analysis. *Osteoporos Int* 16:1330–1338.

Expert Panel on Detection Evaluation and Treatment of High Blood Cholesterol in Adults. 2001. Executive summary of the third report of the National Cholesterol Education Program (NCEP) Expert Panel on Detection, Evaluation, and Treatment of High Blood Cholesterol in Adults (Adults Treatment Panel III). *JAMA* 285:2486–2497.

Goeree, R., O'Brien, B., and Pettitt, D. 1996. An assessment of the burden of illness due to osteoporosis in Canada. *J Soc Obstet Gynaecol Can* 18S:15–24.

Hu, G. and Root, M. 2005. Building prediction models for coronary heart disease by synthesizing multiple longitudinal research findings. *Eur J Cardiovasc Prev Rehabil* 12:459–464.

Hui, S.L., Slemenda, C.W., and Johnston, C.C., Jr. 1988. Age and bone mass as predictors of fracture in a prospective study. *J Clin Invest* 81:1804–1809.

Hui, S.L., Slemenda, C.W., and Johnston, C.C., Jr. 1989. Baseline measurement of bone mass predicts fracture in white women. *Ann Intern Med* 111:355–361.

Janghorbani, M., Van Dam, R.M., Willett, W.C., et al. 2007. Systematic review of type 1 and type 2 diabetes mellitus and risk of fracture. *Am J Epidemiol* 166:495–505.

Kanis, J.A. 2002. Diagnosis of osteoporosis and assessment of fracture risk. *Lancet* 359:1929–1936.

Kanis, J.A., Black, D., Cooper, C., et al. 2002. A new approach to the development of assessment guidelines for osteoporosis. *Osteoporos Int* 13:527–536.

Kanis, J.A., Borgstrom, F., De Laet, C., et al. 2005a. Assessment of fracture risk. *Osteoporos Int* 16:581–589.

Kanis, J.A., and Glüer, C.C. 2000. An update on the diagnosis and assessment of osteoporosis with densitometry. Committee of Scientific Advisors, International Osteoporosis Foundation. *Osteoporos Int* 11:192–202.

Kanis, J.A., Johansson, H., Johnell, O., et al. 2005b. Alcohol intake as a risk factor for fracture. *Osteoporos Int* 16:737–742.

Kanis, J.A., Johansson, H., Odén, A., et al. 2004a. A family history of fracture and fracture risk: A meta-analysis. *Bone* 35:1029–1037.

Kanis, J.A., Johansson, H., Odén, A., et al. 2004b. A meta-analysis of prior corticosteroid use and fracture risk. *J Bone Miner Res* 19:893–899.

Kanis, J.A., Johnell, O., Odén, A., et al. 2001. Ten year probabilities of osteoporotic fractures according to BMD and diagnostic thresholds. *Osteoporos Int* 12:989–995.

Kanis, J.A., Johnell, O., Odén, A., et al. 2005c. Smoking and fracture risk: A meta-analysis. *Osteoporos Int* 16:155–162.

Leslie, W.D., Metge, C., Salamon, E.A., et al. 2002. Bone mineral density testing in healthy postmenopausal women. The role of clinical risk factor assessment in determining fracture risk. *J Clin Densitom* 5:117–130.

Leslie, W.D., Metge, C., and Ward, L. 2003. Contribution of clinical risk factors to bone density-based absolute fracture risk assessment in postmenopausal women. *Osteoporos Int* 14:334–338.

Melton, L.J. 1995. How many women have osteoporosis now? *J Bone Miner Res* 10:175–177.

National Center for Health Statistics. *Plan and Operation of the Third National Health and Nutrition Examination Survey, 1988–94*. Hyattsville, MD: National Center for Health Statistics; 1994. http://www.cdc.gov/nchs/data/series/sr_01/sr01_032.pdf (Vital and Health Statistics, Series 1: Programs and Collection Procedures, no. 32) (DHHS publication no. (PHS) 94-1308) (GPO no. 017-022-01260-0).

Royal College of Physicians. 1999. *Osteoporosis: Clinical Guidelines for the Prevention and Treatment*, Royal College of Physicians, London.

Samsa, G., Hu, G., and Root, M. 2005. Combining information from multiple data sources to create multivariable risk models: Illustration and preliminary assessment of a new method. *J Biomed Biotechnol* 2:113–123.

Part VI

Conclusion

35 Nutrition and Bone Health
Promotion of Bone Gain and Prevention of Bone Loss across the Life Cycle

John J.B. Anderson, Philip J. Klemmer, and Sanford C. Garner

CONTENTS

INTRODUCTION

Healthy bone development and maintenance result primarily from good dietary intakes and regular physical activities throughout life. Overwhelmingly, the strict approach of dietary prevention of osteoporosis has involved supplementation with calcium and/or vitamin D, or a combination of the two micronutrients, as well as other nutrients or plant chemicals. A broad spectrum of supplements, including multiple micronutrients, has not been studied in prospective clinical trials for the prevention of osteoporosis. More recently, several reports have supported skeletal benefits of these supplements in older adults, primarily postmenopausal women, who were supplemented with one or another micronutrient, with soy isoflavones, and with small combinations of nutrients. Yet, a consensus of the skeletal benefits of both nutrients and non-nutrient plant molecules has not yet been established. Therefore, this chapter attempts to review a few of the nutritional issues that raise concerns about skeletal health, and it points to areas where further clinical investigation is needed.

Environmental factors have been estimated to explain only about 15% to 50% of the variation of bone measurements (Ralston and Uitterlinden, 2010). Diet and physical activity, two major lifestyle factors, each make respective contributions of 7% to 25%, and of this percentage, diet may represent slightly less of a contribution than does physical activity, based on one meta-analysis (Welten et al., 1994). Therefore, the contribution of diet to bone health needs also to be considered along with physical activity and possibly other factors that impact positively or negatively on bone.

TABLE 35.1
Optimal Nutrient Intakes for Bone Health across the Life Cycle

- Optimal calcium intakes (from diet and any supplements) are recommended. A calcium intake, up to a total of 2500 mg/day, appears to be safe in most individuals; 2500 is the tolerable upper limit of safety for calcium.
- Adequate vitamin D is essential for optimal calcium absorption, especially when calcium intake is below recommended levels.
- Adequate intakes of vitamin K are recommended.
- Phosphorus intakes in minimal amounts, that is, avoidance of foods processed with phosphate-containing salts, and limited intakes of phosphate-containing soft drinks.
- Adequate intakes of other micronutrients, for example, iron, vitamin A, vitamin C, and others, are recommended.
- Adequate intakes of macronutrients, including protein and omega-3 fatty acids from fish and plant oils.
- Sufficient intakes of phytochemicals via foods (plants) rather than from supplements.

TABLE 35.2
Optimal Physical Activities for Bone Health across the Life Cycle

- Aerobic activities, especially walking for older adults
- Strength and weight-bearing activities
- Isometric exercises

Only in recent decades has physical activity been recognized as a significant factor impacting favorably on bone development and growth in early life and helping to maintain bone during the later years of life. In fact, the quantitative benefit of activities that favorably affect bone health may be equal or even exceed the positive effects of a healthy diet. Bone health depends heavily on both regular physical activities and wholesome dietary intakes.

This brief closing chapter highlights the effects of calcium, vitamin D, and other nutrients on bone measurements, especially of older adults, and it also focuses on the prevention of osteoporotic fractures, especially those involving the proximal femur or hip, through healthy eating practices and regular physical activities and exercise early as well as in later life (Tables 35.1 and 35.2). The major issues of this review of the current state of bone research cover the topics calcium, phosphate, and vitamins D and K; acid–base balance, protein, and potassium; other micronutrients, including antioxidants; physical activity, and bone development and maintenance; and vascular calcification in late life.

EFFECTS OF DIETARY CALCIUM, PHOSPHATE, VITAMIN D, AND VITAMIN K ON SKELETAL DEVELOPMENT AND MAINTENANCE

Peak bone mass in white females and males results from healthy diets that contain adequate amounts of calcium, vitamin D, and other nutrients. Paradoxically, peak bone mass in African American children may be achieved at calcium intake levels substantially lower than those of their white counterparts (see also Chapters 24 and 25). Limited understanding of the mechanism for black–white differences in skeletal accrual exists, but one likely hypothesis relates to a reduction in parathyroid hormone (PTH) action on bone. In this scenario, fewer remodeling cycles occur, and the bone tissue is able to incorporate more mineral in association with the matrix, and bone mass increases and becomes more dense (see Chapter 29).

Supplement studies have shown that the gains of bone mass, that is, bone mineral content, of children are not maintained after the supplements are stopped and that bone losses may quickly offset the earlier gains (Slemenda et al., 1992; Lloyd et al., 1994) (see also Chapter 25). Supplementation alone may not be as effective in promoting gain in bone mass if the individual is already consuming an adequate amount of calcium, that is, near or above the recommended intake. The mechanism of increased bone mass by intake of calcium may partly result from suppression of PTH and the resulting decrease in the rate of bone remodeling that accompanies PTH suppression. Whites do not, however, obtain the same gains in bone mass and density as do blacks (see Chapter 29).

Elevated phosphate intake has been proposed to have a negative effect on the maintenance of bone mass in adults, and it may also impact on skeletal growth and development. Absorbed phosphate ions have been shown to increase serum PTH concentrations in adults (see Chapters 9 and 26). Further long-term studies are needed to establish whether high consumption of phosphate contributes to chronic bone loss. With the new knowledge about the actions of fibroblast growth factor 23 (FGF 23) in reducing both renal tubular reabsorption and intestinal phosphate absorption of phosphate ions impacting on the actions of PTH, the role of phosphatonins in regulating renal phosphate reabsorption need to be considered alongside of calcium homeostasis and the maintenance of bone mineral density (BMD) in human subjects (Quarles, 2008). FGF 23 also reduces renal production of $1,25(OH)_2$vitamin D. If an elevated FGF 23 is indeed associated with cardiovascular diseases, especially in elderly subjects, then concentrations of this hormone may prove to be useful in the assessment of risks of cardiovascular disease as well as osteoporosis.

The gains of BMD in postmenopausal women receiving a calcium supplement alone over a period of 2 years or more compared with those on placebo is small in those with good dietary calcium intakes (Riis et al., 1987). Skeletal benefits, including reduction of hip fractures, have been observed when calcium supplements have been administered with vitamin D (Chapuy et al., 1992; Dawson-Hughes et al., 1997). Whether vitamin K given along with vitamin D and calcium will provide any additional improvement of bone mass of older adults remains to be determined. Although men have been investigated less than women, older men may also require modest increments in the same three nutrients as do women for the maintenance of bone health late in life.

In older individuals, calcium supplements are widely recommended by physicians for improving BMD. Concern has been raised that higher amounts of calcium from supplements may also increase the risk of arterial calcification among the elderly and those with reduced renal function. See below for further insight into this issue of arterial calcification and its increasing concern with prevalence in older adults.

Vitamin D alone has little or no benefit for skeletal improvement in bone mineral measurements and reduction of fractures; calcium must be given along with vitamin D. Why supplements of vitamin D are administered along with calcium to achieve skeletal benefits, as long as serum 25-hydroxyvitamin D (25OHD) is adequate, remains unclear. In one large population study in Australia, annual oral intakes of vitamin D (50,000 IU) actually increased falls and fractures in older women (Sanders et al., 2010). Calcium intakes of both the treatment group and the placebo group in this study were comparable. The vitamin D status, as indicated by serum 25OHD measurement, remains a physiological enigma. The 25OHD metabolite is not hormonally active, and it requires renal activation to form $1,25(OH)_2D$, the active hormonal form that facilitates intestinal calcium absorption by the small intestine at low calcium intakes and organic matrix formation in bone via osteoblasts. The serum 25OHD concentrations are an order of magnitude greater than serum $1,25(OH)_2D$. Furthermore, serum concentrations of 25OHD are never rate limiting in the enzymatic activation of renal 1-alpha-hydroxylase that generates $1,25(OH)_2D$. An increase in serum 25OHD, whether derived from skin biosynthesis or dietary sources, does not *per se* increase the synthesis of $1,25(OH)_2D$ (see Chapter 10). The well-established definitions of true deficiency, insufficiency, and normal status of vitamin D by 25OHD cut points seem to be less meaningful unless dietary calcium intake is considered in conjunction with vitamin D status. Clearly, vitamin D is needed for skeletal health, but its beneficial effects on bone are derived from the combined intake of both calcium and vitamin D, whether from diet alone or from a combination of diet and supplements. Extraskeletal benefits of vitamin D, such as effects on muscle strength, are quite well established.

Vitamin K supplementation to improve bone health is increasingly being recommended by investigators (see Chapter 12). In fact, vitamin K, vitamin D, and calcium as a supplemental package make considerable sense for older adults if dosages per day are not excessive. Besides vitamin K effects on the coagulation system, it also has other actions that favorably affect the health of the elderly. Several forms of vitamin K exist, but they all seem to act similarly, when taken in appropriate amounts, on bone and arteries. The protein formed by vitamin K–enzyme activation is matrix gla protein (MGP), also known as bone gla protein, and its function in bone matrix is thought to be the enhancement of calcification, that is, modification of soft bone tissue to hard bone. In arterial walls, the active form of MGP acts to block or slow calcification when the intake of vitamin K is adequate; if inadequate, high serum concentrations of the inactive form of MGP permit calcification in arterial walls. This view may be overly simplistic, but vitamin K deficiency seems to be at least one culprit in the arterial calcification process.

Vitamin K and vitamin D, that is, the active form, may operate synergistically in cells to synthesize MGP, which improves bone health and inhibits, at least in part, calcification in arterial walls. Adequate dietary consumption of vitamin K supports the protective action of MGP in the arteries while promoting bone calcification, a process enhanced by sufficient intakes of both vitamin D and calcium.

In summary, a healthy diet needs to supply these with all the nutrients in amounts required for bone growth and retention. If the typical diet does not meet these needs, nutrient supplements in appropriate doses—even possibly individualized in the future—become with may be required to fill in the gaps of inadequate intakes of specific nutrients, if bone health is to be optimally supported.

EFFECTS OF ACID–BASE BALANCE AND PROTEIN ON BONE DEVELOPMENT AND MAINTENANCE

The pH of extracellular fluids and blood is rigorously defended by the combined actions of the kidneys and lungs, as well as by interconnected buffer systems, which include the skeletal system. Each day, a 70-kg person generates approximately 70 mmol of hydrogen ions (H^+) from food and metabolic pathways. In the face of this acid load, extracellular pH is maintained at the physiological level of 7.40 by means of extracellular bicarbonate and intracellular buffer systems, which are in equilibrium with each other and with the buffer system established within the bone envelope. The carbon dioxide generated by the union of protons (H^+) and bicarbonate buffers is promptly discharged by the lungs by an immediate increase in the compensatory mechanism of the brain that responds by increasing the minute ventilatory volume. The brainstem regulates this ventilatory response by sensing small increases in H^+ in the cerebrospinal fluid. Serum bicarbonate stores would rapidly be depleted if only this immediate short-term buffer system were operative. Fortunately, the distal tubule maintains bicarbonate homeostasis.

The kidneys provide long-term acid–base homeostasis by actively secreting H^+ and providing the regeneration of bicarbonate ions that were lost in the extracellular fluids in the formation of carbon dioxide and water. The distal renal tubule actively secretes H^+ against an electrochemical gradient into the lumen where it combines with filtered buffers, chiefly $HPO_4^=$, to form titratable acid, that is, $H_2PO_4^-$.

Approximately 50% of the proton load each day, ~35 mmol, is excreted as titratable acidity. The remaining 35 mmol of H^+ is excreted as urinary ammonium ions (NH_4^+). In contrast to this fixed titratable acid excretion (at maximum capacity), an extra acid load from dietary sources, that is, animal proteins, challenges the kidneys; the response is up to a 10-fold increase in NH_4^+ urinary excretion by the healthy kidneys above baseline. This enhanced capacity to excrete acid is diminished or lost in the presence of chronic kidney disease. Combined titratable acidity plus ammonium excretion (net acid excretion) not only facilitates H^+ excretion (and balances pH in blood and other extracellular fluids), but it also enables the regeneration of sufficient quantities of bicarbonate ions that have been lost in the initial buffering of H^+ in the extracellular compartments. The ability of the kidneys to adapt to variable H^+ loads explains the tight regulation of arterial pH at 7.40 across low-acid vegetarian diets as well as higher acid diets containing meats, eggs, and dairy proteins. The urinary excretion of $SO_4^=$, derived from the oxidation of sulfur-containing amino acids, provides the majority of the acid load following consumption of animal proteins.

The distal renal tubule responds to organic acid loads by increasing urinary calcium excretion or hypercalciuria. Because no compensatory increase in intestinal calcium absorption follows, large organic loads from diets rich in animal proteins have the potential for causing negative calcium balance. In growing children, the theoretical potential exists for poor skeletal growth because of hypercalciuria. In practice, growing children who consume adequate amounts of protein typically accrue bone in a healthy pattern and do not suffer from hypercalciuria. This issue, however, is of greater concern for postmenopausal women who ingest diets high in animal proteins but low in calcium. Generally, urinary calcium excretion increases exponentially with an increase in urine net acid excretion (Lemann et al., 2003). Very few studies have examined high-protein, low-calcium diets in osteoporotic patients. In contrast, patients with chronic kidney disease, an estimated 29 million Americans, have major defects in H^+ excretion, which leads to excessive acid buffering in the skeleton and rarefaction of bone, that is, osteopenia or osteoporosis. Patients with impaired distal tubular H^+ excretion may result in kidney stones in adults and growth retardation in children. The administration of alkali therapy, that is, bicarbonate, alleviates both maladies.

EFFECTS OF OTHER MICRONUTRIENTS, INCLUDING ANTIOXIDANTS, ON BONE DEVELOPMENT AND MAINTENANCE

Adequate nutrition plays a major role in the prevention and treatment of osteoporosis; the nutrients of greatest importance are calcium and vitamin D, but a number of micronutrients, both minerals and vitamins, also may impact bone health either positively or negatively. These include vitamin A (Chapter 11), vitamin C (Chapter 14), iron (Chapter 13), copper (Chapters 13 and 14), and omega-3 fatty acids (Chapter 16).

Vitamin A and its associated forms (retinol, retinyl esters, retinal, and retinoic acids) are a family of essential, fat-soluble, diet-derived compounds that support vision, reproduction, cell differentiation, immune system regulation, and bone growth (see Chapter 11). In general prospective studies in humans indicated that excessive intake of vitamin A is associated with increased risk of fracture, but the level of intake at which the fracture risk increases has not yet been determined. Although vitamin A intakes slightly above the Dietary Reference Intake have been shown to be associated with reduced bone density and increased risk of hip fractures, the provitamin A precursor beta-carotene has not been shown to cause bone toxicity in either humans or laboratory animals.

Vitamin A (retinol acting through retinoic acid) has been demonstrated in many animal studies to cause adverse effects on the skeleton through increased bone resorption and decreased bone formation. Vitamin A has little or no effect, however, on mineralization in either humans or animals. High vitamin A intakes in humans were shown to increase the size of osteocyte lacunae and the area of resorptive surfaces.

Vitamin C and the trace elements iron and copper are required for collagen formation and maturation. Vitamin C (Chapter 14) is an essential cofactor for collagen formation and synthesis of the modified amino acids, hydroxyproline and hydroxylysine. Some evidence supports an association between vitamin C and bone mass, with low vitamin C intakes being associated with a faster rate of bone loss. The underlying mechanisms by which iron and copper deficiency could affect bone strength are not known but most likely relate the role of these elements in collagen synthesis and cross-linking. Copper has a role in collagen formation as part of the enzyme lysyl oxidase (a cuproenzyme), which is the rate-limiting enzyme in collagen strengthening. Iron (ferrous) ions also play an essential role in hydroxylation reactions essential to collagen maturation and cross-linking together with ascorbic acid (vitamin C), molecular oxygen, and α-ketoglutarate. Prolyl hydroxylase catalyzes formation of hydroxyproline from proline, and lysyl hydroxylase catalyzes hydroxylation of lysine. A lack of lysine–hydroxylysine cross-linking weakens collagen.

BMD and content measured by DXA have been reported to decrease in both humans and animals with iron deficiency. One study of female military recruits reported an increase in the incidence of stress fractures in iron-deficient recruit compared with those who were iron replete (Moran et al., 2008). In addition, some, but not all, animal studies of iron deficiency have demonstrated decreased femoral breaking strength, smaller cortical areas, and larger medullary areas.

Other micronutrients with impacts on bone quality include the B vitamins; sodium, magnesium, and fluoride; and the trace elements boron, zinc, and silicon (Chapter 14). These micronutrients affect bone health in different ways. Sodium increases calcium excretion by the kidney; and higher salt intake has been shown to be related to increased circulating PTH and greater rates of bone resorption in postmenopausal women. Some evidence supports a positive relationship between BMD and magnesium intake, but little evidence suggests that magnesium is needed to prevent osteoporosis. Fluoride ions interact with mineralized tissue in a number of ways, including incorporation into the chemical structure of hydroxyapatite bone mineral, mainly at the crystal surfaces, but fluoride dietary supplements at 1 ppm do not appear to benefit skeletal health in adults.

Three B vitamin (folate, B_{12}, or B_6) deficiencies can increase serum homocysteine, which has been linked to hip fracture in older men and women. However, the association of low BMD or osteoporosis with low intakes of vitamin B_{12} might simply reflect overall poor nutrition (Dhonukshe-Rutten et al., 2003; Tucker et al., 2005), which could contribute to the risk of fracture. Although boron and zinc have been suggested to affect bone health, little evidence exists that links intake of these elements with osteoporosis. A role for silicon in bone health has been proposed, but the biological mechanism is not known. An effect of silicon on collagen has been proposed, but little supporting data exist.

Evidence is now accumulating to support a role for omega-3 fatty acids in modulating interactions between muscle and bone in the development and maintenance of bone health (Chapter 16). Muscle and bone interact in ways that determine the development and maintenance, that is, modeling and remodeling, of the skeleton. The strain produced by muscles on long bones to which they are attached controls the shape and density of the bones. Muscle loss is followed by osteopenia at all ages. Evidence from a number of studies supports a role for lipids in development and maintenance of bone mass. Although omega-6 fatty polyunsaturated acids (PFAs) have a potential negative effect on bone, the omega-3 fatty acids (e.g., DHA and EPA) increase bone formation in growing rodents, perhaps by lowering levels of PGE_2. In addition, the omega-3 PFA DHA attenuates loss of bone and muscle mass associated with skeletal unloading in rodent models. Omega-3 PFAs have been shown to reduce the loss of muscle in cancer patients (cachexia) and in advanced aging, and they support bone growth directly. The endocannabinoid system, which consists of endogenous arachidonic-acid-derived ligands for the G-protein-coupled receptors, is also involved in bone cell differentiation and mature functioning of the skeletal system.

PHYSICAL ACTIVITY AND BONE DEVELOPMENT AND MAINTENANCE

Physical activities, including different types of programmed exercises, have been experimentally found to be positively associated with increases in bone density and improvements of bone structure and microarchitectural quality. What has not been so clear from the reported studies is the long-term sustainability of exercise-induced gains in bone mass and structure into late life. Several chapters in this book (Chapters 5, 21, 22, 23, and 32) provide careful and detailed reviews relating exercise or exercise and diet to bone health.

Another recent review supports the long-term benefits of moderate exercise during growth early in life on the adult skeleton (Karlsson et al., 2008). The retention of these gains from exercises during adulthood, however, is only partial during late life when elders are no longer engaged in their physical activities. So, the take-home message is that moderate activities of some type must be continued throughout life to maintain bone mass and quality as optimally as possible, even if some loss of bone mass does occur in late life, and such physical activity should greatly help prevent fractures (Table 35.2). Cessation of such usual activities definitely leads to bone loss and increased risk of fracture.

Diet–exercise interactions also influence bone development and maintenance. Optimal intakes of the bone-building nutrients, energy, protein, minerals, and vitamins support growth, but modestly lower intakes than optimal intakes coupled with regular physical activity may also contribute sufficiently to bone development and maintenance. Although research has focused in any depth on only a few of the essential nutrients, results suggest that calcium is more efficiently utilized by the skeleton by active children during the growth years and also during adulthood. Protein also needs to be consumed, along with energy, in reasonable amounts for the development of the bone matrix.

Exercise intervention studies that target two of the following, that is, strength, balance, flexibility, and endurance, have resulted in reductions in both the risk of falls and the annual rate of falls that lead to fractures (Gillespie et al., 2009).

In summary, exercise programs, including sports activities and dance, have robust effects on the gains of bone mass starting early in childhood through adolescence, the consolidation of bone during the early adult decades, and the maintenance of bone during the later adult years. Also, regular activities are considered to improve bone strength and microarchitectural structure of bone. The net effect of such activities in the elderly is reductions in falls and fractures. Additional prospective randomized controlled trials are needed to determine which types of activities provide the biggest benefits during late adulthood and delay or reduce the risk of osteoporosis and fractures.

VASCULAR CALCIFICATION IN LATE LIFE

In 1863 at Charitie Hospital in Berlin, Virchow first reported the presence of calcium salts and, less often, fully formed bone within arteries and heart valves in autopsy cases. The physiological basis for this pathological observation remained an enigma for almost the next 130 years until Demer and colleagues (Bostrom et al., 1993) identified in these lesions the presence of osteogenic transcription factors and components of bone osteoid (organic matrix) in the subintimal calcifications of patients with atherosclerosis. Prior to this seminal study, vascular calcification was regarded as a passive response to injury rather than an actively regulated process resulting from the progression of atherosclerosis. Arterial stiffening was associated with the calcification (see also Chapters 33 and 8).

In recent years, investigations have been undertaken to identify the factors which may promote or inhibit arterial calcification. For example, in the population suffering from advanced kidney disease (CKD Stages 4 and 5), hyperphosphatemia has been linked to quantitative measurements of arterial calcification (Blacher et al., 1999). In addition, Giachelli and colleagues (2001) have identified a cellular mechanism by which hyperphosphatemia may promote the phenotypic transformation of arterial smooth muscle cells into bone-forming osteoblastic cells. Several controlled experimental studies (Chertow et al., 2002; Block et al., 2005) in dialysis patients have suggested that calcium loading may also contribute to vascular calcification and cardiovascular events in CKD patients. In the general elderly population, many individuals have CKD without being aware that either hyperphosphatemia or calcium loading may be contributing to their decline in cardiovascular health. The traditional Framingham risk factors for CVDs, that is, smoking, diabetes mellitus type 2, lipid abnormalities, hypertension, and physical inactivity, may also be contributing to the promotion of arterial calcification.

Because of cost and concerns about radiation exposure, quantitative measurement of coronary artery calcification (CAC) by means of computerized tomography is unlikely to become a commonly available clinical tool for further identifying CVD risk or for monitoring the efficacy of therapeutic interventions. As a research tool, however, quantitative measurement of the CAC score provides a rich database for population-based studies of late-life calcification. In elderly populations, many unanswered questions remain regarding the physiological basis for the inverse relationship between BMD and measures of arterial calcification. Oxidized low-density lipoprotein cholesterol has been proposed as a possible mediator of both osteopenia and vascular calcification in patients not suffering from renal disease (Demer, 2002). Further research using randomized controlled trials or prospective designs is needed to establish the optimal range of total calcium intakes that have the least effect on the arterial calcification process but will support healthy bone remodeling in late life. This important public health question deserves greater attention in the future as many populations across much of the world are aging out.

CONCLUSIONS

The best prevention against osteoporotic fractures is to build an optimal skeletal mass, containing strong microarchitectural components in both trabecular and compact bone tissues, during the preadolescent and adolescent years, that is, peak bone mass during the growth years, and then maintain the amassed bone tissue through good dietary and health practices during the remainder of life. Finally, excessive supplemental intakes of calcium and perhaps vitamin D by elderly individuals may not improve bone mass or density, unless individuals have clinically established insufficient or deficient intakes of one or more of the major bone-supportive nutrients. On the other hand, excessive intakes of calcium and perhaps vitamin D, especially when coupled with reduced renal function, may contribute to increases in arterial calcification throughout the body, a relatively newly recognized adverse effect of excessive calcium from foods and supplements and from unhealthy dietary practices that contribute to atherosclerosis.

Many questions and uncertainties remain about the specific dietary and exercise effects on skeletal development and maintenance. The impacts of modern genetics, especially of epigenetics, should help further understandings of this complex array of factors that influence the skeleton at all stages of life. Overall bone health typically accompanies skeletal muscle mass so that the linkages of the skeletal and muscle systems hold hidden keys to preventing or delaying bone loss late in life and forestalling fractures.

REFERENCES

Blacher, J., Guerin, A.P., Pannier, B., et al. 1999. Impact of aortic stiffness on survival in end-stage renal disease. *Circulation* 99: 2434–2439.

Block, G.A., Spiegel, D.M., Ehrlich, J., et al. 2005. Effects of sevelamer and calcium on coronary artery calcification in patients new to hemodialysis. *Kidney Int* 68: 1815–1824.

Bostrom, K., Watson, K.E., Horn, S., et al. 1993. Bone morphogenic protein expression in human atherosclerotic lesions. *J Clin Invest* 91: 1800–1809.

Chapuy, M.C., Arlot, M.E., Duboeuf, F., et al. 1992. Vitamin D_3 and calcium to prevent hip fractures in elderly women. *New Engl J Med* 327: 1637–1642.

Chertow, G.M., Burke, S.K., and Raggi, P. 2002. Sevelamer attenuates the progression of coronary and aortic calcification in hemodialysis patients. *Kidney Int* 62: 245–252.

Dawson-Hughes, B., Harris, S., Krall, E., et al. 1997. Effect of calcium and vitamin D supplementation on bone density in men and women 65 years of age or older. *New Engl J Med* 337: 670–676.

Demer, L.L. 2002. Vascular calcification and osteoporosis: Inflammatory responses to oxidized lipids. *Int J Epidemiol* 31: 737–741.

Dhonukshe-Rutten, R.A., Lips, M., de Jong, N., et al. 2003. Vitamin B-12 status is associated with bone mineral content and bone mineral density in frail elderly women but not in men. *J Nutr* 133:801–807.

Giachelli, C.M., Jono, S., Shioi, A., et al. 2001. Vascular calcification and inorganic phosphate. *Am J Kidney Dis* 38 (Suppl 1): S34–S37.

Gillespie, L.D., Robertson, M.C., Gillespie, W.J., et al. 2009. Interventions for preventing falls in older people living in the community [Review]. *The Cochrane Library Issue* 4.

Karlsson, M.K., Nordqvist, A., and Karlsson, C. 2008. Sustainability of exercise-induced increases in bone density and structure. *Food Nutr Res* 52. DOI: 10.3402/fnr.v52i0.1872.

Lemann, J., Jr., Bushinsky, D.A., and Hamm, L.L. 2003. Bone buffering of acid and base in humans. *Am J Physiol Renal Physiol* 285: F811–F832.

Lloyd, T., Rollings, N., Andon, M.B., et al. 1994. Enhanced bone gain in early adolescence due to calcium supplementation does not persist in late adolescence. *J Bone Miner Res* 11:S154. [Abstract]

Moran, D.S., Israeli, E., Evans, R.K., et al. 2008. Prediction model for stress fracture in young female recruits during basic training. *Med Sci Sports Exerc* 40: S636–S644.

Quarles, L.D. 2008. Endocrine functions of bone mineral metabolism regulation. *J Clin Invest* 118: 3820–3828.

Ralston, S.H., and Uitterlinden, A.G. 2010. Genetics of osteoporosis. *Endocr Rev* 31. DOI:10.1210/er.2009.0044.

Riis, B., Thomson, K., and Christiansen, C. 1987. Does calcium supplementation prevent postmenopausal bone loss? A double-blind, controlled clinical trial. *New Engl J Med* 316: 173–177.

Sanders, K.M., Stuart, A.L., Williamson, E.J., et al. 2010. Annual high-dose oral vitamin D and falls and fractures in older women. *JAMA* 303: 1815–1822.

Slemenda, C.W., Christian, J.C., Williams, C.J., et al. 1992. Genetic determinants of bone mass in adult women: A reevaluation of the twin model and the potential importance of gene interaction on heritability estimates. *J Bone Miner Res* 6:561–567.

Tucker, K.L., Hannan, M.T., Qiao, N., et al. 2005. Low plasma vitamin B12 is associated with lower BMD: The Framingham Osteoporosis Study. *J Bone Miner Res* 20: 152–158.

Virchow, R. 1863. *Cellular pathology: As based upon physiological and pathological histology.* Dover, New York, NY, pp. 404–408. Unabridged reprinting, 1971.

Welten, D.C., Kemper, H.C.G., Post, G.B., et al. 1994. Weight-bearing activity during youth is a more important factor for peak bone mass than calcium intake. *J Bone Miner Res* 14: 1089–1095.

Index

Note: Page numbers followed by "*f*" and "*t*" refer to figures and tables, respectively.